Total carbs minus fiber = net carbs

**MORE LISTINGS. MORE CHOICES.
MORE ESSENTIAL COUNTS FOR
CARBOHYDRATES AND FIBER
THAN ANY OTHER REFERENCE!**

Are you counting carbs? Watching your fiber intake? Or just taking charge of your health—at last? It's easier than ever to keep track of what you eat with **The Corinne T. Netzer Carbohydrate and Fiber Counter**. Whether you're following a specific diet or just watching your carbohydrate and fiber grams, here is the most comprehensive, easy-to-use reference on the market today. Discover essential counts for those new high-fiber cereals…the latest carb-controlled options…the tempting new offerings at your health food store…the most exotic ethnic cuisines—including Indian, Japanese, Thai, and Mexican.

Now you can know *exactly* how many grams of carbohydrates and fiber you're eating every day—whether you're preparing a quick dinner for your family or grabbing a snack on the run—with the indispensable reference you can't afford to miss!

**THE
CORINNE T. NETZER
CARBOHYDRATE AND FIBER
COUNTER**

THE CORINNE T. NETZER CARBOHYDRATE AND FIBER COUNTER

Corinne T. Netzer

A Dell Book

THE CORINNE T. NETZER CARBOHYDRATE AND FIBER COUNTER
A Dell Book / May 2006

Published by Bantam Dell
A Division of Random House, Inc.
New York, New York

Dell is a registered trademark of Random House, Inc., and the colophon is
a trademark of Random House, Inc.

ISBN-10: 0-440-24295-9
ISBN-13: 978-0-440-24295-6

Printed in the United States of America
Published simultaneously in Canada

www.bantamdell.com

OPM   10   9   8   7   6   5   4   3   2   1

**For
Chris Healy**

Introduction

The Corinne T. Netzer Carbohydrate and Fiber Counter is important to you in three ways: if you are counting carbs, if you are trying to increase your fiber intake, or if you want to determine the net carbs in a food (subtract the fiber count from the carbohydrate count and you have the figure for net carbs).

No matter what your aim or interest in carbohydrates and/or fiber might be, the information on all the foods—whether it be generic or brand name, fresh or frozen, even a fast-food favorite—can be found here.

Because this book is alphabetized, there is no index. I have tried to cross-reference as many items as possible; however, space does not allow this in every instance. If you do not find the item you are seeking in one place, please look for it under a category—i.e., if you don't find "apple pie" under "Apple," look for it under "Pie."

If you are making comparisons, remember to only compare foods that are similar in measure. Eight ounces is not necessarily equivalent to one eight-ounce cup. Eight ounces is a measure of how much the food weighs, while an eight-ounce cup is a measure of how much space the food occupies. For example, a cup of popcorn weighs about an ounce, thus eight ounces of popcorn would fill quite a few cups.

The data contained herein is derived from information supplied by the various food producers, processors, distributors, and food chains, and from the United States Department of Agriculture. As we go to press, this information is the most complete and accurate available.

Good luck and good eating.

C.T.N.

Abbreviations and Symbols in This Book

"	inch
<	less than
>	more than
approx.	approximately
cont.	container
diam.	diameter
lb.	pound(s)
n.a.	not available
oz.	ounce(s)
pkg.	package(s)
pkt.	packet(s)
tbsp.	tablespoon(s)
tsp.	teaspoon(s)
*	prepared according to basic package directions

THE
CORINNE T. NETZER
CARBOHYDRATE
AND FIBER
COUNTER

A

Food and Measure	carb. (gms)	fiber (gms)
Abalone, meat only, raw, 4 oz.	6.8	0
Abiyuch, ½ cup, 4 oz.	20.1	6.0
Abruzzese sausage (*Boar's Head*), 1 oz.	<1.0	0
Acerola, fresh:		
10 fruits	3.7	.5
peeled, 1 cup	7.5	1.1
Acerola juice, fresh, 8 fl. oz.	11.6	.7
Acorn squash:		
raw:		
(*Frieda's*), ¾ cup, 3 oz.	9.0	2.0
4'' squash, 15.2 oz.	44.9	6.6
cubed, 1 cup	14.6	2.1
baked, cubed, ½ cup	14.9	4.5
boiled, mashed, ½ cup	10.8	3.2
Adobo fresco, 1 tbsp.	3.3	.3
Adobo sauce (*Doña Maria*), 2 tbsp.	10.0	2.0
Adobo seasoning (*Goya*), ¼ tsp.	0	0
Aduki beans, canned (*Eden*), ½ cup	19.0	5.0
Abzuki beans:		
dry (*Arrowhead Mills*), ¼ cup	26.0	5.0
boiled, ½ cup	28.5	8.4
Aioli, see "Mayonnaise"		
Alfalfa seeds (*Shiloh Farms*), 2¼ tsp.	4.0	2.0
Alfalfa sprouts (*Jonathan's*), 1 cup	3.0	2.0
Alfredo sauce, jar, ¼ cup:		
(*Classico* di Roma/di Sorrento)	3.0	0
creamy or creamy garlic (*Bertolli*)	3.0	0
Parmesan (*Ragú* Classic)	3.0	0
tomato, sun-dried (*Classico* di Capri)	4.0	2.0

Food and Measure	carb. (gms)	fiber (gms)
Alfredo sauce, refrigerated:		
(*Buitoni* Family Size/Light/Portobello), ¼ cup	5.0	0
(*DiGiorno*), ¼ of 10-oz. cont.	3.0	0
Alfredo sauce mix, dry, creamy garlic		
(*McCormick*), 2 tbsp.	4.0	0
Allspice, 1 tsp.	1.4	.4
Almond, shelled:		
(*Beer Nuts*), 1 oz.	6.0	3.0
(*Fisher*), 1 oz.	6.0	3.0
(*Planters*), 1 oz.	5.0	3.0
(*Planters* Salted), 1 oz.	6.0	3.0
raw (*Shiloh Farms*), 1 oz., about 24 kernels	7.0	4.0
raw (*Tree of Life*), ¼ cup	7.0	3.0
coated, see "Candy"		
dried, 1 oz.	5.8	3.1
dry-roasted, salted, 1 oz.	6.9	3.9
dry-roasted, tamari (*Eden* Organic), 3 tbsp., 1 oz.	8.0	4.0
honey-roasted, 1 oz.	7.9	3.9
oil-roasted, salted, 1 oz.	4.5	3.2
sliced (*Planters*), 1.2 oz.	6.0	4.0
sliced (*Shiloh Farms*), ¼ cup	7.0	4.0
slivered (*Planters*), 2-oz. pkg.	11.0	6.0
slivered, ¼ cup	6.9	3.7
smoked (*Planters*), 1 oz.	6.0	3.0
toasted, 1 oz.	6.5	3.2
Almond butter:		
(*Kettle Roaster Fresh*), 1 oz.	6.0	0
all varieties (*Tree of Life*), 2 tbsp.	7.0	4.0
Almond flour (*Shiloh Farms*), 1 oz.	6.0	3.0
Almond meal, 1 oz.	8.2	n.a.
Almond paste, see "Pastry filling"		
Amaranth, whole grain:		
(*Arrowhead Mills*), ¼ cup	31.0	7.0
(*Shiloh Farms*), ¼ cup	36.0	6.0
1 oz.	18.8	4.3
Amaranth flakes, see "Cereal, ready-to-eat"		
Amaranth flour (*Arrowhead Mills*), ⅓ cup	20.0	2.0

Food and Measure	carb. (gms)	fiber (gms)
Amaranth leaves, ½ cup:		
raw, trimmed	.6	n.a.
boiled, drained	2.7	n.a.
Amaranth seeds (*Arrowhead Mills*), ¼ cup	29.0	3.0
Amaretto syrup (*Ferrara*), 2 oz.	32.0	0
Anasazi beans, dry (*Arrowhead Mills*), ¼ cup	26.0	6.0
Anchovy, fresh, without added ingredients	0	0
Anchovy, canned, in olive oil	0	0
Anchovy paste (*Reese's*), 1 tbsp.	0	0
Andouille sausage, see "Sausage"		
Angel-hair pasta:		
dry, see "Pasta"		
refrigerated, plain (*Buitoni*), 1¼ cups	43.0	2.0
Angel-hair pasta entree, frozen, 10-oz. pkg.:		
(*Lean Cuisine Everyday Favorites*)	48.0	3.0
marinara (*Smart Ones*)	42.0	4.0
Angel-hair pasta entree mix, spicy tomato		
(*Near East*), 1 cup*	41.0	4.0
Anise seeds, 1 tsp.	1.1	.3
Antelope, meat only, without added ingredients	0	0
Apple, fresh:		
(*Del Monte*), 5.4-oz. apple	22.0	5.0
(*Dole/Dole* Cameo), 5.4-oz. apple	22.0	5.0
(*Frieda's* Lady Apple), 5 oz.	21.0	3.0
raw, with peel, 2¾'' apple	21.1	3.7
raw, with peel, sliced, ½ cup	8.4	3.0
raw, peeled, 2¾'' apple	19.0	2.4
raw, peeled, sliced, ½ cup	8.2	1.0
cooked, peeled, sliced, boiled, ½ cup	11.7	2.0
Apple, can or jar:		
baked, sliced, in syrup (*Lucky Leaf/Musselman's*		
Dutch), ½ cup	41.0	3.0
fried (*Lucky Leaf*), ½ cup	43.0	0
fried, seasoned (*Glory*), ½ cup	21.0	1.0
rings, spiced (*Lucky Leaf/Musselman's*), 1 ring	9.0	0
sliced (*Lucky Leaf/Musselman's*), ½ cup	12.0	1.0
sliced, sweetened, drained, ½ cup	17.0	1.7

Food and Measure	carb. (gms)	fiber (gms)
Apple, dried:		
(*Sunsweet*), ¼ cup, 1.4 oz.	27.0	3.0
dehydrated, ½ cup	28.1	7.4
dehydrated, diced (*AlpineAire*), 1 oz.	26.0	2.0
sulfured, 1 ring	4.2	4.2
sulfured, ½ cup	28.3	7.5
Apple, frozen:		
½ cup unheated	10.7	1.6
seasoned (*Stouffer's* Harvest), ½ of 12-oz. pkg.	42.0	3.0
Apple, sour, drink mixer (*Rose's* Cocktail Infusions), 1.5 fl. oz.	16.0	0
Apple butter, 1 tbsp.:		
(*Apple Time/Lucky Leaf/Musselman's*)	8.0	0
(*Eden* Organic)	4.0	1.0
(*R.W. Knudsen*)	9.0	0
(*Shiloh Farms*)	3.0	0
(*Smucker's* Cider)	11.0	0
cherry (*Eden* Organic)	6.0	1.0
Apple cider, see "Apple juice"		
Apple cider, alcoholic (*Hard Core* Crisp), 12 fl. oz.	19.0	0
Apple cinnamon glaze (*Litehouse*), 2 tbsp.	17.0	0
Apple drink, 8 fl. oz.:		
(*Lincoln*)	31.0	0
(*Mott's* Light Juice Beverage)	15.0	0
cocktail (*Langers* Diet)	14.0	0
cocktail (*Langers* Low Carb)	7.0	0
Apple dumpling, frozen (*Pepperidge Farm*), 3-oz. piece	33.0	1.0
Apple juice, 8 fl. oz., except as noted:		
(*After the Fall* Organic)	22.0	0
(*Apple Time/Lincoln/Lucky Leaf/Musselman's*)	31.0	0
(*Capri Sun Fruit Waves* Apple Splash), 6.75 fl. oz.	23.0	0
(*Eden* Organic)	23.0	0
(*Hood*)	31.0	0
(*Langers* Cider/Juice/Harvest)	28.0	0
(*Lucky Leaf* 120% Vitamin C), 5.5-oz. can	21.0	0
(*Martinelli's Gold Medal* Juice/Cider)	35.0	0
(*Minute Maid*)	28.0	0
(*Minute Maid*), 6.75-fl.-oz. box	23.0	0

Food and Measure	carb. (gms)	fiber (gms)
(*Minute Maid*), 12-fl.-oz. bottle	41.0	0
(*Mott's* Natural)	27.0	0
(*Mott's* Original)	29.0	0
(*Musselman's* 120% Vitamin C), 5.5-oz. can	20.0	0
(*Nantucket Nectars* Cider/Pressed)	25.0	<1.0
(*Nantucket Nectars* Cloudy Organic)	29.0	0
(*Ocean Spray*)	28.0	0
(*R.W. Knudsen* Natural/Organic/Cider & Spice)	25.0	0
(*Santa Cruz Organic/Organic* Cider & Spice)	30.0	0
(*Seneca*)	28.0	0
(*S&W*)	30.0	0
(*Walnut Acres*)	29.0	0
frozen* (*Cascadian Farm*)	29.0	0
frozen* (*Minute Maid*)	28.0	0
sparkling:		
(*Lucky Leaf/Musselman's Cider*)	36.0	0
(*Martinelli* Cider)	35.0	0
(*Martinelli* Juice), 10 fl. oz.	43.0	1.0
(*R.W. Knudsen* Crisp/Organic)	28.0	0
Apple juice blend, 8 fl. oz.:		
apricot (*R.W. Knudsen*)	30.0	0
cherry (*Eden* Organic)	30.0	1.0
cranberry (*R.W. Knudsen*)	25.0	0
grape (*Juicy Juice*)	29.0	0
grape (*Mott's*)	32.0	0
punch (*Mott's*)	30.0	0
sparkling, all varieties (*Martinelli*)	27.0	0
Applesauce, ½ cup, except as noted:		
natural/unsweetened:		
(*Apple Time*)	13.0	2.0
(*Apple Time*), 4-oz. cup	12.0	2.0
(*Eden* Organic)	15.0	2.0
(*Langers*)	13.0	2.0
(*Lucky Leaf/Musselman's* Lite/Natural)	13.0	2.0
(*Lucky Leaf/Musselman's* Natural), 4-oz. cup	12.0	2.0
(*Mott's/Mott's* Organics)	14.0	1.0
(*Mott's* Single Serve), 1 cont.	12.0	1.0
(*Musselman's* Organic)	12.0	2.0

Food and Measure	carb. (gms)	fiber (gms)
(*Santa Cruz Organic*)	13.0	2.0
(*Tree of Life*)	15.0	2.0
cinnamon (*Apple Time*)	12.0	2.0
cinnamon (*Musselman's* Natural)	13.0	2.0
cinnamon (*Santa Cruz Organic*)	19.0	2.0
Granny Smith (*Mott's* Healthy Harvest Single Serve), 1 cont.	13.0	1.0
sweetened:		
(*Lucky Leaf/Musselman's*)	22.0	2.0
(*Mott's* Original)	29.0	1.0
(*Mott's* Original Organics)	27.0	1.0
(*Musselman's* Organic), 4-oz. cup	20.0	2.0
chunky (*Musselman's* Homestyle)	25.0	2.0
cinnamon (*Lucky Leaf/Musselman's*)	25.0	2.0
cinnamon (*Lucky Leaf/Musselman's*), 4-oz. cup	20.0	2.0
cinnamon (*Mott's*)	29.0	1.0
cinnamon (*Mott's* Single Serve), 1 cont.	25.0	1.0
Golden Delicious, Granny Smith, or McIntosh (*Musselman's*)	22.0	2.0
Applesauce fruit blend:		
all varieties (*Santa Cruz Organic*), ½ cup or 4 oz.	13.0	2.0
cherry (*Eden Organic*), ½ cup	17.0	3.0
cherry (*Lucky Leaf/Musselman's* Lite), 4-oz. cup	15.0	1.0
orange, raspberry, or strawberry (*Lucky Leaf/ Musselman's* Lite), 4-oz. cup	14.0	1.0
peach (*Lucky Leaf/Musselman's* Lite), 4-oz. cup	14.0	2.0
strawberry (*Eden* Organic), ½ cup	13.0	2.0
strawberry (*Mott's* Single Serve), 1 cont.	23.0	1.0
Apricot, fresh:		
(*Del Monte*), 3 medium, 4 oz.	11.0	1.0
(*Dole*), 3 medium, 4 oz.	11.0	1.0
3 medium, 12 per lb.	11.8	2.5
pitted, halves, ½ cup	8.6	1.9
pitted, sliced, ½ cup	9.2	2.0
Apricot, can or jar, halves, except as noted:		
in juice, with liquid, ½ cup	15.1	2.0
in extra light syrup (*Del Monte* Lite), ½ cup	16.0	1.0
in light syrup, ½ cup:		

Food and Measure	carb. (gms)	fiber (gms)
(*Del Monte Orchard Select*)	21.0	1.0
with liquid	20.9	2.0
chunks (*S&W* Sun)	22.0	1.0
almond flavor (*Del Monte*)	22.0	1.0
in heavy syrup, ½ cup:		
(*Del Monte*)	26.0	1.0
with liquid	27.7	2.1
whole, peeled (*S&W*)	29.0	1.0
Apricot, dried:		
(*Express*), 1.4 oz., about 5 pieces	22.0	3.0
(*Shiloh Farms* California), 8 pieces, 1.4 oz.	31.0	1.0
(*Shiloh Farms* Turkish), 5 pieces, 1.1 oz.	20.0	3.0
(*Sun•Maid Fast Fruit*), ¼ cup, 1.4 oz.	24.0	3.0
(*Sunsweet* California), 5 pieces, 1.4 oz.	24.0	4.0
(*Sunsweet* Mediterranean), 6 pieces, 1.4 oz.	24.0	3.0
dehydrated, ½ cup	49.3	n.a.
sulfured, ½ cup	40.1	5.9
Apricot, frozen, sweetened, ½ cup	30.4	2.1
Apricot juice:		
(*Ceres*), 8 fl. oz.	30.0	0
(*Walnut Acres*), 8 fl. oz.	32.0	0
Apricot nectar:		
(*Goya*), 6 fl. oz.	29.0	0
(*Goya*), 8 fl. oz.	31.0	0
(*Goya*), 12 fl. oz.	53.0	1.0
(*R.W. Knudsen*), 8 fl. oz.	30.0	0
(*Santa Cruz Organic*), 8 fl. oz.	27.0	0
(*S&W*), 8 fl. oz.	15.0	1.0
(*S&W*), 12 fl. oz.	53.0	1.0
Apricot-orange drink (*Snapple* Snaprlcot), 8 fl. oz.	30.0	0
Arame, see "Seaweed"		
Arby's, 1 serving:		
breakfast:		
biscuit, plain	26.0	<1.0
add butter or Swiss cheese	0	0
add egg	2.0	2.0
biscuit, bacon or ham	27.0	<1.0
biscuit, sausage	26.0	<1.0

Food and Measure	carb. (gms)	fiber (gms)
croissant, bacon or sausage and egg	31.0	<1.0
croissant, ham and cheese	30.0	<1.0
sourdough, egg and cheese	31.0	1.0
sourdough, egg and ham or bacon and cheese	33.0	1.0
sandwiches:		
beef, roast:		
beef 'n cheddar	44.0	2.0
Big Montana	41.0	3.0
giant	41.0	2.0
junior or regular	34.0	2.0
super	48.0	3.0
chicken:		
breast fillet	48.0	3.0
bacon 'n Swiss	49.0	2.0
roast, club	39.0	2.0
Market Fresh:		
BLT	75.0	6.0
chicken salad	78.0	9.0
roast turkey, ranch 'n bacon	75.0	5.0
roast beef 'n Swiss	74.0	6.0
roast ham 'n Swiss	74.0	5.0
roast turkey 'n Swiss	74.0	5.0
Market Fresh wraps:		
BLT	48.0	31.0
chicken, Southwest	45.0	30.0
chicken club	52.0	31.0
roast turkey, ranch 'n bacon	48.0	30.0
Market Fresh salads:		
chicken club	32.0	5.0
add buttermilk ranch dressing	4.0	0
add light dressing	13.0	<1.0
Martha's Vineyard	23.0	4.0
add sliced almonds	2.0	1.0
add raspberry vinaigrette	16.0	0
Santa Fe	40.0	5.0
add ranch dressing	4.0	0
add seasoned tortilla strips	10.0	.5

Food and Measure	carb. (gms)	fiber (gms)
sides:		
chicken fingers, 4-pack	42.0	3.0
chicken fingers, combo	89.0	5.0
fries, curly:		
large	73.0	7.0
medium	47.0	5.0
small	39.0	4.0
add cheddar sauce	4.0	0
fries, home-style:		
large	82.0	6.0
medium	55.0	4.0
small	44.0	3.0
potato cakes, 2 cakes	26.0	2.0
Sidekickers:		
Jalapeño Bites, large, 10 pieces	58.0	4.0
Jalapeño Bites, regular, 5 pieces	29.0	2.0
mozzarella sticks, large, 8 pieces	76.0	4.0
mozzarella sticks, regular, 4 pieces	38.0	2.0
onion petals, large	88.0	5.0
onion petals, regular	35.0	2.0
sauces/condiments:		
Arby's Sauce, pkt.	4.0	0
BBQ dipping sauce, 1 oz.	10.0	0
Bronco Berry Sauce, 2 oz.	30.0	0
buttermilk ranch dressing, 2 oz.	3.0	0
honey mustard dipping sauce, 1 oz.	5.0	0
Horsey Sauce, pkt.	3.0	0
ketchup, pkt.	4.0	0
mayo, pkt.	0	0
mayo, light, pkt.	1.0	0
marinara sauce, 2.5 oz.	4.0	1.0
red ranch sauce, pkt.	5.0	0
Tangy Southwest Sauce, 2 oz.	5.0	0
three pepper sauce, pkt.	3.0	0
shakes:		
chocolate, large	110.0	<1.0
chocolate, regular	83.0	0

Food and Measure	carb. (gms)	fiber (gms)
Jamocha, large	107.0	<1.0
Jamocha, regular	81.0	0
strawberry, large	107.0	<1.0
strawberry, regular	81.0	0
vanilla, large	107.0	0
vanilla, regular	82.0	0
desserts:		
chocolate cookie	26.0	1.0
cinnamon roll, see "*T.J. Cinnamons*"		
turnover, apple or cherry, without icing	35.0	2.0
turnover icing	29.0	0
Arctic char, without added ingredients	0	0
Arrowhead:		
raw, 1 medium corm, 2⅝''	2.4	<1.0
boiled, drained, 1 medium corm, .4 oz.	1.9	<1.0
Arrowroot, raw, sliced, ½ cup	8.0	.8
Arrowroot flour, ¼ cup	28.2	1.1
Artichoke, globe, fresh:		
raw:		
(*Dole*), 1 medium, 2 oz. edible	6.0	3.0
4.5-oz. choke	13.5	6.9
5.7-oz. choke	17.0	8.9
boiled, drained, 1 medium, 4.2 oz.	13.4	6.5
hearts, boiled, drained, ½ cup	9.4	4.5
Artichoke, canned (see also "Artichoke, marinated"), in water: bottoms or small (*Fanci Food*),		
3 pieces, 4.6 oz.	3.0	2.0
hearts:		
(*Cento*), 2 pieces, 2.8 oz.	6.0	1.0
(*Pompeian*), 4.5 oz.	6.0	4.0
(*Progresso*), 2 pieces, 2.9 oz.	6.0	1.0
(*Vigo*), 2 pieces, 2.8 oz.	6.0	1.0
Artichoke, frozen, hearts:		
(*Birds Eye*), 12 pieces, 3 oz.	7.0	5.0
(*C&W*), ½ cup, 3 oz.	4.0	5.0
9-oz. pkg.	19.8	9.9
Artichoke, Jerusalem, see "Jerusalem artichoke"		

Food and Measure	carb. (gms)	fiber (gms)
Artichoke, marinated, in jars:		
(*Fanci Food* Hot/Quartered/Salad), 1 oz.	2.0	.5
(*Pompeian*), 1 oz.	2.0	.5
(*Progresso*), 2 pieces, 1.1 oz.	2.0	0
quarters (*S&W*), 2 pieces, 1 oz.	2.0	1.0
Artichoke dip, 2 tbsp.:		
(*Victoria*)	2.0	1.0
spinach (*Fiesta*)	12.0	0
Artichoke paste (*Cucina Aromatica*), 1 oz.	3.5	2.8
Arugula, fresh:		
baby (*Ready Pac*), 3 oz.	5.0	3.0
10 leaves	.7	.3
½ cup	.4	.2
Asparagus, fresh:		
raw, spears, trimmed:		
(*Dole*), 5 medium, 3.3 oz.	4.0	2.0
4 small, 1.8 oz.	2.6	1.2
purple (*Frieda's*), 3 oz.	4.0	1.0
boiled, 4 spears, ½''-diam. base	2.5	1.3
boiled, drained, cuts, ½ cup	3.8	1.9
Asparagus, can or jar:		
all styles (*Del Monte*), ½ cup	3.0	1.0
spears (*Green Giant*), 4.5 oz., approx. 5 spears	3.0	1.0
spears, white (*Fanci Food*), ½ cup	3.0	2.0
cuts (*Green Giant/Green Giant* Low Sodium), ½ cup	3.0	1.0
drained, ½ cup	3.0	2.0
Asparagus, frozen:		
boiled, drained, 1 cup	8.8	2.9
spears:		
(*Birds Eye*), 7 spears, 3 oz.	3.0	0
(*C&W*), 7 spears, 3 oz.	3.0	2.0
(*Seabrook Farms*), 7 spears, 3 oz.	3.0	2.0
4 spears, 2 oz.	2.4	1.1
cuts:		
(*Birds Eye*), ¾ cup	3.0	0
(*Cascadian Farm*), ⅔ cup	3.0	1.0
(*Green Giant*), ⅔ cup	3.0	2.0

Food and Measure	carb. (gms)	fiber (gms)
Asparagus beans, see "Winged beans"		
Asparagus combination, frozen (*Birds Eye* Stir-fry),		
2 cups frozen, 1 cup*	15.0	2.0
Atemoya (*Frieda's*), 3 oz.	20.0	4.0
Au Bon Pain, 1 serving:		
breakfast:		
bagel, with egg and bacon or cheese or		
cheese and bacon	63.0	3.0
yogurt, large:		
all flavors, with fruit and granola	112.0	5.0
blueberry or strawberry with fruit	75.0	1.0
vanilla, with fruit	64.0	2.0
yogurt, small:		
plain, low fat	36.0	0
all flavors, with fruit and granola	56.0	2.0
bagels:		
plain	61.0	3.0
apple, Dutch	98.0	5.0
asiago cheese	59.0	3.0
cinnamon crisp	96.0	3.0
cinnamon raisin	71.0	3.0
everything	63.0	3.0
French toast	76.0	3.0
honey 9-grain	75.0	6.0
jalapeño cheddar	56.0	2.0
sesame seed	62.0	3.0
cake and pastry:		
apple crumble	62.0	1.0
apple strudel	56.0	1.0
blonde, with nuts	57.0	2.0
butter crumb	96.0	2.0
cheese Danish, sweet	54.0	1.0
cheesecake brownie	55.0	1.0
cherry Danish	52.0	1.0
cherry strudel	49.0	1.0
chocolate chip brownie	61.0	2.0
cinnamon roll	67.0	2.0
crème de fleur	71.0	1.0

Food and Measure	carb. (gms)	fiber (gms)
lemon Danish	57.0	1.0
pecan brownie	55.0	3.0
pecan roll	112.0	4.0
raspberry crumb	94.0	2.0
rocky road brownie	49.0	2.0
cookies:		
butterscotch chip with pecans	42.0	1.0
chocolate chip	40.0	1.0
confetti, with *M&M's*	37.0	1.0
cranberry almond macaroon, chocolate dipped	42.0	3.0
oatmeal raisin	42.0	2.0
shortbread	35.0	1.0
shortbread, chocolate dipped	52.0	1.0
shortbread, white chocolate dipped	46.0	2.0
toffee, English	26.0	1.0
croissants:		
plain	44.0	2.0
almond	63.0	3.0
apple	47.0	2.0
cheese, sweet	52.0	1.0
chocolate	61.0	3.0
cinnamon raisin	69.0	3.0
ham and cheese	46.0	2.0
raspberry	55.0	2.0
spinach and cheese	32.0	2.0
muffins:		
apple spice	65.0	3.0
banana walnut	60.0	3.0
berry, triple, low fat	61.0	2.0
blueberry	76.0	5.0
carrot nut	71.0	4.0
chocolate cake, low fat	74.0	4.0
chocolate chunk	83.0	5.0
corn	64.0	2.0
cranberry blueberry	76.0	5.0
cranberry walnut	69.0	5.0
raisin bran	100.0	12.0
scone, cinnamon	88.0	2.0

Food and Measure	carb. (gms)	fiber (gms)
scone, orange	62.0	2.0
bread, artisan:		
baguette, 2 oz.	30.0	1.0
baguette, 3.5-oz. piece	53.0	1.0
baguette, honey multigrain, 2 oz.	30.0	2.0
baguette, honey multigrain, 3.5-oz. piece	53.0	3.0
bread bowl, 9.24 oz.	127.0	6.0
chocolate cherry, 2 oz.	31.0	2.0
cranberry raisin nut loaf, 2 oz.	28.0	2.0
ficelle, 2 oz.	34.0	1.0
focaccia, 4.5 oz.	58.0	2.0
lahvash, 3.8 oz.	55.0	4.0
multigrain, 1 slice	31.0	2.0
rosemary-garlic bread stick, 2.3 oz.	33.0	2.0
rye, Bavarian, 1 slice	49.0	4.0
sun-dried tomato loaf, 2 oz.	27.0	2.0
white, French country, 2-oz. slice	27.0	1.0
white roll, soft, 4.7 oz.	65.0	2.0
cream cheese, 2 oz.:		
plain	4.0	0
honey walnut	12.0	0
smoked salmon or vegetable	3.0	0
sun-dried tomato	5.0	0
soup, 8 oz.:		
black bean	27.0	14.0
black-eye pea	34.0	12.0
broccoli cheddar	13.0	2.0
chicken chili	28.0	5.0
chicken Florentine	17.0	1.0
chicken noodle	11.0	0
clam chowder	18.0	0
corn and green chili bisque	17.0	2.0
curried rice lentil	18.0	4.0
Italian wedding	12.0	2.0
minestrone	14.0	3.0
onion, French	11.0	2.0
pasta e fagioli	24.0	5.0

Food and Measure	carb. (gms)	fiber (gms)
pepper, Mediterranean	30.0	7.0
potato, baked stuffed	20.0	1.0
potato leek	17.0	2.0
pumpkin, harvest	15.0	4.0
red bean, rice, sausage	28.0	11.0
split pea with ham	23.0	8.0
tomato basil bisque	18.0	3.0
tomato Florentine	10.0	1.0
tomato lentil	19.0	6.0
tomato rice	15.0	2.0
tortilla, Southwest	17.0	3.0
vegetable, garden	7.0	2.0
vegetable, Southwest	23.0	4.0
vegetable, Tuscan	20.0	3.0
vegetable beef barley	11.0	2.0
vegetarian chili	30.0	15.0
wild mushroom bisque	12.0	2.0
salad, without dressing:		
Caesar	23.0	4.0
chef's salad	9.0	4.0
chicken, Mediterranean	13.0	5.0
chicken, Thai	14.0	6.0
chicken Caesar	24.0	4.0
chicken pesto	14.0	5.0
garden, large	19.0	5.0
garden, small	10.0	3.0
Gorgonzola walnut	10.0	7.0
tuna garden	11.0	5.0
tuna niçoise	19.0	5.0
turkey Cobb	23.0	6.0
salad dressing, 2.5 oz.:		
balsamic vinaigrette	9.0	0
blue cheese	3.0	0
Caesar	6.0	0
honey mustard, lite	26.0	0
Mediterranean	4.0	0
olive oil vinaigrette, lite	7.0	0

Food and Measure	carb. (gms)	fiber (gms)
Parmesan peppercorn or lite ranch	5.0	0
raspberry vinaigrette	19.0	0
Thai peanut	24.0	0
sandwiches:		
basil goat cheese	67.0	6.0
beef, roast, and Gorgonzola	86.0	8.0
beef, roast, and Swiss	57.0	2.0
chicken breast, chili Dijon, with cheddar	52.0	4.0
chicken club, grilled, chili dressing	64.0	4.0
chicken mozzarella	73.0	6.0
chicken salad, Asian	50.0	3.0
chicken tarragon	71.0	4.0
chicken tarragon, on ficelle	35.0	0
chocolate cherry	92.0	4.0
honey Dijon Cordon Bleu	71.0	3.0
pork, pulled, BBQ	18.0	6.0
portobello, roasted, and goat cheese	63.0	6.0
steak and Gorgonzola, on onion roll	76.0	6.0
tomato and mozzarella on ficelle	40.0	0
tuna, spicy, on multigrain	72.0	8.0
turkey, guacamole and Swiss, on baguette	77.0	6.0
turkey club, hickory smoked	59.0	3.0
turkey tenderloin	67.0	6.0
the Tuscan	60.0	3.0
sandwiches, baked:		
chicken, grilled, and blue cheese	64.0	3.0
mozzarella, tomato, basil pesto, and onion	66.0	3.0
tuna, cheddar, and red pepper	62.0	3.0
turkey, roasted, cranberry, and cheese	80.0	3.0
sandwich filling:		
beef, roast	1.0	0
Brie cheese	0	0
capicola, hot	1.0	0
cheddar, Gorgonzola, or provolone cheese	1.0	0
chicken breast	1.0	0
chicken tarragon	1.0	0
cranberry cheese	6.0	0

Food and Measure	carb. (gms)	fiber (gms)
ham	2.0	0
hummus	8.0	2.0
mozzarella cheese	3.0	0
olive tapenade, 2 oz.	1.0	1.0
red peppers, roasted	4.0	1.0
salami, Genoa	0	0
Swiss cheese	0	0
tarragon mayo sauce	2.0	0
tomato spread	4.0	0
tuna salad mix	3.0	0
turkey breast	4.0	0
wraps:		
chicken Caesar	63.0	5.0
chopped Cobb	65.0	6.0
fields and feta	90.0	14.0
Mediterranean	80.0	9.0
tuna, Southwest	68.0	7.0
Au jus gravy, canned (*Campbell's*), ¼ cup	0	0
Au jus gravy mix, ¼ cup*:		
(*Lawry's*)	4.0	0
(*McCormick* Natural Style)	1.0	0
Aubergine, see "Eggplant"		
Auntie Anne's:		
pretzels, 1 piece:		
almond, with or without butter	72.0	2.0
cinnamon sugar	74.0	2.0
cinnamon, with butter	83.0	3.0
garlic	66.0	2.0
garlic with butter	68.0	2.0
Glazin' Raisin	104.0	3.0
Glazin' Raisin, with butter	107.0	4.0
jalapeño	58.0	2.0
jalapeño, with butter	59.0	2.0
maple crumb, with or without butter	112.0	3.0
original, with or without butter	72.0	3.0
Parmesan herb	74.0	4.0
Parmesan herb, with butter	72.0	9.0

Food and Measure	carb. (gms)	fiber (gms)
sesame	63.0	3.0
sesame, with butter	64.0	7.0
sour cream and onion, with or without butter	66.0	2.0
whole wheat, with or without butter	72.0	7.0
pretzel dips:		
caramel	27.0	0
cheese	4.0	0
chocolate flavor	24.0	1.0
cream cheese, light	1.0	0
cream cheese, strawberry	4.0	0
marinara	4.0	0
mustard, sweet	8.0	0
salsa cheese, hot	4.0	0
pretzel dog	25.0	1.0
pretzel stix, plain, with or without butter, 4 pieces	48.0	2.0
Smart Bites, 1 piece	2.0	1.0
Smart Bites, 15 pieces	30.0	15.0
Dutch Ice, 14 oz.:		
cherry, wild	48.0	0
grape	43.0	0
kiwi-banana	44.0	0
lemonade	77.0	0
mocha	74.0	0
orange crème	64.0	0
piña colada	53.0	0
raspberry, blue	38.0	0
strawberry	50.0	0
Dutch Latte, 14 oz.:		
caramel	49.0	0
coffee	38.0	0
mocha	47.0	0
Dutch shake, 14 oz.:		
chocolate	75.0	0
coffee	77.0	0
strawberry	78.0	0
vanilla	58.0	0
Dutch smoothie, 14 oz.:		
cherry, wild	41.0	0

Food and Measure	carb. (gms)	fiber (gms)
grape	36.0	0
kiwi-banana	38.0	0
lemonade	53.0	0
mocha	50.0	0
orange crème	46.0	0
piña colada	44.0	0
raspberry, blue	34.0	0
strawberry	40.0	0
lemonade	43.0	0
lemonade, strawberry	48.0	0
Australian blue squash (*Frieda's*), ¾ cup, 3 oz.	7.0	1.0
Avocado:		
(*Del Monte*), ⅓ medium, 1.1 oz.	3.0	3.0
all varieties, cubed, 1 cup	12.8	10.1
California, pulp from 1 medium, 6.1 oz.	14.9	11.8
California, pureed, ½ cup	9.9	7.8
Florida, pureed, ½ cup	9.0	6.4
seedless (*Frieda's* Cocktail), 1.4-oz. fruit	3.0	2.0
Avocado dip (see also "Guacamole"),		
(*Litehouse*), 2 tbsp.	2.0	0
A&W, 1 serving:		
sandwiches:		
cheeseburger	43.0	3.0
cheeseburger deluxe	43.0	4.0
cheeseburger deluxe, double	47.0	4.0
cheeseburger deluxe, bacon	44.0	4.0
cheeseburger deluxe, bacon double	47.0	4.0
cheeseburger Jr.	41.0	3.0
chicken, crispy	57.0	5.0
chicken, grilled	37.0	4.0
hamburger	39.0	3.0
hamburger deluxe	40.0	4.0
hamburger Jr.	37.0	3.0
hot dogs:		
plain	22.0	1.0
cheese dog	25.0	1.0
coney (chili)	24.0	2.0
coney (chili) cheese	27.0	2.0

Food and Measure	carb. (gms)	fiber (gms)
chicken strips, 3 pieces	32.0	2.0
dipping sauce, 1 oz.:		
barbecue	10.0	0
honey mustard	12.0	0
ranch	2.0	0
sweet and sour	12.0	0
fries:		
cheese	50.0	4.0
chili	49.0	5.0
chili cheese	51.0	5.0
regular, kids	45.0	4.0
regular, large	61.0	6.0
onion rings	45.0	2.0

B

Food and Measure	carb. (gms)	fiber (gms)
Babaganoush, see "Eggplant appetizer"		
Bacon, raw or pan-fried, 3 medium slices,		
20 slices per lb.	.1	0
Bacon, Canadian:		
(*Boar's Head*), 2 oz.	0	0
(*Hormel*), 2 oz.	0	0
(*Hormel Pillow Pack*), 22 slices, 2 oz.	2.0	0
pizza (*Hormel*), 22 slices, 2 oz.	1.0	0
unheated, 2 oz.	1.9	0
Bacon, Irish (*Dawn Irish Gold*), 2 slices, 2 oz.	1.0	0
Bacon, Italian, .5 oz.	0	0
"Bacon," vegetarian, frozen:		
(*Morningstar Farms* Breakfast Strips), 2 slices	2.0	<1.0
(*Worthington Stripples*), 2 slices	2.0	<1.0
Canadian style (*Yves*), 1.3 oz.	1.0	1.0
Bacon bits, 1 tbsp.	0	0
"Bacon" bits, imitation:		
(*Bac 'n Pieces*), 1 tbsp.	2.0	0
chips or bits (*Bac-Os*), 1 tbsp.	2.0	0
Bacon dip:		
and cheddar (*Kraft*), 2 tbsp.	3.0	0
horseradish (*Cabot*), 2 tbsp.	1.0	0
Bacon grease, ¼ cup	0	0
Bagel, 1 piece:		
plain:		
(*Pepperidge Farm*)	54.0	3.0
(*Sara Lee*), 2.2 oz.	33.0	1.0
(*Sara Lee*), 3.4 oz.	52.0	2.0
(*Thomas'*), 3.7 oz.	56.0	3.0

Food and Measure	carb. (gms)	fiber (gms)
mini (*Pepperidge Farm*)	22.0	1.0
mini (*Thomas'*), 1.7 oz.	26.0	1.0
plain, onion, poppy, or sesame, 2 oz.	30.4	1.3
apple cinnamon (*Sara Lee*), 4 oz.	64.0	3.0
banana walnut (*Sara Lee*), 4 oz.	61.0	4.0
blueberry:		
(*Sara Lee* Deluxe), 3.4 oz.	53.0	2.0
(*Sara Lee* Toaster Size), 2.2 oz.	34.0	1.0
(*Thomas'*), 3.7 oz.	59.0	3.0
mini (*Sara Lee*), 1 oz.	15.0	<1.0
swirl, mini (*Pepperidge Farm*)	24.0	<1.0
brown sugar cinnamon, mini (*Pepperidge Farm*)	24.0	2.0
cinnamon raisin:		
(*Pepperidge Farm*)	57.0	3.0
(*Sara Lee* Deluxe), 3.4 oz.	55.0	4.0
(*Sara Lee* Toaster Size), 2.2 oz.	33.0	1.0
cranberry orange (*Sara Lee*), 4 oz.	64.0	3.0
egg, 2 oz.	30.2	1.3
everything (*Pepperidge Farm*)	55.0	3.0
everything (*Thomas'*), 3.7 oz.	54.0	3.0
honey wheat (*Sara Lee*), 3.4 oz.	50.0	4.0
multigrain (*Pepperidge Farm*)	55.0	5.0
multigrain (*Thomas'*), 3.7 oz.	57.0	4.0
oat bran, 2 oz.	30.4	2.1
onion:		
(*Sara Lee*), 2.2 oz.	33.0	1.0
(*Sara Lee* Deluxe), 3.4 oz.	51.0	2.0
(*Thomas'*), 3.7 oz.	56.0	3.0
sesame seed (*Thomas'*), 3.7 oz.	53.0	3.0
sun-dried tomato and basil (*Sara Lee*), 4 oz.	61.0	2.0
whole wheat (*Sara Lee* Heart Healthy), 3.3 oz.	47.0	6.0
whole wheat (*Thomas'*), 3.7 oz.	55.0	1.0
Bagel, with cream cheese, ½ of 6.4-oz. pkg.:		
plain or chive cream cheese (*Philadelphia* To-Go)	34.0	2.0
strawberry (*Philadelphia* To-Go)	37.0	2.0
Baked beans, ½ cup:		
(*Allens* Homestyle)	29.0	5.0
(*Allens* Original)	29.0	8.0

Food and Measure	carb. (gms)	fiber (gms)
(*Bush's* Bold & Spicy)	24.0	5.0
(*Bush's* Boston)	32.0	6.0
(*Bush's* Country)	33.0	7.0
(*Bush's* Homestyle)	28.0	8.0
(*Bush's* Original)	29.0	7.0
bacon, maple cured:		
(*Allens*)	27.0	4.0
(*Bush's*)	28.0	7.0
(*S&W* Sweet Bacon)	29.0	6.0
barbecue:		
(*Allens*)	29.0	5.0
(*Bush's*)	32.0	6.0
(*S&W* Country)	28.0	6.0
(*S&W* Ranch Recipe)	25.0	8.0
brown sugar and bacon (*Campbell's*)	28.0	6.0
honey mustard (*S&W*)	28.0	6.0
maple sugar (*S&W*)	29.0	6.0
onion (*Allens*)	25.0	4.0
onion (*Bush's*)	26.0	6.0
with pork:		
(*Campbell's*)	27.0	7.0
(*Wagon Master*)	23.0	9.0
(*Wagon Master* 1 lb.)	21.0	6.0
sorghum and mustard (*Eden* Organic)	27.0	7.0
vegetarian:		
(*Allens*)	28.0	4.0
(*Amy's*)	24.0	6.0
(*Bush's*)	24.0	6.0
(*S&W*)	24.0	8.0
Baking mix (see also "Biscuit mix"), all purpose:		
(*Bisquick* Original), ⅓ cup	26.0	0
(*Bisquick* Reduced Fat), ⅓ cup	27.0	<1.0
(*Don's Chuck Wagon*), ¼ cup	21.0	1.0
(*"Jiffy"*), ¼ cup	22.0	1.0
whole wheat (*Hodgson Mill* Insta-Bake), ⅓ cup	29.0	3.0
Baking powder:		
(*Calumet*), ⅛ tsp.	0	0
1 tsp.	1.1	0

Food and Measure	carb. (gms)	fiber (gms)
Baking soda, 1 tsp.	0	0
Baklava pastry, frozen (*Athens/Apollo*), 2 pieces, 2 oz.	26.0	<1.0
Balsam pear, ½ cup, except as noted:		
(*Frieda's* Bittermelon), 1 cup, 3 oz.	3.0	2.0
leafy-tips raw	.8	.6
leafy-tips boiled, drained	2.0	.6
pods, raw, ½'' pieces	1.7	1.3
pods, boiled, drained, ½'' pieces	2.7	1.2
Bamboo shoots, fresh, slices:		
raw, ½ cup	4.0	.7
boiled, drained, ½ cup	1.2	<1.0
Bamboo shoots, canned, drained, ½ cup	2.1	2.0
Banana (see also "Plantain"), fresh:		
(*Chiquita*), 1 medium, 4.4 oz.	29.0	4.0
(*Dole*), 1 medium, 4.4 oz.	29.0	4.0
(*Frieda's* Baby Nino/Burro), 3-oz. piece	20.0	1.0
1 medium, 8¾'' long	26.7	2.7
sliced, ½ cup	17.6	1.8
mashed, ½ cup	26.4	2.7
red (*Frieda's*), 5 oz.	33.0	2.0
red, 7¼'' long	30.7	n.a.
Banana, dried:		
(*Frieda's*), 1.2-oz. piece	33.0	2.0
dehydrated, ¼ cup	22.1	1.9
Banana chips:		
(*SunRidge Farms*), 1 oz.	12.0	1.0
(*Tree of Life*), ¼ cup	27.0	4.0
Banana drink blend, 8 fl. oz.:		
(*After the Fall Banana Casablanca*)	37.0	0
(*Snapple* Go Bananas)	30.0	0
mango carrot (*Nantucket Nectars*)	30.0	0
Banana milk drink, see "Milk, flavored"		
Banana squash (*Frieda's*), ¾ cup, 3 oz.	7.0	1.0
Barbecue beans, see "Baked beans"		
Barbecue coating mix, see "Chicken coating mix"		
Barbecue rub (*D.L. Jardine's* 5-Star Ranch), 1 tbsp.	3.0	0
Barbecue sauce (see also "Grilling sauce"), 2 tbsp., except as noted:		

Food and Measure	carb. (gms)	fiber (gms)
(*Annie's Natural* Organic Original)	9.0	0
(*Bilardo Brothers* Original)	5.0	1.0
(*Bull's-Eye* Original)	13.0	0
(*D.L. Jardine's* Chick'n Lik'n)	7.0	0
(*D.L. Jardine's* 5-Star), 1 tbsp.	10.0	<1.0
(*D.L. Jardine's* Killer)	6.0	<1.0
(*D.L. Jardine's* Texas Pecan)	7.0	1.0
(*Hunt's* Original)	9.0	<1.0
(*Hunt's* Original Bold)	13.0	<1.0
(*KC Masterpiece*)	15.0	0
(*Kraft Carb Well*)	3.0	0
(*Kraft* Char-Grill)	13.0	0
(*Kraft* Original)	9.0	0
(*Kraft* Original Easy Squeeze)	11.0	0
(*Kraft* Steakhouse)	14.0	0
(*Kraft Thick 'n Spicy* Original)	12.0	0
(*Litehouse*)	11.0	0
(*Lloyd's* Original)	11.0	0
(*Neera's* Southwest Sizzler), 2 tsp.	5.0	0
(*Silver Dollar City* Original)	11.0	0
(*Silver Dollar City* Ozark Recipe)	14.0	0
(*Woody's* Cook-in' Concentrate)	4.0	1.0
(*World Harbors*)	16.0	0
all varieties (*Maull's*)	13.0	0
Asian (*San-J*)	7.0	0
Cajun (*Kraft Thick 'n Spicy*)	12.0	0
concentrate, all varieties (*Watkins*), 2 tsp.	5.0	0
bacon, hickory (*Kraft Thick 'n Spicy*)	13.0	0
brown sugar, spicy (*Kraft Thick 'n Spicy*)	15.0	0
chipotle, hot (*Annie's Naturals* Organic)	9.0	0
chipotle, smoky (*Texas Longhorn*)	8.0	0
garlic, (*Pain is Good* Garlic-Que)	8.0	0
garlic, roasted (*Kraft*)	12.0	0
hickory:		
(*Bull's-Eye* Smoke-house)	13.0	0
(*Hunt's*)	13.0	<1.0
brown sugar (*Hunt's*)	16.0	1.0
brown sugar (*KC Masterpiece*)	15.0	0

Food and Measure	carb. (gms)	fiber (gms)
honey (*Hunt's*)	12.0	<1.0
smoke (*Kraft*)	9.0	0
smoke (*Kraft Thick 'n Spicy*)	12.0	0
smoke, w/onion bits (*Kraft*)	11.0	0
smoke, sweet (*Bull's-Eye*)	15.0	0
sweet (*Silver Dollar City*)	11.0	0
honey:		
(*Kraft Thick 'n Spicy*)	13.0	0
mustard (*Hunt's*)	12.0	1.0
mustard (*Kraft*)	13.0	0
roasted garlic (*Kraft*)	11.0	0
smoke (*Bull's-Eye*)	11.0	0
and spice (*Bilardo Brothers*)	7.0	1.0
spicy (*Bull's-Eye*)	12.0	0
spicy (*Kraft*)	14.0	0
teriyaki (*KC Masterpiece*)	14.0	0
hot:		
(*Bilardo Brothers*)	8.0	1.0
(*Kraft*)	9.0	0
spicy (*Bull's-Eye*)	13.0	0
and spicy (*Hunt's*)	11.0	<1.0
jalapeño (*Texas Longhorn* Rodeo)	8.0	0
jerk, Jamaican (*Pain is Good*)	14.0	0
Kansas City style:		
(*Cowtown*)	11.0	0
(*Cowtown* Night of the Living)	10.0	0
(*Kraft*)	11.0	0
maple, smoky (*Annie's Naturals* Organic)	9.0	0
mesquite:		
(*Bull's-Eye* Texas Style)	13.0	0
(*D.L. Jardine's*)	6.0	<1.0
(*Hunt's*)	9.0	<1.0
(*Kraft*)	9.0	0
smoke (*Kraft Thick 'n Spicy*)	12.0	0
onion, grilled, w/garlic (*Bull's-Eye*)	14.0	1.0
onion bits (*Kraft*)	11.0	0
Polynesian (*Sagawa's*)	13.0	0
Southern style (*Pain is Good*)	14.0	0

Food and Measure	carb. (gms)	fiber (gms)
Southern style, vinegar (*Bilardo Brothers*)	5.0	1.0
St. Louis style (*Silver Dollar City*)	9.0	0
sweet and mild (*Silver Dollar City*)	11.0	0
sweet and sour (*Woody's*)	17.0	1.0
tangy (*Silver Dollar City*)	7.0	0
teriyaki (*Kraft*)	12.0	0
Barbecue seasoning (*McCormick*), ¼ tsp.	0	0
Barley:		
dry, ¼ cup:		
(*Shiloh Farms*)	35.0	6.0
pearled (*Arrowhead Mills*)	32.0	8.0
pearled	38.9	7.8
cooked, pearled, ½ cup	22.2	3.0
Barley flakes (*Arrowhead Mills*), ⅓ cup	28.0	5.0
Barley flour:		
(*Arrowhead Mills*), ⅓ cup	19.0	4.0
(*Shiloh Farms*), ¼ cup	19.0	3.0
Barley grits (*Shiloh Farms*), ¼ cup	35.0	6.0
Barley malt syrup (*Eden* Organic), 1 tbsp.	14.0	0
Barley miso, see "Miso"		
Basella, see "Vine spinach"		
Basil, fresh:		
1 oz.	1.2	.3
5 medium leaves	.1	.1
chopped, 2 tbsp.	.2	.2
Basil, dried:		
ground, 1 tbsp.	2.7	.5
ground, 1 tsp.	.9	.2
Baskin-Robbins, 4-oz. scoop, except as noted:		
ice cream:		
banana nut	27.0	1.0
black walnut	25.0	1.0
butter pecan	24.0	1.0
chocolate	33.0	0
chocolate *World Class*	33.0	0
chocolate almond	32.0	1.0
chocolate chip	28.0	1.0
chocolate chip cookie dough	36.0	1.0

Food and Measure	carb. (gms)	fiber (gms)
chocolate eclair	35.0	0
chocolate fudge	35.0	0
chocolate ribbon	31.0	0
crème brûlée	41.0	0
fudge brownie	35.0	1.0
German chocolate cake	36.0	1.0
gold medal ribbon	34.0	0
Jamoca	26.0	0
Jamoca almond fudge	31.0	1.0
mint chocolate chip	28.0	1.0
nutty coconut	28.0	1.0
Oreo cookies 'n cream	32.0	1.0
peanut butter chocolate	31.0	1.0
pistachio almond	25.0	1.0
pralines 'n cream	34.0	0
Reese's peanut butter cup	31.0	0
rocky road	36.0	1.0
strawberry, very berry	28.0	0
strawberry shortcake	34.0	0
tiramisu	32.0	0
vanilla or French vanilla	26.0	0
ice cream, light:		
berries 'n banana	25.0	1.0
caramel turtle	37.0	0
chocolate, mad about	35.0	1.0
chocolate chip or chocolate chocolate chip	30.0	1.0
chocolate cookie	34.0	1.0
espresso 'n cream	32.0	1.0
pineapple coconut	27.0	0
tin roof sundae	34.0	1.0
frozen yogurt, ½ cup:		
low fat:		
Maui brownie madness	39.0	1.0
perils of praline	37.0	1.0
Raspberry Cheese Louise	36.0	1.0
vanilla, nonfat	32.0	0
soft serve:		
chocolate	25.0	1.0

Food and Measure	carb. (gms)	fiber (gms)
peppermint	24.0	0
red raspberry	25.0	0
Truly Free, no sugar:		
butter pecan	17.0	1.0
café mocha	18.0	1.0
chocolate	15.0	0
strawberry or vanilla	17.0	1.0
vanilla, nonfat	23.0	0
ice, daiquiri, margarita, or watermelon	34.0	0
sherbet, blue raspberry, orange, or rainbow	34.0	0
sherbet, red raspberry	36.0	0
sundae, 1 serving:		
banana royale	91.0	5.0
banana split	168.0	7.0
hot fudge, 2-scoop	62.0	0
hot fudge, 3-scoop	86.0	0
Bold Breeze, 16 oz.:		
kiwi	87.0	3.0
kiwi, creamy	107.0	3.0
strawberry citrus	89.0	2.0
strawberry citrus, creamy	109.0	3.0
wild mango	84.0	2.0
wild mango, creamy	104.0	2.0
Cappuccino Blast, 16 oz.:		
cappuccino	43.0	0
low fat or nonfat	45.0	0
with whipped cream	67.0	0
chocolate	81.0	0
mocha	57.0	0
mocha, with whipped cream	58.0	0
Mintopia	63.0	0
turtle	92.0	0
shake, 16 oz.:		
chocolate, with chocolate	81.0	1.0
chocolate, with vanilla	85.0	0
vanilla	81.0	0
shake, espresso, 24 oz.	80.0	0
Bass, all varieties, without added ingredients	0	0

Food and Measure	carb. (gms)	fiber (gms)
Batter and breading mix (see also specific listings), seasoned, ¼ cup, except as noted:		
(*Old Bay Better Batter*)	13.0	0
(*Old Bay Dip & Crisp*)	15.0	0
all purpose:		
batter (*Don's Chuck Wagon*)	20.0	1.0
batter or breading (*Golden Dipt* Fry Easy)	20.0	0
beer batter (*Golden Dipt* Fry Easy)	19.0	0
Cajun (*Golden Dipt Oven Easy*)	11.0	0
garlic and herb (*Golden Dipt Oven Easy*), 3 tbsp.	13.0	0
lemon and pepper (*Golden Dipt Oven Easy*)	12.0	0
tempura (*Golden Dipt* Fry Easy)	20.0	0
Bay leaf, dried, crumbled, 1 tsp.	.3	<1.0
Bean dip, 2 tbsp., except as noted:		
(*Fritos* Original)	5.0	1.0
(*Pace*), ½ cup	15.0	4.0
black bean:		
(*D.L. Jardine's* Texas Pate)	5.0	2.0
(*Fritos*)	6.0	2.0
(*Garden of Eatin'* Baja)	5.0	1.0
mild or spicy (*Guiltless Gourmet*)	5.0	2.0
jalapeño (*Fritos* Hot)	5.0	1.0
jalapeño lime (*Synder's*)	5.0	n.a.
pinto bean, with cheese, salsa		
(*Cedarlane* 5-Layer Mexican)	4.0	1.0
red bean, spicy chipotle (*Garden of Eatin'*)	5.0	2.0
Bean dishes, see specific bean listings		
Bean salad (see also "Beans, mixed"):		
dill sauce (*S&W* Provençal Recipe), ½ cup	14.0	3.0
three bean (*Green Giant*), ½ cup	20.0	4.0
Bean sauce, Asian:		
black bean (*Ka•Me*), 1 tbsp.	3.0	0
black bean, garlic (*Lee Kum Kee*), 1 tbsp.	4.0	1.0
brown bean, spicy (*House of Tsang*), 1 tsp.	3.0	0
Bean sprouts, fresh, see specific listings		
Beans, see specific listings		
Beans, baked, see "Baked beans"		

Food and Measure	carb. (gms)	fiber (gms)
Beans, mixed (see also "Bean salad"), canned, ½ cup:		
(*Bush's*)	19.0	6.0
(*S&W* New York Deli Style)	17.0	6.0
(*S&W* San Antonio)	20.0	6.0
(*S&W* Santa Fe)	21.0	6.0
(*Westbrae Natural* Organic)	19.0	5.0
(*Westbrae Natural* Organic Soup Beans)	19.0	6.0
seasoned (*Glory* Crock Pot Beans)	25.0	7.0
Beans, snap or string, see "Green bean" and "Snap bean"		
Beans and franks:		
(*Hormel*), 7.5-oz. can	32.0	5.0
(*Kid's Kitchen*), 1 cup	37.0	7.0
Beans and rice, see "Rice dishes" and "Rice entree"		
Bear, meat only, without added ingredients	0	0
Béarnaise sauce, in jars (*Reese*), 2 tbsp.	1.0	0
Béarnaise sauce mix (*McCormick*), 1 tsp.	1.0	0
Beaver, meat only, without added ingredients	0	0
Bee pollen (*Tree of Life*), 1 tsp.	3.4	0
Beechnuts, dried, shelled, 1 oz.	9.5	n.a.
Beef, meat only, without added ingredients	0	0
Beef, canned, see "Beef entree, can or pkg." and specific listings		
Beef, corned (see also "Beef lunch meat"), brisket, cooked, 4 oz.	.5	0
Beef, corned, canned:		
(*Hormel*), 2 oz.	0	0
(*Libby's*), 2 oz.	0	0
hash, see "Beef hash"		
Beef, dried (see also "Beef jerky"):		
(*Hormel/Hormel Pillow Pack*), 10 slices, 1 oz.	1.0	0
cured, 1 oz.	.4	0
Beef, frozen or refrigerated, raw, boneless, marinated, sirloin, 4 oz.:		
peppercorn (*Always Tender*)	2.0	0
tequila lime (*Always Tender*)	3.0	0
teriyaki (*Always Tender*)	4.0	0

Food and Measure	carb. (gms)	fiber (gms)
Beef, frozen or refrigerated, cooked:		
back ribs, split, with barbecue sauce (*Lloyd's*),		
2 ribs with sauce, 7.5 oz.	25.0	0
barbecue, shredded (*Hormel*), 5 oz.	10.0	0
barbecue shredded, with original sauce (*Lloyd's*), ¼ cup	11.0	0
brisket, barbecued, sliced (*Hormel*), 5 oz.	23.0	0
pot roast, in gravy (*Tyson*), 5 oz.	2.0	0
roast (*Hormel*), 5 oz.	3.0	0
roast, in brown gravy (*Tyson*), 5 oz.	5.0	0
shredded, Southwestern (*Hormel*), 2 oz.	2.0	0
steak, breaded, fingers (*Tyson*), 2 pieces, 3.2 oz.	13.0	1.0
steak, breaded, country fried (*Tyson*), 3.2-oz. patty	17.0	1.0
steak, sliced, and gravy (*Hormel*), 5 oz.	3.0	0
steak, strips, seasoned (*Tyson*), 3 oz.	1.0	0
teriyaki (*Simply Simmered*), 5 oz.	10.0	1.0
tips (*Hormel*), 5 oz.	5.0	1.0
tips, in gravy (*Tyson*), 5 oz.	5.0	0
"Beef," vegetarian (see also "Burger, vegetarian"):		
canned (*Worthington Prime Stakes*), 3.2-oz. piece	7.0	1.0
frozen/refrigerated:		
(*Loma Linda* Swiss Stake), 3.2-oz. piece	9.0	3.0
(*Worthington Stakelets*), 2.5-oz. piece.	7.0	2.0
corned (*Worthington*), 3 slices, 2 oz.	5.0	0
ground (*Quorn*), ⅔ cup, 3 oz.	5.0	4.0
ground, regular or Mexican		
(*Yves* The Good Ground), 1.9 oz.	5.0	3.0
meatballs (*Yves* The Good Ground), 2.1 oz.	7.0	3.0
smoked (*Worthington*), 3 slices, 2 oz.	7.0	<1.0
strips (*Lightlife*), 3 oz.	6.0	4.0
Beef dinner, frozen, 1 pkg.:		
pot roast:		
(*Healthy Choice*), 11 oz.	39.0	6.0
(*Stouffer's* Homestyle), 16 oz.	43.0	7.0
(*Swanson Hungry-Man*), 18.5 oz.	47.0	7.0
ribs, boneless, barbecue sauce (*Healthy Choice*), 11 oz.	47.0	8.0
roasted:		
mushroom (*Healthy Choice*), 11 oz.	28.0	5.0

Food and Measure	carb. (gms)	fiber (gms)
oven (*Healthy Choice*), 10.15 oz.	33.0	5.0
slow, and gravy (*Stouffer's* Homestyle), 14 oz.	41.0	8.0
Salisbury steak:		
(*Healthy Choice*), 12.5 oz.	45.0	5.0
(*Lean Cuisine Dinnertime Selections*), 15.5 oz.	35.0	6.0
(*Stouffer's* Homestyle), 16 oz.	49.0	5.0
(*Swanson Hungry-Man*), 16.25 oz.	47.0	3.0
with redskin mashed potato (*Healthy Choice*), 8 oz. . . .	21.0	3.0
steak, country fried (*Stouffer's* Homestyle), 16 oz.	52.0	4.0
steak, Southwest, mesquite (*Stouffer's* Homestyle),		
14 oz.	50.0	8.0
steak tips Dijon (*Lean Cuisine Dinnertime Selections*),		
12 oz.	44.0	5.0
Stroganoff (*Healthy Choice*), 11 oz.	40.0	7.0
tips, portobello (*Healthy Choice*), 11.25 oz.	28.0	3.0
"Beef" dinner, vegetarian, frozen, Salisbury steak		
(*Amy's* Country Dinner), 11-oz. pkg.	60.0	8.0
Beef entree, can or pkg.:		
hash, see "Beef hash"		
pot roast (*Hormel* Bowl), 10 oz.	20.0	2.0
roast, with gravy (*Hormel*), ½ cup	3.0	3.0
roast, with potatoes (*Hormel* Bowl), 10 oz.	25.0	2.0
Salisbury steak (*Hormel* Bowl), 10 oz.	25.0	3.0
stew:		
(*Dinty Moore* Bowl), 10 oz.	22.0	2.0
(*Dinty Moore* Can), 1 cup	17.0	2.0
(*Dinty Moore* Can), 7.5-oz. can	15.0	2.0
(*Dinty Moore* Cup), 1 cont.	14.0	2.0
(*Dinty Moore* Steakhouse Can), 1 cup	16.0	2.0
(*Hormel* Meal), 1 cont.	14.0	2.0
Beef entree, freeze-dried, 1 serving:		
patty, flame-broiled (*Mountain House*), ½ pouch	26.0	3.0
rotini (*AlpineAire*)	59.0	3.0
stew:		
(*Mountain House* Can/Four), 1 cup	24.0	3.0
(*Mountain House* Double), ½ pouch	37.0	4.0
(*Mountain House* Single)	37.0	4.0

Food and Measure	carb. (gms)	fiber (gms)
Stroganoff flavor:		
(*AlpineAire*)	40.0	2.0
(*Mountain House* Can/Four), 1 cup	31.0	2.0
(*Mountain House* Double), ½ pouch	30.0	3.0
(*Mountain House* Single)	46.0	2.0
with beef and rice (*Instant Gourmet*)	67.0	5.0
tamale pie (*AlpineAire* Western)	50.0	7.0
teriyaki (*Mountain House*), ½ pouch	55.0	4.0
teriyaki (*Mountain House* Can), 1 cup	44.0	3.0
Beef entree, frozen (see also "Beef, frozen or refrigerated, cooked"), 1 pkg., except as noted:		
chipped, creamed (*Stouffer's* 11 oz.), 4.4 oz.	9.0	0
chow mein (*Shanghai*), ⅓ of 24-oz. pkg.	29.0	3.0
and broccoli:		
garlic (*Lean Cuisine* Cafe Classics), 9 oz.	16.0	3.0
Hunan (*Lean Cuisine Everyday Favorites*), 8.5 oz.	36.0	1.0
spicy (*Michelina's Yu Sing* Bowls), 11 oz.	78.0	2.0
spicy, with rice (*Uncle Ben's* Rice Bowl), 12 oz.	62.0	1.0
stir-fry (*Shanghai*), ⅕ of 44-oz. pkg.	42.0	4.0
broccoli and (*Stouffer's Skillet Sensations*), ⅓ of 25-oz. pkg.	29.0	2.0
fajita, see "Fajita"		
home style (*Stouffer's Skillet Sensations*), 7.1 oz.	19.0	2.0
Merlot (*Healthy Choice*), 10 oz.	26.0	7.0
Oriental (*Healthy Choice*), 10.6 oz.	27.0	8.0
Oriental (*Lean Cuisine* Cafe Classics), 9.25 oz.	31.0	2.0
pepper steak:		
(*Smart Ones Bistro Selections*), 10 oz.	32.0	4.0
green (*Stouffer's* Homestyle), 10.5 oz.	30.0	2.0
and rice (*Michelina's* Authentico), 8 oz.	43.0	1.0
and rice (*Michelina's Lean Gourmet*), 8 oz.	43.0	1.0
peppercorn (*Lean Cuisine* Cafe Classics), 8.75 oz.	25.0	3.0
peppercorn, fillet (*Smart Ones Bistro Selections*), 9.5 oz.	24.0	4.0
picadillo (*Ethnic Gourmet*), 10 oz.	36.0	3.0
pie (*Swanson*), 7 oz.	42.0	3.0
portobello (*Lean Cuisine* Cafe Classics), 9 oz.	25.0	2.0
pot roast:		
(*Lean Cuisine* Cafe Classics), 9 oz.	23.0	2.0

	carb. (gms)	fiber (gms)
(*Smart Ones* Higher Protein), 9 oz.	9.0	2.0
(*Stouffer's* Homestyle), 8⅞ oz.	24.0	3.0
with potato (*Michelina's Signature*), 10 oz.	35.0	4.0
Yankee (*Stouffer's Skillet Sensations*), ⅓ of 24-oz. pkg.	24.0	4.0
roast/roasted:		
with gravy (*Smart Ones Bistro Selections*), 9 oz.	19.0	3.0
oven (*Lean Cuisine* Cafe Classics), 9.25 oz.	18.0	2.0
portobello (*Smart Ones* Higher Protein), 9 oz.	9.0	2.0
Salisbury steak:		
(*Boston Market*), 16 oz.	44.0	4.0
(*Lean Cuisine* Cafe Classics), 9.5 oz.	26.0	3.0
(*Michelina's* Authentico), 8 oz.	22.0	2.0
(*Michelina's Lean Gourmet*), 8.5 oz.	23.0	2.0
(*Michelina's Signature*), 10.5 oz.	35.0	2.0
(*Smart Ones*), 9.5 oz.	25.0	4.0
(*Smart Ones* Higher Protein), 9 oz.	9.0	2.0
(*Stouffer's* Homestyle), 9⅝ oz.	27.0	1.0
(*Swanson* Angus), 13 oz.	24.0	3.0
shepherd's pie (*Ian's* Natural), ½ of 9.5-oz. pkg.	23.0	2.0
sirloin, and Asian vegetables		
(*Smart Ones* Higher Protein), 9 oz.	11.0	3.0
sirloin, roasted, with noodles (*Michelina's*		
Lean Gourmet/Authentico), 8 oz.	30.0	2.0
spicy (*Contessa* Minute Meal Bowl), 10.5 oz.	52.0	4.0
steak:		
and garlic potatoes (*Birds Eye Voila!*), 1 cup*	22.0	5.0
grilled, roasted garlic sauce (*Healthy Choice*), 10 oz.	46.0	6.0
grilled whiskey (*Healthy Choice*), 9.5 oz.	46.0	6.0
and portobello mushrooms (*Stouffer's* Bowl Cuisine),		
11 oz.	33.0	4.0
strips, grilled, with onion, peppers (*Swanson Hungry-Man*		
Steakhouse), 20 oz.	75.0	6.0
steak, with dipping sauce:		
barbecue (*Healthy Choice*), 13 oz.	51.0	8.0
teriyaki (*Healthy Choice*), 14 oz.	74.0	6.0
zesty (*Healthy Choice*), 13 oz.	37.0	6.0
stew:		
(*Green Giant* Complete Skillet Meal), ¼ of 32-oz. pkg.	27.0	4.0

Food and Measure	carb. (gms)	fiber (gms)
(*Stouffer's* Bowl Cuisine), 11 oz.	32.0	5.0
and vegetable (*Michelina's* Homestyle Bowls), 11 oz.	31.0	4.0
stir-fry (*Contessa*), 1¾ cups*	28.0	4.0
Stroganoff:		
(*Michelina's Lean Gourmet*), 8 oz.	38.0	2.0
(*Stouffer's* Homestyle), 9¾ oz.	34.0	2.0
(*Stouffer's Skillet Sensations* 40 oz.), 7.25 oz.	24.0	3.0
teriyaki (*Healthy Choice*), 9.5 oz.	46.0	5.0
teriyaki, and rice (*Lean Cuisine Skillet Sensations*),		
⅓ of 24-oz. pkg.	31.0	2.0
teriyaki steak:		
(*Lean Cuisine* Cafe Classics Bowl), 10.5 oz.	47.0	4.0
(*Michelina's Yu Sing* Bowls), 11 oz.	64.0	3.0
(*Stouffer's Skillet Sensations*), ⅓ of 23.5-oz. pkg.	33.0	2.0
tips, Southern (*Lean Cuisine* Cafe Classics), 8.75 oz.	36.0	3.0
tips, steak, portobello (*Lean Cuisine* Cafe Classics),		
7.5 oz.	13.0	3.0
and vegetables:		
(*Ethnic Gourmet* Bulgogi), 10 oz.	36.0	2.0
(*Smart Ones* Bowls), 11 oz.	40.0	3.0
teriyaki (*Birds Eye Voila!* Reduced Carb), 1 cup*	15.0	4.0
teriyaki steak (*Green Giant* Complete Skillet Meal),		
¼ of 32-oz. pkg.	53.0	3.0
"Beef" entree, vegetarian, frozen, 1 pkg.:		
pepper steak (*Hain Vegetarian Classics*), 10 oz.	41.0	9.0
Santa Fe veggie beef (*Yves* The Good Bowl), 10.5 oz.	57.0	5.0
Beef entree mix, see "Hamburger entree mix"		
Beef gravy, ¼ cup:		
(*Boston Market* Classic)	4.0	0
(*Campbell's/Campbell's* Fat Free)	3.0	0
roast, slow (*Franco-American/Franco-American* Fat Free)	3.0	0
with roasted garlic (*Campbell's*)	4.0	0
savory (*Heinz* Home Style)	4.0	0
Beef gravy mix, and herb (*McCormick*), ¼ cup*	3.0	0
Beef hash, canned, 1 cup, except as noted:		
corned beef:		
(*Armour*)	23.0	2.0

Food and Measure	carb. (gms)	fiber (gms)
(*Castleberry*)	25.0	3.0
(*Mary Kitchen*)	22.0	2.0
(*Mary Kitchen*), 7.5-oz. can	20.0	2.0
(*Mary Kitchen* 50% Less Fat)	25.0	3.0
roast beef (*Mary Kitchen*)	22.0	2.0
Beef hash, freeze-dried, roast beef		
(*AlpineAire* All American), 2 oz.	28.0	3.0
Beef jerky, 1 oz.:		
(*Pemmican* Homestyle Tender Original)	3.0	1.0
(*Pemmican* Long Lasting Original)	5.0	0
(*Pemmican* Premium Cut Original)	4.0	1.0
hot and spicy or peppered (*Pemmican* Long Lasting)	4.0	0
kippered, original, peppered, or teriyaki (*Pemmican*)	2.0	0
kippered, sweet and hot (*Pemmican*)	6.0	0
shredded, original, peppered, or teriyaki (*Pemmican*)	3.0	1.0
steak tips (*Pemmican*)	5.0	0
teriyaki (*Pemmican* Long Lasting)	6.0	0
Beef liver, see "Liver"		
Beef lunch meat (see also "Bologna," etc.), 2 oz., except as noted:		
corned:		
(*Black Bear* Brisket)	2.0	0
(*Boar's Head*)	0	0
(*Dietz & Watson* Brisket)	0	0
(*Healthy Choice*)	0	0
(*Healthy Deli*)	2.0	0
(*Hormel*)	0	0
(*Sara Lee*)	0	0
(*Sara Lee* Sliced), 2 slices, 1.8 oz.	1.0	0
(*Tyson* Bag), 2 slices, 2.25 oz.	0	0
London broil (*Black Bear*)	0	0
London Broil (*Dietz & Watson*)	0	0
oven roasted:		
(*Boar's Head* Top Round No Salt)	0	0
(*Healthy Deli* Zero Carb)	0	0
Italian style (*Healthy Deli*)	1.0	0
Cajun style (*Boar's Head*)	0	0

Food and Measure	carb. (gms)	fiber (gms)
pepper seasoned (*Boar's Head* Eye Round)	0	0
roast/roasted:		
(*Dietz & Watson* Cap Off)	0	0
(*Hansel 'n Gretel*)	2.0	0
(*Hatfield Deli Choice*)	0	0
(*Sara Lee*)	1.0	0
(*Sara Lee* Sliced), 2 slices, 1.6 oz.	0	0
(*Tyson* Bag), 2 slices, 2.25 oz.	1.0	0
extra lean (*Alpine Lace* 97% Fat Free)	1.0	0
eye round, Italian, or marinated (*Dietz & Watson*)	0	0
Italian style (*Boar's Head*)	1.0	0
medium (*Healthy Choice*)	1.0	0
peppered (*Sara Lee*)	1.0	0
seasoned (*Hormel*)	0	0
seasoned (*Williams* Black Angus)	0	0
teriyaki, eye round (*Dietz & Watson*)	0	0
top round (*Boar's Head* Low Sodium)	<1.0	0
whole muscle (*Healthy Choice*), 2 slices, 1.6 oz.	1.0	0
Beef pie, see "Beef entree, frozen"		
Beef pocket/sandwich, frozen, 1 piece, 4.5 oz., except as noted:		
barbecue sauce with (*Lean Pockets*)	47.0	3.0
cheeseburger (*Lean Pockets*)	42.0	3.0
cheeseburger (*White Castle*), 2 pieces, 3.7 oz.	23.0	6.0
hamburger (*White Castle*), 2 pieces	23.0	5.0
Philly cheese steak:		
(*Croissant Pockets*)	33.0	3.0
(*Lean Pockets*)	40.0	3.0
sub (*Michelina's Hot Subs*), 2.1 oz.	36.0	1.0
steak fajita (*Lean Pockets*)	39.0	3.0
Beef potato puffs, frozen (*Goya*), 1 piece	18.0	3.0
Beef sausage, see "Sausage" and specific listings		
Beef seasoning, and pork (*Lawry's* Perfect Blend),		
¼ tsp.	0	0
Beef seasoning mix (see also specific listings):		
pot roast (*McCormick Bag 'n Season*), 1 tsp.	1.0	0
stew:		
(*Adolph's Meal Makers*), 1 tsp.	3.0	0

Food and Measure	carb. (gms)	fiber (gms)
(*Lawry's*), 1 tsp.	2.0	0
(*McCormick*), 2 tsp.	2.0	0
(*McCormick Bag 'n Season*), 1 tsp.	1.0	0
Stroganoff (*Lawry's*), 1 tbsp.	5.0	0
Stroganoff (*McCormick*), 2 tsp.	3.0	0
Swiss steak (*McCormick Bag 'n Season*), 1 tsp.	2.0	0
Beef stew, see "Beef entree"		
Beef-tomato drink, see "Tomato-beef drink"		
Beefalo, meat only, without added ingredients	0	0
Beefsteak leaf, pickled, see "Shiso leaf powder"		
Beer:		
regular, 12 fl. oz.	13.2	0
light, 12 fl. oz.	4.8	0
Beerwurst, pork and beef, 2 oz.	2.4	.5
Beet, fresh:		
raw:		
(*Frieda's*), ½ cup, 3 oz.	8.0	2.0
2 medium, 2'' diam.	15.6	4.6
trimmed, sliced, ½ cup	6.5	1.9
boiled, drained, 2 medium, 2'' diam.	10.0	1.7
broiled, drained, sliced, ½ cup	8.5	1.4
Beets, canned:		
whole (*Freshlike Small*), 3 pieces., 4.4 oz.	9.0	2.0
whole or sliced (*S&W*), ½ cup	8.0	2.0
whole or sliced, with liquid, ½ cup	8.3	1.4
sliced, ½ cup:		
(*Del Monte*)	8.0	2.0
(*Freshlike Small*)	9.0	2.0
(*Veg-All*)	8.0	1.0
Harvard (*Greenwood Sweet & Tangy*), ½ cup	27.0	1.0
Harvard, with liquid, ½ cup	22.4	1.0
pickled:		
(*Greenwood*), 1 oz.	6.0	0
(*S&W*), 1 oz.	4.0	1.0
sliced (*Del Monte*), ½ cup	19.0	2.0
sliced (*Freshlike Selects*), 4 pieces, 1 oz.	4.0	0
with liquid, ½ cup	18.5	3.0

Food and Measure	carb. (gms)	fiber (gms)
Beet greens, ½ cup:		
raw, 1'' pieces	.8	.7
boiled, drained, 1'' pieces	3.9	2.1
Berliner, pork and beef, 1 oz.	.7	0
Berries, mixed, frozen:		
(*Cascadian Farm* Harvest), 1 cup	16.0	4.0
(*C&W* Medley), 1 cup	14.0	2.0
(*Tree of Life*), ¾ cup	16.0	3.0
Berry drink blend, 8 fl. oz., except as noted:		
(*Bolthouse Farms* Berry Boost Smoothie)	30.0	4.0
(*Minute Maid Coolers*), 6.75-fl.-oz. pouch	26.0	0
(*SoBe Black & Blue*)	31.0	0
(*V8 Splash*)	27.0	0
(*V8 Splash* Smoothies Wild Berry Creme)	30.0	0
kiwi (*Minute Maid*)	29.0	0
kiwi (*Minute Maid*), 12-fl.-oz. bottle	43.0	0
punch:		
(*Minute Maid*)	32.0	0
(*Nantucket Nectars* Maine)	27.0	0
frozen* (*Minute Maid*)	30.0	0
Berry juice, 8 fl. oz.:		
(*After the Fall* Oregon)	32.0	0
(*Juicy Juice*)	30.0	0
(*L&A*)	30.0	0
(*Langers*)	30.0	0
nectar (*Santa Cruz Organic*)	30.0	0
Biryani paste, see "Curry paste"		
Biscuit, plain or buttermilk, 2-oz. pc.	27.5	.7
Biscuit, frozen or refrigerated, 1 piece, except as noted:		
(*Grands!* Extra Rich)	26.0	<1.0
(*Grands!* Original Homestyle/*Butter Tastin'*)	24.0	<1.0
(*Pillsbury Butter Tastin'* Golden Homestyle/*Butter Tastin'* Golden Layers)	14.0	0
(*Pillsbury Butter Tastin'* Microwave)	24.0	<1.0
(*Pillsbury Butter Tastin'* Oven Baked)	22.0	<1.0
(*Pillsbury Country*)	29.0	<1.0
(*Pillsbury Easy Split* Oven Baked Extra Large)	34.0	1.0

Food and Measure	carb. (gms)	fiber (gms)
buttermilk:		
(*Grands!*)	24.0	<1.0
(*Grands!* Flaky Layers)	23.0	<1.0
(*Grands!* Reduced Fat)	25.0	<1.0
(*Perfect Portions*)	25.0	<1.0
(*Pillsbury*)	29.0	<1.0
(*Pillsbury* Microwave)	24.0	<1.0
(*Pillsbury* Oven Baked)	22.0	<1.0
(*Pillsbury Golden Homestyle/Golden Layers*)	14.0	0
(*Pillsbury 1869*)	12.0	0
(*Rhodes*)	25.0	<1.0
cheddar garlic (*Pillsbury* Oven Baked)	20.0	<1.0
cinnamon sugar (*Pillsbury Golden Layers*)	16.0	<1.0
corn, golden (*Grands!*)	28.0	<1.0
flaky:		
(*Grands!* Original/*Butter Tastin'*)	23.0	<1.0
(*Grands!* Original Reduced Fat)	25.0	<1.0
(*Pillsbury* Layers), 3 pieces	28.0	1.0
(*Pillsbury* Oven Baked)	20.0	0
flaky or honey butter (*Pillsbury Golden Layers*)	14.0	0
Southern style (*Grands!*)	24.0	<1.0
Southern style (*Pillsbury* Oven Baked)	22.0	<1.0
wheat (*Grands!* Reduced Fat)	27.0	2.0
Biscuit mix (see also "Baking mix"), ⅓ cup, except as noted:		
(*Kentucky Kernel*), ¼ cup	28.0	1.0
buttermilk (*Bisquick* Complete)	21.0	0
buttermilk ("*Jiffy*")	29.0	<1.0
cheese, three (*Bisquick* Complete)	21.0	0
cheese garlic (*Bisquick* Complete)	22.0	0
cinnamon swirl (*Bisquick* Complete)	26.0	0
honey butter (*Bisquick* Complete)	24.0	0
Bison, meat only, without added ingredients	0	0
Bitter melon, see "Balsam pear"		
Bitters (*Angostura*), 2 tbsp.	14.0	0
Black bean, dried:		
dry (*Goya*), ¼ cup	23.0	15.0
boiled, ½ cup	20.4	7.5
turtle, dry (*Arrowhead Mills*), ¼ cup	27.0	10.0

Food and Measure	carb. (gms)	fiber (gms)
turtle, dry (*Shiloh Farms*), ¼ cup	28.0	9.0
turtle, boiled, ½ cup	22.4	4.9
Black bean, canned (see also "Refried beans"), ½ cup:		
(*Allens*)	19.0	8.0
(*Bush's*)	20.0	7.0
(*Eden* Organic)	18.0	6.0
(*Progresso*)	17.0	7.0
(*S&W/S&W* 50% Less Salt)	17.0	6.0
(*Westbrae Natural* Organic)	19.0	5.0
(*Zapata*)	19.0	7.0
Caribbean (*Eden* Organic)	20.0	7.0
Caribbean (*S&W*)	23.0	7.0
with rice (*Glory*)	16.0	2.0
seasoned (*Trappey's*)	20.0	7.0
Black bean, mix, instant (*Fantastic*), ⅓ cup	29.0	7.0
Black bean dish, frozen, and rice, seasoned		
(*Glory* Savory Accents), ½ cup	16.0	2.0
Black bean entree, frozen, and sausage		
(*Glory* Savory Singles), 11-oz. pkg.	41.0	8.0
Black bean sauce, see "Bean sauce"		
Blackberry, fresh, ½ cup	9.2	3.6
Blackberry, canned, in syrup, ½ cup	29.6	4.4
Blackberry, dried (*Frieda's* Marionberry), ⅓ cup, 1.4 oz.	32.0	2.0
Blackberry, frozen:		
(*Cascadian Farm*), 1 cup	22.0	7.0
unsweetened, ½ cup	11.8	3.8
Blackberry syrup (*Smucker's*), ¼ cup	52.0	0
Black-eyed peas (see also "Cowpeas"):		
fresh (*Frieda's*), ⅓ cup, 3 oz.	21.0	11.0
dry (*Shiloh Farms*), ¼ cup	23.0	10.0
mature, boiled, ½ cup	17.9	5.6
Black-eyed peas, canned, ½ cup:		
(*Allens* Dry)	18.0	4.0
(*Allens/East Texas Fair*)	21.0	6.0
(*Bush's*)	19.0	4.0
(*Eden* Organic)	16.0	4.0
with bacon:		
(*Allens*)	20.0	5.0

Food and Measure	carb. (gms)	fiber (gms)
or bacon and jalapeño (*Bush's*)	18.0	5.0
or bacon and pork (*Trappey's*)	19.0	5.0
and pork (*Sunshine*)	20.0	5.0
with rice (*Glory*)	17.0	3.0
seasoned (*Glory* Southern)	25.0	5.0
with snaps (*Allens/East Texas Fair*)	20.0	5.0
with snaps (*Bush's*)	17.0	5.0
Black-eyed peas, frozen, ½ cup:		
(*McKenzie's*)	21.0	4.0
boiled, drained	20.2	4.3
seasoned, and rice (*Glory* Savory Accents)	17.0	3.0
Blackened seasoning (*Old Bay*), ½ tsp.	0	0
Blimpie, 1 serving:		
café sandwiches, 6'':		
Cable Car Club	36.0	2.0
Fisherman's Wharf tuna melt	35.0	3.0
Golden Gate Gourmet	40.0	2.0
Union Square Veggie	39.0	2.0
cold subs, 6'':		
Blimpie Best	52.0	3.3
Buffalo Chicken	50.0	3.0
club or tuna	50.5	3.3
ham and cheese	51.5	3.3
roast beef or turkey	49.0	3.3
seafood	58.0	3.8
grilled subs, 6'':		
beef, turkey, and cheddar	49.0	2.7
Cuban	50.4	2.7
pastrami special	52.0	3.3
Reuben	55.0	2.4
ultimate club	51.0	2.7
hot subs, 6''		
BLT	49.0	3.3
Buffalo Chicken	50.0	2.7
chicken, grilled	50.0	3.3
ChikMax	71.0	8.0
meatball	55.0	1.7
pastrami	53.0	3.3

Food and Measure	carb. (gms)	fiber (gms)
steak and onion melt	49.0	3.0
MexiMax	65.0	7.3
VegiMax	60.0	8.3
wraps:		
BLT, ultimate	60.0	3.0
beef and cheddar	57.0	3.0
chicken Caesar	56.0	3.0
Italian, zesty	74.0	3.0
Southwestern	54.0	3.0
steak and onion	64.0	3.0
breads:		
ciabatta	43.0	2.0
regular, 6":		
honey oat	49.0	4.2
Parmesan, zesty	44.0	1.8
rye, marbled	55.0	3.4
wheat	55.0	3.4
wheat, poppy	42.0	3.8
wheat, sesame	41.0	3.9
white	43.0	1.7
white, poppy	44.0	1.8
white, sesame	43.0	1.9
wrap, spinach/herb	49.0	2.0
wrap, traditional	51.0	2.0
dressing/toppings:		
cheese, cheddar, provolone, or Swiss, 1 slice	0	0
dressing, 1.5 oz.:		
Blimpie	24.0	0
blue cheese or Caesar	2.0	0
Dijon honey	8.0	0
Italian, fat-free	5.0	0
Italian, light	2.0	0
Parmesan peppercorn	2.0	0
ranch, light	8.0	0
Thousand Island	11.0	0
guacamole	7.4	1.4
oil and vinegar for 6" sub	.5	0
pesto, 1 oz.	1.0	0

Food and Measure	carb. (gms)	fiber (gms)
sides, 5 oz.:		
coleslaw	13.0	1.0
macaroni salad	25.0	1.0
potato salad	19.0	1.0
potato salad, mustard	21.0	1.0
soup, 8 oz.:		
broccoli cheese	15.0	3.0
chicken noodle	18.0	1.0
chicken rice	21.0	2.0
chili grande	30.0	18.0
potato, cream of	24.0	3.0
tomato basil ravioli	22.0	<1.0
vegetable, garden	14.0	3.0
vegetable beef	13.0	2.0
salad, regular:		
antipasto	10.0	2.7
chef	9.0	3.0
Chili Olé	42.0	3.0
grilled chicken, Caesar dressing	8.6	2.6
Roast Beef 'n Bleu	29.0	0
seafood	16.0	3.2
tuna	8.0	2.7
turkey, Zesto Pesto	31.0	0
Blintz, frozen, 1 piece:		
apple (A&B Famous), 2.5 oz.	28.0	1.0
apple raisin (Empire), 2.2 oz.	16.0	1.0
cheese:		
(A&B Famous), 3 oz.	30.8	1.0
(Empire), 2.2 oz.	13.0	2.0
(Golden), 2.2 oz.	13.0	2.0
(Kineret), 2.2 oz.	12.0	0
potato:		
(A&B Famous), 2.5 oz.	12.9	0
(Empire), 2.2 oz.	15.0	2.0
(Kineret), 2.2 oz.	12.0	0
Blintz, nondairy, frozen, "cheese," 1 piece:		
(Tofutti Mintz's Blintzes)	15.0	0
with apple, blueberry, or cherry (Tofutti Pillows)	16.0	0

Food and Measure	carb. (gms)	fiber (gms)
Blood sausage, 1 oz.	.4	0
Bloody Mary drink mixer:		
(*Angostura*), 8 fl. oz.	15.0	0
(*Mr & Mrs T*), 11.5-fl.-oz. can	13.0	0
(*Pace*), 8 fl. oz.	10.0	2.0
(*Sacramento*), 8 fl. oz.	13.0	3.0
spicy (*D.L. Jardine's* Red Snapper), 3 fl. oz.	5.0	0
spicy (*Pain is Good* Original/Cajun/Jamaican), 1 fl. oz. ...	1.0	0
Bloody Mary seasoning (*Angostura*), 1 tsp.	0	0
Blue squash, see "Australian blue squash"		
Blueberry, fresh, ½ cup	10.2	2.0
Blueberry, canned, in heavy syrup:		
(*S&W*), ⅓ cup	16.0	6.0
½ cup	28.2	1.9
Blueberry, dried:		
(*Frieda's*), ¼ cup, 1.4 oz.	33.0	4.0
wild (*Hodgson Mill*), ¼ cup, 1.4 oz.	32.0	6.0
wild (*Shiloh Farms*), ⅓ cup	38.0	2.0
Blueberry, freeze-dried (*AlpineAire*), .5 oz.	12.0	0
Blueberry, frozen:		
(*Cascadian Farm*), 1 cup	22.0	4.0
(*C&W*), ¾ cup	17.0	4.0
(*Tree of Life*), 1 cup	20.0	2.0
unsweetened, ½ cup	9.4	2.1
sweetened, ½ cup	25.2	2.4
Blueberry glaze (*Litehouse*), 3 tbsp.	18.0	0
Blueberry juice, 8 fl. oz.:		
(*After the Fall* Maine Coast)	31.0	0
(*R.W. Knudsen* Just Blueberry)	24.0	0
(*Walnut Acres*)	31.0	<1.0
Blueberry juice concentrate (*Tree of Life*), 8 tsp.	31.0	0
Blueberry nectar, 8 fl. oz.:		
(*R.W. Knudsen*)	30.0	0
banana (*Nantucket Nectars*)	28.0	1.0
Blueberry syrup (*Smucker's*), ¼ cup	52.0	0
Blueberry-chickpea spread (*Cedar's* Mediterranean),		
2 tbsp.	11.0	2.0
Blueberry-cranberry drink (*Langers*), 8 fl. oz.	34.0	0

Food and Measure	carb. (gms)	fiber (gms)
Bluefish, without added ingredients	0	0
Boar, wild, meat only, without added ingredients	0	0
Bob Evans, 1 serving:		
breakfast combos:		
country biscuit	71.0	4.0
eggs Benedict	35.0	2.0
fruit yogurt plate	96.0	8.0
pot roast hash	37.0	4.0
sausage, lite	48.0	4.0
sausage gravy, bowl	26.0	0
sausage gravy, cup	14.0	0
sunshine skillet	35.0	4.0
breakfast omelet:		
regular, plain	1.0	0
cheese	3.0	1.0
farmer's market	11.0	1.0
ham or sausage and cheese	2.0	0
Southwest chicken	5.0	1.0
Western	6.0	1.0
Egg Beaters, plain	2.0	0
cheese	4.0	1.0
farmer's market	12.0	1.0
ham or sausage and cheese	3.0	1.0
Southwest chicken	5.0	2.0
Western	7.0	2.0
breakfast items:		
bacon, 1 piece	0	0
bacon, Canadian, 1 piece	0	0
egg, hard-boiled, 1 egg	1.0	0
eggs, scrambled	1.0	0
French toast, stuffed, 9.9 oz.	55.0	3.0
French toast, stuffed, 6.6 oz.	38.0	2.0
fruit cup	42.0	4.0
grits	29.0	2.0
ham, smoked, 1 piece	2.0	0
home fries	28.0	4.0
hotcake, 1 piece:		
blueberry	32.0	2.0

Food and Measure	carb. (gms)	fiber (gms)
buttermilk	28.0	1.0
cinnamon	41.0	1.0
multigrain	34.0	2.0
mush, 1 slice	14.0	0
oatmeal, bowl	34.0	5.0
sausage, regular or light, 1 link or patty	0	0
sirloin steak	3.0	0
strawberry yogurt	28.0	1.0
waffle, Belgian, 1 piece	57.0	2.0
burgers/sandwiches:		
bacon cheeseburger	31.0	1.0
big BLT	30.0	2.0
BLT, plain	26.0	2.0
Bob's BLT	48.0	0
cheese, grilled	25.0	2.0
cheeseburger, plain	31.0	1.0
chicken:		
fried, club	40.0	2.0
fried, plain	39.0	2.0
grilled, club	31.0	2.0
grilled, plain	30.0	2.0
chicken salad, plain	55.0	3.0
haddock	65.0	0
hamburger, plain	30.0	1.0
pot roast	62.0	1.0
turkey bacon melt	56.0	3.0
lunch savors:		
pulled pork sandwich	54.0	3.0
steak tips and noodles	48.0	3.0
stir-fry chicken	55.0	5.0
stir-fry vegetables	55.0	4.0
lunch savors salad:		
Cobb, grilled chicken	9.0	3.0
Frisco, fried chicken	26.0	4.0
Frisco, grilled chicken	9.0	3.0
spinach, country	11.0	4.0
Wildfire, fried chicken	74.0	8.0
Wildfire, grilled chicken	57.0	8.0

Food and Measure	carb. (gms)	fiber (gms)
salads, farm-fresh:		
chicken salad	77.0	12.0
Cobb, grilled chicken	15.0	6.0
Frisco salad, fried chicken	40.0	6.0
Frisco salad, grilled chicken	1.0	6.0
side, garden	26.0	2.0
side, garden, without croutons	5.0	2.0
side, specialty	16.0	2.0
side, specialty, without croutons	5.0	2.0
spinach, country	13.0	5.0
Wildfire, fried chicken	88.0	11.0
Wildfire, grilled chicken	68.0	10.0
salad dressing, 3 oz.[1]:		
bleu cheese	6.0	0
colonial	23.0	0
French	19.0	0
honey mustard	16.0	0
hot bacon	35.0	0
Italian, lite	8.0	0
ranch	3.0	0
ranch, lite	5.0	0
Thousand Island	14.0	0
vinegar and oil	0	0
Wildfire ranch	18.0	0
soup, hearty:		
bean, bowl	23.0	7.0
bean, cup	16.0	5.0
cheddar potato, bowl	31.0	2.0
cheddar potato, cup	25.0	1.0
sausage chili, bowl	26.0	10.0
sausage chili, cup	19.0	7.0
vegetable beef, bowl	23.0	4.0
vegetable beef, cup	13.0	2.0
dinner:		
catfish, grilled, 1 piece	4.0	4.0
chicken, fried	9.0	1.0

[1] Dinner portion; divide by 2 for the 1.5-oz. side portion.

Food and Measure	carb. (gms)	fiber (gms)
chicken, grilled	0	0
chicken, grilled, with barbecue sauce	27.0	2.0
chicken, grilled, with garlic butter	15.0	2.0
chicken-n-noodles	32.0	2.0
chicken pot pie	46.0	2.0
chicken strip, 1 piece	9.0	0
chicken tender, 1 piece	0	0
cod, lemon pepper, 1 piece	15.0	0
meat loaf	14.0	1.0
noodles, buttered	35.0	2.0
pork chop	2.0	0
pork chop, with barbecue sauce	29.0	2.0
pork chop, with garlic butter	16.0	2.0
roast beef, open face	24.0	1.0
salmon, plain	12.0	1.0
shrimp, fried, plain	8.0	0
spaghetti, marinara	104.0	10.0
spaghetti, meatballs	116.0	13.0
spaghetti, meatballs, seniors	59.0	7.0
steak, country fried	26.0	0
steak, country fried, with gravy	31.0	0
steak Monterey	7.0	1.0
steak tips and noodles	94.0	7.0
steak tips and noodles, seniors	47.0	3.0
stir-fry chicken	84.0	6.0
stir-fry chicken, seniors	55.0	5.0
stir-fry vegetables	99.0	12.0
strip steak	12.0	1.0
strip steak, with garlic butter	15.0	2.0
turkey and dressing	41.0	4.0
side items:		
applesauce	26.0	2.0
baked potato, plain	54.0	6.0
baked potato, loaded	57.0	7.0
bread dressing	36.0	0
broccoli florets	8.0	5.0
broccoli florets, cheddar	14.0	5.0
carrots, glazed	21.0	4.0

Food and Measure	carb. (gms)	fiber (gms)
coleslaw	18.0	2.0
corn, buttered	18.0	2.0
cottage cheese	4.0	0
fries	35.0	3.0
fruit dish	23.0	2.0
green beans with ham	5.0	2.0
mushrooms, grilled	10.0	5.0
onion rings	49.0	1.0
potatoes, mashed	15.0	1.0
rice pilaf	32.0	1.0
vegetables, garden, grilled	23.0	7.0
garnish/condiments:		
cranberry relish	13.0	1.0
garlic herb butter	2.0	1.0
gravy, beef	5.0	0
gravy, chicken	4.0	0
gravy, country	6.0	0
hollandaise sauce	6.0	0
onion ring garnish	12.0	1.0
bread/rolls:		
banana nut	30.0	1.0
biscuit	36.0	0
cranberry nut	25.0	1.0
dinner roll	34.0	1.0
English muffin	28.0	2.0
garlic bread	16.0	1.0
Kaiser bun	30.0	1.0
mini bun	20.0	1.0
pumpkin bread	27.0	1.0
sourdough bread	26.0	0
Texas toast	12.0	1.0
wheat bread	13.0	2.0
white bread	12.0	1.0
desserts:		
apple dumpling	119.0	5.0
berry cobbler	85.0	5.0
blackberry cobbler	87.0	0
hot fudge cake	108.0	5.0

Food and Measure	carb. (gms)	fiber (gms)
pie, 1 slice:		
apple, no sugar	52.0	2.0
caramel pecan silk	69.0	2.0
cherry supreme	46.0	2.0
coconut cream	67.0	2.0
French silk	82.0	2.0
pecan	94.0	1.0
pumpkin	69.0	3.0
Reese's cup	78.0	1.0
Reese's sundae	104.0	3.0
vanilla ice cream, à la mode or 1 serving	19.0	0
Bockwurst, raw, 1 oz.	.1	0
Bok choy, see "Cabbage, Chinese"		
Bologna (see also "Ham bologna," etc.), 2 oz., except as noted:		
(*Boar's Head* 28% Lower Sodium)	0	0
(*Deli Delight*)	4.0	0
(*Hansel 'n' Gretel* Classic)	3.0	0
(*Hatfield Deli Choice*)	2.0	0
(*Johnsonville* Country Style Ring)	1.0	0
(*Oscar Mayer*), 1 oz.	1.0	0
(*Oscar Mayer* Light), 1 oz.	2.0	0
beef:		
(*Boar's Head*)	0	0
(*Deli Delight*)	4.0	0
(*Hansel 'n' Gretel*)	4.0	0
(*Hatfield Deli Choice*)	2.0	0
(*Healthy Deli* Zero Carb)	0	0
(*Johnsonville* Hearty Ring)	1.0	0
(*Oscar Mayer*), 1 oz.	1.0	0
(*Oscar Mayer* Light), 1 oz.	2.0	0
(*Tyson*), .9-oz. slice	1.0	0
lean (*Hebrew National*)	1.0	0
garlic (*Boar's Head*)	1.0	0
German:		
(*Hansel & Gretel*)	3.0	0
(*Hatfield Deli Choice*)	2.0	0
(*Healthy Deli* Zero Carb)	0	0

Food and Measure	carb. (gms)	fiber (gms)
Lebanon (*Boar's Head*)	3.0	0
pork and beef (*Boar's Head*)	<1.0	0
"Bologna," vegetarian, frozen, slices:		
(*Worthington Bolono*), 3 slices, 2 oz.	3.0	2.0
(*Yves*), 2.2 oz.	4.0	1.0
Boniato (*Frieda's*), 3 oz.	24.0	3.0
Bonito, meat only, raw, 4 oz.	.5	0
Bonito flakes (*Eden*), 2 tbsp.	0	0
Borage:		
raw, 1" pieces, ½ cup	1.4	<1.0
boiled, drained, 4 oz.	4.0	<2.0
Boston Market, 1 serving:		
entree, chicken:		
crispy baked country, with gravy	33.0	5.0
garlic, rotisserie:		
½ with skin	4.0	0
¼ dark, with skin	2.0	0
¼ dark, without skin	1.0	0
¼ white, with or without skin and wing	2.0	0
pastry top pot pie	57.0	2.0
Tuscan, rotisserie:		
½ spicy	8.0	1.0
¼ spicy, dark or white	4.0	1.0
entree, other:		
cod, baked	11.0	0
ham, honey glazed	10.0	0
meat loaf, 2 slices	22.0	2.0
meat loaf, with beef gravy, 2 slices	27.0	2.0
meat loaf, with chunky tomato, 2 slices	30.0	3.0
turkey, rotisserie	3.0	0
sides, cold, coleslaw	29.0	10.0
sides, cold, cranberry	25.0	<1.0
sides, hot:		
apples, cinnamon	56.0	3.0
butternut squash	25.0	6.0
corn, sweet	30.0	2.0
green bean casserole	9.0	2.0
green beans	6.0	2.0

Food and Measure	carb. (gms)	fiber (gms)
macaroni and cheese	33.0	1.0
pasta, penne	29.0	2.0
potato, mashed	30.0	2.0
potato, mashed, with gravy	32.0	3.0
potato, new garlic dill	25.0	2.0
poultry gravy	2.0	0
spinach, creamed	11.0	2.0
spinach, sauteed	8.0	5.0
squash casserole	20.0	3.0
stuffing, savory	27.0	2.0
sweet potato casserole	39.0	2.0
vegetables, steamed	6.0	2.0
sandwiches, with cheese:		
chicken, with sauce	68.0	5.0
meat loaf	102.0	7.0
turkey, with sauce	68.0	5.0
salads:		
Caesar, entree	17.0	3.0
Caesar, side	13.0	<1.0
chicken Caesar	19.0	3.0
chicken, Asian	57.0	8.0
chicken, Asian, without dressing and noodles	22.0	7.0
fruit salad	16.0	1.0
soup:		
chicken noodle, cup	8.0	0
tortilla, with toppings	18.0	2.0
tortilla, without toppings	7.0	1.0
desserts:		
apple pie, 1 slice	66.0	3.0
brownie, chocolate	88.0	6.0
brownie, caramel pecan	114.0	6.0
cake, chocolate	86.0	2.0
cake, molten fudge	34.0	1.0
chocolate chip cookie	51.0	2.0
chocolate Mania	36.0	1.0
corn bread	21.0	0
oatmeal cookie	47.0	2.0

Bouillon (see also "Bouillon concentrate"):
beef:

Food and Measure	carb. (gms)	fiber (gms)
(*Herb-Ox*), 1 cube	0	0
(*Herb-Ox* Instant), 1 tsp.	0	0
(*Herb-Ox* Instant Broth/Seasoning), 1 pkt.	0	0
(*Herb-Ox* Instant Low Sodium), 1 pkt.	2.0	0
(*Knorr*), ½ cube	<1.0	0
(*Maggi* Instant), 1 tsp.	0	0
(*Tyson*), 1 cube or 1 tsp.	0	0
chicken:		
(*Herb-Ox*), 1 cube	0	0
(*Herb-Ox* Instant), 1 tsp.	0	0
(*Herb-Ox* Instant Broth/Seasoning), 1 pkt.	0	0
(*Herb-Ox* Instant Broth/Seasoning Low Sodium), 1 pkt.	2.0	0
(*Knorr*), ½ cube	<1.0	0
(*Maggi* Instant), 1 tsp.	1.0	0
(*Tyson*), 1 cube or tsp.	1.0	0
garlic (*Herb-Ox*), 1 cube	0	0
tomato (*Doña Maria*), 1 tsp.	1.0	0
fish (*Knorr*), ½ cube	0	0
ham (*Knorr*), ½ cube	<1.0	0
vegetable:		
(*Herb-Ox*), 1 cube	0	0
(*Knorr* Vegetarian), ½ cube	1.0	0
(*Morga*), ½ cube	1.3	0
(*Maggi* Vegetarian), 1 cube	1.0	0
Bouillon concentrate, liquid:		
beef (*Bovril*), 2 tsp.	1.0	0
beef (*Home Again* Base), 1 tsp.	1.0	0
beef flavor (*Savory Basics* Stock), 1 tsp.	1.0	0
chicken:		
(*Bovril*), 2 tsp.	2.0	0
(*Home Again* Base), 1 tsp.	<1.0	0
(*Home Again* Base No MSG), 1 tsp.	2.0	0
(*Savory Basics* Stock), 1 tsp.	1.0	0
chicken flavor (*Home Again* Stock), 1 tsp.	2.0	0

Food and Measure	carb. (gms)	fiber (gms)
ham (*Home Again* Base), ¾ tsp.	1.0	0
vegetable (*Savory Basics* Stock), 2 tsp.	3.0	0
Bow-tie pasta, see "Pasta, dry"		
Bow-tie pasta entree, frozen, and chicken		
(*Lean Cuisine* Cafe Classics), 9.5 oz.	31.0	3.0
Boysenberry, fresh, see "Blackberry"		
Boysenberry, frozen, unsweetened, ½ cup	8.1	2.6
Boysenberry nectar (*R.W. Knudsen*), 8 fl. oz.	35.0	0
Boysenberry syrup (*Smucker's*), ¼ cup	52.0	0
Brains, braised or fried, without added ingredients	0	0
Bran, see "Cereal" and specific grains		
Bratwurst, cooked, 1 link, except as noted:		
(*Boar's Head*), 4 oz.	0	0
(*Johnsonville* Brat Bites Precooked), 6 links, 2 oz.	1.0	0
(*Johnsonville* Heat & Serve), 2.7 oz.	3.0	0
(*Johnsonville* Oktoberfest), 4 oz.	1.0	0
(*Johnsonville* Original/Beer 'n Bratwurst/Savory Onion),		
3 oz.	1.0	0
(*Johnsonville* Precooked/Stadium Style), 2.7 oz.	2.0	0
(*Organic Valley*), 3 oz.	2.0	0
beef, smoked (*Johnsonville*), 2.7 oz.	2.0	0
cheddar (*Johnsonville*), 3 oz.	2.0	0
chicken, with wild rice (*Bilinski*), 2 oz.	2.0	0
garlic and honey (*Johnsonville*), 3 oz.	5.0	0
hot and spicy (*Johnsonville*), 3 oz.	2.0	0
smoked (*Johnsonville*), 2.7 oz.	2.0	0
turkey (*Shady Brook Farms*), 3 oz.	1.0	0
"Bratwurst," vegetarian, frozen (*Boca*), 2.5-oz. link	6.0	1.0
Bratwurst burger, grilled (*Johnsonville*), 2.5-oz. piece	1.0	0
Braunschweiger (see also "Liverwurst"), 2 oz.:		
(*Black Bear*)	2.0	0
(*Boar's Head* Lite)	1.0	0
(*Hansel 'n' Gretel*)	4.0	0
(*Oscar Mayer*)	1.0	0
Brazil nuts, shelled:		
(*Shiloh Farms*), ¼ cup	5.0	2.0
8 medium or 6 large, 1 oz.	3.6	1.6

Food and Measure	carb. (gms)	fiber (gms)
Bread, 1 slice, except as noted:		
banana swirl (*Pepperidge Farm*)	15.0	<1.0
buttermilk:		
(*Earth Grains*)	20.0	<1.0
(*Pillsbury*)	15.0	0
sweet (*Pepperidge Farm Farmhouse*)	22.0	1.0
cinnamon swirl (*Pepperidge Farm*)	14.0	2.0
cinnamon swirl raisin (*Pepperidge Farm*)	14.0	1.0
French (*Pepperidge Farm* Hot & Crusty Thin Sliced),		
2 slices	29.0	1.0
French toast swirl:		
brown sugar cinnamon (*Pepperidge Farm*)	25.0	1.0
maple syrup cinnamon (*Pepperidge Farm*)	25.0	2.0
vanilla, French (*Pepperidge Farm*)	23.0	<1.0
garlic (*Pepperidge Farm* Hot & Crusty), 2 slices, ½"	21.0	1.0
grain, whole (*Healthy Choice*)	18.0	3.0
honey (*Earth Grains*)	19.0	2.0
Indian flatbread, see "Chapati"		
Italian (*Arnold Carb Counting*)	8.0	2.0
Italian (*Pepperidge Farm*)	15.0	1.0
kamut (*Shiloh Farms* Organic)	18.0	3.0
multigrain:		
(*Arnold Carb Counting*)	9.0	3.0
(*Earth Grains*)	19.0	5.0
(*Pepperidge Farm* Natural Whole Grain)	15.0	3.0
(*Sara Lee* Heart Healthy)	19.0	2.0
(*Sara Lee* Heart Healthy Plus)	14.0	4.0
(*Sara Lee* Heart Healthy Plus with Honey)	19.0	5.0
(*Shiloh Farms* Organic Sandwich)	17.0	3.0
crunchy (*Pepperidge Farm* Natural Whole Grain)	15.0	3.0
5-grain (*Shiloh Farms* Organic/No Salt)	19.0	4.0
7-grain (*Healthy Choice*)	18.0	3.0
7-grain (*Pepperidge Farm Carb Style*)	8.0	3.0
7-grain (*Pepperidge Farm Farmhouse*)	20.0	2.0
7-grain (*Pepperidge Farm Light Style*), 3 slices	27.0	2.0
7-grain (*Shiloh Farms* Organic/No Salt)	19.0	3.0
9-grain (*Pepperidge Farm* Natural Whole Grain)	15.0	3.0

Food and Measure	carb. (gms)	fiber (gms)
10-grain, sprouted (*Shiloh Farms* Organic), 2 slices	26.0	5.0
12-grain (*Pepperidge Farm Farmhouse*)	21.0	3.0
soft (*Healthy Choice*)	12.0	2.0
oat:		
crunchy (*Pepperidge Farm Farmhouse*)	19.0	2.0
honey (*Pepperidge Farm* Natural Whole Grain)	15.0	2.0
nut (*Earth Grains*)	20.0	1.0
nutty (*Pepperidge Farm Farmhouse*)	21.0	3.0
oatmeal:		
(*Arnold Bakery Light*), 2 slices	19.0	4.0
(*Pepperidge Farm*)	11.0	1.0
(*Pepperidge Farm Light Style*), 3 slices	27.0	2.0
soft (*Pepperidge Farm Farmhouse*)	21.0	1.0
pita, 1 piece:		
(*Garden of Eatin' Bible Bread*)	31.0	2.0
(*Garden of Eatin' Bible Bread* Very Low Salt)	30.0	1.0
spelt (*Shiloh Farms*)	29.0	4.0
white (*Sahara*)	32.0	2.0
whole wheat (*Sahara*)	27.0	5.0
whole wheat (*Shiloh Farms*)	31.0	3.0
potato (*Earth Grains*)	20.0	<1.0
potato (*Pepperidge Farm Farmhouse* Golden)	22.0	1.0
pumpernickel:		
(*Arnold* Real Jewish)	16.0	1.0
(*Pepperidge Farm* Family)	15.0	2.0
(*Pepperidge Farm* Party), 5 slices	24.0	3.0
(*Rubschlager Rye-Ola*)	20.0	3.0
with whole kernels (*Mestemacher* Westphalian)	16.0	3.0
rye:		
(*Arnold* Melba Thin), 2 slices	21.0	1.0
(*Arnold Carb Counting*)	9.0	3.0
(*Pepperidge Farm* Party), 5 slices	25.0	3.0
(*Shiloh* Rich n Rye), 2 slices	27.0	5.0
(*Wild's* Party), 3 slices	14.0	2.0
black (*Rubschlager Rye-Ola*)	20.0	3.0
with seeds (*Levy's* Real Jewish)	17.0	1.0
with seeds (*Pepperidge Farm*)	15.0	2.0

Food and Measure	carb. (gms)	fiber (gms)
with seeds or seedless (*Arnold* Real Jewish)	15.0	1.0
seedless (*Pepperidge Farm*)	15.0	1.0
rye, soy (*Rubschlager Rye-Ola*)	20.0	3.0
rye/pumpernickel (*Arnold* Deli Swirl)	15.0	1.0
rye/pumpernickel (*Pepperidge Farm* Deli Swirl)	15.0	1.0
sourdough (*Pepperidge Farm Farmhouse*)	20.0	1.0
spelt (*Shiloh Farms* Organic)	21.0	2.0
sunflower, rye (*Rubschlager Rye-Ola*)	19.0	3.0
wheat:		
(*Pepperidge Farm Farmhouse* Butter-topped)	21.0	1.0
(*Pepperidge Farm Farmhouse* Hearty Country)	21.0	2.0
(*Pillsbury*)	15.0	1.0
(*Sara Lee* Classic)	13.0	2.0
(*Sara Lee* Delightful)	9.0	2.0
(*Shiloh Farms* Homestyle Organic), 2 slices	29.0	<1.0
buttermilk (*Pepperidge Farm Farmhouse*)	21.0	1.0
dark (*Pepperidge Farm* Whole Grain German)	15.0	3.0
honey (*Sara Lee*)	14.0	1.0
honey, soft (*Healthy Choice*)	12.0	2.0
sesame (*Pepperidge Farm Farmhouse*)	19.0	2.0
wheat, whole:		
(*Arnold Carb Counting*)	9.0	3.0
(*Earth Grains*)	19.0	5.0
(*Lifeworks*), 2 slices	27.0	3.0
(*Pepperidge Farm* Thin Sliced)	11.0	2.0
(*Pepperidge Farm* Very Thin Sliced), 3 slices	21.0	3.0
(*Pepperidge Farm Carb Style*)	8.0	3.0
(*Pepperidge Farm Farmhouse*)	19.0	3.0
(*Sara Lee* Heart Healthy)	19.0	2.0
(*Sara Lee* Heart Healthy Plus)	14.0	4.0
(*Sara Lee* Heart Healthy Plus with Honey)	19.0	5.0
(*Sara Lee* Homestyle/Homestyle Wide Pan)	20.0	2.0
(*Shiloh Farms* Organic), 2 slices	26.0	4.0
(*Shiloh Farms* Organic No Salt), 2 slices	26.0	3.0
honey (*Earth Grains*)	20.0	5.0
stone ground (*Earth Grains*)	19.0	2.0
stone ground, whole grain (*Pepperidge Farm*)	16.0	2.0
wheat berry (*Earth Grains*)	20.0	1.0

Food and Measure	carb. (gms)	fiber (gms)
wheat berry (*Pepperidge Farm Farmhouse*)	20.0	2.0
white:		
(*Arnold* Country Classics)	19.0	<1.0
(*Arnold Brick Oven*), 2 slices	25.0	1.0
(*Arnold Brick Oven* Big Slice)	17.0	<1.0
(*Lifeworks*), 2 slices	28.0	2.0
(*Pepperidge Farm* Canadian)	16.0	<1.0
(*Pepperidge Farm* Sandwich), 2 slices	23.0	<1.0
(*Pepperidge Farm* Sandwich Family/Large), 2 slices ...	27.0	0
(*Pepperidge Farm* Toasting)	16.0	0
(*Pepperidge Farm* Very Thin Sliced), 3 slices	24.0	1.0
(*Pepperidge Farm Carb Style*)	8.0	3.0
(*Pepperidge Farm Farmhouse* Butter-topped)	21.0	<1.0
(*Pepperidge Farm Farmhouse* Country)	20.0	2.0
(*Pepperidge Farm Farmhouse* Hearty)	22.0	1.0
(*Pillsbury*)	15.0	1.0
(*Sara Lee* Classic)	15.0	<1.0
(*Sara Lee* Delightful)	18.0	4.0
honey (*Pillsbury*)	15.0	0
honey (*Sara Lee*)	22.0	<1.0
Bread, brown, canned (*B&M*), ½'' slice	29.0	2.0
Bread, frozen, ready-to-bake:		
challah (*Kineret*), ⅛ loaf, 2 oz.	27.0	<1.0
challah, round (*Kineret* Holiday), ⅛ loaf, 2 oz.	25.0	<1.0
cheese, mini (*Pepperidge Farm*), 2 slices, ¼''	21.0	1.0
dough, sweet, see "Dough, sweet"		
dough, wheat or white (*Rhodes*), 1.8 oz.	24.0	2.0
French, crusty (*Pillsbury*), ⅕ loaf	28.0	<1.0
garlic:		
(*Pepperidge Farm*), 2 slices, ½''	24.0	2.0
5 cheese (*Pepperidge Farm*), 2 slices, ½''	24.0	2.0
mini (*Pepperidge Farm*), 2 slices, ½''	25.0	1.0
mozzarella (*Pepperidge Farm*), 2 slices, ¼''	22.0	2.0
Parmesan (*Pepperidge Farm*), 2 slices, ½''	23.0	2.0
Italian (*Pillsbury* Country), ⅛ loaf	21.0	<1.0
Italian, with garlic (*Pillsbury*), 1¼'' slice, ½ tsp. spread ..	21.0	<1.0
Texas toast, 1 slice:		
5 cheese (*Pepperidge Farm*)	18.0	1.0

Food and Measure	carb. (gms)	fiber (gms)
garlic (*Pepperidge Farm*)	18.0	2.0
mozzarella/Monterey jack (*Pepperidge Farm*)	20.0	<1.0
Parmesan (*Pepperidge Farm*)	14.0	<1.0
Bread, mix (see also "Bread mix, sweet"), dry mix, ¼ cup, except as noted:		
barley, with soy (*Hodgson Mill*)	23.0	2.0
cheese and herb (*Hodgson Mill*)	21.0	<1.0
focaccia (*Buitoni*), 1 serving	21.0	0
multigrain, 9, with soy (*Hodgson Mill*)	22.0	3.0
potato, with soy (*Hodgson Mill*)	23.0	<1.0
rye, caraway, with soy (*Hodgson Mill*)	22.0	3.0
white, with soy (*Hodgson Mill* Wholesome)	22.0	1.0
whole wheat, honey (*Hodgson Mill*)	22.0	2.0
Bread mix, sweet:		
banana (*Betty Crocker* Quick), ¹⁄₁₂ pkg.*	25.0	0
banana (*Produce Partners*), 2 tbsp. mix	32.0	0
carrot (*Produce Partners*), ½ cup mix	60.0	0
cinnamon streusel (*Betty Crocker* Quick), ¹⁄₁₄ pkg.*	28.0	0
corn:		
(*Glory* Homestyle), 1.2-oz. square*	24.0	2.0
(*Hodgson Mill*), ¼ cup mix	28.0	3.0
(*Kentucky Kernel*), ¼ cup	24.0	0
jalapeño (*Hodgson Mill*), ¼ cup mix	21.0	1.0
cranberry orange (*Betty Crocker* Quick), ¹⁄₁₂ pkg.*	29.0	0
gingerbread, whole wheat (*Hodgson Mill*), ¼ cup mix	24.0	2.0
lemon poppy seed (*Betty Crocker* Quick), ¹⁄₁₂ pkg.*	25.0	0
Bread crumbs, ¼ cup or 1 oz.:		
plain (*Arnold* All Purpose)	19.0	1.0
plain (*Progresso*)	19.0	1.0
garlic and herb (*Progresso*)	18.0	1.0
Italian (*Contadina*)	19.0	1.0
Italian (*Progresso*)	20.0	1.0
Parmesan (*Progresso*)	19.0	1.0
Bread cubes, see "Stuffing"		
Bread dough, see "Bread, frozen"		
Bread stick:		
plain:		
(*Colonna*), 2 pieces	14.0	0

Food and Measure	carb. (gms)	fiber (gms)
(*Stella D'oro*/*Stella D'oro* No Salt), 1 piece	7.0	0
mini (*Stella D'oro*), 4 pieces	12.0	1.0
cracked pepper, mini (*Stella D'oro*), 4 pieces	11.0	0
garlic, roasted (*Stella D'oro*), 1 piece	8.0	0
sesame (*Stella D'oro*), 1 piece	7.0	1.0
sesame, mini (*Stella D'oro*), 4 pieces	11.0	1.0
Bread stick, frozen or refrigerated:		
(*Pillsbury* Soft), 2 pieces	25.0	<1.0
(*Rhodes*), 1/6 pkg.	32.0	1.0
corn bread (*Pillsbury* Twists), 1 piece	17.0	1.0
garlic (*Pepperidge Farm*), 1 piece	25.0	1.0
garlic with herbs (*Pillsbury*), 2 pieces, 1/2 tsp. spread	24.0	<1.0
Parmesan, with garlic (*Pillsbury*), 2 pieces, 1/2 tsp. spread	24.0	<1.0
Breadfruit, raw, 1/2 cup	29.8	5.4
Breadfruit seeds:		
raw, 1 oz.	8.3	1.5
boiled, shelled, 1 oz.	9.1	1.4
roasted, shelled, 1 oz.	11.4	1.7
Breading mix, see "Batter and breading mix" and specific listings		
Breadnut tree seeds, dried, 1 oz.	22.5	4.2
Breakfast dish, see "Egg breakfast," "Tofu breakfast" and specific listings		
Breakfast pocket/sandwich (see also "Burrito, breakfast" and "Taco, breakfast"), frozen, 1 piece:		
bacon and sausage (*Toaster Scrambles*)	14.0	0
bagel, sausage/egg/cheese (*Jimmy Dean*), 4.8 oz.	33.0	1.0
biscuit:		
bacon, egg, and cheese (*Jimmy Dean*), 3.6 oz.	27.0	1.0
double sausage, egg, and cheese (*Swanson Hungry-Man*), 6 oz.	35.0	1.0
sausage, egg, and cheese (*Jimmy Dean*), 4.5 oz.	28.0	1.0
cheese, egg, and bacon (*Toaster Scrambles*)	14.0	0
cheese, egg, and ham or sausage (*Toaster Scrambles*)	14.0	0
croissant, sausage, egg, and cheese (*Aunt Jemima*), 4.1 oz.	22.0	<1.0
croissant, sausage, egg, and cheese (*Jimmy Dean*), 4.8 oz.	24.0	1.0

Food and Measure	carb. (gms)	fiber (gms)
English muffin:		
ham and cheese (*Smart Ones*), 4 oz.	28.0	2.0
sausage, egg, and cheese (*Jimmy Dean*), 4.6 oz.	28.0	1.0
veggie, with cheese (*Morningstar Farms*)	35.0	5.0
French toast:		
(*Pop•Tarts*)	34.0	<1.0
sausage, egg, and cheese (*Aunt Jemima*), 4.7 oz.	26.0	1.0
pocket, egg and cheese:		
bacon (*Hot Pockets*), 4.5 oz.	32.0	2.0
bacon (*Hot Pockets*), 2.25 oz.	20.0	1.0
bacon (*Lean Pockets*), 2.25 oz.	21.0	2.0
ham (*Hot Pockets*), 2.25 oz.	17.0	1.0
sausage (*Croissant Pockets*), 4.5 oz.	34.0	3.0
sausage (*Hot Pockets*), 2.25 oz.	19.0	1.0
sausage (*Lean Pockets*), 2.25 oz.	19.0	2.0
tofu scramble (*Amy's*), 4.5 oz.	23.0	<1.0
wrap, bacon or ham, egg, and cheddar		
(*Jimmy Dean*) 4.3 oz.	23.0	<1.0
Breakfast syrup, see "Pancake syrup"		
Brewer's yeast flakes (*Louis Labs*), 1.1 oz.,		
2 rounded tbsp.	13.0	6.0
Broad beans, fresh:		
raw, ½ cup	6.4	2.3
boiled, drained, 4 oz.	11.5	<3.0
Broad beans, mature:		
dry:		
(*Frieda's* Fava), ¾ cup, 3 oz.	50.0	21.0
(*Shiloh Farms* Fava), ¼ cup	22.0	12.0
peeled (*Frieda's* Habas), ½ cup, 3 oz.	17.0	4.0
boiled, ½ cup	16.7	4.6
Broad beans, mature, canned, ½ cup:		
(*Progresso* Fava Beans)	20.0	5.0
with liquid	15.9	4.7
Broccoli, fresh:		
raw:		
(*Dole*), 1 medium stalk, 5.2 oz.	8.0	5.0
8.7-oz. stalk	7.9	4.5
chopped, ½ cup	2.3	1.3

Food and Measure	carb. (gms)	fiber (gms)
boiled, drained, 1 stalk, 6.3 oz.	9.1	5.2
boiled, drained, chopped, ½ cup	3.9	2.3
Broccoli, Chinese, see "Kale, Chinese"		
Broccoli, freeze-dried, chopped (*AlpineAire*), ¼ oz.	4.0	2.0
Broccoli, frozen:		
spears:		
(*Birds Eye*), 2 spears, 3.1 oz.	4.0	2.0
(*Green Giant*), 3.5 oz., approx. 3 spears	4.0	2.0
(*Green Giant Select*), 3 oz., approx. 3 spears	4.0	2.0
baby (*Birds Eye*), 4 spears, 3 oz.	4.0	2.0
10-oz. pkg.	15.2	8.5
spears or chopped, boiled, drained, 1 cup	9.8	5.5
florets:		
(*Cascadian Farm* Bag), ⅔ cup	4.0	2.0
(*Cascadian Farm* Box), 1⅓ cups	4.0	2.0
(*C&W*), 5 pieces, 3 oz.	4.0	2.0
(*Green Giant Select*), 1⅓ cups	4.0	2.0
baby (*Birds Eye*), 1 cup	4.0	2.0
cuts:		
(*Birds Eye* Tender), 1 cup	4.0	2.0
(*Cascadian Farm*), ⅔ cup	4.0	2.0
(*Green Giant/Green Giant* Boil-in-Bag), 1 cup	4.0	2.0
(*Tree of Life*), 1 cup	4.0	2.0
chopped:		
(*Green Giant*), ¾ cup	4.0	2.0
baby (*Birds Eye*), ¾ cup	4.0	2.0
10-oz. pkg.	3.6	8.5
in butter sauce, spears (*Green Giant*), 4 oz.,		
approx. 3 spears	6.0	2.0
in cheese sauce:		
(*Birds Eye*), ½ cup	8.0	1.0
(*Green Giant*), ⅔ cup	9.0	2.0
cheddar (*Cascadian Farm* Bag), ½ cup	7.0	3.0
cheddar (*Cascadian Farm* Box), ⅔ cup	7.0	2.0
three cheese (*Green Giant*), ½ cup cooked	5.0	2.0
creamed (*C&W*), ½ cup	7.0	2.0
Broccoli combinations, frozen:		
carrots, water chestnuts (*Birds Eye*), 1 cup	6.0	2.0

Food and Measure	carb. (gms)	fiber (gms)
carrots, water chestnuts (*Green Giant Select*), ⅔ cup	5.0	2.0
cauliflower (*Birds Eye*), 1 cup	4.0	2.0
cauliflower, carrots:		
(*Green Giant Select*), ⅔ cup	4.0	2.0
cheese sauce (*Green Giant*), ½ cup cooked	7.0	2.0
cheese sauce (*Green Giant* Boil-in-Bag), ⅔ cup	9.0	2.0
corn, peppers (*Birds Eye*), ¾ cup	11.0	1.0
green beans, onion, pepper (*Birds Eye*), 1 cup	5.0	2.0
peppers, onion, mushrooms (*Birds Eye*), 1 cup	4.0	1.0
red peppers, sugar snaps, water chestnuts (*C&W*),		
1 cup	6.0	2.0
Broccoli dish, frozen:		
nuggets (*Dr. Praeger's*), 4 pieces, 1.4 oz.	5.0	1.0
pancake (*Dr. Praeger's*), 1.3-oz. piece	5.0	<1.0
pancake (*Dr. Praeger's* Bombay), 1.3-oz. piece	8.0	1.0
Broccoli entree, frozen, pot pie (*Amy's*), 7.5 oz.	46.0	4.0
Broccoli rabe, fresh:		
(*Andy Boy*), ⅕ bunch, 3 oz.	3.0	2.0
(*Frieda's* Rapini), 3 oz.	4.0	0
cooked (*Ready Pac*), ½ cup	3.0	2.0
Broccoli rabe, frozen (*Seabrook Farms*), 1 cup	4.0	2.0
Broccoli snack rolls, frozen (*Health is*		
Wealth Munchees), 2 pieces, 1 oz.	10.0	1.0
Broccoli sprouts (*Jonathan's*), 1 cup	5.0	4.0
Broccoli-cheese pocket sandwich, frozen		
(*Amy's*), 4.5-oz. piece	37.0	3.0
Broiling sauce, see "Grilling sauce"		
Brown gravy, with onion (*Campbell's*), ¼ cup	4.0	<1.0
Brown gravy mix, ¼ cup*:		
(*Lawry's*)	4.0	0
(*McCormick*)	3.0	0
Brownie, 1 piece, except as noted:		
(*Hostess* Bites), 3 pieces, 1.3 oz.	21.0	1.0
chocolate chip:		
(*Awrey's* Decadent), 1.6 oz.	27.0	<1.0
(*Awrey's* Low Fat), 1.3 oz.	27.0	<1.0
peanut butter (*Awrey's*), 1.6 oz.	25.0	<1.0
fudge (*Entenmann's*), ½ piece, 1.5 oz.	25.0	1.0

Food and Measure	carb. (gms)	fiber (gms)
fudge (*Little Debbie*) 1.5 oz.	39.0	1.0
wheat free (*Foods by George*), ⅛ slice	28.0	1.0
Brownie, frozen, chocolate fudge, triple (*Sara Lee*), 7-oz. piece	12.0	1.0
Brownie, mix, ¹⁄₂₀ pkg.*, except as noted:		
(*Betty Crocker* Supreme Original)	27.0	0
with caramel, walnuts (*Betty Crocker* Supreme Turtle)	23.0	0
chocolate:		
dark (*Betty Crocker* Supreme)	25.0	0
fudge, dark (*Betty Crocker*)	24.0	0
fudge, dark (*Duncan Hines* Family), ¹⁄₁₈ pkg.*	25.0	<1.0
German (*Betty Crocker*)	29.0	1.0
milk, chunk (*Duncan Hines* Chocolate Lovers), ¹⁄₁₆ pkg.*	25.0	1.0
triple (*Duncan Hines* Decadence), ¹⁄₁₆ pkg.*	25.0	1.0
walnut (*Duncan Hines* Chocolate Lovers), ¹⁄₁₆ pkg.*	24.0	2.0
chocolate chunk (*Betty Crocker* Supreme/Supreme Triple)	25.0	1.0
chocolate chunk, walnut (*Betty Crocker* Supreme)	24.0	1.0
frosted (*Betty Crocker* Supreme)	31.0	1.0
fudge:		
(*Betty Crocker*)	23.0	0
(*Betty Crocker* Low Fat), ¹⁄₁₈ pkg.*	27.0	1.0
(*Betty Crocker* Pouch), ⅑ pkg.*	27.0	1.0
(*"Jiffy"*), ⅕ cup mix	28.0	<1.0
chewy (*Duncan Hines* Family Style)	24.0	<1.0
peanut butter (*Betty Crocker* Supreme)	23.0	0
pecan (*Betty Crocker* Supreme)	22.0	1.0
walnut (*Betty Crocker* Supreme)	22.0	0
with whole wheat flour, flax seeds (*Hodgson Mill*), 3 tbsp. mix	28.0	2.0
Brownie à la mode, see "Ice cream dessert"		
Browning sauce:		
(*GravyMaster*), ¼ tsp.	<1.0	0
(*Kitchen Bouquet*), 1 tsp.	3.0	0
Bruegger's:		
bagels, 1 piece:		
plain	61.0	4.0
blueberry, cinnamon raisin, or cranberry orange	68.0	4.0

Food and Measure	carb. (gms)	fiber (gms)
chocolate chip	69.0	4.0
cinnamon sugar	71.0	6.0
everything, garlic, or onion	62.0	4.0
honey grain	64.0	5.0
jalapeño	63.0	4.0
poppy	61.0	4.0
pumpernickel	64.0	5.0
rosemary olive oil	62.0	4.0
salt, sesame, or sun-dried tomato	61.0	4.0
cream cheese, 2 tbsp.:		
plain	4.0	0
plain, light	3.0	0
bacon scallion	4.0	0
chive	2.0	0
garden veggie	3.0	0
garden veggie, light	2.0	0
herb garlic, light	3.0	0
honey walnut	5.0	0
jalapeño	3.0	0
olive pimento	2.0	0
smoked salmon	2.0	0
strawberry, light, or wildberry	4.0	0
breakfast sandwich, egg and cheese, plain or with bacon, ham, or sausage	66.0	4.0
deli sandwich:		
chicken breast	62.0	4.0
chicken salad, mayo	67.0	4.0
ham, honey mustard	77.0	4.0
turkey, mayo	65.0	4.0
filling only, hummus, 2 tbsp.	4.0	2.0
filling only, tuna salad, 2.5 oz.	6.0	0
specialty sandwich:		
chicken fajita	74.0	5.0
garden veggie	80.0	7.0
Leonardo da Veggie	69.0	4.0
smoked salmon	66.0	4.0
turkey, herby	73.0	4.0
turkey, Santa Fe	71.0	4.0

Food and Measure	carb. (gms)	fiber (gms)
desserts:		
Blondie bar	42.0	2.0
brownie, chocolate chunk	39.0	2.0
brownie, mint	34.0	0
Bruegger Bar	47.0	3.0
cappuccino bar	45.0	1.0
lemon bar	39.0	0
oatmeal cranberry mountain	49.0	3.0
pecan chocolate chunk bar	32.0	1.0
raspberry sammies	36.0	1.0
Bruschetta, frozen, pesto, mozzarella, tomato (*Cedarlane*), 1.25-oz. piece	10.0	.5
Bruschetta topping, olive (*Delallo*), 2 tbsp.	1.0	0
Brussels sprouts, fresh:		
raw (*Dole*), 4 pieces, 3 oz.	6.0	3.0
raw, ½ cup	3.9	1.8
boiled, 7-oz. piece	1.8	.9
boiled, drained, ½ cup	6.8	3.4
Brussels sprouts, frozen:		
(*Birds Eye*), 10 pieces, 3 oz.	8.0	3.0
(*Birds Eye* Tender), 6 pieces, 3 oz.	8.0	3.0
(*C&W* Petite), 3 oz., approx. 10 pieces	5.0	3.0
in butter sauce (*Green Giant*), ½ cup cooked	6.0	3.0
boiled, drained, ½ cup	6.5	1.4
Brussels sprouts combination, frozen, cauliflower, carrots (*Birds Eye*), 1 cup	7.0	2.0
Buckwheat, grain:		
1 oz.	20.3	2.8
¼ cup	30.4	4.3
Buckwheat flour:		
(*Arrowhead Mills*), ⅓ cup	20.0	6.0
(*Hodgson Mill*), ⅓ cup	33.0	2.0
(*Shiloh Farms*), ¼ cup	21.0	3.0
¼ cup	21.2	3.0
Buckwheat groats, dry, except as noted:		
(*Arrowhead Mills*), ¼ cup	31.0	4.0
(*Shiloh Farms*), ¼ cup	30.0	3.0

Food and Measure	carb. (gms)	fiber (gms)
roasted:		
(*Shiloh Farms* Kasha), ¼ cup	30.0	3.0
(*Wolff's* Kasha), ¼ cup	35.0	2.0
1 oz.	21.2	.8
roasted, cooked, 1 cup	39.5	4.5
Buffalo wing sauce, see "Wing sauce"		
Bulgur:		
dry:		
(*Shiloh Farms*), ¼ cup	33.0	4.0
(*Shiloh Farms* Organic), ⅓ cup	33.0	4.0
¼ cup	26.6	6.4
cooked, 1 cup	33.8	8.2
Bulgur salad, see "Tabouli"		
Bun, see "Roll"		
Bun, sweet, frozen or refrigerated, 1 piece:		
caramel (*Pillsbury*)	24.0	<1.0
cinnamon, plain:		
(*Rhodes*)	42.0	1.0
(*Rhodes Anytime!*)	39.0	1.0
giant (*Rhodes*)	37.0	1.0
cinnamon, with frosting*:		
(*Rhodes Anytime!*)	51.0	1.0
(*Sara Lee* Deluxe)	41.0	1.0
giant (*Rhodes*)	44.0	1.0
cinnamon, with icing:		
(*Grands!*)	53.0	1.0
(*Grands!* Reduced Fat)	54.0	1.0
(*Pillsbury* Bakery Style)	92.0	2.0
(*Pillsbury* Oven Baked)	46.0	1.0
(*Pillsbury* Reduced Fat)	24.0	<1.0
buttercream or cream cheese icing (*Grands!*)	52.0	1.0
regular or cream cheese (*Pillsbury*)	23.0	<1.0
cinnamon, toaster, mini (*Eggo Toaster*		
Swirlz), 1 set, 4 pieces	20.0	<1.0
cinnamon raisin, with icing (*Pillsbury*)	26.0	<1.0
orange, plain (*Rhodes*)	42.0	1.0
orange, plain (*Rhodes Anytime!*)	39.0	1.0

Food and Measure	carb. (gms)	fiber (gms)
orange, with frosting* (*Rhodes*)	49.0	1.0
orange, with frosting* (*Rhodes Anytime!*)	51.0	1.0
orange, with icing (*Pillsbury*)	25.0	<1.0
strawberry, toaster, mini (*Eggo Toaster Swirlz*), 1 set, 4 pieces	19.0	<1.0
Burbot, without added ingredients	0	0
Burdock root:		
raw:		
(*Frieda's* Gobo Root), ¾ cup, 3 oz.	15.0	3.0
7.3-oz. piece	13.6	5.1
pieces, ½ cup	10.3	1.9
boiled, 1" pieces, ½ cup	13.2	1.1
Burger, see "Beef pocket/sandwich"		
Burger, vegetarian:		
canned:		
(*Loma Linda* Redi-Burger), ⅝" slice, 3 oz.	7.0	4.0
(*Loma Linda* Vege-Burger), ¼ cup	2.0	2.0
(*Worthington Burger*), ¼ cup	3.0	1.0
frozen, crumbles (*Morningstar Farms Grillers*), ⅔ cup ...	4.0	2.0
frozen, ground (*Boca*), 2 oz.	6.0	3.0
mix (*Fantastic* Nature's Burger), ¼ cup	30.0	5.0
mix, tofu (*Fantastic*), 3 tbsp.	13.0	1.0
Burger patty, vegetarian, frozen, 1 piece, 2.5 oz., except as noted:		
(*Boca* Original Vegan)	6.0	4.0
(*Garden Gourmet* Veggie Patties), 2.6 oz.	6.0	4.0
(*Morningstar Farms Better 'n Burgers*)	6.0	3.0
(*Morningstar Farms Garden Veggie Patties*), 2.4 oz.	9.0	4.0
(*Morningstar Farms Grillers* Original), 2.25 oz.	5.0	2.0
(*Morningstar Farms Harvest Burgers*), 3.2 oz.	8.0	5.0
(*Yves* The Good Burger Original), 2.6 oz.	7.0	3.0
(*Yves* Veggie Authentic), 2.6 oz.	9.0	7.0
(*Yves* Veggie Chick'n), 2.6 oz.	5.0	2.0
all American (*Amy's*)	15.0	3.0
all American (*Boca*)	9.0	3.0
black bean, spicy (*Morningstar Farms*), 2.75 oz.	16.0	5.0
Bombay (*Dr. Praeger's*), 2.75 oz.	9.5	4.0

Food and Measure	carb. (gms)	fiber (gms)
California:		
(*Amy's*)	19.0	5.0
(*Dr. Praeger's*), 2.75 oz.	9.5	4.0
(*Dr. Praeger's* Family Pack), 3.8 oz.	12.0	5.0
char-broiled (*Garden Gourmet* Veggie Patties), 2.6 oz.	2.0	4.0
cheeseburger (*Boca*)	5.0	3.0
Chicago (*Amy's*)	20.0	3.0
fajita (*Morningstar Farms*), 2.25 oz.	7.0	3.0
garlic, roasted (*Boca*)	6.0	4.0
Italian (*Dr. Praeger's*), 2.75 oz.	9.5	4.0
onion, roasted (*Boca*)	10.0	4.0
Philly cheese steak burgers (*Morningstar Farms*), 2.25 oz.	6.0	3.0
pizza burger (*Dr. Praeger's*), 3.1 oz.	11.5	4.0
pizza burger, tomato and basil (*Morningstar Farms*), 2.4 oz.	7.0	7.0
portobello and peppers (*Morningstar Farms*), 2.4 oz.	9.0	3.0
prime (*Morningstar Farms Grillers*)	5.0	2.0
savory (*Yves*), 2.6 oz.	18.0	4.0
soy or Tex-Mex (*Dr. Praeger's*), 2.75 oz.	9.5	4.0
Texas (*Amy's*)	14.0	3.0
vegetable, grilled (*Boca*)	6.0	4.0
Burger King, 1 serving:		
breakfast:		
Croissan'wich:		
egg and cheese, with or without bacon or ham	26.0	<1.0
sausage and cheese	24.0	1.0
sausage, egg, and cheese	26.0	1.0
Croissan'wich, double:		
ham and bacon or double ham and bacon	27.0	<1.0
ham or bacon and sausage	27.0	1.0
sausage, double	26.0	2.0
enormous omelet sandwich	44.0	3.0
French toast sticks, 5 pieces	46.0	2.0
hash brown rounds, small	23.0	2.0
hash brown rounds, medium	38.0	4.0
jam, grape or strawberry	7.0	0
syrup	21.0	0

Food and Measure	carb. (gms)	fiber (gms)
burgers/sandwiches:		
Angus burger	62.0	3.0
Angus burger, bacon and cheese	64.0	3.0
Angus burger, low carb	2.0	<1.0
bacon cheeseburger	31.0	1.0
bacon cheeseburger, double	32.0	2.0
BK Veggie Burger, with or without mayo	46.0	7.0
cheeseburger	31.0	1.0
cheeseburger, double	32.0	2.0
Double Whopper, with or without mayo	52.0	4.0
Double Whopper, with cheese	53.0	4.0
Double Whopper, with cheese, low carb	5.0	<1.0
Double Whopper, low carb	3.0	<1.0
hamburger	30.0	1.0
hamburger double	30.0	1.0
Whopper, with or without mayo	52.0	4.0
Whopper, with cheese	53.0	4.0
Whopper, with cheese, low carb	5.0	<1.0
Whopper, low carb	3.0	<1.0
Whopper Jr., with or without mayo	31.0	2.0
Whopper Jr., with cheese	32.0	2.0
Whopper Jr., with cheese, low carb	2.0	0
Whopper Jr., low carb	1.0	0
sandwiches:		
BK Big Fish/BK Big Fish spicy	69.0	4.0
BK Big Fish spicy, without tartar sauce	68.0	4.0
chicken, without mayo	52.0	3.0
Chicken Whopper, without mayo	48.0	4.0
Chicken Whopper, low carb	3.0	1.0
Tendercrisp chicken	70.0	6.0
Tendercrisp chicken, spicy	71.0	6.0
Tendercrisp chicken, spicy, without sauce or mayo	70.0	6.0
Chicken Tenders:		
4 pieces	10.0	0
5 pieces	13.0	<1.0
6 pieces	15.0	<1.0
8 pieces	20.0	<1.0

Food and Measure	carb. (gms)	fiber (gms)
dipping sauce:		
barbecue or honey mustard	9.0	0
honey flavored	23.0	0
ketchup, 1 pkt.	3.0	0
onion ring	3.0	<1.0
ranch	1.0	0
sweet and sour	10.0	0
sides:		
bacon, 1 strip	0	0
fries:		
king	76.0	6.0
large	63.0	5.0
medium	46.0	4.0
small	29.0	2.0
onion rings:		
king	70.0	5.0
large	60.0	5.0
medium	40.0	3.0
small	22.0	2.0
salad, without dressing or toast:		
chicken Caesar	9.0	1.0
chicken Caesar, *Tendercrisp*	25.0	4.0
garden	4.0	<1.0
garden, chicken	12.0	.0
garden, chicken *Tendercrisp*	28.0	.0
garden, shrimp	13.0	.0
shrimp Caesar	9.0	.0
salad dressing and toast:		
garden ranch/garlic Caesar	7.0	0
honey mustard	18.0	0
onion vinaigrette	8.0	0
tomato balsamic vinaigrette	9.0	0
toast, garlic Parmesan	9.0	0
shakes:		
vanilla, large	113.0	<1.0
vanilla, medium	76.0	0
vanilla, small	57.0	0

Food and Measure	carb. (gms)	fiber (gms)
shakes, syrup added:		
chocolate, large	133.0	2.0
chocolate, medium	97.0	2.0
chocolate, small	65.0	<1.0
strawberry, large	131.0	<1.0
strawberry, medium	96.0	0
strawberry, small	64.0	0
Icee, cherry or *Coca-Cola,* medium	40.0	0
dessert, pie:		
Dutch apple	45.0	1.0
Hershey's sundae	31.0	1.0
Burrito (see also "Burrito, breakfast"), frozen, 1 piece:		
bean/cheese:		
(*Amy's*), 6 oz.	43.0	6.0
(*El Monterey*), 4 oz.	24.0	4.0
(*El Monterey*), 5 oz.	43.0	5.0
(*El Monterey*), 8 oz.	69.0	8.0
(*El Monterey* XX Large!), 10 oz.	87.0	9.0
(*Reser's*), 5 oz.	51.0	5.0
bean and rice (*Amy's*), 6 oz.	48.0	5.0
bean, rice, and cheese (*Cedarlane* Low Fat), 6 oz.	48.0	7.0
beef:		
grilled fajita (*El Monterey Supreme*), 5 oz.	48.0	2.0
steak, shredded (*El Monterey* Carb Friendly), 5 oz.	26.0	14.0
taco seasoned (*El Monterey*), 4 oz.	32.0	2.0
beef and bean:		
(*El Monterey*), 4 oz.	34.0	3.0
(*El Monterey* XX Large!), 10 oz.	86.0	9.0
(*El Monterey* Red Hot XX Large!), 10 oz.	86.0	9.0
(*El Monterey/El Monterey* Red Hot), 5 oz.	42.0	4.0
(*El Monterey/El Monterey* Red Hot), 8 oz.	68.0	7.0
beef and bean, green chili:		
(*El Monterey*), 4 oz.	35.0	3.0
(*El Monterey*), 5 oz.	41.0	4.0
(*El Monterey* XX Large!), 10 oz.	84.0	7.0
beef and bean, red chili:		
(*El Monterey*), 4 oz.	35.0	3.0
(*El Monterey*), 5 oz.	42.0	4.0

Food and Measure	carb. (gms)	fiber (gms)
(*El Monterey*), 8 oz.	66.0	6.0
(*El Monterey* XX Large!), 10 oz.	84.0	8.0
beef and cheese, shredded (*El Monterey Supreme*), 5 oz.	37.0	1.0
black bean, rice (*Amy's* Especial), 6 oz.	45.0	3.0
black bean, vegetable (*Amy's*), 6 oz.	44.0	4.0
chicken (*El Monterey*), 4 oz.	32.0	1.0
chicken, grilled (*El Monterey Supreme*), 5 oz.	44.0	2.0
chicken and cheese, chipotle (*El Monterey* Carb Friendly), 5 oz.	26.0	14.0
steak, char-broiled (*El Monterey*), 5 oz.	39.0	1.0
vegetable and cheese (*Cedarlane*), 6 oz.	48.0	3.0
Burrito, breakfast, frozen, 1 piece:		
(*Amy's*), 6 oz.	38.0	5.0
egg, cheese, salsa, bacon (*El Monterey Supreme*), 4.5 oz.	36.0	1.0
egg sausage (*El Monterey Supreme*), 4.5 oz.	34.0	1.0
Burrito entree, frozen, grande, chili verde sauce or salsa roja (*Cedarlane*), ½ of 10-oz. pkg.	27.0	2.0
Burrito entree kit (*Old El Paso* Dinner Kit), 1 burrito*	27.0	1.0
Burrito seasoning mix:		
(*Chi-Chi's* Fiesta), pkg.	6.0	1.0
(*Lawry's*), 2 tsp.	4.0	<1.0
(*McCormick*), 1 tbsp.	5.0	0
Burrito snack rolls, frozen (*Health is Wealth Munchees*), 10 pieces, 5 oz.	53.0	6.0
Butter, salted or unsalted:		
regular, 1 stick or 4 oz.	0	0
whipped, 1 stick or ½ cup	<.1	0
Butter, flavored, 1 tbsp.:		
garlic, roasted, with oil (*Land O Lakes*)	0	0
honey (*Downey's*)	11.0	0
honey (*Land O Lakes*)	4.0	0
Butter beans (see also "Lima beans"), canned, ½ cup:		
(*Bush's* Speckled)	19.0	5.0
(*McKenzie's*)	20.0	4.0
(*S&W*)	19.0	5.0
baby (*Allens*)	22.0	6.0
baby (*Bush's*)	19.0	5.0
green (*Sunshine*)	22.0	6.0

Food and Measure	carb. (gms)	fiber (gms)
large:		
(*Allens*)	20.0	7.0
(*Bush's*)	18.0	5.0
white, with sausage (*Trappey's*)	21.0	6.0
seasoned (*Glory*)	20.0	5.0
Butter flavor seasoning, 1 tsp.:		
(*Butter Buds*)	2.0	0
(*Molly McButter* Light Sodium)	2.0	0
(*Molly McButter* Natural)	1.0	0
cheese or roasted garlic (*Molly McButter*)	1.0	0
Butterbur, fresh:		
raw, .2-oz. stalk	.2	<1.0
boiled, drained, 4 oz.	2.4	n.a.
Butterbur, canned, chopped, ½ cup	.2	n.a.
Buttercup squash (*Frieda's*), ¾ cup, 3 oz.	7.0	1.0
Butterfish, without added ingredients	0	0
Buttermilk, see "Milk"		
Butternut, dried:		
in shell, 1 lb.	14.8	5.8
shelled, 1 oz.	3.4	1.3
Butternut squash:		
raw (*Frieda's*), ¾ cup, 3 oz.	7.0	1.0
raw, cubed, ½ cup	8.1	1.1
baked, cubed, ½ cup	10.7	2.9
Butternut squash, frozen:		
12-oz. pkg.	49.0	4.4
boiled, drained, mashed, ½ cup	12.1	n.a.
Butterscotch baking chips (*Hershey's Bake Shoppe*), 1 tbsp.	10.0	0
Butterscotch syrup (*Smucker's Sundae Syrup*), 2 tbsp.	25.0	0
Butterscotch topping, 2 tbsp.:		
(*Hershey's*)	27.0	0
(*Smucker's* Spoonable)	30.0	0
caramel (*Smucker's* Special Recipe)	30.0	<1.0

C

Food and Measure	carb. (gms)	fiber (gms)
Cabbage, fresh:		
raw, 5¾''-diam. head, approx. 2.5 lbs.	49.3	20.9
raw, shredded, ½ cup	1.9	.8
boiled, drained, shredded, ½ cup	3.4	2.1
Cabbage, can or jar:		
red, sweet and sour (*Greenwood*), ½ cup	24.0	0
seasoned (*Glory* Country), ½ cup	6.0	2.0
Cabbage, Chinese, fresh:		
bok choy:		
raw (*Frieda's/Frieda's* Baby), 3 oz.	2.0	1.0
raw, whole, 1 lb.	8.7	4.0
raw, shredded, ½ cup	.8	.4
boiled, drained, shredded, ½ cup	1.5	1.4
Napa, raw (*Frieda's*), 1 cup, 3 oz.	3.0	1.0
pe-tsai:		
raw, whole, 1 lb.	13.6	4.2
raw, shredded, ½ cup	1.2	.4
boiled, drained, shredded, ½ cup	1.4	1.0
Cabbage, freeze-dried, (*AlpineAire*), .9 oz.	13.0	5.0
Cabbage, frozen, seasoned (*Glory* Savory Accents Country), ½ cup	7.0	2.0
Cabbage, marinated, see "Kim chee"		
Cabbage, mustard, raw (*Frieda's* Gai Choy), 1 cup, 3 oz.	4.0	2.0
Cabbage, Napa, see "Cabbage, Chinese"		
Cabbage, red, fresh:		
raw, whole, 1 lb.	22.2	7.3
raw, shredded (*Fresh Express*), 1 cup	4.0	1.0

Food and Measure	carb. (gms)	fiber (gms)
raw, shredded, ½ cup	2.1	.7
boiled, drained, shredded, ½ cup	3.5	1.5
Cabbage, savoy, fresh:		
raw (*Frieda's Salad Savoy*), ⅔ cup, 3 oz.	5.0	3.0
raw, whole, 1 lb.	22.1	11.2
raw, shredded, ½ cup	2.1	1.1
boiled, drained, shredded, ½ cup	4.0	n.a.
Cabbage, stuffed, entree, frozen (*Lean Cuisine Everyday Favorites*), 9.5-oz. pkg.	26.0	4.0
Cabbage, Tuscan (*Frieda's*), ⅔ cup, 3 oz.	5.0	2.0
Cactus pads, fresh:		
raw (*Frieda's*), ¾ cup, 3 oz.	4.0	1.0
raw, sliced, 1 cup	2.9	2.0
cooked, 1 cup	4.9	3.0
cooked, 1 pad	1.0	.6
Cactus pads, canned:		
(*Doña María* Nopalitos), 2 tbsp.	1.0	0
(*La Costeña* Nopalitos), 1 cup	4.0	2.0
in escabeche (*Royal Crown* Nopalitos), ⅔ cup	1.0	2.0
sliced (*Embasa* Nopalitos), 2 tbsp.	1.0	2.0
Cactus pear, see "Prickly pear"		
Cajun seasoning:		
(*Luzianne*), ¼ tsp.	0	0
(*McCormick*), ¼ tsp.	0	0
(*McCormick 1 Step*), 1 tsp.	1.0	0
Cake:		
banana crunch (*Entenmann's*), ⅛ cake	32.0	<1.0
butter (*Entenmann's Sunshine*), ⅙ cake	44.0	0
butter loaf (*Entenmann's*), ⅙ cake	31.0	0
butter cream, French (*Awrey's Dessert*), ⅑ cake	37.0	<1.0
carrot (*Entenmann's Deluxe*), ⅑ cake	30.0	1.0
chocolate (*Bill Knapp's*), ⅛ cake	54.0	1.0
chocolate chip, Swiss (*Entenmann's*), ⅑ cake	45.0	<1.0
chocolate fudge (*Entenmann's*), ⅛ cake	40.0	2.0
crumb cake:		
(*Entenmann's Ultimate*), ⅒ cake	33.0	<1.0
chocolate chip, filled (*Entenmann's*), ⅑ cake	49.0	1.0

Food and Measure	carb. (gms)	fiber (gms)
raspberry almond (*Entenmann's* Ultimate), ¹⁄₁₀ cake	30.0	<1.0
wheat free (*Foods by George*), ⅑ cake	36.0	<1.0
golden, fudge iced (*Entenmann's*), ⅛ cake	41.0	1.0
lemon coconut (*Entenmann's*), ⅛ cake	38.0	<1.0
lemon crunch (*Entenmann's*), ⅑ cake	49.0	<1.0
marble loaf (*Entenmann's*), ⅛ cake	27.0	<1.0
pound, wheat free (*Foods by George*), 2.7-oz. slice	35.0	<1.0
raisin loaf (*Entenmann's*), ⅛ cake	35.0	1.0
sour cream loaf (*Entenmann's*), ⅛ cake	26.0	0
Cake, frozen (see also "Cheesecake"):		
carrot:		
(*Mrs. Smith's*), ⅙ cake	37.0	1.0
(*Pepperidge Farm* Dessert Classics), ⅑ cake	32.0	1.0
(*Smart Ones*), 3.2-oz. piece	33.0	2.0
chocolate chip (*Kineret*), 2 slices, 2 oz.	27.0	0
chocolate, ⅛ cake:		
chunk (*Pepperidge Farm* 3 Layer)	41.0	<1.0
decadence (*Pepperidge Farm* Dessert Classics)	32.0	1.0
German (*Pepperidge Farm* 3 Layer)	31.0	<1.0
layer, double (*Sara Lee*)	33.0	2.0
chocolate fudge:		
(*Pepperidge Farm* 3 Layer), ⅛ cake	31.0	1.0
double (*Smart Ones*), 2.7-oz. piece	20.0	2.0
stripe (*Pepperidge Farm* 3 Layer), ⅛ cake	31.0	<1.0
coffee cake:		
butter streusel (*Sara Lee*), ⅙ cake	25.0	1.0
crumb (*Sara Lee*), ⅛ cake	30.0	1.0
pecan (*Sara Lee*), ⅙ cake	23.0	1.0
coconut layer (*Pepperidge Farm* 3 Layer), ⅛ cake	35.0	<1.0
coconut layer (*Sara Lee*), ⅛ cake	33.0	1.0
devil's food (*Pepperidge Farm* 3 Layer), ⅛ cake	34.0	<1.0
golden layer (*Pepperidge Farm* 3 Layer), ⅛ cake	33.0	<1.0
golden layer fudge (*Sara Lee*), ⅛ cake	34.0	1.0
guava (*Pepperidge Farm* 3 Layer), ⅛ cake	36.0	<1.0
mango (*Pepperidge Farm* 3 Layer), ⅛ cake	35.0	<1.0
marble (*Kineret*), 2 slices, 2 oz.	25.0	0

Food and Measure	carb. (gms)	fiber (gms)
pineapple, golden (*Pepperidge Farm* Dessert Classics),		
⅒ cake	34.0	1.0
pound cake:		
(*Sara Lee* Free & Light), ¼ cake	39.0	1.0
butter (*Sara Lee*), ¼ cake	37.0	1.0
butter (*Sara Lee* Family Size), ⅙ cake	34.0	1.0
strawberry swirl (*Sara Lee*), ¼ cake	44.0	1.0
red, white, and blue (*Pepperidge Farm* 3 Layer), ⅛ cake	35.0	<1.0
strawberry stripe (*Pepperidge Farm* 3 Layer), ⅛ cake	32.0	<1.0
tiramisu (*Ritch & Famous*), 2.7-oz. piece	34.0	<1.0
vanilla layer (*Pepperidge Farm* 3 Layer), ⅛ cake	35.0	<1.0
vanilla layer (*Sara Lee*), ⅛ cake	32.0	0
Cake, mix, 1/12 cake*, except as noted:		
angel food:		
(*Betty Crocker*)	32.0	0
(*Duncan Hines*)	31.0	0
confetti (*Betty Crocker*)	34.0	0
banana (*Duncan Hines*)	36.0	0
Boston cream pie, with filling and frosting		
(*Duncan Hines Signature Dessert*), ⅙ cake*	59.0	1.0
butter pecan (*SuperMoist*)	35.0	0
carrot (*SuperMoist*), ⅒ cake*	42.0	0
chocolate:		
butter recipe (*SuperMoist*)	35.0	2.0
double swirl (*SuperMoist*)	35.0	1.0
German (*SuperMoist*)	36.0	0
milk (*SuperMoist*)	34.0	1.0
chocolate chip (*SuperMoist*)	35.0	0
chocolate fudge (*SuperMoist*)	35.0	1.0
dark (*Duncan Hines*)	36.0	1.0
chocolate silk torte, with filling, frosting		
(*Duncan Hines Signature Dessert*), ⅙ cake*	65.0	2.0
devil's food:		
(*Duncan Hines*)	35.0	1.0
(*"Jiffy"*), ⅕ pkg.	40.0	1.0
(*SuperMoist*)	35.0	2.0
fudge, butter recipe (*Duncan Hines*), ⅒ cake*	43.0	1.0
fudge marble (*Duncan Hines*)	35.0	<1.0

Food and Measure	carb. (gms)	fiber (gms)
fudge marble (*SuperMoist*), 1/10 cake*	42.0	0
funnel cake (*Golden Dipt* Fry Easy Batter mix), 1/4 cup	23.0	0
gingerbread (*Betty Crocker*), 1/8 cake*	39.0	0
golden, butter recipe (*Duncan Hines*), 1/10 cake*	43.0	0
lemon (*SuperMoist*)	35.0	0
lemon or orange (*Duncan Hines*)	36.0	0
orange with filling, glaze (*Duncan Hines Signature Desserts* Dreamsicle)	57.0	<1.0
pineapple:		
(*Duncan Hines*)	36.0	0
(*SuperMoist*)	35.0	0
upside-down (*Betty Crocker*), 1/6 cake*	64.0	0
pound (*Betty Crocker*), 1/8 cake*	45.0	0
rainbow chip (*SuperMoist*), 1/10 cake*	41.0	0
rainbow swirl (*SuperMoist*)	35.0	0
sour cream white (*SuperMoist*), 1/10 cake*	41.0	0
strawberry or spice (*Duncan Hines*)	36.0	0
strawberry or spice (*SuperMoist*)	35.0	0
vanilla, French (*SuperMoist*)	35.0	0
white (*SuperMoist*)	34.0	0
white or yellow (*Duncan Hines*)	36.0	0
white or yellow (*"Jiffy"*), 1/5 pkg.	41.0	<1.0
yellow (*SuperMoist*)	35.0	0
yellow, butter recipe (*SuperMoist*)	36.0	0
Cake, snack (see also "Danish," "Donuts," and specific listings), 1 piece, except as noted:		
caramel cookie bar (*Little Debbie*), 1.2 oz.	22.0	0
chocolate, with crème:		
(*Devil Dogs*), 1.6 oz.	26.0	<1.0
(*Ding Dongs*), 2 pieces, 2.8 oz.	47.0	2.0
(*Drake's* Swiss Rolls), 3 oz.	48.0	2.0
(*Hostess HoHos*), 3 oz.	50.0	2.0
(*Little Debbie Devil Squares*), 1.7 oz.	29.0	0
(*Ring Dings*), 2 pieces, 2.7 oz.	43.0	2.0
(*Suzy Q's*), 2 oz.	35.0	1.0
with coconut (*Sno Balls*), 1.8 oz.	32.0	1.0
chocolate chip crème pie (*Little Debbie*), 1.2 oz.	23.0	<1.0

Food and Measure	carb. (gms)	fiber (gms)
coffee cake:		
(*Drake's*), 1.2 oz.	20.0	0
(*Drake's* Low Fat), 1.2 oz.	21.0	0
(*Little Debbie*), 2 pieces, 2.2 oz.	42.0	0
crumb cake:		
(*Entenmann's*), 3 oz.	47.0	<1.0
apple (*Entenmann's*), 4 oz.	63.0	1.0
raspberry almond (*Entenmann's*), 4 oz.	60.0	1.0
cupcake:		
(*Hostess* Baseballs), 1.6 oz.	31.0	0
chocolate (*Hostess*), 1.8 oz.	30.0	1.0
chocolate, with crème (*Yankee Doodles*), 2 pieces, 2 oz.	33.0	<1.0
golden (*Hostess*), 1.9 oz.	33.0	0
orange (*Hostess*), 1.9 oz.	35.0	0
fudge cake, frosted (*Little Debbie*), 1.5 oz.	25.0	<1.0
golden, with crème:		
(*Sunny Doodles*), 2 pieces, 2 oz.	33.0	0
(*Twinkies*), 1.5 oz.	25.0	0
jelly crème pie (*Little Debbie*), 1.2 oz.	23.0	0
maple crème pie (*Little Debbie*), 1.2 oz.	23.0	<1.0
marble cake (*Entenmann's*), 2.75 oz.	25.0	1.0
oatmeal crème pie (*Little Debbie*), 1.2 oz.	26.0	<1.0
pecan swirls (*Drake's*), 1 oz.	16.0	0
pound cake (*Entenmann's*), 2.75 oz.	37.0	<1.0
Cake, snack, mix (see also specific listings), ⅑ pkg., except as noted:		
banana walnut (*Betty Crocker Snackin' Cake*)	31.0	0
chocolate chip/chunk (*Betty Crocker Snackin' Cake*)	32.0	1.0
cinnamon swirl (*Betty Crocker Snackin' Cake*)	34.0	0
lemon (*Betty Crocker Sunkist* Supreme Dessert Bar), ⅟₁₆ pkg.*	24.0	0
Calabaza (*Frieda's*), ½ cup, 3 oz.	2.0	1.0
Calamari, see "Squid"		
Calamari dish, frozen, breaded, fried:		
(*Contessa*), 13 pieces or 2 oz., 2 tbsp. sauce	16.0	0
rings (*Fisherman's Pride*), 20 pieces, 4 oz.	20.0	1.0
Calves liver, see "Liver"		

Food and Measure	carb. (gms)	fiber (gms)
Camote, see "Boniato"		
Camouflage melon (*Frieda's*), 1 cup, 5 oz.	13.0	1.0
Candy:		
almond, coated:		
carob (*Tree of Life*), 1.4 oz.	20.0	1.0
chocolate (*Brach's* Supremes), 11 pieces, 1.4 oz.	22.0	2.0
chocolate (*Planter's*), 12 pieces., 1.4 oz.	19.0	2.0
chocolate, candy (*M&M's*), 1.3-oz. pkg.	21.0	2.0
yogurt (*Tree of Life*), 1.4 oz.	20.0	2.0
almond paste, see "marzipan," below		
bridge mix (*Brach's*), 16 pieces, 1.4 oz.	26.0	>1.0
butter rum (*LifeSavers*), 2 pieces	5.0	0
butter toffee crème (*Creme Savers*), .5 oz.	13.0	0
butterscotch (*Brach's*), 3 pieces, .6 oz.	17.0	0
butterscotch disks (*Star Brites*), 3 pieces, .6 oz.	16.0	0
candy corn (*Brach's*), 26 pieces, 1.4 oz.	35.0	0
caramel:		
(*Brach's Milk Maid*), 4 pieces, 1.4 oz.	30.0	0
(*Sugar Babies*), 30 pieces, 1.6 oz.	41.0	0
(*Sugar Daddy* Junior), 3 pieces., 1.3 oz.	35.0	0
(*Sugar Daddy* Large), 1.7 oz.	43.0	0
egg (*Cadbury*), 1.4-oz. piece	24.0	0
rolls (*Brach's Milk Maid*), 5 pieces, 1.3 oz.	28.0	0
caramel, chocolate coated:		
(*Brach's Milk Maid*), 18 pieces, 1.4 oz.	28.0	0
(*Milk Duds*), 13 pieces, 1.4 oz.	28.0	0
(*Mini Rolo Bites*), 19 pieces., 1.4 oz.	26.0	<1.0
(*Rolo*), 1.7-oz. pkg.	31.0	0
clusters (*Brach's*), 3 pieces, 1.6 oz.	23.0	1.0
clusters (*Pot of Gold*), 3 pieces, 1.6 oz.	24.0	1.0
cookie bar (*Twix*), 2 bars	37.0	1.0
dark chocolate (*Milky Way*), 5 pieces	29.0	1.0
milk chocolate (*Milky Way*), 5 pieces	30.0	0
peanut, nougat, white chocolate (*Zero*), 1.8-oz. bar	36.0	<1.0
carob chips (*Tree of Life*), 50 pieces, .5 oz.	9.0	1.0
cashew, chocolate coated (*Planters*), 13 pieces,		
1.4 oz.	21.0	1.0
cherry, chocolate covered (*Cella's*), 2 pieces, 1 oz.	19.0	<1.0

Food and Measure	carb. (gms)	fiber (gms)
cherry, dried, chocolate coated (*Harvest Sweets*), 1.25 oz.	24.0	1.0
cherry flavor:		
(*Twizzlers* Bites), 17 pieces, 1.4 oz.	32.0	0
(*Twizzlers* Nibs), 2.25-oz. pkg.	51.0	0
(*Twizzlers Pull-n-Peel*), 1.2-oz. piece	25.0	0
(*Twizzlers* twists), 4 pieces, 1.6 oz.	36.0	0
chocolate, coffee crunch (*Mauna Loa* Kona), 1.75-oz. bar .	29.0	4.0
chocolate, cookies and cream (*Hershey's*), 1.5 oz.	26.0	0
chocolate, dark:		
(*Cadbury Royal Dark*), 10 blocks, 1.4 oz.	24.0	3.0
(*Dove*), 1.3-oz. bar	22.0	2.0
(*Dove Promises*), 5 pieces, 1.4 oz.	24.0	2.0
(*Hershey's Kisses Rich*), 9 pieces, 1.5 oz.	25.0	3.0
(*Hershey's Special Dark*), 1.4 oz.	25.0	3.0
almond (*Hershey's Nuggets Special Dark*), 4 pieces, 1.3 oz.	20.0	3.0
honey almond nougat (*Toblerone*), 1.2 oz.	20.0	2.0
mint (*Cadbury Royal Dark*), 10 blocks, 1.4 oz.	24.0	3.0
orange (*Terry's*), 1.6 oz.	28.0	3.0
raspberry (*Hershey's Nuggets*), 4 pieces, 1.4 oz.	24.0	3.0
chocolate, milk:		
(*Brach's Stars*), 10 pieces, 1.3 oz.	24.0	0
(*Cadbury Dairy Milk*), 10 blocks, 1.4 oz.	24.0	<1.0
(*Dove*), 1.3-oz. bar	22.0	1.0
(*Dove Promises*), 5 pieces, 1.4 oz.	24.0	1.0
(*Hershey's*), 1.5 oz.	25.0	1.0
(*Hershey's Hugs*), 9 pieces, 1.4 oz.	23.0	0
(*Hershey's Kisses*), 9 pieces, 1.4 oz.	24.0	1.0
(*Hershey's Nuggets*), 4 pieces, 1.4 oz.	24.0	1.0
(*Hershey's Swoops*), 1.25-oz. cup	20.0	<1.0
(*Milka*), 1/3 bar, 1.2 oz.	20.0	1.0
(*Nestlé*), 1/4 of 5-oz. bar	23.0	<1.0
(*Symphony*), 1.5 oz.	24.0	<1.0
(*Terry's*), 1.6 oz.	27.0	0
almond (*Cadbury Roast Almond*), 10 blocks, 1.4 oz.	21.0	1.0
almond (*Hershey's*), 1.4 oz.	20.0	1.0
almond (*Hershey's Kisses*), 9 pieces, 1.4 oz.	21.0	1.0

Food and Measure	carb. (gms)	fiber (gms)
almond (*Hershey's Nuggets*), 4 pieces, 1.3 oz.	20.0	1.0
almond toffee (*Symphony*), 1.5 oz.	22.0	1.0
candy coated (*M&M's*), 1.7-oz. pkg.	34.0	1.0
candy coated (*M&M's* Fun Size), .7-oz. pkg.	15.0	1.0
candy coated, minis (*M&M's*), 1.1-oz. tube	21.0	1.0
caramel (*Caramello*), 6 blocks, 1.5 oz.	27.0	<1.0
caramel filled (*Hershey's Kisses*), 8 pieces, 1.3 oz.	24.0	0
crème egg (*Cadbury*), 1.4-oz. piece	25.0	<1.0
crisps (*Crunch*), ¼ of 5-oz. bar	24.0	<1.0
crisps (*Krackel*), 1.4-oz. bar	28.0	<1.0
crisps, with caramel (*Crunch*), 1.52-oz. bar	29.0	<1.0
crispy, candy coated (*M&M's*), 1.5-oz. pkg.	31.0	1.0
fruit and nut (*Cadbury Fruit & Nut*), 10 blocks, 1.4 oz. .	25.0	1.0
fruit and nut (*Chunky*), ¼ of 5-oz. bar	21.0	1.0
honey almond nougat (*Toblerone*), 1.76-oz. bar	32.0	1.0
honey almond nougat (*Toblerone*), 1.23-oz. bar	23.0	1.0
macadamia (*Mauna Loa*), 1.75-oz. bar	27.0	1.0
macadamia, crisps (*Mauna Loa*), 1.75-oz. bar	29.0	<1.0
mint (*Hershey's Kisses*), 9 pieces, 1.4 oz.	24.0	1.0
orange (*Terry's*), 1.6 oz.	27.0	1.0
peanut butter chips (*Butterfinger*), ⅕ bar, 1.4 oz.	27.0	<1.0
raisins and almonds, extra creamy (*Hershey's Nuggets*), 4 pieces, 1.4 oz.	23.0	1.0
raspberry crème (*Cadbury*), 10 blocks, 1.4 oz.	23.0	0
strawberry crème (*Hershey's Kisses*), 9 pieces, 1.5 oz. .	24.0	0
toffee and almonds, extra creamy (*Hershey's Nuggets*), 4 pieces, 1.4 oz.	21.0	1.0
chocolate, white, with honey almond nougat (*Toblerone*), 1.2 oz.	20.0	0
chocolate assortment:		
(*Pot of Gold*), 1.1-oz. box	21.0	<1.0
(*Pot of Gold* Premium), 1.5 oz.	26.0	1.0
(*Pot of Gold* Sugar Free), 1.5 oz.	22.0	1.0
caramel (*Pot of Gold*), 1.5 oz.	27.0	<1.0
crèmes (*Pot of Gold*), 1.4 oz.	32.0	<1.0
mint (*Pot of Gold*), 1.4 oz.	26.0	1.0
nut (*Pot of Gold*), 1.5 oz.	21.0	1.0
chocolate caramel crème (*Creme Savers*), .5 oz.	13.0	0

Food and Measure	carb. (gms)	fiber (gms)
chocolate chews:		
(*Tootsie Roll* Midgees), 6 pieces, 1.4 oz.	28.0	0
(*Tootsie Roll* Midgees Small), 12 pieces, 1.3 oz.	25.0	0
chocolate thins, 1.3 oz.:		
cherry jubilee (*Andes*), 8 pieces	22.0	<1.0
crème de menthe (*Andes*), 8 pieces	22.0	0
mint parfait (*Andes*), 8 pieces	21.0	0
toffee crunch (*Andes*), 8 pieces	23.0	0
chocolate twists (*Twizzlers*), 4 pieces, 1.5 oz.	34.0	<1.0
cinnamon:		
(*Brach's* Imperials), 52 pieces, .5 oz.	15.0	0
disks (*Star Brites*), 3 pieces, .6 oz.	16.0	0
hard (*Brach's*), 3 pieces, .6 oz.	17.0	0
circus peanuts (*Brach's*), 6 pieces, 1.5 oz.	39.0	0
coconut, with chocolate:		
(*Almond Joy Swoops*), 1.25-oz. cup	21.0	<1.0
(*Mounds*), 1.7-oz. bar	29.0	2.0
almond (*Almond Joy*), 1.6-oz. bar	27.0	2.0
chocolate chocolate (*Almond Joy*), 1.6-oz. bar	25.0	3.0
piña colada (*Almond Joy*), 1.6-oz. bar	25.0	2.0
coconut, Neapolitan (*Brach's* Sundaes), 3 pieces, 1.3 oz. .	28.0	1.0
cotton candy:		
(*Charms Fluffy Stuff*), .6-oz. bag	17.0	0
(*Charms Fluffy Stuff*), 1.1-oz. bag	30.0	0
(*Jays*), 2 oz.	56.0	0
cranberry, chocolate coated, dark (*Cape Cod*), 1¼ oz. . . .	23.0	2.0
crèmes, assorted (*Rich & Dreamy*), 3 pieces, 1.7 oz.	36.0	>1.0
crèmes, egg (*Cadbury*), 1.4-oz. piece	28.0	0
dulce de leche (*Hershey's Kisses*), 8 pieces, 1.3 oz.	24.0	0
fruit flavor, assorted:		
(*Brach's* Jube Jels), 12 piece, 1.4 oz.	34.0	0
(*Jolly Rancher Stix*), .6-oz. pkg.	17.0	0
(*LifeSavers* Fruit Slices), 1.4 oz.	36.0	0
(*Mason Dots*), 12 pieces, 1.5 oz.	35.0	0
(*Wild 'n Fruity* Rainbow Bears), 4 pieces, 1.6 oz.	38.0	0
all varieties, except sours (*Skittles*), 2.2-oz. bag	54.0	0
chews (*Jolly Rancher*), 6 pieces, 1.14 oz.	33.0	0
chews (*Starburst*), 2.1-oz. pkg.	48.0	0

Food and Measure	carb. (gms)	fiber (gms)
chews (*Tootsie Frooties*), 12 pieces, 1.3 oz.	29.0	0
chews (*Tootsie Roll*), 6 pieces, 1.4 oz.	28.0	0
chews, sour (*Twizzlers Sourz*), 1.8-oz. pkg.	41.0	<1.0
chews, tangy (*Wild 'n Fruity*), 12 pieces, 1.4 oz.	32.0	0
gummy (*Brach's*), 13 pieces, 1.4 oz.	25.0	0
gummy (*Jolly Rancher*), 10 pieces, 1.4 oz.	29.0	0
gummy (*LifeSavers*), 1.4 oz.	30.0	0
gummy (*Wild 'n Fruity* Bears/Worms), 5 pieces, 1.4 oz.	32.0	0
gummy, sour (*Wild 'n Fruity* Fish), 8 pieces, 1.4 oz. ...	26.0	0
gummy, sour (*Wild 'n Fruity* Worms), 5 pieces, 1.6 oz. .	36.0	0
slices (*Brach's*), 3 pieces, 1.6 oz.	38.0	0
sours (*Jolly Rancher Screaming Sours*),		
16 pieces, 1.4 oz.	34.0	0
sours (*Skittles*), 1.8-oz. bag	44.0	0
fruit flavor, hard:		
(*Jolly Rancher*), 3 pieces, .6 oz.	17.0	0
(*Jolly Rancher* Sugar Free), 4 pieces, .6 oz.	13.0	0
(*LifeSavers*), 2 pieces	5.0	0
(*LifeSavers* Sours), .5 oz.	15.0	0
(*LifeSavers* Fusions), .5 oz.	15.0	0
(*Wild 'n Fruity*), 3 pieces, .6 oz.	18.0	0
(*Jolly Rancher Rocks*), 1.1 oz.	30.0	0
(*Starburst*), 3 pieces, .5 oz.	13.0	0
and crème (*CremeSavers*), .5 oz.	13.0	0
sour balls (*Charms*), 1 piece	5.0	0
squares (*Charms*), 2 pieces, .2 oz.	6.0	0
fudge, double (*Hershey's Kisses*), 9 pieces, 1.5 oz.	25.0	1.0
ginger, chocolate (*SunRidge Farms*), ¼ cup, 1.8 oz.	25.0	6.0
ginger, hard (*Gin-Gins*), 3 pieces, .3 oz.	8.0	0
gum, chewing, 1 piece, except as noted:		
(*Abra Cabubble*)	10.0	0
(*Bubble Yum*)	6.0	0
(*Bubble Yum* Sugarless)	3.0	0
(*Big Red/Juicy Fruit/Wrigley's Spearmint/*		
Doublemint/Winterfresh)	2.0	0
(*Skittles*), 2 pieces	2.0	0
all varieties:		
(*Freedent*)	2.0	0

Food and Measure	carb. (gms)	fiber (gms)
(*Orbit/Eclipse* Sugar Free), 2 pieces	2.0	0
except bubble (*Extra* Sugar Free)	2.0	0
bubble (*Extra* Sugar Free)	1.0	0
jelly beans:		
(*Jelly Belly*), 35 pieces, 1.4 oz.	37.0	0
(*Jolly Rancher* Assorted), 1.4 oz.	34.0	0
(*Jolly Rancher* Bold Smoothie), 1.4 oz.	35.0	0
(*Smucker's*), 25 pieces, 1.4 oz.	37.0	0
(*Starburst*), ¼ cup, 1.5 oz.	38.0	0
licorice:		
(*Crows*), 12 pieces, 1.5 oz.	35.0	0
(*Kookaburra*), 4 pieces, 1.4 oz.	31.0	0
(*Twizzlers*), 4 pieces, 1.6 oz.	34.0	0
(*Twizzlers* Bites), 18 pieces, .4 oz.	30.0	0
(*Twizzlers* Nibs), 2.25-oz. pkg.	48.0	0
candy coated (*Good & Plenty*), 1.75-oz. pkg.	43.0	0
chews (*SunRidge Farms*), ¼ cup, 1.4 oz.	27.0	<1.0
lollipop, 1 piece, except as noted:		
(*Charms* Sweet/Sour), .6 oz.	17.0	0
(*Charms* Blow Pop), .6 oz.	16.0	0
(*Charms* Blow Pop Junior), .5 oz.	14.0	0
(*Charms* Blow Pop Super), 1.3 oz.	35.0	0
(*Jolly Rancher* Assorted), .6 oz.	16.0	0
(*Jolly Rancher* Filled), .6 oz.	15.0	0
(*LifeSavers*), .4 oz.	10.0	0
(*Starburst* Fruit Chew), .5 oz.	13.0	0
(*Tootsie Roll* Pop), .6 oz.	15.0	0
(*Tootsie Roll* Pop Miniature), 3 pieces, .5 oz.	13.0	0
(*Tootsie Roll* Pop Small), .45 oz.	11.0	0
macadamia nuts, coated:		
butter candy glaze (*Mauna Loa*), 1 oz.	10.0	1.0
butter corn crunch (*Mauna Loa*), 1 oz.	18.0	1.0
chocolate, dark (*Mauna Loa*), 9 pieces, 1.3 oz.	18.0	3.0
chocolate, milk (*Mauna Loa*), 1 oz., ¼ cup	15.0	1.0
chocolate, milk (*Mauna Loa* Deluxe), 4 pieces, 1.3 oz.	19.0	1.0
chocolate, milk (*Mauna Loa Mountains*), 4 pieces, 1.3 oz.	21.0	1.0

Food and Measure	carb. (gms)	fiber (gms)
chocolate milk, candy (*Mauna Loa*), 1.4 oz.	25.0	1.0
chocolate, milk, toffee (*Mauna Loa*), 7 pieces, 1.4 oz. .	23.0	1.0
malt balls, coated:		
carob (*SunRidge Farms*), ¼ cup, 1.9 oz.	34.0	0
carob (*Tree of Life*), 1.4 oz.	28.0	0
chocolate (*Brach's Malts*), 15 pieces, 1.4 oz.	30.0	1.0
chocolate (*Whoppers*), ¾-oz. pkg.	16.0	0
chocolate, candy (*Whoppers Robin Eggs*),		
24 pieces, 1.4 oz.	31.0	0
marshmallows:		
(*Kraft Jet-Puffed*), 1 oz.	23.0	0
all flavors (*Kraft FunMallows*), 1.1 oz.	24.0	0
crème (*Kraft*), .4 oz.	10.0	0
toasted coconut (*Kraft*), 1 oz.	21.0	0
marzipan (*Biermann*), .42-oz. piece	10.0	1.0
mint:		
(*Brach's* Kentucky), 7 pieces, .6 oz.	16.0	0
(*Brach's Ice Blue Mint Coolers*), 3 pieces, .6 oz.	17.0	0
(*BreathSavers*), 1 piece	2.0	0
(*LifeSavers Cryst-O-Mint/Pep-O-Mint/ Wint-O-Green*),		
2 pieces	5.0	0
dessert (*Brach's*), 14 pieces, .5 oz.	15.0	0
peppermint, cool (*Hain*), 6 pieces	2.0	0
peppermint or spearmint (*Star Brites* Starlight),		
3 pieces, .5 oz.	15.0	0
mint, chocolate coated (see also "peppermint," below)		
(*Junior Mints*), 16 pieces, 1.4 oz.	30.0	<1.0
nonpareils (*Brach's Sprinkles*), 17 pieces, 1.4 oz.	29.0	1.0
nonpareils (*Sno•Caps*), ¼ cup, 1.4 oz.	30.0	2.0
nougat, jelly (*Brach's*), 5 pieces, 1.4 oz.	34.0	0
nougat, with chocolate:		
(*Milky Way*), 2-oz. bar	41.0	1.0
(*Milky Way* Fun Size), 2 bars, 1.4 oz.	28.0	0
(*Milky Way* Miniature), 5 pieces, 1.5 oz.	30.0	0
(*Milky Way Pop'ables*), 13 pieces, 1.4 oz.	28.0	0
(*3 Musketeers*), 2.13-oz. bar	46.0	1.0
(*3 Musketeers* Fun Size), 2 bars, 1.2 oz.	25.0	1.0
(*3 Musketeers* Miniature), 7 pieces, 1.5 oz.	31.0	1.0

Food and Measure	carb. (gms)	fiber (gms)
chocolate (*Charleston Chew*), 1.9-oz. bar	43.0	<1.0
chocolate chews (*3 Musketeers Chewlicious*), .8-oz. bar	18.0	0
dark (*Milky Way Midnight*), 1.76-oz. bar	36.0	1.0
dark (*Milky Way Midnight* Fun Size), 2 bars, 1.4 oz. ...	28.0	1.0
dark (*Milky Way Midnight* Miniature), 5 pieces, 1.4 oz. .	29.0	1.0
strawberry (*Charleston Chew*), 1.9-oz. bar	43.0	0
vanilla (*Charleston Chew*), 1.9-oz. bar	44.0	0
vanilla (*Charleston Chew* Mini), 13 pieces, 1.4 oz.	29.0	0
orange slices (*Brach's*), 2 pieces, 1.3 oz.	32.0	0
peanut bar:		
(*Planters*), 1.6 oz.	22.0	2.0
(*Planters* Carb Well), 1.23 oz.	16.0	2.0
chocolate (*Chew-ets/Peanut Chews*), 3 pieces, 1 oz. ..	17.0	<1.0
peanut butter, with chocolate:		
(*Brach's* Meltaways), 3 pieces, 1.3 oz.	19.0	1.0
(*Butterfinger*), 2.1-oz. bar	43.0	1.0
(*Butterfinger* King), 1/3 bar, 1.25 oz.	25.0	<1.0
(*Butterfinger* Minis), 4 bars, 1.4 oz.	29.0	<1.0
(*Butterfinger* Crisp), 1.76-oz. bar	33.0	1.0
(*Butterfinger* Crisp Minis), 4 bars, 1.6 oz.	29.0	1.0
(*5th Avenue*), 2-oz. bar	35.0	2.0
(*Reese's Bites*), 16 pieces, 1.4 oz.	23.0	1.0
(*Reese's Peanut Butter Cups*), 1.5 oz.	23.0	1.0
(*Reese's Pieces*), 1.5-oz. pkg.	26.0	1.0
(*Reese's Swoops*), 1.25-oz. cup	17.0	2.0
candy coated (*M&M's*), 1.6-oz. pkg.	26.0	2.0
coconut (*Zagnut*), 1.75-oz. bar	31.0	2.0
cookie bar (*Twix*), 2 bars	28.0	2.0
dark (*Reese's Peanut Butter Cups*), 1.5 oz.	22.0	2.0
fudge (*Reese's Peanut Butter Cups*), 1.5 oz.	22.0	2.0
nougat (*Reese's Fast Break*), 2-oz. bar	34.0	2.0
nuts (*Reese's NutRageous*), 1.8-oz. bar	27.0	2.0
white chocolate (*Reese's Peanut Butter Cups*), 1.5 oz. .	22.0	1.0
peanut caramel bar:		
(*Baby Ruth*), 2.1-oz. bar	37.0	2.0
(*PayDay*), 1.8-oz. bar	28.0	2.0
(*Snickers*) 2.1-oz. bar	35.0	1.0
(*Snickers* Fun Size), 2 bars, 1.4 oz.	24.0	1.0

Food and Measure	carb. (gms)	fiber (gms)
(*Snickers* Miniature), 4 pieces, 1.3 oz.	22.0	1.0
(*Snickers Crunchier*) 1.55-oz. bar	25.0	1.0
(*Snickers Pop'ables*), 13 pieces, 1.4 oz.	24.0	1.0
(*Whatchamacallit*), 1.6-oz. bar	29.0	<1.0
honey roasted (*PayDay*), 1.8-oz. bar	30.0	2.0
peanuts, coated:		
butter toffee (*Fisher*), ¼ cup, 1 oz.	17.0	1.0
butter toffee (*Old Dominion*), 1 oz.	16.0	2.0
butter toffee, maple (*Brach's* Maple Nut Goodies),		
7 pieces, 1.5 oz.	30.0	1.0
candy (*M&M's*), 1.7-oz. pkg.	30.0	2.0
candy (*M&M's* Fun Size), .7-oz. pkg.	13.0	1.0
carob (*Tree of Life*), 1.4 oz.	20.0	<1.0
chocolate (*Brach's* Double Dippers), 15 pieces,		
1.4 oz.	23.0	2.0
chocolate (*Goobers*), ¼ cup, 1.4 oz.	22.0	2.0
chocolate (*Mr. Goodbar*), 1.7-oz. bar	27.0	2.0
chocolate (*Mr. Goodbar Bites*), 25 pieces, 1.4 oz.	21.0	1.0
chocolate clusters (*Brach's*), 3 pieces, 1.4 oz.	21.0	2.0
French burnt (*Brach's*), 31 pieces, 1.4 oz.	29.0	1.0
yogurt (*Tree of Life*), 1.4 oz.	19.0	<1.0
pecan caramel clusters, chocolate:		
(*Nestlé* Turtles), 4 pieces, 1.5 oz.	25.0	1.0
(*Pot of Gold*), 3 pieces, 1.6 oz.	24.0	1.0
(*Russell Stover* Pecan Delights Sugar-Free),		
2 pieces, 1.2 oz.	17.0	3.0
peppermint, with chocolate:		
(*Brach's* Mint Patties), 3 pieces, 1.3 oz.	29.0	0
(*York* Pattie), 1.4-oz. piece	32.0	<1.0
(*York Bites*), 15 pieces, 1.4 oz.	33.0	<1.0
(*York Swoops*), 1.25-oz. cup	21.0	2.0
pretzel, caramel, peanut chocolate (*Take 5*), 1.5-oz. bar	25.0	1.0
pretzel, coated:		
chocolate, milk (*Synders* Dips), 1 oz.	18.0	n.a.
chocolate, white (*Synders* Dips), 1 oz.	19.0	n.a.
chocolate, white (*Hershey's Bites*), 23 pieces, 1.4 oz.	25.0	1.0
yogurt (*SunRidge Farms*), 8 pieces, 1.4 oz.	27.0	0
yogurt (*Tree of Life*), 1.4 oz.	28.0	0

Food and Measure	carb. (gms)	fiber (gms)
raisins, coated:		
carob (*SunRidge Farms*), ¼ cup, 2.1 oz.	41.0	1.0
carob (*Tree of Life*), 1.4 oz.	28.0	<1.0
chocolate (*Brach's California*), 35 pieces, 1.4 oz.	28.0	1.0
chocolate (*Raisinets*), ¼ cup, 1.4 oz.	32.0	1.0
yogurt (*SunRidge Farms*), 1.4 oz.	29.0	<1.0
yogurt (*Tree of Life*), 1.4 oz.	27.0	<1.0
root beer (*Brach's Barrels*), 3 pieces, .6 oz.	17.0	0
soy nuts, coated, chocolate (*GeniSoy*), 1 oz.	15.0	2.0
soy nuts, coated, praline (*GeniSoy*), 1 oz.	18.0	2.0
spearmint (*Brach's Leaves*), 5 pieces, 1.4 oz.	34.0	0
spice drops (*Brach's*), 12 pieces, 1.4 oz.	33.0	0
strawberry twists (*Twizzlers*), 4 pieces, 1.6 oz.	36.0	0
toffee, 3 pieces, .6 oz.:		
coffee (*Brach's Special Treasures*)	14.0	0
fruit and cream (*Brach's Special Treasures*)	13.0	0
golden (*Brach's Special Treasures*)	15.0	0
toffee, with chocolate:		
(*Heath*), 1.4-oz. bar	24.0	<1.0
(*Health Bites*), 15 pieces, 1.4 oz.	25.0	<1.0
(*Skor*), 1.4-oz. bar	24.0	<1.0
truffles:		
(*Truffelettes*), 4 pieces, 1.1 oz.	14.0	1.4
assorted (*Pot of Gold*), 1.5 oz.	27.0	1.0
chocolate, dark (*Harry and David*), 2 pieces, 1.3 oz.	19.0	2.0
cookies and cream bar (*Milka*), ⅓ bar, 1.2 oz.	19.0	1.0
wafer, with chocolate:		
(*KitKat*), 1.5-oz. bar	27.0	<1.0
(*KitKat Bites*), 15 pieces, 1.4 oz.	25.0	<1.0
mint (*KitKat*), 1.5-oz. bar	27.0	<1.0
peanut butter (*ReeseSticks*), 1.5 oz.	23.0	1.0
triple chocolate (*KitKat*), 1.5-oz. bar	26.0	1.0
white chocolate (*KitKat*), 1.5-oz. bar	26.0	0
walnuts, glazed (*Emerald Original*), 1 oz.	12.0	1.0
Cane juice, dehydrated (*Tree of Life Organic*), 1 level tsp.	3.0	0
Cane syrup, 1 tbsp.	13.4	0
Cannellini beans, see "Kidney beans"		

Food and Measure	carb. (gms)	fiber (gms)
Cannelloni entree, frozen, cheese (*Lean Cuisine Everyday Favorites*), 9⅛-oz. pkg.	30.0	3.0
Cannoli shell (*Ferrara*), .5-oz. shell	8.0	0
Cantaloupe:		
(*Del Monte*), ¼ medium	12.0	1.0
(*Dole*), ¼ medium	12.0	1.0
½ of 5″ melon	22.3	2.1
cubed, 1 cup	13.4	1.3
Cantaloupe, dried (*SunRidge Farms*), ¼ cup, 1.4 oz.	34.0	1.0
Caper berries (*Haddon House*), ½ oz.	1.0	0
Capers (*Goya*), 1 tbsp.	1.0	0
Capicola, see "Ham lunch meat"		
Capon, see "Chicken"		
Caponata, see "Eggplant appetizer"		
Cappuccino, see "Coffee, flavored, mix" and "Coffee, iced"		
Carambola, fresh:		
(*Frieda's* Starfruit), 5 oz.	11.0	4.0
1 medium, 4.7 oz.	9.9	3.4
sliced, ½ cup	1.0	1.5
Carambola, dried (*Frieda's* Starfruit), ⅓ cup, 1.4 oz.	29.0	1.0
Caramel dip, see "Fruit dip"		
Caramel syrup, 2 tbsp.:		
(*Hershey's Classic Caramel* Sundae)	25.0	0
(*Smucker's Sundae Syrup*)	25.0	0
Caramel topping, 2 tbsp.:		
(*Hershey's Classic Caramel*)	27.0	0
(*Smucker's*)	31.0	0
(*Smucker's Magic Shell*)	14.0	0
(*Smucker's Plate Scapers*)	25.0	0
butterscotch, see "Butterscotch topping"		
dulce de leche (*Smucker's*)	23.0	0
dulce de leche (*Smucker's* Spoonable)	25.0	0
hot (*Smucker's* Spoonable)	29.0	0
Caraway seeds, 1 tsp.	1.1	<1.0
Cardamom, ground:		
1 tsp.	1.4	.5
1 tbsp.	4.0	1.6

Food and Measure	carb. (gms)	fiber (gms)
Cardoon:		
raw (*Frieda's*), 1 cup, 3 oz.	4.0	1.0
raw, shredded, ½ cup	4.4	1.4
boiled, drained, 4 oz.	6.0	n.a.
Caribou, meat only, without added ingredients	0	0
Carissa:		
1 medium, .8 oz.	2.7	n.a.
sliced, ½ cup	10.2	n.a.
Carl's Jr., 1 serving:		
breakfast items:		
burrito	37.0	1.0
Croissant Sunrise Sandwich, with or without bacon	29.0	0
Croissant Sunrise Sandwich, with sausage	31.0	0
eggs, scrambled, with bacon	69.0	5.0
eggs, scrambled, with sausage	72.0	5.0
French Toast Dips, 6 pieces, without syrup	59.0	0
French Toast Dips, 9 pieces, without syrup	88.0	1.0
French toast syrup.	21.0	0
jelly or jam	9.0	0
quesadilla	38.0	2.0
sourdough sandwich, with or without bacon or sausage	39.0	2.0
sourdough sandwich, with ham	40.0	2.0
sandwiches:		
Carl's bacon Swiss crispy chicken	91.0	3.0
Carl's crispy chicken, ranch or Western	72.0	3.0
Carl's Catch Fish	58.0	2.0
Charbroiled BBQ Chicken	47.0	4.0
Charbroiled Chicken Club/Santa Fe Chicken	43.0	4.0
chicken, spicy	48.0	2.0
chili burger	57.0	5.0
double sourdough bacon cheeseburger	45.0	2.0
Double Western Bacon Cheeseburger	65.0	2.0
Famous Star burger	50.0	3.0
Famous Star burger, with cheese	51.0	3.0
hamburger	36.0	1.0
sourdough bacon cheeseburger	41.0	2.0
Super Star burger	52.0	3.0
Super Star burger, with double cheese	53.0	3.0

Food and Measure	carb. (gms)	fiber (gms)
The Six Dollar Burger	72.0	6.0
The Western Bacon Six Dollar Burger	79.0	2.0
Western Bacon Cheeseburger	64.0	2.0
side dishes:		
chicken breast strips, 3 pieces	27.0	1.0
chicken breast strips, 5 pieces	45.0	2.0
chicken stars, 6 pieces	15.0	0
chicken stars, 9 pieces	23.0	1.0
chili cheese fries	89.0	9.0
CrissCut Fries	43.0	4.0
fries:		
kids	32.0	3.0
large	80.0	7.0
medium	59.0	5.0
small	37.0	3.0
hash brown nuggets	32.0	3.0
onion rings	53.0	3.0
zucchini	31.0	2.0
potato, baked:		
plain or with margarine	63.0	7.0
bacon or broccoli and cheese	71.0	7.0
sour cream and chive	65.0	7.0
salad:		
Buffalo ranch chicken	42.0	6.0
Charbroiled Chicken Salad-To-Go	17.0	5.0
Garden Salad-To-Go	5.0	2.0
salad croutons, .5 oz.	8.0	0
salad dressing, 2 oz.:		
blue cheese	1.0	0
Buffalo ranch	2.0	0
French, fat free	16.0	0
house	3.0	0
Italian, fat free	4.0	0
Thousand Island	7.0	0
sauce, dipping:		
barbecue	11.0	0
buffalo wing	0	0
honey	22.0	0

Food and Measure	carb. (gms)	fiber (gms)
house	2.0	0
mustard	11.0	0
sweet and sour	12.0	0
desserts:		
chocolate chip cookie	46.0	1.0
chocolate cake	48.0	1.0
strawberry swirl cheesecake	30.0	0
shakes:		
chocolate, medium	148.0	0
chocolate, small	98.0	0
strawberry, medium	133.0	0
strawberry, small	93.0	0
vanilla, medium	115.0	0
vanilla, small	77.0	0
Carnival squash (*Frieda's*), ¾ cup, 3 oz.	7.0	1.0
Carob drink mix, powder, 3 tsp.	11.2	<1.0
Carob flour, 1 cup	91.6	41.0
Carob powder (*Shiloh Farms*), 1 tbsp.	11.0	1.0
Carp, without added ingredients	0	0
Carrot, fresh:		
raw:		
(*Dole*), 7'' long, 1¼'' diam.	8.0	2.0
(*Frieda's* Gold), ⅔ cup, 3 oz.	9.0	3.0
whole, 7'' long, 2.8 oz.	7.3	2.2
shredded (*Fresh Express*), 1 cup, 3 oz.	10.0	3.0
shredded, ½ cup	5.6	1.7
raw, baby:		
(*Mann's*), 3 oz.	9.0	2.0
medium, 2¾'' long	.8	.2
peeled, mini (*Dole*), 3 oz.; ¾ cup	9.0	2.0
boiled, drained, sliced, ½ cup	8.2	2.6
Carrot, can or jar, ½ cup, except as noted:		
baby (*Reese*)	3.0	1.0
crinkle sliced (*Freshlike*)	11.0	3.0
shredded (*Hengstenberg* Salad), ¼ cup	3.0	1.0
sliced:		
(*Allens* Tiny)	8.0	3.0
(*Del Monte*)	8.0	3.0

Food and Measure	carb. (gms)	fiber (gms)
(*S&W*)	8.0	1.0
(*Veg-All* Tender)	5.0	2.0
with liquid	6.2	1.1
drained	4.0	1.1
honey (*Glory*)	13.0	2.0
honey glazed (*Del Monte Savory Sides*)	18.0	1.0
Carrot, dehydrated, diced (*AlpineAire*), ¾ oz.	2.0	2.0
Carrot, frozen:		
baby or sliced (*Birds Eye*), ⅔ cup	7.0	2.0
crinkle cut (*Dr. Praeger's*), ⅔ cup	7.0	2.0
round (*C&W* Parisienne), ⅔ cup	10.0	3.0
sliced, boiled, drained, ½ cup	6.0	2.6
Carrot, glazed, frozen:		
(*Green Giant*), ½ cup cooked	7.0	2.0
honey (*Green Giant* Boil-in-Bag), 1 cup	13.0	2.0
Carrot, pickled, in jars (*Hogue Farms*), 5 pieces, 1.1 oz.	7.0	1.0
Carrot drink blend, 8 fl. oz.:		
with fruit juices (*AriZona* Crazy Cocktail)	38.0	.8
orange mango (*Nantucket Nectars*)	30.0	0
Carrot juice, 8 fl. oz.:		
(*Bolthouse Farms*)	14.0	<1.0
(*Hain*)	16.0	0
(*Hollywood*)	27.0	1.0
Carvel, 1 serving:		
ice cream, ½ cup:		
chocolate	22.0	0
chocolate, nonfat	28.0	0
vanilla	21.0	0
vanilla, nonfat or sugar free	25.0	0
sherbet, ½ cup	31.0	0
sundaes:		
caramel	73.0	0
caramel apple	88.0	2.0
cherries, Bordeaux	69.0	1.0
banana barge	132.0	7.0
fudge, bittersweet	69.0	1.0
fudge, hot	65.0	1.0
fudge, nonfat	84.0	0

Food and Measure	carb. (gms)	fiber (gms)
fudge brownie	109.0	5.0
strawberry	58.0	1.0
strawberry, nonfat	63.0	1.0
strawberry shortcake	96.0	2.0
turtle	195.0	3.0
coladas, 16 fl. oz.:		
banana or strawberry	68.0	0
peach or raspberry	69.0	0
piña colada	61.0	0
Creammachino, 16 fl. oz.:		
caramel cream	74.0	0
classic	13.0	0
mocha fudge	61.0	1.0
drinks, fountain:		
Carvelanche with topping	71.0	<1.0
Carvelanche, nonfat, fruit	82.0	0
Fizzlers, regular	75.0	1.0
ice cream soda	63.0	0
ice cream soda, chocolate	68.0	1.0
ice cream soda, nonfat	68.0	8.0
shake, nonfat:		
chocolate	104.0	0
mocha	97.0	0
vanilla	62.0	0
shake, thick:		
chocolate	96.0	0
chocolate, reduced fat	100.0	<1.0
vanilla	79.0	0
vanilla, reduced fat	84.0	<1.0
smoothies, 16 fl. oz.:		
banana or raspberry	79.0	0
berry, Staten Island	80.0	0
berry, Times Square	75.0	0
cooler, Grand Central	73.0	0
Casaba melon:		
1/10 of 7¾'' melon	10.2	1.3
cubed, 1 cup	10.5	1.4

Food and Measure	carb. (gms)	fiber (gms)
Cashew, 1 oz., except as noted:		
(*Beer Nuts*)	8.0	1.0
(*Frito Lay* Salted)	8.0	1.0
(*Kettle*)	8.0	1.0
(*Planters* Fancy/Whole)	8.0	1.0
raw, whole, ¼ cup (*Shiloh Farms*)	11.0	1.0
dry-roasted, 18 medium, 1 oz.	9.3	.9
dry-roasted, whole or halves, 1 cup	44.8	4.1
halves and pieces (*Planters*)	7.0	1.0
honey-roasted (*Planters*)	11.0	1.0
oil-roasted, 18 medium, 1 oz.	8.1	1.1
oil-roasted, whole or halves, 1 cup	37.1	4.9
Cashew butter (*Kettle Roaster Fresh*), 1 oz.	9.0	0
Cashew sesame mix, with peanuts (*Planters*), 1 oz.	9.0	2.0
Cassava (see also "Yuca root"), raw:		
14.4-oz. root	155.2	7.3
1 cup	78.4	3.7
Catfish, without added ingredients	0	0
Catfish entree, frozen, strips, fried (*Delta Pride* Country Crisp), 4 oz.	20.0	0
Catjang, boiled, ½ cup	17.5	3.1
Cauliflower, fresh:		
raw:		
(*Dole*), ⅙ medium head, 3.5 oz.	5.0	2.0
florets, 3 pieces	2.9	1.4
1" pieces, ½ cup	2.6	1.3
boiled, drained, 1" pieces, ½ cup	2.6	1.7
green:		
raw, ⅕ head	5.7	3.0
raw, 1" pieces, ½ cup	3.0	1.6
boiled, drained, 1" pieces, ½ cup	3.9	2.0
Cauliflower, frozen:		
florets (*Birds Eye*), 4 pieces, 3 oz.	4.0	1.0
florets (*Green Giant*), 1 cup	3.0	2.0
boiled, drained, 1" pieces, ½ cup	3.4	2.0
in cheese sauce (*Green Giant*), ½ cup	7.0	1.0
in garlic sauce (*Birds Eye*), 1¼ cups	6.0	2.0

Food and Measure	carb. (gms)	fiber (gms)
Cauliflower combinations, frozen, with carrots, snow pea pods (*Birds Eye*), 1 cup	6.0	2.0
Caviar (see also "Roe"), 1 tbsp., except as noted:		
black or red	.6	0
salmon or lumpfish, black, red, or gold (*Romanoff*)	0	0
sturgeon, granular (*Romanoff* Beluga/Osetra/Sevruga), 1 oz.	.9	0
whitefish, black or gold (*Romanoff*)	1.0	0
Caviar spread, see "Taramosalata"		
Cayenne, see "Pepper"		
Ceci beans, see "Garbanzo beans"		
Celeriac, fresh, raw:		
(*Frieda's* Celery Root), ¾ cup, 3 oz.	8.0	2.0
trimmed, ½ cup	7.2	1.4
Celery:		
raw:		
(*Dole*), 2 stalks	2.0	2.0
7½" stalk, 1.6 oz.	1.5	.7
diced, ½ cup	2.2	1.0
boiled, drained, diced, ½ cup	3.0	1.2
Celery, Chinese (*Frieda's* Kahn Choy), 1 cup, 3 oz.	3.0	1.0
Celery, dehydrated (*AlpineAire*), .3 oz.	5.0	1.0
Celery, dried, flake or seed (*Tone's*), 1 tsp.	.9	.3
Celery root, see "Celeriac"		
Celery salt:		
(*McCormick*), ¼ tsp.	0	0
(*Tone's*), 1 tsp.	.6	.2
Cellophane noodles, see "Noodle, Asian"		
Celtus, raw, trimmed:		
1 oz.	1.0	.3
.3-oz. leaf	.3	.1
Cereal, ready-to-eat (see also specific grains), 1 cup, except as noted:		
amaranth flakes (*Arrowhead Mills*)	26.0	3.0
bran:		
(*All-Bran* Original), ½ cup	23.0	10.0
(*All-Bran Bran Buds*), ⅓ cup	24.0	13.0
(*Fiber One*), ½ cup	25.0	14.0

Food and Measure	carb. (gms)	fiber (gms)
(*Post* 100% Bran), ⅓ cup	22.0	9.0
flakes (*Arrowhead Mills*)	22.0	5.0
flakes (*Kellogg's Complete*), ¾ cup	23.0	5.0
flakes (*Malt-O-Meal Balance*), ¾ cup	23.0	3.0
flakes (*Post*), ¾ cup	24.0	5.0
bran, raisin:		
(*Cascadian Farm*)	43.0	6.0
(*Erewhon*)	40.0	6.0
(*General Mills Para su Familia*), 1⅓ cups	42.0	7.0
(*Kellogg's*)	45.0	7.0
(*Kellogg's Raisin Bran Crunch*)	45.0	4.0
(*Malt-O-Meal*)	45.0	8.0
(*Post*)	46.0	8.0
(*Total*)	42.0	5.0
nut (*General Mills*), 1¼ cups	44.0	5.0
buckwheat flakes, maple (*Arrowhead Mills*)	35.0	1.0
corn:		
(*Barbara's Puffins*), ¾ cup	23.0	5.0
(*Boo Berry*)	26.0	0
(*Chex* Corn)	25.0	1.0
(*Cocomotion*), ¾ cup	22.0	<1.0
(*Franken Berry*)	26.0	0
(*French Toast Crunch*), ¾ cup	26.0	1.0
(*Kaboom*), 1¼ cups	25.0	1.0
(*Kellogg's Corn Pops*)	28.0	<1.0
(*Kellogg's Smorz*)	25.0	<1.0
(*Kix*), 1⅓ cups	25.0	1.0
(*Malt-O-Meal Corn Bursts*)	28.0	0
(*Trix*)	26.0	1.0
(*Trix* Reduced Sugar)	26.0	1.0
berry (*Malt-O-Meal Berry Colossal Crunch*), ¾ cup	26.0	1.0
caramel (*Barbara's* Organic Wild Puffs)	25.0	<1.0
cinnamon (*Barbara's Puffins*), ¾ cup	26.0	6.0
cinnamon bun (*Kellogg's Mini Swirlz*)	25.0	1.0
cocoa (*Barbara's* Organic Wild Puffs)	25.0	1.0
cocoa (*Malt-O-Meal Coco-Roos*), ¾ cup	27.0	0
fruity punch (*Barbara's* Organic Wild Puffs)	26.0	1.0
peanut butter (*Barbara's Puffins*), ¾ cup	23.0	2.0

Food and Measure	carb. (gms)	fiber (gms)
puffed (*Arrowhead Mills*)	12.0	2.0
corn and amaranth (*Erewhon Aztec*)	26.0	1.0
corn and rice (*Cinnamon Crunch Crispix*), ¾ cup	26.0	<1.0
corn and rice (*Crispix*)	25.0	<1.0
corn and wheat (*Malt-O-Meal Honey Graham Squares*), ¾ cup	25.0	1.0
cornflakes:		
(*Arrowhead Mills*)	27.0	2.0
(*Barbara's*)	26.0	2.0
(*Erewhon*), 1¼ cups	45.0	3.0
(*General Mills Country*)	25.0	1.0
(*Kellogg's Corn Flakes* Original)	24.0	1.0
(*Malt-O-Meal*)	26.0	1.0
(*New Morning*)	26.0	2.0
(*Organic Promise Cranberry Sunshine*)	26.0	2.0
(*Post Toasties*)	24.0	1.0
(*Total*), 1⅓ cups	23.0	1.0
frosted (*Malt-O-Meal*), ¾ cup	28.0	1.0
frosted (*New Morning*)	27.0	2.0
honey crunch (*Kellogg's Corn Flakes*), ¾ cup	26.0	1.0
granola:		
(*Almond Raisin Crisp Granola*), ½ cup	36.0	6.0
(*Apple Raisin Walnut Granola* Organic), ½ cup	33.0	4.0
(*Apple Sunrise Granola*), ⅓ cup	30.0	3.0
(*Banana Crunch Granola* Organic), ⅔ cup	47.0	4.0
(*Berry Good Granola*), ⅔ cup	44.0	4.0
(*Cascadian Farm* Oats & Honey), ⅔ cup	42.0	3.0
(*Cape Cod Cranberry Granola*), ½ cup	41.0	3.0
(*Honey Crunch Granola*), ½ cup	37.0	4.0
(*Magical Maple Granola*), ½ cup	34.0	3.0
(*Maple Almond Date Granola*), ½ cup	39.0	5.0
(*Outrageous Raspberry Granola*), ½ cup	37.0	4.0
(*Peachy Keen Granola*), ½ cup	33.0	3.0
(*Pecan Splendor Granola*), ½ cup	37.0	5.0
(*Save the Forest Absolutely Nuts* Organic), ⅔ cup	30.0	4.0
(*Save the Forest Raspberry Razzmataz* Organic), ¾ cup	37.0	4.0
(*Shiloh Farms* Apple Pie/Festive Flavors), ½ cup	39.0	5.0
(*Shiloh Farms* Maple Morning), ½ cup	37.0	5.0

Food and Measure	carb. (gms)	fiber (gms)
(*Shiloh Farms* Sunny Honey Oat), ½ cup	36.0	4.0
(*Shiloh Farms* Sunrise Almond), ½ cup	35.0	4.0
cinnamon raisin (*Cascadian Farm*), ⅔ cup	42.0	3.0
nut (*Save the Forest*), ½ cup	35.0	4.0
with raisins (*Kellogg's Crunchy Blends*), ⅔ cup	48.0	3.0
without raisins (*Kellogg's Crunchy Blends*), ½ cup	39.0	3.0
spelt and kamut (*Shiloh* Flaky), ½ cup	45.0	4.0
kamut:		
flakes (*Arrowhead Mills*)	25.0	2.0
flakes (*Erewhon*), ⅔ cup	25.0	4.0
flakes (*Shiloh Farms*), ½ cup	28.0	4.0
puffed (*Arrowhead Mills Puffed Kamut*)	11.0	2.0
millet, puffed (*Arrowhead Mills*)	11.0	1.0
multigrain (see also "granola," above):		
(*Alpen* No Sugar), ⅔ cup	40.0	4.0
(*Alpen* Original), ⅔ cup	41.0	4.0
(*Apple Jacks*)	30.0	1.0
(*Arrowhead Mills Perfect Harvest*)	25.0	5.0
(*Barbara's* Grain Shop), ½ cup	24.0	8.0
(*Barbara's* Honey Crunch'n Oats), ¾ cup	24.0	2.0
(*Basic 4*)	42.0	3.0
(*Blueberry Muesli* Fat Free), ½ cup	39.0	3.0
(*Cascadian Farm* Squares), ¾ cup	25.0	2.0
(*Cascadian Farm Hearty Morning*), ¾ cup	43.0	8.0
(*Cheerios*)	24.0	3.0
(*Chex* Multi-Bran)	46.0	7.0
(*Cocoa Puffs*)	26.0	1.0
(*Cocoa Puffs* Reduced Sugar)	25.0	1.0
(*Cookie Crisp*)	26.0	1.0
(*Count Chocula*)	26.0	1.0
(*Cranberry Muesli* Fat Free), ½ cup	39.0	3.0
(*Froot Loops*)	28.0	1.0
(*Good Friends*)	43.0	12.0
(*Good Friends Cinna-Raisin Crunch*)	41.0	8.0
(*Grape-Nuts*), ½ cup	47.0	6.0
(*Grape-Nuts O's*)	28.0	2.0
(*Heart to Heart*), ¾ cup	25.0	5.0
(*Honey Comb*)	26.0	1.0

Food and Measure	carb. (gms)	fiber (gms)
(*Kashi Medley*), ¾ cup	26.0	3.0
(*Kellogg's Crunchy Blends Just Right*), ¾ cup	43.0	3.0
(*Kellogg's Crunchy Blends Müeslix*), ⅔ cup	40.0	4.0
(*Kellogg's Smart Start* Antioxidants)	43.0	3.0
(*Kellogg's Smart Start* Healthy Heart), 1¼ cups	49.0	5.0
(*Kellogg's Smart Start* Soy Protein)	40.0	4.0
(*Malt-O-Meal Honey Buzzers*), 1⅓ cups	26.0	<1.0
(*Malt-O-Meal Tootie Fruities*)	28.0	1.0
(*New England Natural Muesli* Organic), ½ cup	40.0	8.0
(*Product 19*)	25.0	1.0
(*Reese's Puffs*), ¾ cup	23.0	1.0
(*Seven in the Morning*), ½ cup	47.0	7.0
(*Team Cheerios*)	25.0	2.0
(*Total*), ¾ cup	23.0	3.0
(*Waffle Crisp*)	25.0	1.0
almond (*Honey Bunches of Oats*), ¾ cup	25.0	2.0
banana (*Honey Bunches of Oats*), ¾ cup	26.0	2.0
banana (*Post Selects Banana Nut Crunch*)	44.0	5.0
blueberry (*Post Selects Blueberry Morning*), 1¼ cups	48.0	2.0
brown sugar and oat (*Total*), ¾ cup	23.0	1.0
cranberry almond (*Post Selects Cranberry Almond Crunch*)	43.0	3.0
dates, raisins, walnuts (*Post Fruit & Bran*)	42.0	6.0
flakes (*Arrowhead Mills*)	33.0	3.0
flakes (*Fiber One Honey Clusters*)	47.0	14.0
flakes (*Grape-Nuts*), ¾ cup	24.0	3.0
honey nut (*Clusters*)	46.0	3.0
honey-roasted (*Honey Bunches of Oats*), ¾ cup	25.0	2.0
maple pecan (*Post Selects Maple Pecan Crunch*), ½ cup	39.0	3.0
marshmallow bits (*Oreo O's*)	22.0	1.0
peaches (*Honey Bunches of Oats*), ¾ cup	26.0	1.0
peaches, raisins, almonds (*Post Fruit & Bran*)	42.0	6.0
pecans, crunchy (*Post Selects Great Grains*), ½ cup	38.0	4.0
puffed (*Kashi*)	15.0	1.0
puffed, honey (*Kashi*)	25.0	2.0
raisins, dates, pecans (*Post Selects Great Grains*), ½ cup	40.0	4.0

Food and Measure	carb. (gms)	fiber (gms)
strawberry (*Honey Comb*), 1⅓ cups	26.0	1.0
strawberry (*Honey Bunches of Oats*), ¾ cup	26.0	1.0
oat:		
(*Alpha-Bits*)	27.0	1.0
(*Arrowhead Mills* Organic Nature O's)	25.0	2.0
(*Barbara's* Breakfast O's), 1¼ cups	22.0	3.0
(*Cascadian Farm Purely O's*)	29.0	3.0
(*Cheerios*)	22.0	3.0
(*Fruit-E-O's*)	25.0	2.0
(*Lucky Charms*)	25.0	1.0
(*Malt-O-Meal Marshmallow Mateys*)	25.0	2.0
(*Malt-O-Meal Toasty O's*)	22.0	3.0
(*Oatios* Original)	22.0	3.0
almond (*Oatmeal Crisp*)	42.0	4.0
apple (*Malt-O-Meal Apple Zings*)	30.0	1.0
apple cinnamon (*Barbara's* Toasted O's), ¾ cup	24.0	2.0
apple cinnamon (*Malt-O-Meal Toasty O's*), ¾ cup	25.0	1.0
apple cinnamon (*Oatios*)	18.0	2.0
apple cinnamon (*Oatmeal Crisp*)	45.0	4.0
berry, triple (*Cheerios* Berry Burst)	24.0	2.0
berry, triple (*Oatmeal Crisp*)	45.0	5.0
chocolate (*Lucky Charms*)	26.0	1.0
cocoa or honey almond (*Oatios*)	17.0	2.0
honey almond (*Cascadian Farm*)	24.0	2.0
honey nut (*Barbara's* Toasted O's), ¾ cup	23.0	2.0
honey nut (*Cheerios*)	23.0	2.0
honey nut (*Malt-O-Meal Toasty O's*)	24.0	2.0
with marshmallows (*Alpha-Bits*)	26.0	1.0
raisin (*Oatmeal Crisp*)	44.0	3.0
shredded (*Barbara's* Shredded Spoonfuls), ¾ cup	24.0	4.0
shredded, vanilla almond (*Barbara's*)	42.0	4.0
strawberry (*Cheerios* Berry Burst)	24.0	2.0
strawberry banana (*Cheerios* Berry Burst)	24.0	3.0
oat bran:		
(*Hodgson Mill*), ¼ cup	23.0	6.0
(*Kellogg's Cracklin' Oat Bran*), ¾ cup	35.0	6.0
(*Ultimate Oat Bran*), ⅔ cup	22.0	3.0
flakes (*Kellogg's Complete*), ¾ cup	23.0	4.0

Food and Measure	carb. (gms)	fiber (gms)
oat bran flakes (*Arrowhead Mills*)	24.0	4.0
oat and corn:		
(*Apple Stroodles*), ¾ cup	25.0	1.0
apple cinnamon (*Cheerios*), ¾ cup	25.0	1.0
frosted (*Cheerios*)	25.0	1.0
rice:		
(*Chex* Rice), 1¼ cups	26.0	<1.0
(*Fruity Pebbles*), ¾ cup	24.0	0
(*Rice Krispies*), 1¼ cups	29.0	0
(*Rice Krispies Treats*), ¾ cup	26.0	0
(*Rice Twice*), ¾ cup	26.0	0
(*Tony's Cinnamon Crunchers*), ¾ cup	23.0	<1.0
brown, crisps (*Barbara's*)	25.0	1.0
brown, crispy (*Erewhon*)	25.0	1.0
brown, crispy, with berries (*Erewhon*)	27.0	1.0
brown, crispy (*Erewhon* Gluten Free)	25.0	0
cocoa (*Cocoa Pebbles*), ¾ cup	25.0	0
cocoa (*Kellogg's Rice Krispies*), ¾ cup	27.0	1.0
cocoa, crispy (*New Morning*), ¾ cup	26.0	1.0
crispy (*Malt-O-Meal*), 1¼ cups	29.0	0
flakes (*Arrowhead Mills* Sweetened)	40.0	1.0
fruit (*Malt-O-Meal Fruity Dyno-Bites*), ¾ cup	24.0	0
honey (*Barbara's Puffins*), ¾ cup	25.0	2.0
puffed (*Arrowhead Mills*)	14.0	<1.0
puffed (*Malt-O-Meal*)	13.0	0
rice and corn frosted or honey nut (*Chex*)	26.0	0
rice and wheat:		
(*Organic Promise Strawberry Fields*)	28.0	1.0
banana berry (*Fruit Harvest*), ¾ cup	25.0	1.0
peach strawberry (*Fruit Harvest*), ¾ cup	26.0	1.0
red berries (*Kellogg's Special K*)	25.0	1.0
strawberry blueberry (*Fruit Harvest*), ¾ cup	25.0	1.0
vanilla almond (*Kellogg's Special K*), ¾ cup	25.0	1.0
spelt flakes (*Arrowhead Mills*)	24.0	3.0
wheat:		
(*Barbara's* Organic Crispy Wheats), ¾ cup	25.0	3.0
(*Barbara's* Organic Wild Puffs)	23.0	<1.0
(*Barbara's* SoyEssence), ¾ cup	25.0	5.0

Food and Measure	carb. (gms)	fiber (gms)
(*Chex* Wheat)	40.0	5.0
(*Cinnamon Toast Crunch*), ¾ cup	24.0	2.0
(*Golden Crisp*), ¾ cup	25.0	1.0
(*Golden Grahams*), ¾ cup	25.0	1.0
(*Honey Smacks*), ¾ cup	24.0	1.0
(*Kellogg's Tiger Power*)	21.0	2.0
(*Malt-O-Meal Golden Puffs*), ¾ cup	25.0	<1.0
(*Total* Protein), ¾ cup	11.0	3.0
(*Weetabix*), 2 pieces	28.0	4.0
(*Wheaties*)	24.0	3.0
berries (*Malt-O-Meal Balance*)	26.0	5.0
cinnamon (*Malt-O-Meal Cinnamon Toasters*), ¾ cup	24.0	1.0
flakes (*Cascadian Farm* Wheat Crunch), ¾ cup	25.0	2.0
peanut butter (*Toast Crunch*), ¾ cup	23.0	1.0
whole, flakes (*Erewhon*)	42.0	6.0
whole, with flaxseed (*Uncle Sam*)	38.0	10.0
whole, with flaxseed, berries (*Uncle Sam*)	39.0	10.0
wheat, puffed (*Arrowhead Mills*)	12.0	2.0
wheat, puffed (*Malt-O-Meal*)	11.0	1.0
wheat, shredded:		
(*Arrowhead Mills*)	38.0	6.0
(*Arrowhead Mills* Sweetened)	42.0	5.0
(*Barbara's*), 2 pieces	31.0	5.0
(*Malt-O-Meal Frosted Mini Spooners*)	45.0	6.0
(*Post Shredded Wheat 'n Bran Spoon Size*), 1¼ cups	48.0	8.0
(*Post Shredded Wheat Original*), ⅙ of 10-oz. pkg.	37.0	6.0
(*Post Shredded Wheat Original Spoon Size*)	40.0	6.0
frosted (*Kellogg's Mini-Wheats*), approx. 24 pieces, 1.8 oz.	44.0	5.0
frosted (*Kellogg's Mini-Wheats* Big Bite), approx. 5 pieces, 1.8 oz.	41.0	5.0
frosted (*Kellogg's Mini-Wheats* Bite Size), approx. 24 pieces, 2.1 oz.	48.0	6.0
frosted (*Post Shredded Wheat Spoon Size*)	43.0	5.0
honey nut (*Post Shredded Wheat Spoon Size*)	43.0	4.0
raisin (*Kellogg's Mini-Wheats*), approx. 23 pieces, ¾ cup	42.0	5.0

Food and Measure	carb. (gms)	fiber (gms)
strawberry (*Kellogg's Mini-Wheats*), approx. 23 pieces, ¾ cup	40.0	5.0
vanilla crème, frosted (*Kellogg's Mini-Wheats*), approx. 24 pieces, ¾ cup	43.0	5.0
wheat and rice (*Cinnamon Toast Crunch*), ¾ cup	24.0	1.0
wheat, soy, rice flakes (*Kellogg's Special K Low Carb Lifestyle*), ¾ cup	14.0	5.0
wheat bran, see "bran," above		
Cereal, cooking/hot (see also specific grains), uncooked, except as noted:		
barley (*Arrowhead Mills* Bits O Barley), ¼ cup	34.0	6.0
barley (*Erewhon* Plus), ¼ cup	37.0	4.0
buckwheat, cream of (*Wolff's*), ⅓ cup	21.0	0
bulgur, with soy (*Hodgson Mill*), ¼ cup	22.0	3.0
farina, see "wheat," below		
grits, see "Barley grits" and "Corn grits"		
multigrain:		
(*Country Choice Naturals*), ½ cup	29.0	5.0
(*Kashi* Pilaf), ½ cup*	30.0	6.0
4 grain (*Arrowhead Mills* Plus Flax), ¼ cup	28.0	9.0
7 grain (*Arrowhead Mills*), ⅓ cup	28.0	6.0
7 grain (*Arrowhead Mills* Wheat Free), ¼ cup	30.0	3.0
with flax seeds and soy (*Hodgson Mill*), ⅓ cup	25.0	6.0
oat bran:		
(*Arrowhead Mills*), ⅓ cup	21.0	4.0
(*Shiloh Farms* 12 oz.), ⅓ cup	25.0	6.0
with wheat germ (*Erewhon*), ⅓ cup	31.0	5.0
oat:		
(*Quaker* Old Fashioned/Quick), ½ cup	27.0	4.0
flakes (*Arrowhead Mills*), ⅓ cup	23.0	4.0
steel cut (*Arrowhead Mills*), ¼ cup	27.0	8.0
oatmeal, 1 pkt., except as noted:		
(*Arrowhead Mills* Instant Original)	19.0	2.0
(*Arrowhead Mills* Old-Fashioned), ⅓ cup	23.0	4.0
(*Country Choice Naturals* Instant)	19.0	3.0
(*Malt-O-Meal Big Bowl*)	28.0	4.0
(*Uncle Sam* Instant)	24.0	5.0
with added oat bran (*Erewhon* Instant)	25.0	4.0

Food and Measure	carb. (gms)	fiber (gms)
apple cinnamon (*Country Choice Naturals* Instant)	27.0	3.0
apple cinnamon (*Erewhon* Instant)	24.0	3.0
apple cinnamon (*Fantastic Big Cereal*)	54.0	6.0
apple cinnamon (*Heart to Heart* Instant)	33.0	5.0
apple cinnamon (*Malt-O-Meal Big Bowl*)	41.0	5.0
banana nut barley (*Fantastic Big Cereal*)	55.0	8.0
brown sugar or French vanilla (*Country Choice Naturals* Organic Plus)	32.0	3.0
cinnamon raisin almond (*Arrowhead Mills*)	24.0	3.0
cinnamon spice (*Malt-O-Meal Big Bowl*)	54.0	5.0
cranberry orange (*Fantastic Big Cereal*)	56.0	7.0
maple, golden brown (*Heart to Heart* Instant)	33.0	5.0
maple apple spice (*Arrowhead Mills*)	26.0	3.0
maple brown sugar (*Malt-O-Meal Big Bowl*)	49.0	5.0
maple raisin 3-grain (*Fantastic Big Cereal*)	60.0	8.0
maple spice (*Erewhon* Instant)	25.0	3.0
maple syrup (*Country Choice Naturals* Instant)	32.0	4.0
raisin, dates, walnuts (*Erewhon* Instant)	24.0	3.0
raisin spice (*Heart to Heart* Instant)	33.0	4.0
wheat and berries (*Fantastic Big Cereal*)	56.0	8.0
rice:		
(*Arrowhead Mills* Rice & Shine), ¼ cup	32.0	2.0
(*Cream of Rice*), 1 pkt.	38.0	0
(*Lundberg* Organic Hot 'n Creamy), ⅓ cup	43.0	3.0
almond, sweet (*Lundberg* Hot 'n Creamy), ⅓ cup	40.0	4.0
brown, cream (*Erewhon*), ¼ cup	36.0	1.0
cinnamon raisin (*Lundberg* Hot 'n Creamy), ⅓ cup ...	42.0	4.0
wheat:		
(*Arrowhead Mills* Bear Mush), ¼ cup	32.0	2.0
(*Cream of Wheat* 1, 2½, or 10 Minute), 1 pkt.	25.0	1.0
(*Cream of Wheat* Instant), 1 pkt.	17.0	1.0
(*Farina*), 3 tbsp.	22.0	<1.0
(*Malt-O-Meal* Original), 3 tbsp.	26.0	1.0
(*Malt-O-Meal* Perfect Balance), ⅓ cup	32.0	3.0
apple cinnamon (*Cream of Wheat* Instant), 1 pkt.	29.0	1.0
chocolate (*Malt-O-Meal*), 3 tbsp.	27.0	1.0
cinnamon swirl (*Cream of Wheat* Instant), 1 pkt.	28.0	1.0
cracked (*Hodgson Mill*), ¼ cup	25.0	5.0

Food and Measure	carb. (gms)	fiber (gms)
maple brown sugar (*Cream of Wheat* Instant), 1 pkt. ..	27.0	1.0
maple brown sugar (*Malt-O-Meal*), ¼ cup	37.0	1.0
peaches or strawberries and cream		
(*Cream of Wheat* Instant), 1 pkt.	28.0	1.0
wheat, rye, and flax:		
(*Red River* Original), ¼ cup	27.0	5.7
(*Red River* Ready-to-Serve), 1 pkt.	24.0	5.3
maple brown sugar (*Red River* Ready-to-Serve),		
1 pkt.	29.0	4.5
Cereal crumbs, see "Cornflake crumbs"		
Cereal bar, see "Granola/cereal bar"		
Cervelat, see "Summer sausage"		
Challah, see "Bread, frozen"		
Chapati (*Garden of Eatin'*), 1.3-oz. piece	20.0	2.0
Chayote:		
raw, 1 medium, 7.2 oz.	11.0	6.1
raw, 1'' pieces, ½ cup	3.6	2.0
boiled, drained, 1'' pieces, ½ cup	4.1	2.3
Cheese (see also "Cheese food/product" and "Cheese		
spread"), 1 oz., except as noted:		
all varieties, except Monterey jack (*Land O Lakes*		
Snack'N Cheese To-Go!), ¾ oz.	0	0
American, processed:		
(*Boar's Head* Loaf)	1.0	0
(*Kraft* Singles), ⅔ oz.	1.0	0
(*Kraft* Singles Extra Thick), 1.2 oz.	3.0	0
(*Kraft* Singles/Singles Fat Free), ¾ oz.	2.0	0
(*Kraft Deli Deluxe* Slices)	1.0	0
(*Kraft Deli Deluxe* Slices), ¾ oz.	0	0
(*Land O Lakes* Slices), ¾ oz.	2.0	0
(*Land O Lakes/Land O Lakes* Light)	1.0	0
(*Land O Lakes Naturally Slender*)	1.0	0
(*Sara Lee*)	1.0	0
(*Sara Lee* Slices), .8 oz.	0	0
(*Sargento BurgerCheese*), ⅔-oz. slice	<1.0	0
sharp (*Land O Lakes* Slices)	1.0	0
white (*Hatfield Deli Choice*)	0	0
white or yellow (*Alpine Lace* Reduced Fat)	1.0	0

Food and Measure	carb. (gms)	fiber (gms)
asiago:		
(*BelGioioso*)	0	0
(*Sara Lee*)	0	0
shredded (*Sargento* Extra Fine), 2 tsp.	0	0
(*BelGioioso Auribella/Italico*)	0	0
blend, shredded, ¼ cup (*Cabot* Fancy)	1.0	0
blend, shredded, 4 cheese (*Kraft* Classic Melts), ¼ cup	1.0	0
blue/bleu:		
(*Athenos*)	<1.0	0
(*Point Reyes* Original)	0	0
creamy (*Boar's Head*)	0	0
blue, crumbled:		
(*Athenos*), 3 tbsp.	2.0	<1.0
(*Litehouse* Idaho), ¼ cup, 1.1 oz.	2.0	0
(*Sargento*), ¼ cup	1.0	0
brick (*Land O Lakes*)	1.0	0
Brie	.1	0
butterkase, plain or smoked (*Boar's Head*)	0	0
Camembert	.1	0
caraway	.9	0
Chedarella (*Land O Lakes*)	0	0
cheddar:		
(*Alpine Lace* Reduced Fat)	0	0
(*Boar's Head* Canadian/Vermont)	0	0
(*Kraft* 2% Fat)	1.0	0
(*Land O Lakes*)	0	0
(*Organic Valley*)	<1.0	0
(*Organic Valley*), ¾-oz. slice	0	0
(*Sargento* Slices)	0	0
medium (*Kraft*)	1.0	0
mild (*Cracker Barrel Cracker Cuts*)	0	0
mild (*Kraft* Longhorn)	0	0
mild (*Sara Lee*)	1.0	0
mild (*Sara Lee* Slices), .8 oz.	0	0
mild (*Sargento* Snack Single)	1.0	0
mild (*Sargento* Snack 6-Pack), .8 oz.	0	0
mild (*Sargento* Cubes), 7 pieces, 1.1 oz.	<1.0	0
raw or sharp (*Organic Valley*)	0	0

Food and Measure	carb. (gms)	fiber (gms)
sharp (*Boar's Head*)	<1.0	0
sharp (*Cracker Barrel* Reduced Fat)	1.0	0
sharp (*Cracker Barrel* Slices), ¾ oz.	0	0
sharp (*Kraft*)	0	0
sharp (*Kraft* Singles/Singles Fat Free), ¾ oz.	2.0	0
sharp (*Kraft* Singles 2% Fat), ¾ oz.	1.0	0
sharp (*Kraft Deli Deluxe* Slices), .8 oz.	0	0
sharp, extra (*Cracker Barrel* Reduced Fat)	1.0	0
sharp, extra (*Cracker Barrel Cracker Cuts*)	0	0
sharp, extra (*Land O Lakes* Processed)	1.0	0
sharp or extra sharp (*Cracker Barrel*)	0	0
sharp or extra sharp (*Sara Lee*)	1.0	0
sharp, white (*Cracker Barrel* Vermont/Reduced Fat)	1.0	0
cheddar, shredded, ¼ cup:		
(*Organic Valley*)	1.0	0
(*Sargento* Thick & Hearty/ChefStyle)	1.0	0
fine (*Kraft* Free)	1.0	0
mild (*Sargento/Sargento* Reduced Fat)	1.0	0
mild or sharp, fine (*Kraft/Kraft* 2% Fat)	1.0	0
with tomato, jalapeño, salsa (*Sargento Bistro*)	2.0	0
cheddar, flavored:		
bacon (*Kraft*)	2.0	0
chipotle, horseradish, Parmesan, pepperoni pizza, or smoky bacon (*Cabot*)	1.0	0
garlic, roasted (*Kraft*)	1.0	0
garlic herb, roasted garlic, habañero, Mediterranean, peppercorn, or tomato basil (*Cabot*)	<1.0	0
horseradish (*Boar's Head*)	0	0
cheddar blend, shredded, ¼ cup:		
American (*Kraft* Classic Melts)	1.0	0
jack (*Kraft* Mexican)	1.0	0
jack (*Sargento*)	1.0	0
Monterey jack (*Kraft*)	1.0	0
cheddar Monterey jack, marbled (*Kraft*)	1.0	0
Cheshire	1.4	0
Colby:		
(*Boar's Head* Longhorn)	<1.0	0
(*Kraft*)	1.0	0

Food and Measure	carb. (gms)	fiber (gms)
(*Kraft* Longhorn/2%Fat)	0	0
(*Land O Lakes*)	1.0	0
(*Organic Valley*)	<1.0	0
(*Sara Lee*)	1.0	0
(*Sara Lee* Longhorn Slices)	0	0
(*Sargento* Slices), ¾ oz.	<1.0	0
Colby jack:		
(*Alpine Lace Co-Jack* Reduced Fat)	1.0	0
(*Boar's Head*)	0	0
(*Cabot*)	1.0	0
(*Cracker Barrel Cracker Cuts*)	1.0	0
(*Kraft Deli Deluxe* Slices), .8 oz.	0	0
(*Land O Lakes Co-Jack*)	0	0
(*Sara Lee*)	0	0
(*Sargento* Slices), ⅔ oz.	0	0
(*Sargento* Snacks)	<1.0	0
(*Sargento* Cubes), 7 pieces, 1.1 oz.	<1.0	0
marbled (*Kraft*)	0	0
Colby jack, shredded, ¼ cup or 1 oz.:		
(*Sargento*)	1.0	0
fine (*Kraft*)	1.0	0
cottage, 4%, ½ cup:		
(*Darigold* Large/Small Curd)	5.0	0
(*Friendship*)	3.0	0
(*Hood* Country/Large Curd)	5.0	0
(*Organic Valley*)	3.0	0
chive (*Darigold*)	5.0	0
chive (*Hood*)	5.0	0
pineapple (*Darigold*)	17.0	0
pineapple (*Friendship*)	14.0	0
pineapple (*Hood*)	15.0	0
cottage, 2%, ½ cup:		
(*Breakstone's* Large/Small Curd)	6.0	0
(*Cabot*)	4.0	0
(*Darigold*)	5.0	0
(*Friendship* Pot Style)	3.0	0
(*Knudsen* Low Fat)	6.0	0
(*Organic Valley*)	4.0	0

Food and Measure	carb. (gms)	fiber (gms)
cottage, 1%, ½ cup:		
(*Friendship*)	3.0	0
(*Friendship* No Salt)	4.0	0
(*Hood/Hood* No Salt)	6.0	0
black pepper and herbs (*Hood*)	6.0	0
chive and toasted onion (*Hood*)	5.0	0
peaches (*Hood*)	18.0	0
pineapple (*Friendship*)	16.0	0
pineapple and cherry (*Hood*)	6.0	0
strawberries (*Hood*)	19.0	0
cottage, nonfat, ½ cup:		
(*Breakstone's*)	8.0	0
(*Cabot*)	5.0	0
(*Darigold*)	6.0	0
(*Friendship*)	4.0	0
(*Hood*)	7.0	0
(*Knudsen Free*)	7.0	0
peach (*Friendship*)	15.0	0
pineapple (*Friendship*)	16.0	0
pineapple (*Hood*)	16.0	0
cream cheese, 2 tbsp., except as noted:		
(*Boar's Head*)	2.0	0
(*Organic Valley* Bar), 1 oz.	1.0	0
(*Organic Valley* Tub)	2.0	0
(*Philadelphia* Bar)	1.0	0
(*Philadelphia* Bar Fat Free)	2.0	0
(*Philadelphia* Light)	2.0	0
(*Philadelphia* ⅓ Less Fat) Tub/Tub Fat Free	1.0	0
berries or brown sugar cinnamon (*Philadelphia* Swirls)	4.0	0
chive and onion (*Philadelphia*)	2.0	0
garlic herb (*Philadelphia* Swirls)	3.0	0
honey nut (*Philadelphia*)	4.0	0
pineapple (*Philadelphia*)	4.0	0
salmon (*Philadelphia*)	1.0	0
strawberry (*Philadelphia*)	4.0	0
strawberry (*Philadelphia* Light)	6.0	0
vegetable, garden (*Philadelphia*)	2.0	0

Food and Measure	carb. (gms)	fiber (gms)
cream cheese, whipped, 2 tbsp.:		
(*Philadelphia*)	1.0	0
berry, mixed (*Philadelphia*)	3.0	0
chive (*Philadelphia*)	<1.0	0
cinnamon brown sugar (*Philadelphia*)	3.0	0
garlic and herb or ranch (*Philadelphia*)	1.0	0
Edam (*Boar's Head*)	0	0
Edam (*Sara Lee*)	0	0
farmer (*Friendship/Friendship* No Salt)	0	0
farmer, kefir, 2 tbsp. (*Lifeway*)	4.0	0
farmer, kefir, 2 tbsp. (*Lifeway* Lite)	2.0	0
feta:		
(*Alpine Lace* Reduced Fat)	1.0	0
(*Athenos* Mild/Traditional/Traditional Reduced Fat)	<1.0	0
(*Boar's Head*)	1.0	0
(*Organic Valley*)	1.0	0
(*Shiloh Farms* Goat)	0	0
basil tomato or peppercorn (*Athenos*)	<1.0	<1.0
garlic herb (*Athenos*)	0	0
feta, crumbled, ¼ cup:		
(*Athenos* Mild/Traditional Reduced Fat)	1.0	<1.0
(*Athenos* Traditional)	2.0	<1.0
basil tomato (*Athenos/Athenos* Reduced Fat)	2.0	<1.0
garlic herb (*Athenos*)	1.0	1.0
peppercorn (*Athenos*)	2.0	<1.0
(*Finlandia Lappi*)	<1.0	0
fontina (*BelGioioso*)	0	0
fontina (*Denmark's Finest*)	0	0
(*Gjetost*)	11.0	0
Gloucester, double (*Boar's Head*)	0	0
goat:		
(*Shiloh Farms* Just Jack)	<1.0	0
hard type	.6	0
semisoft type	.7	0
soft type	.3	0
chive (*Shiloh Farms* Chive 'n Jack)	0	0
garlic and herbs (*Maitre D'*)	0	0
tomato basil (*Shiloh Farms*)	0	0

Food and Measure	carb. (gms)	fiber (gms)
gorgonzola:		
(*Athenos*)	<1.0	0
(*BelGioioso CreamyGorg*)	0	0
crumbled (*Athenos*), 3 tbsp.	2.0	1.0
Gouda:		
(*Boar's Head*)	0	0
(*Finlandia Naturals/Sandwich Naturals*)	<1.0	0
(*Sara Lee*)	0	0
aged (*Rembrandt*)	0	0
smoked (*Sara Lee*)	0	0
Gruyère	.1	0
havarti:		
(*Finlandia Naturals/Sandwich Naturals*)	<1.0	0
(*Land O Lakes*)	0	0
cream, all varieties (*Boar's Head*)	0	0
regular or dill (*Sara Lee*)	0	0
Italian, shredded, ¼ cup:		
(*Maggio*)	<1.0	0
4 cheese (*Organic Valley*)	1.0	0
4 cheese (*Sargento* Reduced Fat)	1.0	0
5 cheese (*Kraft*)	1.0	0
6 cheese (*Sargento*)	1.0	0
with garlic (*Sargento*)	1.0	0
jalapeño jack (*Tree of Life* Organic)	1.0	0
Jarlsberg:		
(*Jarlsberg/Jarlsberg Lite*)	0	0
(*Sargento Jarlsberg* Slices), .8 oz.	<1.0	0
Kasseri (*BelGioioso*)	0	0
Limburger	.1	0
mascarpone (*BelGioioso*)	0	0
mascarpone (*BelGioioso* Tiramisu)	0	0
Mexican, mild, jalapeño (*Kraft* Singles), ¾ oz.	2.0	0
Mexican, shredded, ¼ cup:		
(*Maggio*)	1.0	0
(*Sargento/Sargento* Reduced Fat/Thick & Hearty)	1.0	0
4 cheese (*Kraft/Kraft* 2% Fat)	1.0	0
Monterey jack:		
(*Boar's Head*)	0	0

Food and Measure	carb. (gms)	fiber (gms)
(*Cabot*)	<1.0	0
(*Kraft*)	0	0
(*Kraft* 2% Fat)	1.0	0
(*Kraft* Singles), ¾ oz.	1.0	0
(*Land O Lakes*)	0	0
(*Land O Lakes Snack'n Cheese To-Go!*), ¾ oz.	0	0
(*Organic Valley*)	0	0
(*Sara Lee*)	0	0
(*Sara Lee* Slices) .8 oz.	0	0
(*Sargento* Slices), ¾ oz.	0	0
(*Tree of Life* Organic)	1.0	0
hot pepper (*Land O Lakes*)	0	0
jalapeño (*Boar's Head*)	0	0
jalapeño (*Land O Lakes*)	1.0	0
jalapeño (*Sara Lee*)	1.0	0
jalapeño (*Sara Lee* Slices), .8 oz.	0	0
semisoft (*Tree of Life*)	0	0
Monterey jack, shredded, ¼ cup:		
(*Colby*)	1.0	0
(*Kraft*)	1.0	0
(*Sargento*)	1.0	0
Monterey jack and Colby, see "Colby jack," above		
mozzarella:		
(*Alpine Lace* Reduced Fat)	1.0	0
(*BelGioioso* Fresh)	0	0
(*Boar's Head* Low Moisture)	1.0	0
(*Kraft* Low Moisture)	1.0	0
(*Kraft* Singles), ¾ oz.	1.0	0
(*Kraft Deli Deluxe* Slices), ¾ oz.	0	0
(*Land O Lakes*)	1.0	0
(*Organic Valley*)	<1.0	0
(*Polly-O* Fresh)	0	0
(*Sara Lee* Slices), .8 oz.	1.0	0
(*Sargento* Slices 8 oz.), ¾ oz.	0	0
(*Sargento* Slices 12 oz.), ¾ oz.	1.0	0
(*Sargento Twirls*), .8-oz. piece	<1.0	0
(*Tree of Life/Tree of Life* Organic)	1.0	0
whole or part skim (*Maggio*)	1.0	0

Food and Measure	carb. (gms)	fiber (gms)
whole, part skim, or nonfat (*Polly-O*)	1.0	0
nonfat (*Kraft* Singles), ¾ oz.	2.0	0
mozzarella, shredded, ¼ cup:		
(*Cabot*)	1.0	0
(*Kraft*)	1.0	0
(*Maggio*)	1.0	0
(*Organic Valley*)	1.0	0
(*Polly-O/Polly-O* Lite/Nonfat/Part Skim)	1.0	0
(*Sargento* ChefStyle Whole/Fancy)	1.0	0
(*Sargento* Reduced Fat)	<1.0	0
(*Sargento* Thick & Hearty)	1.0	0
asiago, with roasted garlic (*Sargento Bistro*)	2.0	0
Parmesan, fine (*Polly-O*)	1.0	0
provolone (*Sargento*)	0	0
provolone, Romano, Parmesan (*Polly-O*)	1.0	0
with sun-dried tomato and basil (*Sargento Bistro*)	1.0	0
Muenster:		
(*Alpine Lace* Reduced Fat)	1.0	0
(*Boar's Head/Boar's Head* Low Sodium)	0	0
(*Finlandia/Finlandia Naturals/Sandwich Naturals*)	<1.0	0
(*Land O Lakes*)	0	0
(*Organic Valley*)	1.0	0
(*Sara Lee*)	0	0
(*Sara Lee* Slices), .8 oz.	0	0
(*Sargento* Slices), ¾ oz.	0	0
nacho, shredded, ¼ cup (*Sargento*)	1.0	0
Neufchâtel (*Philadelphia*)	1.0	0
Parmesan (*BelGioioso/BelGioioso American Grana/ Vegetarian*)	0	0
Parmesan (*Sara Lee*)	1.0	0
Parmesan, grated, 2 tsp.:		
(*Kraft* Reduced Fat)	2.0	0
(*Rienzi*)	0	0
(*Sara Lee*)	0	0
(*Tree of Life*)	0	0
plain or with Romano (*Kraft*)	0	0
plain or with Romano (*Polly-O*)	0	0
plain or with Romano (*Sargento*)	0	0

Food and Measure	carb. (gms)	fiber (gms)
Parmesan, shredded, ¼ cup:		
(*Kraft*)	1.0	0
(*Organic Valley*)	0	0
(*Sara Lee*)	1.0	0
(*Tree of Life*)	1.0	0
mozzarella and Romano (*Sargento Angel Hair*)	1.0	0
Romano and asiago (*Kraft*)	1.0	0
pepato (*BelGioioso*)	0	0
pepper, hot (*Alpine Lace* Reduced Fat American)	1.0	0
pepper, hot (*BelGioioso Peperoncino*)	0	0
pepper jack:		
(*Cabot*)	<1.0	0
(*Kraft*)	1.0	0
(*Kraft* Singles), ¾ oz.	2.0	0
(*Kraft Deli Deluxe* Slices), .8 oz.	0	0
(*Land O Lakes C-Jack*)	0	0
(*Organic Valley*)	0	0
shredded, with habañero (*Sargento*), ¼ cup	<1.0	0
pimento (*Kraft* Singles), ¾ oz.	2.0	0
pizza, shredded, ¼ cup:		
(*Maggio*)	1.0	0
(*Sargento Double Cheese*)	1.0	0
4 cheese (*Kraft*)	1.0	0
mozzarella and cheddar or provolone (*Kraft*)	1.0	0
Port du Salut	.2	0
provolone:		
(*Alpine Lace* Reduced Fat)	1.0	0
(*Boar's Head* 42% Lower Sodium)	1.0	0
(*Hatfield Deli Choice*)	1.0	0
(*Kraft Deli Deluxe* Slices)	0	0
(*Organic Valley*)	1.0	0
(*Sara Lee*)	1.0	0
(*Sargento* Slices), ⅔ oz.	0	0
(*Tree of Life*)	1.0	0
medium, mild, or sharp (*BelGioioso*)	0	0
sharp, picante (*Boar's Head*)	1.0	0
smoke (*Land O Lakes*)	1.0	0
smoked (*Sara Lee* Slices), .8 oz.	0	0

Food and Measure	carb. (gms)	fiber (gms)
ricotta, ¼ cup:		
(*Polly-O* Lite)	3.0	0
(*Polly-O* Original)	2.0	0
(*Sargento* Light)	3.0	0
whole (*BelGioioso Ricotta con Latte*)	0	0
whole, part skim, or nonfat (*Maggio*)	3.0	0
whole or part skim (*Sargento*)	3.0	0
part skim (*Polly-O*)	2.0	0
nonfat (*Polly-O*)	3.0	0
nonfat (*Sargento*)	5.0	0
Romano:		
(*BelGioioso*)	0	0
shredded (*Sara Lee*)	1.0	0
shredded (*Maggio*), 1 tbsp.	0	0
Romano, grated:		
(*Kraft*), 2 tsp.	0	0
(*Maggio*), 1 tbsp.	2.0	0
(*Sara Lee*), 2 tsp.	0	0
(*Tree of Life*), 2 tsp.	0	0
Roquefort	.6	0
string:		
(*Maggio*)	<1.0	0
(*Organic Valley*)	<1.0	0
(*Organic Valley* Stringles)	1.0	1.0
(*Polly-O* String-Ums/String-Ums Reduced Fat)	1.0	0
(*Sargento* Snacks)	<1.0	0
(*Sargento* Snacks Light), ¾-oz. slice	<1.0	0
Swiss:		
(*Alpine Lace* Reduced Fat)	1.0	0
(*Alpine Lace* Reduced Fat), 1.2-oz. slice	0	0
(*Boar's Head* Gold Label Imported)	<1.0	0
(*Boar's Head* Lacey)	0	0
(*Boar's Head* Natural No Salt)	<1.0	0
(*Cabot* Slices)	1.0	0
(*Finlandia/Finlandia Heavenly Light/Naturals*)	<1.0	0
(*Hatfield Deli Choice*), 1.2-oz. slice	1.0	0
(*Kraft* Singles Deli Deluxe Aged/Deli Thin)	0	0
(*Kraft* Singles/Singles Fat Free/2% Milk), ¾ oz.	2.0	0

Food and Measure	carb. (gms)	fiber (gms)
(*Kraft* Singles 2% Milk Deli Deluxe), ¾ oz.	0	0
(*Kraft Deli Deluxe* Slices)	1.0	0
(*Kraft Deli Deluxe* Slices), ⅔ oz.	0	0
(*Land O Lakes*)	1.0	0
(*Sara Lee* Slices), .8 oz.	0	0
(*Sara Lee* Specialty)	1.0	0
(*Sargento* Aged/Thin Slices), ⅔ oz.	0	0
(*Sargento* Reduced Fat Slices), ¾ oz.	1.0	0
(*Sargento* Thick Sliced)	1.0	0
(*Tree of Life*)	1.0	0
smoked (*Williams*)	0	0
Swiss, baby:		
(*Boar's Head*)	<1.0	0
(*Cracker Barrel*)	0	0
(*Land O Lakes*)	1.0	0
(*Organic Valley*)	0	0
(*Sara Lee*)	1.0	0
(*Sara Lee* Slices), .8 oz.	0	0
(*Sara Lee* Specialty)	0	0
(*Sargento* Slices), ⅔ oz.	0	0
Swiss, shredded, ¼ cup (*Kraft*)	1.0	0
Swiss, shredded, ¼ cup (*Sargento*)	<1.0	0
Swiss and American, processed (*Land O Lakes*)	1.0	0
Swiss and cheddar, smoky (*Kraft*)	1.0	0
Cheese, freeze-dried:		
cheddar, powder (*AlpineAire*), 1 oz.	0	0
cottage (*Mountain House*), ½ cup	3.0	0
"Cheese," substitute and nondairy:		
American (*Tofutti*), .7-oz. slice	2.0	0
American (*Yves* The Good Slice), .7-oz. slice	0	0
cheddar style (*Yves* The Good Slice), .7-oz. slice	1.0	0
cheddar style, shredded (*Yves* The Good Shreds), 1 oz.	0	0
cream "cheese," 2 tbsp.:		
plain, except nonhydrogenated (*Tofutti Better Than Cream Cheese*)	1.0	0
plain, nonhydrogenated (*Tofutti Better Than Cream Cheese*)	13.0	0

Food and Measure	carb. (gms)	fiber (gms)
flavored, all varieties (*Tofutti Better Than Cream Cheese*)	1.0	0
garlic, roasted (*Tofutti*), .7-oz. slice	2.0	0
mozzarella style:		
(*Tofutti*), .7-oz. slice	2.0	0
(*Yves* The Good Slice), .7-oz. slice	0	0
shredded (*Yves* The Good Shreds), 1 oz.	1.0	0
Cheese appetizer/snack, frozen:		
jalapeño (*Health is Wealth Munchees*), 2 pieces, 1 oz.	10.0	1.0
sticks, mozzarella, breaded:		
(*Health is Wealth*), 2 pieces, 1.3 oz.	14.0	0
(*Ian's Natural*), 2 pieces, 1.3 oz.	10.0	0
three cheese (*Athens* Tyropita), 2 pieces, 2 oz.	9.0	0
Cheese dip, 2 tbsp.:		
(*Cheez Whiz* Light)	6.0	0
(*Cheez Whiz* Original)	4.0	0
(*D.L. Jardine's* Queso Caliente/Loco)	4.0	0
(*Snyder's*)	3.0	0
beef or chicken and cheese (*Chi-Chi's*)	2.0	0
cheddar:		
jalapeño (*Fritos*)	4.0	0
jalapeño (*Litehouse*)	1.0	0
mild (*Fritos*)	3.0	0
mild (*Snyder's*)	3.0	0
chili (*Fritos*)	3.0	0
Monterey jack (*Tostitos* Party Bowl)	4.0	0
nacho (*Kaukauna*)	4.0	0
nacho, nondairy, mild or spicy (*Road's End Organics Chreese*)	3.0	<1.0
onion, French (*Kaukauna*)	4.0	0
salsa con queso:		
(*Cheez Whiz*)	4.0	0
(*Chi-Chi's*)	3.0	0
(*Pace*)	4.0	1.0
(*Tostitos*)	5.0	<1.0
flame-roasted (*Snyder's*)	4.0	0
medium (*Taco Bell*)	2.0	0

Food and Measure	carb. (gms)	fiber (gms)
mild (*Taco Bell*)	3.0	0
veggie ranch (*Kaukauna*)	3.0	0
Cheese dip kit:		
cheddar (*Sargento Cheese Dips!*), 3.75-oz. pkg.:		
with bagel chips, ranch	24.0	<1.0
with butter pretzels	47.0	2.0
with tortilla chips	26.0	1.0
cheese (*Handi-Snacks*):		
with bread sticks (*Premium*), 1.1 oz.	13.0	0
with crackers (*Ritz*), 1 oz.	10.0	0
with pretzel sticks (*Mr. Salty*), 1 oz.	12.0	0
Cheese entree, frozen (see also "Spinach entree" and specific listings), 1 pkg.:		
matter paneer (*Amy's* Whole Meal), 10 oz.	54.0	6.0
shahi paneer (*Ethnic Gourmet*), 12 oz.	52.0	4.0
Cheese food/product (see also "Cheese" and "Cheese spread"), 1 oz., except as noted:		
(*Velveeta*)	3.0	0
(*Velveeta* Light)	4.0	0
(*Velveeta* Slices), ¾ oz.	1.0	0
(*Velveeta* Slices Extra Thick), 1.2 oz.	2.0	0
jack, with jalapeño (*Land O Lakes*)	1.0	0
jalapeño (*Land O Lakes*)	2.0	0
Mexican (*Velveeta*)	3.0	0
onion or pepperoni (*Land O Lakes*)	2.0	0
shredded (*Velveeta*), ¼ cup, 1.3 oz.	3.0	0
Cheese salt (*Watkins*), ¼ tsp.	0	0
Cheese sandwich, frozen, grilled (*Smucker's Uncrustables*), 1.75-oz. piece	17.0	<1.0
Cheese sauce, ¼ cup:		
jalapeño (*Zapata*)	4.0	0
mild (*Zapata*)	7.0	0
Cheese sauce, cooking, in jars, ¼ cup:		
Alfredo (*Ragú Cheese Creations!* Classic)	3.0	0
cheddar, double (*Ragú Carb Options*)	2.0	0
cheddar, double (*Ragú Cheese Creations!*)	3.0	0
Cheese sauce mix, four, Italian (*McCormick*), 1⅓ tbsp. mix	5.0	0

Food and Measure	carb. (gms)	fiber (gms)
"Cheese" sauce mix, nondairy, dry, ⅓ pkt.:		
Alfredo or cheddar style, gluten free		
(*Road's End Organics Chreese*)	5.0	1.0
cheddar or mozzarella style (*Road's End*		
Organics Chreese)	6.0	1.0
Cheese spread (see also "Cheese," and "Cheese Food/		
Product"), 2 tbsp., except as noted:		
(*Kraft* Manchego Singles), ¾-oz. slice	1.0	0
(*Viola*), 1 oz.	<1.0	0
all varieties (*Kaukauna* Log)	4.0	1.0
bacon (*Kraft*)	1.0	0
bacon, smoky (*Kaukauna/WisPride* Ball)	4.0	1.0
beef and onion (*Kaukauna* Ball)	5.0	0
blue cheese (*Kraft Roka*)	2.0	0
cheddar, sharp:		
(*Kaukauna* Ball)	4.0	1.0
(*WisPride* Lite)	5.0	0
double (*WisPride* Cup/Log)	4.0	.0
extra (*Kaukauna/WisPride*)	3.0	0
extra (*Kaukauna/WisPride* Ball)	4.0	0
or smoky (*Kaukauna/WisPride*)	3.0	0
or smoky (*Kaukauna/WisPride* Lite)	5.0	0
or smoky (*WisPride* Log)	4.0	1.0
cheddar cream cheese (*Kaukauna/WisPride* Ball)	3.0	1.0
feta, original or sun-dried tomato (*Athenos*)	<1.0	0
garlic herb (*Kaukauna/WisPride*)	2.0	0
garlic herb (*Kaukauna/WisPride* Ball)	5.0	1.0
horseradish (*Kaukauna/WisPride*)	3.0	0
horseradish (*Kaukauna/WisPride* Ball)	4.0	1.0
nacho (*Easy Cheese*)	3.0	0
onion, Vidalia (*Kaukauna* Ball)	3.0	0
pimento or olive and pimento (*Kraft*)	3.0	0
pineapple (*Kraft*)	4.0	0
port wine:		
(*Kaukauna/WisPride*)	3.0	0
(*Kaukauna/WisPride* Lite)	5.0	0
(*Kaukauna/WisPride* Ball)	4.0	1.0
ranch cream cheese (*Kaukauna/WisPride* Ball)	6.0	1.0

Food and Measure	carb. (gms)	fiber (gms)
sharp (*Kraft Old English*)	1.0	0
Swiss:		
(*Kaukauna* Ball)	2.0	0
(*WisPride* Ball/Log)	2.0	1.0
almond (*Kaukauna*)	3.0	0
sharp, double (*WisPride* Log)	4.0	1.0
vegetable, garden (*Kaukauna/WisPride*)	2.0	0
vegetable, garden (*WisPride* Ball)	5.0	1.0
Cheese sticks, see "Cheese appetizer/snack"		
Cheeseburger, see "Beef pocket/sandwich"		
Cheesecake, fresh, French style (*Entenmann's*		
Deluxe), ⅕ cake	46.0	1.0
Cheesecake, dried, see "Dessert, freeze-dried"		
Cheesecake, frozen or refrigerated:		
(*Baby Watson*), ⅙ of 18-oz. cake	19.0	0
(*Mother's Kitchen*), ⅙ of 60-oz. cake	29.0	<1.0
(*Sara Lee* Original), ¼ of 17-oz. cake	38.0	1.0
amaretto (*Impromptu Gourmet*), 1 slice	30.0	1.0
caramel fudge (*Impromptu Gourmet*), 1 slice	38.0	1.0
cherry (*Sara Lee* Original), ¼ of 19-oz. cake	55.0	2.0
chocolate swirl (*Atkins*), ⅛ of 24-oz. cake	19.0	0
dulce de leche (*Impromptu Gourmet*), 1 slice	36.0	1.0
French style:		
(*Sara Lee* Classic), ⅕ of 23.5-oz. cake	41.0	1.0
(*Smart Ones*), 3.9-oz. piece	28.0	2.0
chocolate (*Sara Lee*), ⅕ of 21-oz. cake	52.0	2.0
strawberry (*Sara Lee*), ⅙ of 26-oz. cake	43.0	1.0
New York style:		
(*Impromptu Gourmet*), 1 slice	33.0	1.0
(*Sara Lee*), ⅙ of 30-oz. cake	35.0	1.0
(*Smart Ones*), 2.5-oz. piece	21.0	1.0
chocolate swirl (*Sara Lee*), ⅛ of 28-oz. cake	45.0	1.0
pumpkin (*Atkins*), ⅛ of 24-oz. cake	18.0	1.0
raspberry swirl (*Atkins*), ⅛ of 24-oz. cake	19.0	0
strawberry (*Sara Lee* Original), ¼ of 19-oz. cake	49.0	2.0
vanilla (*Atkins*), ⅛ of 24-oz. cake	19.0	0
Cheesecake mix, dry:		
(*Jell-O* No Bake Homestyle), ⅙ pkg.	44.0	1.0

Food and Measure	carb. (gms)	fiber (gms)
(*Jell-O* No Bake Real), ⅙ pkg.	42.0	1.0
cherry or strawberry (*Jell-O* No Bake), ⅑ pkg.	42.0	1.0
strawberry swirl (*Jell-O* No Bake Reduced Fat), ⅛ pkg.	39.0	1.0
Cheesecake snack:		
bars, 1 piece:		
marble brownie (*Philadelphia* Snack Bars), 1.5 oz.	20.0	1.0
strawberry (*Philadelphia* Snack Bars), 1.5 oz.	22.0	0
bites, all varieties (*Philadelphia* Snack Bites), 1-oz. piece	15.0	0
bites, chocolate dipped:		
(*Sara Lee* Original), ½ of 7.75-oz. pkg.	8.0	0
praline pecan (*Sara Lee*), ½ of 7.75-oz. pkg.	8.0	1.0
Cherimoya (see also "Custard apple"):		
(*Frieda's*), 5 oz.	34.0	3.0
1 medium, 1.9 lb.	131.3	3.1
Cherries jubilee topping (*Lucky Leaf/Musselman's*), ¼ cup	20.0	1.0
Cherry, fresh:		
(*Del Monte*), 1 cup, 4.9 oz.	22.0	3.0
(*Dole*), 1 cup, approx. 21 pieces	22.0	3.0
sour, red, ½ cup, with pits	6.3	.6
sour, red, ½ cup, red, pitted	9.4	.9
sweet, with pits, ½ cup	12.0	1.7
sweet, 10 medium	11.3	1.6
Cherry, canned, ½ cup:		
dark, pitted in extra heavy syrup (*S&W*)	34.0	1.0
dark, pitted in heavy syrup (*Del Monte*)	24.0	<1.0
red, tart, pitted, in water (*Lucky Leaf/Musselman's*)	12.0	1.0
sour, pitted:		
in water	10.9	1.3
in light syrup	24.3	1.0
in heavy syrup	29.8	1.0
sweet, with liquid:		
in water	14.6	1.9
in juice	17.3	1.9
in light syrup	21.8	1.9
Cherry, dried:		
bing (*Frieda's*), ¼ cup, 1.4 oz.	26.0	3.0
bing (*Shiloh Farms*), ⅓ cup, 1.6 oz.	35.0	9.0

Food and Measure	carb. (gms)	fiber (gms)
sour/tart:		
(*Eden* Montmorency), ¼ cup, 1.6 oz.	36.0	3.0
(*Frieda's*), ⅓ cup, 1.4 oz.	33.0	2.0
(*Shiloh Farms*), ⅓ cup, 1.4 oz.	31.0	4.0
Cherry, frozen:		
unsweetened, sweet (*Cascadian Farm*), 1 cup	24.0	3.0
unsweetened, ½ cup	8.5	1.2
sweetened, ½ cup	29.0	2.7
Cherry, maraschino, 1 piece:		
red or green mint (*S&W*)	3.0	0
with stems (*Great Expectations*)	2.0	0
Cherry, West Indian, see "Acerola"		
Cherry butter (*Eden* Organic), 1 tbsp.	9.0	1.0
Cherry drink:		
(*Minute Maid Coolers*), 6.75-fl-oz. pouch	28.0	0
black (*Ocean Spray*), 8 fl. oz.	33.0	0
black (*R.W. Knudsen* Concentrate), 8 fl. oz.	31.0	0
Cherry juice, 8 fl. oz.:		
(*Juicy Juice*)	30.0	0
(*Walnut Acres*)	34.0	0
black:		
(*L&A*)	45.0	0
(*R.W. Knudsen*)	43.0	0
(*R.W. Knudsen* Just Cherry)	44.0	0
cider (*R.W. Knudsen*)	31.0	0
tart (*Eden* Organic Montmorency)	33.0	0
tart (*R.W. Knudsen* Just Cherry)	32.0	0
Cherry juice blend, berries (*Ceres* Secret		
of the Valley), 8 fl. oz.	30.0	0
Cherry juice concentrate:		
(*Eden* Organic), 2 tbsp.	26.0	0
black (*Tree of Life*), 8 tsp.	28.0	0
Cherry syrup, maraschino (*Trader Vic's*), 1 fl. oz.	23.0	0
Chervil, dried, 1 tsp.	.3	.1
Chestnut, Chinese, shelled:		
dried, 1 oz.	22.7	<1.0
boiled or steamed, 1 oz.	9.6	<1.0
roasted, 1 oz.	14.9	<1.0

Food and Measure	carb. (gms)	fiber (gms)
Chestnut, European:		
raw, in shell, 1 lb.	152.8	27.2
raw, shelled, with peel, 1 cup, 13 pieces	66.0	11.7
dried, peeled, 1 oz.	23.3	<2.0
boiled, 1 oz.	7.9	<1.0
roasted, peeled, 1 oz.	15.0	3.3
roasted, peeled, 1 cup, 17 kernels	75.7	16.7
Chestnuts, European, in jars (*Minerve*),		
4 whole, 1.1 oz.	12.0	2.0
Chestnut spread (*Faugier*), 2 tbsp.	20.0	0
Chia seeds, dried (*Shiloh Farms*), 3 tbsp.	13.0	10.0
Chick peas, see "Garbanzo beans"		
Chicken, meat only, without added ingredients	0	0
Chicken, canned, chunk, 2 oz.:		
all varieties (*Hormel*)	0	0
all varieties (*Tyson*)	0	0
breast (*Swanson*)	1.0	0
white and dark (*Swanson*)	0	0
Chicken, freeze-dried, cooked, diced:		
(*AlpineAire*), ½ oz.	0	0
(*Mountain House*), ¾ cup	0	0
Chicken, frozen or refrigerated, raw, 4 oz., except as noted:		
all cuts, without added ingredients	0	0
whole, fryer, rotisserie, dark or white, all		
seasoning varieties (*Perdue*)	1.0	0
whole, roasting:		
garlic, toasted, dark or white (*Perdue*)	1.0	0
honey, dark or white (*Perdue*)	4.0	0
breast, boneless, marinated:		
(*Always Tender*)	2.0	0
Italian (*Always Tender*)	3.0	0
lemon pepper (*Always Tender*)	5.0	0
teriyaki (*Always Tender*)	8.0	0
breast, boneless, skinless, sandwich steaks		
(*Bell & Evans*), 2 oz.	<1.0	0
breast, breaded:		
broccoli and cheese stuffed (*Tyson*), 6-oz. piece	22.0	1.0
Cordon Bleu (*Tyson*), 6-oz. piece	19.0	0

Food and Measure	carb. (gms)	fiber (gms)
garlic Parmesan (*Bell & Evans*)	12.0	<2.0
Kiev (*Tyson*), 6-oz. piece	20.0	0
breast tenders, breaded (*Bell & Evans*)	13.0	1.0
breast tenders, breaded coconut (*Bell & Evans*)	16.0	<1.0
nuggets (*Bell & Evans*)	13.0	1.0
patties, breaded (*Bell & Evans*)	13.0	<1.0
patties, breaded with mozzarella (*Bell & Evans*)	11.0	0
tenders, see "breast tenders," above		
thigh (*Tyson Individually Fresh Frozen*), 5-oz. piece	1.0	0
Chicken, frozen or refrigerated, cooked		
(see also "Chicken entree, frozen"):		
all cuts, without added ingredients, 4 oz.	0	0
whole, roasted (*Tyson*), 3 oz.	1.0	0
whole, roasted, seasoned, 3 oz.:		
garlic, toasted, dark or light (*Perdue*)	1.0	0
honey, dark or white (*Perdue*)	3.0	0
lemon pepper (*Tyson*)	1.0	0
barbecue sauce with, shredded, ¼ cup:		
honey hickory sauce (*Lloyd's*)	12.0	0
original sauce (*Lloyd's*)	11.0	0
bites, breaded (*Tyson*), 13 pieces, 3 oz.	15.0	1.0
breast, bone-in, roasted, half (*Tyson*), 5.1-oz. piece	1.0	0
breast, bone-in, skinless, roasted (*Tyson*), 3.75-oz. piece .	1.0	0
breast, carved, ½ cup, 2.5 oz.:		
grilled, Italian or honey roasted (*Perdue Short Cuts*) ...	3.0	0
grilled, lemon pepper or Southwest (*Perdue Short Cuts*)	2.0	0
roasted (*Perdue Short Cuts* Original)	2.0	0
breast, diced, roasted (*Tyson*), 3 oz.	2.0	1.0
breast cutlet, breaded, white, 3 oz.:		
(*Perdue/Perdue* Homestyle Low Fat)	14.0	0
Italian (*Perdue*)	15.0	<1.0
breast cuts, (*Louis Rich*), 3 oz.	1.0	0
breast cuts, honey-roasted (*Louis Rich*), 3 oz.	3.0	0
breast fillets:		
breaded (*Tyson*), 4.6-oz. piece	20.0	0
char-grilled (*Perdue Short Cuts*), 2.4-oz. piece	2.0	0
with gravy (*Hormel*), 6 oz.	4.0	0

Food and Measure	carb. (gms)	fiber (gms)
honey-roasted (*Perdue Short Cuts*), 2.4-oz. piece	5.0	0
mesquite (*Tyson*), 3 oz.	1.0	0
teriyaki (*Hormel*), 5.7 oz.	30.0	0
teriyaki (*Hormel* Family Pack), 6 oz.	35.0	0
teriyaki (*Tyson*), 3.1 oz.	7.0	0
breast medallions, in Marsala sauce (*Tyson*), 5 oz.	4.0	0
breast medallions, in sesame sauce (*Tyson*), 5 oz.	22.0	0
chunks, with sauce:		
Alfredo (*Simply Simmered*), 1 cup	8.0	<1.0
garlic (*Simply Simmered*), 5 oz.	10.0	3.0
marinara (*Simply Simmered*), 5 oz.	9.0	3.0
sesame or sweet and sour (*Simply Simmered*), 5 oz. . . .	26.0	5.0
Szechuan (*Simply Simmered*), 5 oz.	16.0	5.0
teriyaki (*Simply Simmered*), 5 oz.	23.0	1.0
drumstick, roasted (*Tyson*), 3 pieces, 5.8 oz.	2.0	0
fillet, breaded, Italian style (*Barber Foods*), 3.5-oz. piece . .	14.0	<1.0
fingers, breaded:		
(*Barber Foods* All American), 3.3-oz. piece	15.0	<1.0
(*Ian's Natural*), 3 oz., approx. 3 pieces	14.0	0
Buffalo (*Barber Foods*), 3.3-oz. piece	18.0	<1.0
Italian (*Barber Foods*), 3.3-oz. piece	15.0	<1.0
meatballs, Italian style (*Tyson*), 6 pieces, 3 oz.	6.0	2.0
nuggets:		
(*Barber Foods* All American), 4 pieces, 3 oz.	12.0	0
(*Health is Wealth*), 4 pieces, 3 oz.	9.0	0
(*Ian's* Natural Allergen Free), 3 oz., approx. 5 pieces . . .	14.0	0
(*Tyson* Bag/Box), 5 pieces, 3.25 oz.	16.0	0
breast (*Perdue* Individually Frozen), 5 pieces, 3.4oz. . . .	15.0	1.0
cheddar and bacon (*Barber Foods*), 3 pieces, 2.8 oz. . .	8.0	0
golden brown (*Perdue*), 5 pieces, 3.4 oz.	14.0	0
ham and cheese (*Barber Foods*), 3 pieces, 2.8 oz.	8.0	0
pizza stuffed (*Barber Foods*), 3 pieces, 2.8 oz.	7.0	0
Southern style (*Tyson*), 6 pieces, 3 oz.	11.0	1.0
white (*Perdue*), 3 oz.	14.0	0
white (*Perdue Fun Shapes*), 4 pieces, 2.7 oz.	12.0	0
white, and cheese (*Perdue*), 5 pieces, 3 oz.	14.0	0
patties, breaded:		
(*Health is Wealth*), 3-oz. piece	9.0	0

Food and Measure	carb. (gms)	fiber (gms)
(*Ian's* Natural), 3.5-oz. piece	16.0	0
breast (*Tyson*), 2.6-oz. piece	12.0	1.0
breast, Southern style (*Tyson*), 2.6-oz. piece	10.0	1.0
popcorn:		
(*Tyson*), 9 pieces, 3 oz.	21.0	1.0
(*Tyson Popcorn Chicken Bites*), 6 pieces, 3.1 oz.	22.0	2.0
white (*Perdue*), 3 oz.	11.0	0
sticks, all varieties (*Barber Foods*), 3 pieces, 2.8 oz.	15.0	<1.0
strips:		
Buffalo (*Tyson*), 2 pieces, 3.5 oz.	21.0	1.0
crispy (*Tyson*), 2 pieces, 3.3 oz.	13.0	1.0
fajita (*Tyson* Bag), 3 oz.	1.0	1.0
fajita (*Tyson* Box), 3 oz.	1.0	0
Southwest (*Hormel*), 2 oz.	3.0	0
strips, breast, 3 oz.:		
(*Perdue*)	12.0	0
(*Perdue Kick'N Chicken* Original)	14.0	0
(*Tyson*)	1.0	0
barbecue (*Perdue Kick'N Chicken*)	16.0	0
Buffalo (*Perdue*)	12.0	0
fajita (*Tyson*)	3.0	0
grilled (*Louis Rich*)	1.0	0
grilled (*Tyson*)	2.0	0
hot and spicy (*Perdue Kick'N Chicken*)	13.0	0
Italian or Southwest (*Louis Rich*)	1.0	0
Southwest (*Tyson*)	2.0	0
tenderloin, breaded:		
(*Perdue*), 3 oz.	13.0	0
(*Perdue* Individually Frozen), 3 oz.	15.0	0
(*Tyson*), 2.4-oz. piece	12.0	1.0
Southern (*Tyson*), 2.4-oz. piece	9.0	1.0
spicy (*Tyson*), 2.4-oz. piece	13.0	0
white (*Perdue* Low Fat), 3 oz.	15.0	0
tenders, breast:		
(*Health is Wealth*), 3 pieces, 3 oz.	11.0	0
(*Tyson*), 5 pieces, 3 oz.	15.0	0
honey battered (*Tyson*), 5 pieces, 3 oz.	13.0	2.0
with rib meat (*Tyson* Box), 5 pieces, 3 oz.	13.0	2.0

Food and Measure	carb. (gms)	fiber (gms)
thigh, roasted (*Tyson*), 3.6-oz. piece	1.0	1.0
wings:		
barbecue (*Tyson*), 3 pieces, 3.2 oz.	7.0	0
Buffalo, hot (*Tyson*), 4 pieces, 3.4 oz.	1.0	1.0
honey (*Tyson* Bag), 4 pieces, 3.4 oz.	9.0	0
honey (*Tyson* Box), 3 pieces, 3.5 oz.	13.0	15.0
hot (*Tyson* Wings of Fire), 3 pieces, 3.5 oz.	14.0	16.0
hot and spicy (*Perdue* Individually Frozen)	1.0	0
hot and spicy (*Tyson*), 3 pieces, 3 oz.	1.0	1.0
hot and spicy (*Tyson* Box), 3 pieces, 3.4 oz.	1.0	0
split, Buffalo (*Perdue Wingsters*), 3 oz.	3.0	0
"Chicken," vegetarian:		
canned:		
(*Worthington FriChik* Original), 2 pieces, 3.2 oz.	3.0	1.0
diced, drained (*Worthington* Chik), ¼ cup	2.0	1.0
sliced (*Worthington* Chik), 3 slices, 3.2 oz.	3.0	2.0
frozen/refrigerated:		
cutlets (*Quorn*), 2.4-oz. piece	5.0	2.0
cutlet, garlic and herb (*Quorn*), 3.5-oz. piece	20.0	4.0
drumsticks (*GardenGourmet*), 1.8-oz. piece	10.0	2.0
fingers (*Health is Wealth*), 2 oz.	5.0	1.0
fried, with gravy (*Loma Linda*), 2 pieces, 2.9 oz.	5.0	2.0
Italian marinara (*Morningstar Farms*),		
1 piece and 1 pkt. sauce, 5 oz.	29.0	2.0
nuggets (*Boca* Chik'n Original), 3 oz.	18.0	2.0
nuggets (*Dr. Praeger's*) 2 pieces, 1.3 oz.	9.0	1.0
nuggets (*Health is Wealth*), 3 pieces, 2.2 oz.	13.0	2.0
nuggets (*Loma Linda*), 5 pieces, 3 oz.	14.0	2.0
nuggets (*Morningstar Farms* Chik'n), 4 pieces, 3 oz. . .	18.0	2.0
nuggets (*Quorn*), 3–4 pieces, 3 oz.	18.0	3.0
patties (*Boca* Chik'n), 2.5-oz. piece	14.0	1.0
patties (*Health is Wealth*), 3-oz. piece	15.0	2.0
patties (*Morningstar Farms Chik Patties*), 2.5-oz. piece .	16.0	2.0
patties (*Quorn*), 2.6-oz. piece	12.0	3.0
patties (*Worthington Crispy Chik Patties*), 2.5-oz. piece	16.0	2.0
patties, Parmesan ranch (*Morningstar Farms*		
Chik Patties), 2.5-oz. piece	17.0	2.0
patties, spicy (*Boca* Chik'n), 2.5-oz. piece	14.0	2.0

Food and Measure	carb. (gms)	fiber (gms)
roll (*Worthington* Meatless Chicken), ⅜'' slice, 2 oz. ...	2.0	1.0
slices (*Worthington* Meatless Chicken), 3 slices, 2 oz. ..	2.0	1.0
sticks (*Worthington ChikStiks*), 1.7-oz. piece	4.0	2.0
strips (*Lightlife*), 3 oz.	6.0	4.0
tenders (*Quorn*), 1 cup, 3 oz.	8.0	3.0
tenders, honey mustard (*Morningstar Farms* Chik'n), 2 pieces, 2.9 oz.	20.0	4.0
wings, Buffalo (*Boca* Chik'n Hot & Spicy), 3 oz.	14.0	3.0
wings, Buffalo (*Health is Wealth*), 3 pieces, 2.2 oz.	11.0	3.0
wings, Buffalo (*Morningstar Farms*), 5 pieces, 3 oz. ...	18.0	3.0
Chicken coating mix (see also "Batter and breading mix"), seasoned:		
(*Don's Chuck Wagon* Baking Mix), ¼ cup	21.0	1.0
(*McCormick Bag 'n Season*), 1 tbsp.	3.0	0
(*Oven Fry* Extra Crispy), ⅛ pkg.	10.0	0
(*Oven Fry* Homestyle Flour), ⅛ pkg.	7.0	0
(*Shake 'n Bake* Original), 1/16 of 5.5-oz. pkg.	7.0	0
barbecue glaze (*Shake 'n Bake*), 1/16 pkg.	9.0	0
Buffalo wings (*McCormick Bag 'n Season*), 1 tbsp.	5.0	0
Buffalo wings (*Shake 'n Bake*), 1/16 pkg.	8.0	0
country style (*McCormick Bag 'n Season*), 1 tbsp.	3.0	0
fry mix:		
(*Golden Dipt* Fry Easy Extra Crispy), 1½ tbsp.	9.0	0
(*Golden Dipt* Fry Easy Original Homestyle), 2 tbsp.	9.0	0
(*McCormick* Season Fry), 1 tbsp.	6.0	0
herb and spice (*Golden Dipt* Fry Easy), 2 tbsp.	13.0	0
hot and spicy (*Golden Dipt* Fry Easy), 2 tbsp.	9.0	0
garlic herb (*Shake 'n Bake*), 1/16 pkg.	7.0	0
honey glaze (*Shake 'n Bake* Tangy), 1/16 pkg.	9.0	0
hot and spicy or Italian (*Shake 'n Bake*), 1/16 pkg.	7.0	0
Italian herb (*McCormick Bag 'n Season*), 1 tbsp.	2.0	0
nuggets, crispy (*Shake 'n Bake*), 1/16 pkg.	9.0	0
Oriental (*McCormick Bag 'n Season*), 1 tbsp.	4.0	0
Santa Fe (*McCormick*), 2 tsp.	2.0	0
Southwestern (*McCormick Bag 'n Season*), 1 tbsp.	3.0	0
Chicken dinner, frozen, 1 pkg.:		
asiago portobello (*Healthy Choice*), 12.5 oz.	47.0	6.0
blackened (*Healthy Choice*), 11 oz.	36.0	5.0

Food and Measure	carb. (gms)	fiber (gms)
breaded, country (*Healthy Choice*), 10.6 oz.	55.0	5.0
broccoli Alfredo (*Healthy Choice*), 11.5 oz.	34.0	2.0
fettuccine:		
(*Lean Cuisine Dinnertime Selections*), 13⅝ oz.	51.0	5.0
(*Stouffer's* Homestyle), 16.75 oz.	55.0	6.0
Florentine (*Lean Cuisine Dinnertime Selections*), 13.25 oz.	44.0	6.0
fried (*Swanson Hungry-Man* Classic), 16.5 oz.	75.0	6.0
glazed:		
(*Lean Cuisine Dinnertime Selections*), 13 oz.	39.0	4.0
honey (*Healthy Choice*), 11 oz.	46.0	6.0
Oriental (*Lean Cuisine Dinnertime Selections*), 14 oz. ..	58.0	2.0
grilled:		
with barbecue sauce, smoky (*Healthy Choice*), 12 oz. .	59.0	6.0
lime, Southwestern (*Stouffer's* Homestyle), 14 oz.	67.0	9.0
and penne (*Lean Cuisine Dinnertime Selections*), 14 oz.	46.0	5.0
Tuscan (*Lean Cuisine Dinnertime Selections*), 12.5 oz. .	34.0	3.0
herb, country (*Healthy Choice*), 11.35 oz.	37.0	5.0
mesquite barbecue (*Healthy Choice*), 10.5 oz.	44.0	5.0
parmigiana (*Healthy Choice*), 11 oz.	40.0	6.0
roasted (*Lean Cuisine Dinnertime Selections*), 12.5 oz. ..	48.0	4.0
roasted, breast (*Healthy Choice*), 11 oz.	32.0	7.0
sesame (*Healthy Choice*), 10.8 oz.	38.0	5.0
Southwestern Monterey (*Stouffer's* Homestyle), 14.25 oz.	58.0	4.0
Southwestern smothered (*Stouffer's* Homestyle), 14 oz. ..	61.0	6.0
sweet and sour (*Healthy Choice*), 11 oz.	54.0	3.0
teriyaki (*Healthy Choice*), 11 oz.	37.0	6.0
Chicken entree, can or pkg.:		
à la king (*Swanson*), 10.5-oz. can	20.0	2.0
and dumplings:		
(*Dinty Moore* Can), 1 cup	28.0	1.0
(*Dinty Moore* Can), 7.5-oz. can	24.0	1.0
(*Dinty Moore* Cup), 1 cont.	24.0	1.0
(*Hormel* Bowl), 10 oz.	33.0	2.0
(*Swanson*), 1 cup	26.0	2.0
and noodles (*Dinty Moore* Can), 1 cup	24.0	1.0
and noodles (*Hormel* Bowl), 10 oz.	28.0	2.0
and noodles (*Dinty Moore* Cup), 1 cont.	20.0	1.0
with potatoes (*Hormel* Bowl), 10 oz.	27.0	2.0

Food and Measure	carb. (gms)	fiber (gms)
and rice (*Hormel* Bowl), 10 oz.	30.0	3.0
rice and (*Dinty Moore* Cup), 1 cont.	23.0	1.0
rice and (*Hormel* Cup Fiesta), 7.5 oz.	32.0	2.0
stew (*Dinty Moore* Can), 1 cup	17.0	2.0
Chicken entree, dried, 1 serving:		
(*AlpineAire* Kung Fu)	68.0	4.0
(*AlpineAire* Sierra)	54.0	3.0
(*AlpineAire* Summer)	38.0	2.0
à la king and noodles (*Mountain House*), ½ pouch	42.0	3.0
à la king and noodles (*Mountain House* Can), 1 cup	31.0	2.0
almond (*AlpineAire*)	53.0	5.0
barbecue, Texas (*AlpineAire*)	53.0	7.0
barbecue, Texas (*Instant Gourmet*)	85.0	11.0
breast, grilled (*Mountain House*), ½ pouch	22.0	<1.0
gumbo (*AlpineAire*)	102.0	17.0
gumbo (*Instant Gourmet* New Orleans)	48.0	5.0
noodles and (*Mountain House* Can), 1 cup	34.0	1.0
noodles and (*Mountain House*), ½ pouch	42.0	2.0
Oriental, with vegetables (*Mountain House*), ½ pouch	44.0	3.0
Oriental, with vegetables (*Mountain House* Can), 1 cup	33.0	2.0
Polynesian (*Mountain House*), ½ pouch	44.0	1.0
primavera (*AlpineAire*)	45.0	3.0
rice and:		
(*Mountain House* Can/Four), 1 cup	46.0	2.0
(*Mountain House* Double), ½ pouch	59.0	2.0
(*Mountain House* Single)	74.0	3.0
Mexican (*Mountain House*), ½ pouch	46.0	9.0
vegetables (*AlpineAire*)	55.0	8.0
rotelle (*AlpineAire*)	44.0	2.0
Santa Fe (*Instant Gourmet*)	81.0	13.0
stew (*Mountain House*), ½ pouch	34.0	4.0
stew (*Mountain House* Can), 1 cup	26.0	3.0
teriyaki (*Mountain House*), ½ pouch	49.0	3.0
teriyaki (*Mountain House* Can), 1 cup	42.0	2.0
Chicken entree, frozen (see also "Chicken, frozen or refrigerated, cooked"), 1 pkg., except as noted:		
à la king (*Stouffer's*), 11.5 oz.	45.0	2.0

Food and Measure	carb. (gms)	fiber (gms)
Alfredo:		
(*Birds Eye Voila!*), 1 cup*	26.0	2.0
(*Contessa*), 8 oz.	26.0	2.0
(*Green Giant* Complete Skillet Meal), ¼ of 32-oz. pkg.	35.0	2.0
(*Green Giant* Complete Skillet Meal), ¼ of		
32-oz. pkg. with 2% milk*	37.0	2.0
(*Lean Cuisine Skillet Sensations* 24 oz.), 6.9 oz.	23.0	2.0
(*Stouffer's* Family Style Recipes), ⅐ of 57-oz. pkg.	33.0	3.0
(*Stouffer's Skillet Sensations* 25 oz.), 7.1 oz.	25.0	2.0
Florentine (*Michelina's Lean Gourmet*), 8.5 oz.	38.0	2.0
grilled, with broccoli (*Michelina's* Homestyle		
Bowls), 11 oz.	48.0	3.0
grilled, with broccoli (*Michelina's Signature*), 10 oz.	36.0	3.0
with almonds (*Lean Cuisine* Cafe Classics), 8.5 oz.	38.0	3.0
arroz con pollo (*Jeff Nathan Creations*), 10 oz.	40.0	4.0
baked (*Lean Cuisine* Cafe Classics), 8⅝ oz.	32.0	2.0
baked (*Stouffer's* Homestyle), 8⅞ oz.	21.0	2.0
basil (*Smart Ones Bistro Selections*), 9.5 oz.	34.0	2.0
basil cream sauce (*Lean Cuisine* Cafe Classics), 8.5 oz.	32.0	2.0
basil cream sauce (*Lean Cuisine* Cafe Classics		
Bowl), 10.5 oz.	39.0	3.0
biryani (*Ethnic Gourmet*), 11 oz.	57.0	3.0
with black beans and vegetables (*Smart Ones*		
Santa Fe Higher Protein), 9 oz.	10.0	3.0
breast:		
strips, with mac and cheese (*Healthy Choice*), 8 oz.	35.0	3.0
tenders, barbecue sauce (*Stouffer's* Homestyle), 10 oz.	37.0	3.0
and vegetables (*Healthy Choice*), 10.5 oz.	29.0	6.0
breast, stuffed:		
asparagus and cheese (*Barber Foods*), 6-oz. piece	19.0	<1.0
broccoli and cheese (*Barber Foods*), 6-oz. piece	20.0	<2.0
broccoli and cheese (*Barber Foods* Light), 5.5-oz. piece	15.0	<1.0
Cordon Bleu (*Barber Foods*), 6-oz. piece	14.0	<1.0
Cordon Bleu (*Barber Foods* Light), 5.5-oz. piece	14.0	0
crème brie and apple (*Barber Foods*), 6-oz. piece	12.0	<1.0
Kiev (*Barber Foods*), 6-oz. piece	16.0	<1.0
mashed potato (*Barber Foods*), 6-oz. piece	21.0	<1.0

Food and Measure	carb. (gms)	fiber (gms)
rice and vegetables, skinless (*Barber Foods* Homestyle), 6-oz. piece	26.0	<1.0
scallop and lobster (*Barber Foods*), 6-oz. piece	25.0	<1.0
Caesar, grilled (*Lean Cuisine* Cafe Classics Bowl), 9 oz.	32.0	3.0
cacciatore (*Organic Classics*), 10 oz.	38.0	3.0
Cajun style, and shrimp (*Healthy Choice*), 10.4 oz.	32.0	5.0
carbonara:		
(*Healthy Choice*), 9 oz.	39.0	2.0
(*Lean Cuisine* Cafe Classics), 9 oz.	33.0	2.0
(*Smart Ones Bistro Selections*), 9.5 oz.	33.0	3.0
cheese, three:		
(*Birds Eye Voila!*), 1 cup*	21.0	2.0
(*Lean Cuisine* Cafe Classics), 8 oz.	14.0	2.0
(*Lean Cuisine Skillet Sensations* 24 oz.), 6.9 oz.	28.0	2.0
chow mein (*Contessa*), 1¾ cups*	28.0	4.0
chow mein (*Lean Cuisine Everyday Favorites*), 9 oz.	31.0	2.0
curry, Thai style (*Organic Classics*), 10 oz.	42.0	2.0
with dipping sauce:		
barbecue (*Healthy Choice*), 13 oz.	46.0	5.0
honey mustard (*Healthy Choice*), 13 oz.	49.0	6.0
roasted garlic tomato (*Healthy Choice*), 13 oz.	47.0	5.0
roasted red pepper (*Healthy Choice*), 13 oz.	39.0	7.0
teriyaki (*Healthy Choice*), 14 oz.	59.0	5.0
dumplings:		
(*C&W Ultimate Stir Fry Feast*), 1½ cups with sauce	25.0	3.0
(*C&W Ultimate Stir Fry Feast*), 1½ cups without sauce	20.0	2.0
and dumplings:		
(*Glory* Savory Singles), 11 oz.	40.0	6.0
(*Glory* Savory Singles Family Size), 1 cup	34.0	5.0
(*Stouffer's Skillet Sensations* 24 oz.), 6.9 oz.	22.0	2.0
enchilada, see "Enchilada entree"		
escalloped, and noodles (*Stouffer's*), 10 oz.	29.0	4.0
escalloped, and noodles (*Stouffer's* Family Style Recipes), ⅕ of 40-oz. pkg.	26.0	2.0
fettuccine (see also "Fettucine entree"):		
(*Lean Cuisine Everyday Favorites*), 9.25 oz.	33.0	2.0
(*Smart Ones Bistro Selections*), 10 oz.	39.0	4.0

Food and Measure	carb. (gms)	fiber (gms)
(*Stouffer's* Homestyle), 10.5 oz.	37.0	3.0
primavera (*Michelina's* Authentico), 8 oz.	37.0	3.0
fettuccine Alfredo:		
(*Healthy Choice*), 8.5 oz.	28.0	3.0
(*Uncle Ben's* Pasta Bowl), 12 oz.	47.0	2.0
chicken and broccoli (*Michelina's* Authentico), 8.5 oz.	37.0	2.0
Florentine, baked (*Lean Cuisine* Cafe Classics), 8 oz.	14.0	3.0
fried:		
(*Swanson* Classic), 11.5 oz.	45.0	4.0
breast (*Stouffer's* Homestyle), 8⅞ oz.	37.0	2.0
with mashed potato, gravy (*Michelina's* Authentico), 8 oz.	27.0	2.0
fritters, with mashed potato *Michelina's* Authentico Pop'n), 5.5 oz.	38.0	3.0
garlic:		
(*Lean Cuisine Skillet Sensations*), ⅓ of 24-oz. pkg.	36.0	2.0
(*Stouffer's Skillet Sensations*), ¼ of 23-oz. pkg.	25.0	2.0
golden baked (*Smart Ones Bistro Selections*), 10 oz.	42.0	2.0
roasted (*Lean Cuisine* Cafe Classics), 8⅞ oz.	14.0	2.0
garlic, and vegetables:		
(*Birds Eye Voila!*), 1 cup*	21.0	3.0
and pasta (*Green Giant* Complete Skillet Meal), ¼ of 32-oz. pkg.	31.0	2.0
roasted (*Birds Eye Voila!* Reduced Carb), 1 cup*	13.0	3.0
glazed:		
(*Lean Cuisine* Cafe Classics), 8.5 oz.	27.0	2.0
(*Michelina's Lean Gourmet*/Authentico), 8 oz.	45.0	2.0
(*Smart Ones Bistro Selections*), 8.5 oz.	45.0	5.0
country (*Healthy Choice*), 8.5 oz.	29.0	3.0
white (*Boston Market*), 10 oz.	29.0	2.0
grilled:		
(*Lean Cuisine* Cafe Classics), 9⅜ oz.	15.0	4.0
(*Lean Cuisine* Cafe Classics Fiesta), 8.5 oz.	31.0	3.0
Baja (*Healthy Choice*), 10 oz.	33.0	7.0
basil (*Healthy Choice*), 10.6 oz.	33.0	5.0
Caesar (*Healthy Choice*), 10 oz.	42.0	7.0
Caesar (*Michelina's* Homestyle Bowls), 11 oz.	45.0	3.0

Food and Measure	carb. (gms)	fiber (gms)
garlic herb sauce (*Smart Ones* Higher Protein), 9 oz. ...	9.0	2.0
marinara (*Healthy Choice*), 10 oz.	37.0	5.0
and mashed potato (*Healthy Choice*), 8.5 oz.	22.0	4.0
herb:		
garden (*Birds Eye Voila!*), 1 cup*	40.0	3.0
grilled (*Stouffer's*), 9 oz.	33.0	3.0
and roasted potatoes (*Lean Cuisine Skillet Sensations*),		
⅓ of 24-oz. pkg.	24.0	2.0
honey barbecue sauce (*Organic Classics*), 9 oz.	26.0	4.0
honey Dijon (*Smart Ones*), 8.5 oz.	38.0	2.0
honey Dijon grilled (*Lean Cuisine* Cafe Classics), 8 oz. ...	22.0	2.0
honey ginger (*Michelina's Yu Sing* Bowls), 11 oz.	60.0	3.0
honey mustard (*Lean Cuisine* Cafe Classics), 8 oz.	37.0	1.0
korma (*Ethnic Gourmet*), 11 oz.	34.0	3.0
kung pao (*Ethnic Gourmet*), 12 oz.	61.0	3.0
lemon (*Lean Cuisine Spa Cuisine*), 9 oz.	38.0	2.0
lemon grass (*Lean Cuisine Spa Cuisine*), 9⅜ oz.	29.0	4.0
lemon grass and basil (*Ethnic Gourmet*), 11 oz.	53.0	4.0
lemon pepper, grilled (*Stouffer's*), 9 oz.	27.0	5.0
lo mein (*Green Giant* Complete Skillet Meal),		
¼ of 32-oz. pkg.	30.0	3.0
mandarin (*Healthy Choice*), 10 oz.	43.0	4.0
mandarin (*Lean Cuisine Everyday Favorites*), 9 oz.	46.0	2.0
Margherita (*Healthy Choice*), 10 oz.	25.0	6.0
Marsala:		
(*Lean Cuisine* Cafe Classics), 8⅛ oz.	12.0	3.0
(*Organic Classics*), 9.5 oz.	41.0	3.0
with broccoli (*Smart Ones* Higher Protein), 9 oz.	12.0	3.0
with garlic potatoes (*Michelina's Signature*), 8.5 oz. ...	22.0	2.0
roasted (*Healthy Choice*), 10.4 oz.	23.0	4.0
Massaman (*Ethnic Gourmet*), 11 oz.	44.0	4.0
Mediterranean (*Lean Cuisine* Cafe Classics), 10.5 oz.	38.0	4.0
Mediterranean (*Lean Cuisine Spa Cuisine*), 10.5 oz.	35.0	5.0
noodle, creamy (*Green Giant* Complete Skillet Meal),		
¼ of 32-oz. pkg. with 2% milk*	45.0	3.0
and noodles:		
(*Michelina's* Homestyle Bowls), 11 oz.	43.0	4.0

Food and Measure	carb. (gms)	fiber (gms)
(*Stouffer's* Bowl Cuisine Homestyle), 12 oz.	45.0	5.0
(*Stouffer's Skillet Sensations* 25 oz.), 7.1 oz.	28.0	3.0
rice noodles, Thai (*Smart Ones Bistro Selections*), 9 oz.	39.0	2.0
noodles and (*Michelina's* Zap'ems), 8 oz.	36.0	2.0
nuggets, with dessert (*Ian's* Natural Kids Meal), 8 oz.	60.0	2.0
nuggets, with mac and cheese (*Stouffer's Maxaroni*), 8 oz.	33.0	1.0
orange (*Contessa* Minute Meal Bowl), 10.5 oz.	51.0	2.0
orange, a l' (*Lean Cuisine* Cafe Classics), 9 oz.	35.0	2.0
Oriental:		
(*Healthy Choice*), 8.5 oz.	28.0	7.0
(*Lean Cuisine Skillet Sensations* 24 oz.), 6.9 oz.	23.0	2.0
(*Smart Ones*), 9 oz.	34.0	3.0
Parmesan:		
(*Lean Cuisine* Cafe Classics), 10⅞ oz.	36.0	3.0
(*Smart Ones Bistro Selections*), 11 oz.	32.0	3.0
creamy, with garden vegetables (*Smart Ones* Higher Protein), 9 oz.	12.0	4.0
parmigiana:		
(*Stouffer's* Family Style Recipes), ¼ of 52.5-oz. pkg.	59.0	4.0
(*Stouffer's* Homestyle), 12 oz.	53.0	5.0
with linguine (*Michelina's Signature*), 10 oz.	49.0	4.0
and pasta:		
(*Healthy Choice* Homestyle), 9 oz.	32.0	5.0
bake, and broccoli (*Stouffer's* Family Style Recipes), ⅕ of 40-oz. pkg.	27.0	2.0
Cordon Bleu (*Stouffer's* Family Style Recipes), ¼ of 37-oz. pkg.	34.0	1.0
Italiano (*Contessa*), 1¾ cups*	29.0	2.0
and vegetables (*Smart Ones* Mirabella), 9.2 oz.	30.0	4.0
pasta, cheese sauce (*Green Giant* Complete Skillet Meal), ¼ of 32-oz. pkg. with 2% milk*	39.0	3.0
patties, breaded, with fries (*Michelina's* Authentico Chicken Littles), 5.5 oz.	31.0	2.0
peanut satay (*Ethnic Gourmet*), 11 oz.	51.0	3.0
in peanut sauce (*Lean Cuisine* Cafe Classics/*Spa Cuisine*), 9 oz.	32.0	2.0
pecan (*Lean Cuisine Spa Cuisine*), 9 oz.	34.0	4.0
penne with (*Michelina's* Authentico), 8.5 oz.	48.0	2.0

Food and Measure	carb. (gms)	fiber (gms)
penne with (*Smart Ones Bistro Selections* Penne Pollo), 10 oz.	38.0	3.0
pesto primavera (*Birds Eye Voila!*), 1 cup*	24.0	2.0
piccata:		
(*Healthy Choice*), 9 oz.	40.0	2.0
(*Jeff Nathan Creations*), 12 oz.	24.0	6.0
(*Lean Cuisine* Cafe Classics), 9 oz.	41.0	1.0
lemon herb (*Smart Ones*), 9 oz.	36.0	2.0
pie/pot pie:		
(*Boston Market*), 1 cup	35.0	2.0
(*Ian's* Natural), 9 oz.	82.0	3.5
(*Stouffer's*) 10 oz.	56.0	4.0
(*Stouffer's*), ½ of 16-oz. pkg.	45.0	3.0
(*Swanson*), 7 oz.	40.0	2.0
Alfredo, and broccoli (*Pepperidge Farm*), 1 cup	46.0	4.0
broccoli and (*Pepperidge Farm*), 1 cup	42.0	2.0
Parmesan, chunky (*Pepperidge Farm*), 1 cup	57.0	2.0
primavera, with garlic, herbs (*Pepperidge Farm*), 1 cup	49.0	2.0
roasted (*Pepperidge Farm*), 1 cup	43.0	3.0
portobello, grilled (*Stouffer's*), 9 oz.	26.0	4.0
pot stickers:		
(*C&W Pot Sticker Stir Fry Feast*), 2 cups with sauce	30.0	4.0
(*C&W Pot Sticker Stir Fry Feast*), 2 cups without sauce	23.0	4.0
Oriental style (*Lean Cuisine Everyday Favorites*), 9 oz.	55.0	3.0
primavera:		
(*Lean Cuisine Skillet Sensations,* 24 oz.), 6.9 oz.	28.0	1.0
with spirals (*Michelina's* Authentico), 8 oz.	37.0	3.0
ranchero sauce, spicy (*Smart Ones* Fiesta), 8.5 oz.	35.0	5.0
with rice (see also "Rice entree, frozen"):		
beans and vegetables (*Smart Ones* Southwestern Bowls), 11 oz.	32.0	5.0
cheesy (*Healthy Choice*), 9 oz.	33.0	5.0
savory (*Stouffer's Skillet Sensations*), ⅕ of 40-oz. pkg.	36.0	5.0
and vegetable rice bake (*Stouffer's* Family Recipes, Grandma's), ¼ of 36-oz. pkg.	31.0	1.0
roast/roasted:		
(*Lean Cuisine Everyday Favorites*), 8⅛ oz.	32.0	2.0
Chardonnay (*Healthy Choice*), 10.6 oz.	32.0	4.0

Food and Measure	carb. (gms)	fiber (gms)
herb (*Lean Cuisine* Cafe Classics), 8 oz.	23.0	3.0
herb, creamy (*Healthy Choice*), 10 oz.	35.0	7.0
oven (*Smart Ones Bistro Selections*), 9 oz.	37.0	2.0
with sour cream (*Smart Ones Bistro*		
Selections), 9.5 oz.	19.0	2.0
with stuffing (*Stouffer's* Homestyle), 9 ⅝ oz.	34.0	5.0
and vegetables, with rice (*Uncle Ben's* Rice		
Bowl), 12 oz.	25.0	3.0
rosemary (*Lean Cuisine Spa Cuisine*), 8.25 oz.	29.0	3.0
and sausage (*Birds Eye Voila!* Tuscan Reduced		
Carb), 1 cup*	10.0	4.0
sesame:		
(*Healthy Choice*), 9 oz.	34.0	4.0
(*Lean Cuisine* Cafe Classics), 9 oz.	49.0	2.0
(*Michelina's Yu Sing* Bowls), 11 oz.	67.0	2.0
smoked sausage, rice (*Glory* Savory Singles		
Casserole), 11 oz.	49.0	1.0
stir-fry:		
(*Birds Eye Voila!*), 1 cup*	22.0	2.0
(*Contessa*), 1¾ cups*	15.0	4.0
(*Tyson* Meal Kit), 2¾ cups*	73.0	5.0
with rice (*Uncle Ben's* Rice Bowl), 12 oz.	35.0	3.0
sweet and sour:		
(*Green Giant* Complete Skillet Meal), ¼ of 32-oz. pkg. .	62.0	3.0
(*Lean Cuisine* Cafe Classics), 10 oz.	52.0	1.0
(*Smart Ones* Higher Protein), 9 oz.	13.0	1.0
with rice (*Michelina's Yu Sing* Bowls), 11 oz.	82.0	2.0
with rice (*Uncle Ben's* Rice Bowl), 12 oz.	65.0	2.0
tandoori, with spinach (*Ethnic Gourmet*), 11 oz.	39.0	5.0
tenderloins, with barbecue sauce (*Smart Ones*		
Bistro Selections), 9 oz.	30.0	3.0
teriyaki:		
(*Birds Eye Voila!*), 1 cup*	44.0	2.0
(*Ethnic Gourmet*), 11 oz.	63.0	2.0
(*Green Giant* Complete Skillet Meal), ¼ of 32-oz. pkg. .	45.0	3.0
(*Jeff Nathan Creations*), 12 oz.	48.0	4.0
(*Lean Cuisine* Cafe Classics), 10 oz.	42.0	0
(*Lean Cuisine* Cafe Classics Bowl), 11 oz.	58.0	3.0

Food and Measure	carb. (gms)	fiber (gms)
(*Lean Cuisine Skillet Sensations* 24 oz.), 9.6 oz.	37.0	4.0
(*Michelina's Yu Sing*), 11 oz.	77.0	2.0
(*Stouffer's Skillet Sensations* 25 oz.), 7.1 oz.	24.0	2.0
grilled (*Stouffer's*), 9⅜ oz.	45.0	4.0
with rice (*Michelina's* Authentico), 8.5 oz.	64.0	1.0
with rice (*Uncle Ben's* Rice Bowl), 12 oz.	66.0	3.0
stir-fry (*Lean Cuisine Everyday Favorites*), 10 oz.	49.0	3.0
tetrazzini, Cajun style (*Organic Classics*), 10 oz.	46.0	2.0
Thai:		
pad (*Ethnic Gourmet*), 10 oz.	71.0	3.0
style (*Lean Cuisine*) Cafe Classics), 9 oz.	30.0	2.0
style (*Uncle Ben's* Pasta Bowl), 12 oz.	60.0	6.0
tikka masala (*Ethnic Gourmet*), 11 oz.	37.0	7.0
Tuscany (*Healthy Choice*), 10.6 oz.	42.0	6.0
vegetable stir-fry (*Michelina's* Authentico), 8 oz.	29.0	3.0
vegetables and (*Michelina's Yu Sing* Bowls), 11 oz.	59.0	3.0
vegetables and, spicy Szechuan (*Smart Ones*), 9 oz.	34.0	4.0
and vegetables:		
(*Birds Eye Voila!* Down Home Reduced Carb), 1 cup* .	17.0	4.0
(*Ethnic Gourmet* Thit Ga Kho Tieu), 10 oz.	43.0	1.0
(*Glory* Savory Singles Casserole), 11 oz.	27.0	2.0
(*Lean Cuisine* Cafe Classics), 10.5 oz.	30.0	2.0
(*Smart Ones* Homestyle Higher Protein), 9 oz.	8.0	2.0
fire-grilled (*Smart Ones Bistro Selections*), 10 oz.	45.0	2.0
grilled (*Stouffer's Skillet Sensations*), ⅓ of 25-oz. pkg. .	28.0	2.0
hearty (*Stouffer's* Bowl Cuisine), 12 oz.	30.0	4.0
and potato (*Michelina's Lean Gourmet* French Recipe), 8.5 oz.	23.0	4.0
and rice (*Healthy Choice* Princess), 10.75 oz.	41.0	5.0
stew, hearty (*Organic Classics*), 9.5 oz.	39.0	3.0
teriyaki (*Birds Eye Voila!* Reduced Carb), 1 cup*	15.0	4.0
teriyaki (*Smart Ones* Bowls), 10.5 oz.	48.0	3.0
vindaloo (*Ethnic Gourmet*), 11 oz.	46.0	3.0
with zucchini, creamy (*Smart Ones* Tuscan Higher Protein), 9 oz.	9.0	2.0
"Chicken" entree, vegetarian, frozen (see also "Vegetarian entree, frozen"), 1 pkg., except as noted:		
fire-grilled, and vegetables (*Linda McCartney*), 10 oz.	35.0	4.0

Food and Measure	carb. (gms)	fiber (gms)
with lemon grass and basil (*Ethnic Gourmet*), 11 oz.	58.0	7.0
Szechuan (*Ethnic Gourmet*), 12 oz.	69.0	6.0
tenders, with noodles, Thai (*Quorn* Simply Saute), ½ of 18-oz. pkg.	34.0	8.0
tenders, with rice:		
Indian (*Quorn* Simply Saute), ½ of 18-oz. pkg.	47.0	9.0
Mexican (*Quorn* Simply Saute), ½ of 18-oz. pkg.	61.0	7.0
teriyaki stir-fry, with chick'n (*Cedarlane*), 10 oz.	86.0	4.0
Thai lemon grass chick'n (*Yves* The Good Bowl), 10.5 oz.	49.0	4.0
Chicken entree mix, 1 cup*, except as noted:		
Alfredo (*Annie's* Organic Skillet Meal)	30.0	1.0
basil Parmesan, creamy (*Betty Crocker Cookbook Favorites*)	29.0	1.0
and buttermilk biscuits (*Betty Crocker Complete Meals*), ⅕ pkg.*	41.0	2.0
cheddar and broccoli (*Chicken Helper*)	26.0	1.0
cheddar herb (*Annie's* Organic Skillet Meals)	30.0	1.0
cheese, four (*Chicken Helper*)	26.0	1.0
cheesy, enchilada (*Chicken Helper*)	40.0	<1.0
cheesy, with pasta (*Campbell's Supper Bakes*), ⅙ pkg. mix	28.0	1.0
con queso, and Mexican rice (*Betty Crocker Cookbook Favorites*), ⅕ pkg.*	24.0	1.0
and dumplings (*Chicken Helper*)	27.0	1.0
dumplings and (*Betty Crocker Complete Meals*), ⅕ pkg.* .	33.0	2.0
fettuccine Alfredo:		
(*Betty Crocker Complete Meals*), ⅕ pkg.*	38.0	2.0
(*Betty Crocker Cookbook Favorites*)	27.0	1.0
(*Chicken Helper*)	25.0	1.0
fried rice (*Chicken Helper*)	22.0	1.0
garlic, with pasta (*Campbell's Supper Bakes*), ⅙ pkg. mix	44.0	2.0
herb, rice (*Campbell's Supper Bakes*), ⅙ pkg. mix	40.0	1.0
herb, rice (*Chicken Helper*)	24.0	1.0
lemon, with herb rice (*Campbell's Supper Bakes*), ⅙ pkg. mix	43.0	2.0
Parmesan pasta (*Chicken Helper*)	30.0	1.0
penne, garlic and herb (*Betty Crocker Cookbook Favorites*), ⅕ pkg.*	21.0	2.0

Food and Measure	carb. (gms)	fiber (gms)
and potatoes, au gratin (*Chicken Helper*)	25.0	1.0
roast, with stuffing (*Campbell's Supper Bakes Traditional*), ⅙ pkg. mix	29.0	2.0
Southwestern, with rice (*Campbell's Supper Bakes*), ⅙ pkg. mix	32.0	2.0
and stuffing (*Chicken Helper*)	27.0	1.0
teriyaki (*Chicken Helper*)	36.0	<1.0
Chicken fat, 2 tbsp.	0	0
Chicken frankfurter, see "Frankfurter"		
Chicken giblets, simmered:		
4 oz.	1.1	0
chopped, 1 cup	1.4	0
Chicken gravy, can or jar, ¼ cup:		
(*Campbell's/Campbell's Fat Free*)	3.0	0
(*Heinz Home Style*)	4.0	0
giblet (*Campbell's*)	2.0	0
roast, slow (*Franco-American/Franco-American Fat Free*)	3.0	0
roasted (*Boston Market*)	4.0	0
with roasted garlic (*Campbell's*)	4.0	0
Chicken gravy mix, ¼ cup*		
(*McCormick*)	4.0	0
roasted, and herb (*McCormick*)	3.0	0
Chicken lunch meat, breast, 2 oz., except as noted:		
(*Dietz & Watson Gourmet*)	1.0	0
barbecue (*Boar's Head Bar BQ Sauce Basted*)	3.0	0
browned (*Healthy Choice*)	1.0	0
Buffalo style (*Boar's Head Blazing Buffalo*)	0	0
golden roasted (*Tyson* Bag), 3 slices, 2.25 oz.	1.0	0
honey-roasted (*Tyson* Bag), 2 slices, 1.6 oz.	3.0	0
honey-roasted (*Tyson* Box), 2 slices, 1.8 oz.	3.0	0
oven-roasted:		
(*Boar's Head Golden Classic*)	0	0
(*Healthy Choice Hearty Slices*), 1 oz.	2.0	0
(*Healthy Choice Deli Thin*), 4 slices, 1.8 oz.	3.0	0
(*Sara Lee*)	1.0	0
(*Sara Lee* Sliced), 2 slices, 1.6 oz.	1.0	0
(*Tyson* Bag), 2 slices, 1.6 oz.	1.0	0

Food and Measure	carb. (gms)	fiber (gms)
(*Tyson* Box), 5 slices, 1.8 oz.	2.0	0
(*Tyson* Reseal Bag), 3 slices, 2 oz.	2.0	0
rotisserie style/flavor:		
(*Dietz & Watson*)	1.0	0
(*Sara Lee*)	2.0	0
(*Tyson* Box), 2 slices, 1.8 oz.	2.0	0
seasoned (*Boar's Head Aroastica*)	0	0
skinless (*Healthy Choice*)	1.0	0
smoked:		
(*Tyson* Bag), 2 slices, 1.6 oz.	1.0	0
(*Tyson* Box), 5 slices, 1.8 oz.	1.0	0
(*Tyson* Reseal Bag), 3 slices, 2.25 oz.	1.0	0
hickory (*Boar's Head*)	0	0
honey (*Healthy Choice Deli Thin*), 4 slices, 1.8 oz.	4.0	0
mesquite (*Healthy Choice*)	1.0	0
Chicken pie, frozen, see "Chicken entree, frozen"		
Chicken pocket/sandwich, frozen, 1 piece, 4.5 oz., except as noted:		
(*Pot Pie Express*)	40.0	3.0
(*Pot Pie Express* Value 5 Pack)	36.0	3.0
Alfredo (*Croissant Pockets*)	35.0	3.0
and broccoli (*Pot Pie Express*)	40.0	3.0
and broccoli, cheddar (*Croissant Pockets*)	34.0	3.0
cheese, three, and (*Lean Pockets* Quesadilla)	41.0	3.0
cheddar and broccoli (*Lean Pockets*)	39.0	3.0
fajita (*Lean Pockets*)	38.0	3.0
grilled Caesar (*Michelina's Hot Subs*), 2.1 oz.	38.0	2.0
Parmesan (*Croissant Pockets*)	36.0	3.0
Parmesan (*Lean Pockets*)	43.0	3.0
Chicken salad, refrigerated:		
(*Wampler*), ⅓ cup	9.0	1.0
(*Wampler* Low Fat), ⅓ cup	9.0	0
Chicken salad, freeze-dried, 1 serving:		
almond (*AlpineAire*)	10.0	2.0
Oriental (*AlpineAire*)	16.0	2.0
Chicken salad kit, with crackers:		
(*Bumble Bee*) 2.9-oz. can salad	10.0	0
(*Bumble Bee*), 6 crackers, .6 oz.	12.0	0

Food and Measure	carb. (gms)	fiber (gms)
(*Hormel*), 1 pkg.	16.0	0
(*Tyson* Salad Kit), 1 pkg.	15.0	1.0
Chicken sandwich, see "Chicken pocket/sandwich"		
Chicken sauce, see specific listings		
Chicken sauce mix (see also specific listings),		
dry mix:		
cheese, three (*McCormick*), 1 tbsp.	2.0	0
Dijon (*McCormick*), 1⅔ tbsp.	5.0	0
Italian or Parmesan (*McCormick*), 2 tsp.	3.0	0
herb, country (*McCormick*), 1 tbsp.	4.0	0
lemon herb (*McCormick*), 1 tbsp.	5.0	0
rice, fried (*McCormick*), 1 tbsp.	6.0	0
and rice dInner (*A Taste of Thai*), ¼ pkg.	3.0	0
stir-fry (*McCormick*), 2 tsp.	4.0	0
teriyaki (*McCormick*), 1⅓ tbsp.	5.0	0
Chicken sausage, see "Sausage"		
Chicken seasoning, dry:		
all varieties (*McCormick*), ¼ tsp.	0	0
and poultry (*Lawry's* Perfect Blend), ¼ tsp.	0	0
Chicken seasoning mix, see "Chicken coating mix,"		
"Chicken sauce mix," and specific listings		
Chicken spread (*Underwood*), ¼ cup	3.0	0
Chick-fil-A, 1 serving:		
breakfast:		
bagel, wheat	41.0	2.0
bagel with chicken, egg, and cheese	49.0	3.0
biscuit, buttered	38.0	1.0
biscuit, with bacon or bacon and egg	38.0	1.0
biscuit, with bacon, egg, and cheese	39.0	1.0
biscuit, with egg or egg and cheese	38.0	1.0
biscuit, with sausage or sausage and egg	45.0	1.0
biscuit, with sausage, egg, and cheese	46.0	1.0
biscuit with gravy	44.0	1.0
Chick-fil-A burrito, chicken	39.0	2.0
Chick-fil-A burrito, sausage	40.0	2.0
Chick-fil-A Chick-N-Minis, 3 pieces	28.0	1.0
Chick-fil-A Chick-N-Minis, 4 pieces	37.0	2.0
Chick-fil-A chicken biscuit	44.0	2.0

Food and Measure	carb. (gms)	fiber (gms)
Chick-fil-A chicken biscuit, with cheese	45.0	2.0
hash browns	25.0	3.0
chicken sandwiches:		
chargrilled or chargrilled club, without sauce	33.0	3.0
Chick-fil-A	38.0	1.0
chicken salad	32.0	5.0
chicken deluxe	39.0	2.0
Cool Wraps, chargrilled chicken	54.0	3.0
Cool Wraps, chicken Caesar or spicy chicken	52.0	3.0
chicken dishes:		
chicken fillet	10.0	0
chicken fillet, chargrilled	1.0	0
Chick-N-Strips, 4-pack	14.0	1.0
Chick-fil-A nuggets, 8-pack	12.0	<1.0
dipping sauce, 1 pkt.:		
barbeque	11.0	0
Chick-fil-A Buffalo	1.0	0
honey mustard	10.0	0
honey-roasted barbecue	2.0	0
ranch, buttermilk	1.0	0
Polynesian	13.0	0
sides:		
carrot raisin salad	28.0	2.0
chicken soup, hearty, 1 cup	18.0	1.0
coleslaw, small	17.0	2.0
fruit cup, medium	16.0	2.0
Waffle Potato Fries	34.0	4.0
salad:		
Chick-N Strips	22.0	4.0
garden	9.0	3.0
side salad	4.0	2.0
Southwest	17.0	5.0
salad dressing, 2 tbsp.:		
blue cheese, buttermilk ranch, or Caesar	1.0	0
honey mustard, fat free	14.0	0
Italian, light	2.0	0
raspberry vinaigrette	15.0	0

Food and Measure	carb. (gms)	fiber (gms)
spicy	2.0	0
Thousand Island	5.0	0
salad sides, 1 pkt.:		
croutons	6.0	0
sunflower kernels	3.0	1.0
tortilla strips	9.0	1.0
desserts:		
brownie, fudge nut	45.0	2.0
cheesecake, slice	30.0	2.0
IceDream, small cup	41.0	0
IceDream, small cone	28.0	0
lemon pie, slice	51.0	3.0
Chickpeas, see "Garbanzo beans"		
Chicory, witloof:		
(*Frieda's* Endive), 2 cups, 3 oz.	3.0	3.0
5–7'' head, 1.9 oz.	2.1	1.6
½ cup	1.8	1.4
Chicory greens:		
trimmed, 1 oz.	1.3	1.1
chopped, ½ cup	4.2	3.6
Chicory root:		
1 medium, 2.6 oz.	10.5	n.a.
1'' pieces, ½ cup	7.9	n.a.
Chili (see also "Chili starter"), 1 cup, except as noted:		
with beans:		
(*Bush's* Original)	26.0	7.0
(*Campbell's Chunky* Roadhouse)	25.0	7.0
(*Campbell's Chunky* Sizzlin' Steak)	26.0	7.0
(*Castleberry's*)	26.0	8.0
(*Hormel* Homestyle)	28.0	5.0
(*Hormel* Meal/Meal Hot), 1 cont.	27.0	6.0
(*Hormel/Hormel* Chunky/Hot/Less Salt)	34.0	7.0
(*Hormel/Hormel* Hot), 7.5-oz. can	29.0	6.0
(*Stagg Chunkero*)	27.0	5.0
(*Stagg Classic*)	28.0	5.0
(*Stagg Country*)	30.0	5.0
(*Stagg Fiesta Grill*)	25.0	5.0

Food and Measure	carb. (gms)	fiber (gms)
(*Stagg Laredo*)	27.0	6.0
(*Stagg Quick Draw*)	28.0	6.0
(*Stagg Ranch House*)	26.0	6.0
(*Stagg Rio Blanco*)	20.0	5.0
(*Stagg Silverado*)	33.0	6.0
chunky (*Bush's*)	28.0	8.0
hot (*Bush's*)	26.0	7.0
hot (*Stagg Dynamite Hot*)	31.0	6.0
hot and /spicy (*Hormel*)	33.0	7.0
without beans:		
(*Bush's* Original)	16.0	3.0
(*Hormel* Meal), 1 cont.	15.0	2.0
(*Hormel/Hormel* Hot/Less Salt)	17.0	3.0
(*Stagg Steak House*)	16.0	2.0
chunky (*Hormel*)	22.0	5.0
hot and spicy (*Hormel*)	19.0	3.0
turkey, with beans:		
(*Campbell's Chunky*)	27.0	6.0
(*Health Valley* 99% Fat Free)	34.0	8.0
(*Hormel*)	26.0	5.0
(*Stagg Ranchero*)	31.0	6.0
turkey, without beans (*Hormel*)	17.0	3.0
vegetable/vegetarian:		
(*Hormel*)	38.0	7.0
(*Morningstar Farms* Vegan)	25.0	10.0
(*Stagg Vegetable Garden*)	37.0	7.0
(*Worthington*)	25.0	8.0
bean, four (*Walnut Acres*)	28.0	4.0
black bean (*Amy's*)	31.0	15.0
black bean or 3 bean (*Health Valley* 99% Fat Free)	28.0	12.0
burrito flavor (*Health Valley*)	30.0	11.0
lentil (*Health Valley*)	28.0	11.0
medium, with vegetables (*Amy's*)	29.0	8.0
medium or spicy (*Amy's*)	26.0	7.0
mild or spicy (*Health Valley/Health Valley* No Salt)	30.0	11.0
Chili, frozen or refrigerated (see also "Chili entree, frozen"):		
(*Organic Classics* Our Favorite), 1 cup	31.0	9.0

Food and Measure	carb. (gms)	fiber (gms)
(*P.J.'s Beantowne*), 1 cup	32.0	4.0
two bean vegetable (*Moosewood* Texas), 1 cup	34.0	8.0
Chili, mix, vegetarian, dry:		
(*Fantastic*), ¼ cup	17.0	4.0
black bean or Texas (*Health Valley* Low Fat), ⅓ cup	21.0	6.0
Chili beans (see also "Chili starter" and		
"Mexican beans"), canned, ½ cup:		
(*Bush's*)	20.0	6.0
(*Westbrae Natural* Organic)	19.0	5.0
with chipotle (*S&W* Santa Fe)	21.0	6.0
with jalapeño or red pepper (*Eden* Organic)	21.0	7.0
tomato sauce, zesty (*S&W*)	23.0	6.0
Chili dip (see also "Salsa"), chunky (*La Victoria*), 2 tbsp.	2.0	0
Chili entree, dried, l serving or cont.:		
(*AlpineAire* Mountain)	48.0	13.0
(*Instant Gourmet* Hearty Mountain)	52.0	14.0
with beans (*AlpineAire* Black Bart)	41.0	10.0
mac, with beef (*Mountain House* Can), 1 cup	30.0	5.0
mac, with beef (*Mountain House* Double), ½ pouch	40.0	6.0
Chili entree, frozen, 1 pkg.:		
bean, three (*Lean Cuisine Everyday Favorites*), 10 oz.	40.0	8.0
bean, black (*Michelina's* Authentico), 10 oz.	76.0	10.0
beef and bean, chunky (*Stouffer's* Bowl Cuisine), 11 oz.	32.0	6.0
cheese pie (*Cedarlane Carb Buster* Relleno Pie), 9.5 oz.	9.0	1.0
and corn bread (*Amy's* Whole Meal), 10.5 oz.	59.0	10.0
mac (*Michelina's* Zap'ems), 8 oz.	37.0	3.0
vegetarian (*Yves* Veggie), 10.5 oz.	37.0	14.0
Chili entree, pkg.:		
mac (*Fantastic Carb 'Tastic*), 8-oz. pkg.	19.0	14.0
three-bean (*Fantastic Fast Naturals*), 8-oz. pkg.	28.0	5.0
Chili pepper, see "Pepper, chili"		
Chili pepper paste, see "Thai sauce"		
Chili powder:		
(*McCormick*), ¼ tsp.	0	0
1 tbsp.	4.1	2.6
1 tsp.	1.4	.9
Chili relish, hot, Indian (*Patak's* Chile), 1 tbsp.	0	0
Chili sauce, red (*Las Palmas*), ¼ cup	2.0	.0

Food and Measure	carb. (gms)	fiber (gms)
Chili sauce, black bean, see "Black bean sauce"		
Chili sauce, hot, see "Hot sauce" and "Thai sauce"		
Chili sauce, tomato, 1 tbsp.:		
(*Del Monte*)	5.0	0
(*Heinz*)	4.0	0
(*Red Gold*)	5.0	0
(*Texas Pete*)	<1.0	0
Chili seasoning mix, dry:		
(*Adolph's Meal Makers*), 1 tbsp.	5.0	<1.0
(*Carroll Shelby's* Original Texas Mix), 2 tbsp.	12.0	0
(*D.L. Jardine's* Texas Bag O' Fixins/Chili Works), 3 tbsp.	9.0	0
(*Ducks Unlimited*), 1⅓ tbsp.	5.0	0
(*Lawry's*), 1 tsp.	2.0	0
(*McCormick*), 1⅓ tbsp.	5.0	0
hot (*Wick Fowler's* 2-Alarm Kit), 3 tbsp.	10.0	0
mild (*McCormick*), 1⅓ tbsp.	5.0	0
mild (*Wick Fowler's* False-Alarm Kit), 2 tbsp.	9.0	0
Tex-Mex or hot (*McCormick*), 1⅓ tbsp.	4.0	0
white, chicken (*McCormick*), 1⅓ tbsp.	5.0	0
Chili starter, canned, ½ cup, except as noted:		
(*S&W* Chili Makin's Black Bean/Home Style)	19.0	6.0
(*S&W* Chili Makin's Original)	20.0	5.0
(*S&W* Chili Makin's Santa Fe)	18.0	5.0
Louisiana (*Bush's Chili Magic*)	21.0	5.0
Louisiana (*Bush's Chili Magic*), 1 cup*	16.0	3.0
Texas (*Bush's Chili Magic*)	20.0	5.0
Texas (*Bush's Chili Magic*), 1 cup*	15.0	4.0
Traditional (*Bush's Chili Magic*)	19.0	5.0
Traditional (*Bush's Chili Magic*), 1 cup*	15.0	3.0
Chili-garlic sauce, Vietnamese (*Huy Fong*), 1 tsp.	<1.0	0
Chili-ginger sauce, sweet (*The Ginger People*), 2 tbsp.	15.0	0
Chimichanga, frozen, 1 piece, except as noted:		
bean, taco picante (*El Monterey* XX Large!), ½ of 10-oz. piece	42.0	3.0
beef, shredded (*José Olé*), 5 oz.	42.0	2.0
beef and bean (*El Monterey*), 4 oz.	32.0	3.0
beef and bean (*El Monterey* Red Hot XX Large!), 10 oz.	86.0	9.0

Food and Measure	carb. (gms)	fiber (gms)
beef and cheese:		
mini (*El Monterey* Fiesta Pack), 3 pieces, 4.5 oz.	33.0	1.0
shredded (*El Monterey Supreme*), 5 oz.	35.0	1.0
chicken (*José Olé*), 5 oz.	42.0	2.0
chicken and cheese:		
mini (*El Monterey* Fiesta Pack), 3 pieces, 4.5 oz.	33.0	2.0
Monterey jack (*El Monterey Supreme*), 5 oz.	36.0	2.0
cream cheese jalapeño (*El Monterey* Fiesta Minis),		
4.5 oz.	32.0	1.0
nacho cheese and beef, mini, fried (*El Monterey*		
Cruncheros), 3 pieces, 4.5 oz.	35.0	2.0
Chimichurri sauce, see "Marinade"		
Chipotle sauce (*La Morena*), 2 tbsp.	6.0	0
Chitterlings, pork, simmered, 4 oz.	0	0
Chives:		
fresh, 1 oz.	1.2	.9
fresh, chopped, 1 tbsp.	.1	.1
freeze-dried, ¼ cup	.5	<1.0
Chocolate, see "Candy"		
Chocolate, baking, ½ oz. or 1 tbsp., except as noted:		
(*Nestlé Choco Bake*)	4.0	2.0
bars:		
bittersweet or semisweet (*Baker's*)	7.0	1.0
semisweet (*Hershey's Bake Shoppe*)	9.0	<1.0
semisweet (*Nestlé Toll House*)	9.0	<1.0
sweet (*German's*)	8.0	1.0
unsweetened (*Baker's*)	4.0	2.0
unsweetened (*Hershey's Bake Shoppe*)	4.0	2.0
unsweetened (*Nestlé Toll House*)	5.0	3.0
white (*Baker's* Premium)	8.0	0
white (*Nestlé Toll House*)	8.0	0
chips or morsels:		
(*Guittard* Super Cookie Chip)	9.0	1.0
dark (*Hershey's Bake Shoppe Special Dark*)	9.0	<1.0
milk (*Hershey's Bake Shoppe*)	9.0	0
milk (*Hershey's Bake Shoppe Kisses* Unwrapped),		
9 pieces, 1.4 oz.	4.0	1.0

Food and Measure	carb. (gms)	fiber (gms)
milk (*Hershey's Bake Shoppe Mini Kisses*), 11 pieces, .5oz.	9.0	0
milk (*M&M's Mini*)	10.0	0
milk (*Nestlé Toll House*)	9.0	0
mint or raspberry (*Hershey's Bake Shoppe*)	10.0	0
semisweet (*Guittard*)	10.0	<1.0
semisweet (*Hershey's Bake Shoppe*)	10.0	<1.0
semisweet (*Hershey's Bake Shoppe Mini-chips*)	9.0	0
semisweet (*M&M's Mini*)	9.0	1.0
semisweet (*Nestlé Toll House*)	9.0	<1.0
vanilla (*Guittard* Choc-Au-Lait)	9.0	0
white (*Hershey's Bake Shoppe* Premier)	9.0	0
white (*Nestlé Toll House*)	9.0	0
chunks:		
(*Nestlé Toll House*)	8.0	1.0
milk or white (*Baker's*)	9.0	0
semisweet (*Baker's* Real)	9.0	1.0
wafers, 27 pieces, 1.4 oz.:		
dark, bittersweet (*Guittard* Coucher du Soleil)	18.0	4.0
dark, semisweet (*Guittard* Lever du Soleil)	21.0	3.0
milk (*Guittard* Soleil d'Or)	20.0	1.0
white (*Guittard* Crème Française)	21.0	0
Chocolate dip, see "Fruit dip"		
Chocolate drink:		
(*Yoo-hoo*), 8 fl. oz.	29.0	0
(*Yoo-hoo Lite*), 9 fl. oz.	15.0	0
fudge, double (*Yoo-hoo*), 8 fl. oz.	33.0	0
Chocolate drink mix (see also "Cocoa mix"), 2 tbsp., except as noted:		
(*Hershey's* Milk Mix), 3 tbsp.	23.0	<1.0
(*Nesquik*)	19.0	1.0
(*Nesquik* No Sugar)	7.0	1.0
double (*Nesquik*)	17.0	1.0
Chocolate milk, see "Milk, flavored"		
Chocolate mousse, frozen (*Smart Ones*), 2.7-oz. piece	24.0	4.0
Chocolate sprinkles (*Hershey's* Triple Dessert), 2 tbsp.	12.0	<1.0
Chocolate syrup, 2 tbsp., except as noted:		
(*Fox's U-Bet*)	29.0	0

Food and Measure	carb. (gms)	fiber (gms)
(*Hershey's*)	25.0	<1.0
(*Hershey's* Lite)	12.0	<1.0
(*Nesquik*)	24.0	<1.0
(*Santa Cruz Organic*)	22.0	2.0
(*Smucker's Sundae Syrup*)	26.0	1.0
dark (*Hershey's Special Dark*)	26.0	0
double (*Hershey's* Sundae)	24.0	1.0
malt (*Hershey's Whoppers*)	25.0	<1.0
Chocolate topping, 2 tbsp.:		
(*Hershey's* Shell)	16.0	1.0
(*Smucker's Magic Shell*)	16.0	1.0
(*Smucker's Plate Scapers*)	23.0	1.0
crisps (*Krackel* Shell)	14.0	<1.0
dark (*Smucker's Dove*)	22.0	1.0
fudge (*Smucker's* Micro/Spoonable)	28.0	1.0
fudge (*Smucker's Magic Shell*)	19.0	1.0
fudge, hot:		
(*Hershey's* Fat Free)	23.0	1.0
(*Smucker's* Micro/Spoonable)	24.0	1.0
(*Smucker's* Special Recipe)	22.0	<1.0
(*Smucker's* Spoonable Light)	23.0	2.0
(*Smucker's* Spoonable Sugar Free)	23.0	1.0
milk (*Smucker's Dove*)	21.0	1.0
mocha (*Smucker's* Spoonable)	28.0	<1.0
Chocolate-raspberry spread (*Cedar's* Mediterranean), 2 tbsp.	10.0	1.0
Chorizo:		
(*Fiorucci* Cantimpalo), 1 oz.	1.0	0
pork, spicy (*Battisoni*), 1 oz.	0	0
pork and beef, 2-oz. link	1.0	0
Chorizo, vegetarian (*Soyrizo*), 4 tbsp., 1.9 oz.	5.0	12.0
Chow chow pickle:		
(*Crosse & Blackwell*), 1 tbsp.	1.0	<1.0
sweet, with cauliflower, ¼ cup	16.5	.9
Chrysanthemum garland, 1" pieces:		
raw, ½ cup	.5	.4
boiled, drained, ½ cup	2.2	1.2
Chubs, smoked, see "Whitefish, smoked"		

Food and Measure	carb. (gms)	fiber (gms)
Church's Chicken:		
chicken, 1 piece:		
breast	4.0	0
leg	2.0	0
thigh	5.0	0
wing	8.0	0
chicken, batter and skin removed, 1 piece:		
breast	1.0	0
leg	1.3	0
thigh	3.0	0
wing	2.0	0
Crunchy Tenders, 1 piece	11.0	.4
Tender Crunchers, 6–8 pieces	32.0	1.0
sauces, 1 pkt.:		
barbecue	7.0	0
honey mustard	4.0	0
jalapeño, creamy	1.0	0
Purple Pepper Sauce	12.0	0
sweet and sour	8.0	0
sides, regular:		
coleslaw	8.0	2.0
collard greens	5.0	2.0
corn on cob	24.0	9.0
corn nuggets	30.0	2.0
fries	29.0	2.0
Honey Butter Biscuit	26.0	1.0
Jalapeño Cheese Bombers, 4 pieces	29.0	3.0
jalapeños, 2 whole	2.0	1.0
macaroni and cheese	23.0	1.0
mashed potato/gravy	14.0	1.0
okra, fried	19.0	4.0
rice, Cajun	16.0	<1.0
dessert pie:		
apple	41.0	1.0
lemon, double	39.0	0
strawberry cream cheese	32.0	2.0
Churro, cinnamon:		
(*Bearitos*), ½ cup	20.0	0

Food and Measure	carb. (gms)	fiber (gms)
waffle sticks, crispy (*Tio Pepe's Churros*), 1-oz. piece	14.0	2.0
Chutney, 1 tbsp., except as noted:		
(*Trader Vic's* Calcutta), 2 tbsp.	11.0	0
ginger pineapple (*Neera's*)	7.0	0
mango:		
(*Bombay Brand* Major Grey's), 2 tbsp.	25.0	0
(*Crosse & Blackwell* Major Grey's)	14.0	0
(*Neera's*)	5.0	0
(*Patak's/Patak's* Hot/Lime/Major Grey Ginger)	12.0	0
ginger (*Bombay Brand*), 2 tbsp.	23.0	1.0
hot (*Crosse & Blackwell*)	14.0	0
sweet, mild (*Patak's*)	13.0	0
peach (*Neera's*)	6.0	0
pear cardamom (*Neera's*)	7.0	1.0
tomato (*Neera's*)	5.0	1.0
vegetable, hot (*Neera's*)	2.0	0
Cilantro, see "Coriander"		
Cinnamon, ground, 1 tsp.	2.1	1.4
Cinnamon baking chips (*Hershey's Bake Shoppe*), 1 tbsp.	9.0	0
Cinnamon raisin spread (*Cedar's* Mediterranean), 2 tbsp.	8.0	2.0
Cinnamon sugar (*McCormick*), ¼ tsp.	3.0	0
Cisco, without added ingredients	0	0
Citron, candied, diced (*Seneca* Glacé), 2 tbsp.	18.0	<1.0
Citronella root, see "Lemon grass"		
Citrus drink blend, 8 fl. oz., except as noted:		
(*AriZona Extreme Energy Shot*), 8.3-oz. can	34.0	0
(*Five Alive*)	30.0	0
(*V8 Splash*)	28.0	0
frozen* (*Five Alive*)	29.0	0
frozen*	28.5	0
punch (*Minute Maid*)	32.0	0
tropical (*Minute Maid*), 12-fl.-oz. bottle	44.0	0
Citrus fruit salad, see "Fruit, mixed, can or jar"		
Clam, meat only:		
raw, 4 oz.	2.9	0
raw, 9 large or 20 small, 6.3 oz.	4.6	0
boiled, poached, or steamed, 4 oz.	5.8	0

Food and Measure	carb. (gms)	fiber (gms)
Clam, canned, 2 oz. or ¼ cup, except as noted:		
baby, whole:		
(*Brunswick*)	0	0
(*Bumble Bee/Orleans*)	2.0	0
(*Yankee Clipper*)	2.0	0
boiled (*Crown Prince*), ⅓ cup	1.0	0
chopped or minced:		
(*Bumble Bee/Orleans*)	2.0	0
(*Yankee Clipper*)	3.0	0
arctic or ocean (*Chincoteague*)	1.0	0
sea (*Chincoteague*)	0	0
Clam, smoked, canned, in oil, drained:		
(*Bumble Bee/Orleans*), 2 oz.	1.0	0
baby (*Yankee Clipper*), 1 can drained, 2.3 oz.	2.0	2.0
Clam chowder, see "Soup"		
Clam dip (*Cabot*), 2 tbsp.	1.0	0
Clam dish, frozen:		
fried, breaded (*Mrs. Paul's*), 18 pieces, 3 oz.	26.0	1.0
stuffed, in shell, 2 pieces:		
casino (*Matlaw's*), 1.3 oz.	7.0	<1.0
oreganata (*Matlaw's*), 1.2 oz.	6.0	0
New England style (*Matlaw's*), 3.1 oz.	20.0	2.0
Clam juice:		
(*Orleans*), 1 tbsp.	0	0
ocean (*Chincoteague*), ½ cup	1.0	0
sea (*Chincoteague*), ½ cup	0	0
and tomato, see "Tomato-clam drink"		
Clam sauce, canned:		
red, ½ cup:		
(*Chincoteague*)	8.0	<1.0
(*Progresso*)	8.0	1.0
(*Snow's*)	6.0	0
white, ½ cup:		
(*Chincoteague*)	9.0	0
(*Progresso*)	5.0	0
(*Snow's*)	4.0	0
creamy (*Progresso*)	8.0	0
Clover sprouts (*Jonathan's*), 1 cup	3.0	2.0

Food and Measure	carb. (gms)	fiber (gms)
Cloves, ground:		
1 tbsp.	4.0	<1.0
1 tsp.	1.3	.2
Cobbler, frozen:		
apple:		
(*Sara Lee* Anytime), ½ of 8-oz. pkg.	47.0	1.0
with raisins (*Jeff Nathan Creations*), ½ of 8.5-oz. pkg.	47.0	2.0
blackberry (*Sara Lee* Anytime), ½ of 8-oz. pkg.	48.0	2.0
peach (*Mrs. Smith's*), ⅛ of 32-oz. pkg.	34.0	1.0
peach (*Sara Lee* Anytime), ½ of 8-oz. pkg.	43.0	1.0
Cocktail mixers, see specific listings		
Cocktail sauce, see "Seafood sauce"		
Cocoa, 1 tbsp.:		
(*Shiloh Farms*)	2.0	1.0
Dutch or unsweetened (*Hershey's*)	3.0	1.0
Cocoa mix, 1 pkt., except as noted:		
(*Hershey's Goodnight Hugs*)	27.0	0
(*Hershey's Goodnight Kisses*)	28.0	<1.0
chocolate:		
Dutch (*Hershey's*)	28.0	2.0
raspberry (*Hershey's*)	29.0	<1.0
rich, plain, or with marshmallows (*Hershey's*)	23.0	1.0
Royal or Irish mint (*Country Choice Naturals*), 1 oz.	23.0	<1.0
Royal or Irish mint (*Country Choice Naturals* Soy), 1 oz.	23.0	1.0
vanilla, French (*Hershey's*)	28.0	0
Cocoa-coffee mix (*Trader Vic's Kafe-La-Te*), 2 rounded tsp., ½ oz.	13.0	0
Coconut, fresh, shelled:		
(*Frieda's* White/Young), ¼ cup, 1.4 oz.	6.0	4.0
1 oz.	4.3	2.6
shredded or grated, 1 cup not packed	12.2	7.2
Coconut, cream of:		
(*Goya* Coco Cream of Coconut), 2 tbsp.	22.0	0
(*Vigo*), 2 tbsp.	17.0	0
Coconut, dried:		
flaked, sweetened:		
(*Baker's Angel Flake*), 2 tbsp.	6.0	1.0

Food and Measure	carb. (gms)	fiber (gms)
(*Mounds*), 2 tbsp.	6.0	1.0
⅓ cup	11.8	1.1
shredded (*Shiloh Farms*), 3 tbsp.	4.0	2.0
shredded (*Tree of Life/Tree of Life* Macaroon), 1 oz.	7.0	5.0
toasted, 1 oz.	12.6	1.0
Coconut juice drink (*Foco*), 11.8-fl.-oz. can	29.0	1.0
Coconut milk:		
(*Goya*), 1 tbsp.	1.0	0
(*Port Arthur* Lite), ¼ cup	2.0	0
(*A Taste of Thai/A Taste of Thai* Lite), ⅓ cup	3.0	0
(*Thai Kitchen*), ¼ cup	4.0	0
(*Thai Kitchen* Lite), ¼ cup	1.0	0
Coconut nectar (*R.W. Knudsen*), 8 fl. oz.	26.0	2.0
Coconut water (*Goya*), 12 fl. oz.	31.0	10.0
Cod, Atlantic or Pacific, without added ingredients	0	0
Cod, canned, in Biscayan sauce (*Goya*), ¼ cup	1.0	0
Cod entree, frozen, 5-oz. piece:		
au gratin (*Oven Poppers*)	5.0	1.0
stuffed with broccoli and cheese (*Oven Poppers*)	4.0	1.0
Cod liver oil, 2 tbsp.	0	0
Coffee:		
brewed, 6 fl. oz.	.8	0
instant, regular, 1 rounded tsp.	.7	0
Coffee, flavored, mix (*General Foods International Coffees*), 1⅓ tbsp.:		
café Vienna	12.0	0
cappuccino, Italian	10.0	0
chocolate, white, Swiss	12.0	0
chocolate café, Viennese	10.0	0
crème caramel or hazelnut Belgian café	12.0	0
Suisse mocha, vanilla, or French vanilla nut	10.0	0
Coffee, iced, cappuccino, 10.5 fl. oz.:		
(*AriZona* Shake Double Roast/Rich Chocolaty)	36.0	.5
(*AriZona Kahlua*)	24.0	.5
Coffee, iced, mix (*General Foods International Coffees Cappuccino Coolers*), 1 pkt.:		
chocolate	16.0	1.0
vanilla, French	15.0	0

Food and Measure	carb. (gms)	fiber (gms)
Coffee creamer, see "Creamer"		
Coffee liqueur, 1 fl. oz.:		
53 proof	16.3	0
with cream, 34 proof	6.5	0
Coffee substitute, cereal grain (*Postum*), 1 tsp.	3.0	0
Cold cuts, see "Lunch meat" and specific listings		
Coleslaw, refrigerated:		
(*Blue Ridge Farm's*), 4 oz.	19.0	2.0
(*Reser's* Homestyle), ½ cup	19.0	2.0
Coleslaw blend, see "Salad blend" and "Salad kit"		
Coleslaw dressing, see "Salad dressing"		
Coleslaw seasoning mix (*Produce Partners* Super Slaw), 1 tsp. dry	2.0	0
Collard greens, fresh:		
raw:		
(*Glory*), 2 cups	5.0	3.0
chopped (*Del Monte*), 2 cups	5.0	1.0
chopped, ½ cup	1.3	.7
trimmed, 1 oz.	2.0	1.0
boiled, drained, chopped, ½ cup	3.9	1.3
Collard greens, canned, ½ cup:		
(*Allens* No Salt)	5.0	3.0
(*Bush's*)	4.0	2.0
seasoned (*Allens/Sunshine*)	5.0	1.0
seasoned, Southern (*Glory*)	7.0	3.0
turkey flavor (*Glory*)	6.0	2.0
Collard greens, frozen, chopped, ½ cup:		
(*Seabrook Farms*)	2.0	2.0
boiled, drained	6.1	n.a.
seasoned (*Glory* Savory Accents)	10.0	2.0
Conch, baked or broiled, 4 oz.	1.9	0
Cookie (see also "Cake, snack" and specific listings):		
(*Gamesa Marias*), 8 pieces, 1 oz.	24.0	<1.0
(*Stella D'oro* Angel Wings), 2 pieces, 1.1 oz.	14.0	0
(*Stella D'oro* Anginetti), 4 pieces, 1.1 oz.	22.0	0
(*Stella D'oro* Breakfast Treats), .8 oz.	15.0	0
(*Stella D'oro* Breakfast Treats Mini), 1 oz.	21.0	0
(*Stella D'oro* Margherite), 2 pieces, 1 oz.	20.0	0

Food and Measure	carb. (gms)	fiber (gms)
all varieties (*Health Valley* Fat Free), 3 pieces, 1.2 oz.	24.0	3.0
almond:		
(*Frieda's*), 2 pieces, 1 oz.	19.0	0
(*Stella D'oro* Delight), 1.1 oz.	18.0	1.0
(*Stella D'oro* Toast), 2 pieces, 1 oz.	19.0	1.0
butter, toasted (*Tree of Life* Fat Free), 8-oz. piece	16.0	1.0
animal:		
(*Animalitos*), 14 pieces, 1.1 oz.	25.0	<1.0
(*Austin* Zoo), 16 pieces, 1.1 oz.	25.0	<1.0
chocolate chip (*Barbara's Snackimals*), 10 pieces,		
1.1 oz.	19.0	0
frosted (*Keebler*), 8 pieces, 1.1 oz.	21.0	0
iced (*Keebler*), 6 pieces, 1.1 oz.	23.0	<1.0
oatmeal (*Barbara's Snackimals*), 10 pieces, 1.1 oz.	18.0	1.0
vanilla (*Barbara's*), 8 pieces, 1.1 oz.	18.0	<1.0
vanilla (*Barbara's Snackimals*), 10 pieces, 1.1 oz.	17.0	0
apricot raspberry (*Pepperidge Farm Verona*),		
3 pieces, .9 oz.	22.0	<1.0
anisette:		
(*Stella D'oro* Sponge), 2 pieces, .9 oz.	18.0	0
(*Stella D'oro* Toast), 3 pieces, 1.2 oz.	27.0	0
mini (*Stella D'oro* Toast), 1.2 oz.	27.0	0
arrowroot (*Nabisco*), .2-oz. piece	4.0	0
assortment (*Stella D'oro* Lady Stella), 1 oz.	20.0	1.0
banana walnut (*Stella D'oro* Toast), 2 pieces, .9 oz.	19.0	0
biscotti:		
(*Nonnis* Original), 1-oz. piece	15.0	1.0
almond or chocolate almond (*Stella D'oro*), .7-oz. piece	13.0	1.0
amaretto or chocolate (*Health Valley*), 2 pieces, 1.1 oz.	23.0	3.0
chocolate, chocolate dipped (*Nonnis* Decadence),		
1.2-oz. piece	19.0	1.0
chocolate chunk (*Stella D'oro*), .7-oz. piece	14.0	0
vanilla, French (*Stella D'oro*), .7-oz. piece	15.0	0
blueberry (*Stella D'oro* Toast), 2 pieces, .9 oz.	20.0	0
brownie, fudge (*SnackWell's*), .8 oz.	17.0	0
brownie, fudge, double (*Country Choice*), .8-oz. piece	16.0	<1.0
butter:		
(*Pepperidge Farm Chessmen*), 3 pieces, .9 oz.	18.0	<1.0

Food and Measure	carb. (gms)	fiber (gms)
(*Pepperidge Farm Chessmen* Mini), 9 pieces, 1 oz. ...	21.0	<1.0
Danish, 4 pieces, 1.1 oz.	19.0	1.0
butter pecan (*Pepperidge Farm Chessmen*), 3 pieces, .		
9 oz.	18.0	<1.0
caramel apple bar (*Newtons*), 2 pieces, 1.3 oz.	26.0	0
carob (*Tree of Life* Wheat Free California), .8-oz. piece ...	14.0	6.0
carob chip (*Tree of Life* Monster), ⅕ piece	19.0	1.0
carrot cake (*Tree of Life* Fat Free), .8-oz. piece	13.0	1.0
carrot cake (*Tree of Life* Monster Fat Free), ¼ piece	20.0	2.0
cherries and cheesecake bar (*Newtons*), 2 pieces, 1.3 oz. .	25.0	0
chocolate:		
(*Stella D'oro* Breakfast Treats), .8-oz. piece	15.0	1.0
almond (*Hershey's*), 2 pieces, 1 oz.	16.0	<1.0
double Dutch (*Barbara's*), .6-oz. piece	9.0	<1.0
top (*Carr's Imperials*), 2 pieces, 1 oz.	18.0	1.0
top (*Pepperidge Farm Geneva*), 3 pieces, 1.1 oz.	19.0	1.0
top, dark (*Carr's Imperials*), 2 pieces, 1 oz.	19.0	2.0
wafer (*Famous*), 5 pieces, 1.1 oz.	24.0	1.0
chocolate chip/chunk:		
(*Barbara's*), .6-oz. piece	9.0	<1.0
(*Chips Ahoy!*), 3 pieces, 1.1 oz.	21.0	1.0
(*Chips Ahoy!* Candy Blasts), .5-oz. piece	10.0	0
(*Chips Ahoy!* Chewy), .9-oz. piece	17.0	1.0
(*Chips Ahoy!* Mini), 5 pieces, 1.1 oz.	21.0	1.0
(*Chips Ahoy!* Mini Bite-Size Go-Pack), 1.1 oz.	20.0	1.0
(*Chips Ahoy!* Reduced Fat), 3 pieces, 1.1 oz.	22.0	1.0
(*Famous Amos*), 4 pieces, 1 oz.	20.0	<1.0
(*Grandma's* Homestyle), 1.4-oz. piece	28.0	1.0
(*Grandma's* Mini Bites), 1 pkg.	29.0	1.0
(*Grandma's* Rich'n Chewy), 1 pkg.	39.0	1.0
(*Health Valley* Chunk), .9-oz. piece	15.0	1.0
(*Health Valley* Mini), 4 pieces, 1 oz.	16.0	1.0
(*Health Valley Cafe Creations*), .8-oz. piece	13.0	2.0
(*Keebler Chips Deluxe* Chocolate Lovers/Soft & Chewy),		
6-oz. piece	10.0	0
(*Keebler Soft Batch*), .6-oz. piece	10.0	<1.0
(*Murray* Sugar Free), 3 pieces, 1.1 oz.	20.0	<1.0
(*SnackWell's*), 13 pieces, 1 oz.	22.0	1.0

Food and Measure	carb. (gms)	fiber (gms)
(*Tofutti*), 1.1-oz. piece	19.0	0
almond (*Pepperidge Farm Sanibel*), .9-oz. piece	16.0	<1.0
caramel (*Pepperidge Farm* Soft), 1-oz. piece	21.0	<1.0
chocolate (*Health Valley* Mini), 4 pieces, 1 oz.	16.0	1.0
chocolate (*Health Valley Cafe Creations*), .8-oz. piece	13.0	2.0
coconut (*Keebler Chips Deluxe* Tropical), .5-oz. piece	9.0	0
dark chocolate (*Pepperidge Farm* Soft), 1.1-oz. piece	20.0	0
double (*Health Valley* Chunk), .9-oz. piece	15.0	1.0
double (*Pepperidge Farm Nantucket*), .9-oz. piece	18.0	1.0
fudge (*Grandma's* Homestyle), 1.4-oz. piece	28.0	1.0
macadamia (*Mauna Loa*), 2 pieces, .9 oz.	18.0	1.0
macadamia (*Pepperidge Farm Sausalito*), .9-oz. piece	16.0	0
macadamia (*Pepperidge Farm Sausalito* Mini), 4 pieces, 1 oz.	17.0	0
oatmeal (*Country Choice*), .8-oz. piece	15.0	1.0
oatmeal (*Health Valley*), .8-oz. piece	14.0	1.0
oatmeal and walnuts (*Famous Amos*), 4 pieces, 1 oz.	19.0	1.0
pecan (*Famous Amos*), 4 pieces, 1 oz.	19.0	<1.0
pecan (*Murray* Sugar Free), 3 pieces, 1.1 oz.	19.0	<1.0
pecan (*Pepperidge Farm Chesapeake*), .9-oz. piece	15.0	0
powdered sugar (*Keebler* Danish Wedding), 4 pieces, .9 oz.	18.0	<1.0
rainbow (*Keebler Chips Deluxe*), .6-oz. piece	10.0	<1.0
rainbow, mini (*Keebler Chips Deluxe*), 4 pieces, 1.1 oz.	20.0	0
toffee pecan (*Pepperidge Farm Sedona*), .9-oz. piece	17.0	1.0
walnut (*Country Choice*), .8-oz. piece	16.0	<1.0
wheat free (*Foods by George*), 3.25-oz. piece	57.0	2.0
white chocolate (*Health Valley* Chunk), .9-oz. piece	17.0	1.0
white chocolate, macadamia (*Mauna Loa*), 2 pieces, .9 oz.	18.0	1.0
white chocolate, macadamia (*Pepperidge Farm Tahoe*), .9-oz. piece	17.0	<1.0
white fudge, chunky (*Chips Ahoy!*), .6-oz. piece	10.0	0
chocolate chip sandwich, vanilla crème (*Chips Ahoy! Cremewiches*), 1.1 oz.	22.0	1.0
chocolate sandwich:		
(*Austin Choco Cremes*), 1 pkg.	37.0	2.0
(*Country Choice Cremes*), 2 pieces, 1 oz.	19.0	0

Food and Measure	carb. (gms)	fiber (gms)
(*Emperador*), 2 pieces, .9 oz.	19.0	<1.0
(*Famous Amos* Cremes), 3 pieces, 1.2 oz.	24.0	<1.0
(*Murray* Sugar Free Cremes), 3 pieces, 1 oz.	18.0	<1.0
(*Oreo*), 3 pieces, 1.2 oz.	24.0	1.0
(*Oreo*), 1.5-oz. pkg.	29.0	1.0
(*Oreo* Mini Bite Size), 9 pieces, 1 oz.	21.0	1.0
(*Oreo* Reduced Fat), 3 pieces, 1.2 oz.	26.0	1.0
(*Oreo Carb Well*), .8 oz.	16.0	3.0
(*Oreo Double Stuf*) 2 pieces, 1 oz.	20.0	1.0
(*Pepperidge Farm Bordeaux*), 4 pieces, .9 oz.	19.0	<1.0
(*Pepperidge Farm Bordeaux* Mini), 13 pieces, 1 oz.	21.0	<1.0
(*Pepperidge Farm Brussels*), 3 pieces, 1.1 oz.	20.0	1.0
(*Pepperidge Farm Brussels* Mini), 8 pieces, 1 oz.	19.0	1.0
(*Pepperidge Farm Milano*), 3 pieces, 1.2 oz.	21.0	<1.0
(*Pepperidge Farm Milano* Mini), 6 pieces, 1 oz.	18.0	<1.0
chocolate crème (*Oreo*), 3 pieces, 1.1 oz.	21.0	1.0
chocolate crème, mini (*Oreo*), 9 pieces, 1 oz.	21.0	1.0
chocolate crème, mini (*Oreo*), 1.25-oz. pkg.	25.0	1.0
double (*Health Valley Cookie Cremes*), 2 pieces, .9 oz.	19.0	0
double (*Pepperidge Farm Milano*), 2 pieces, 1 oz.	17.0	<1.0
fudge coated (*Oreo*), .7-oz. piece	13.0	1.0
fudge coated, white (*Oreo*), .75-oz. piece	14.0	0
fudge mint coated (*Oreo*), .6-oz. piece	12.0	1.0
golden, with chocolate crème (*Oreo Uh-Oh!*), 1.2 oz.	24.0	1.0
mint (*Health Valley Cookie Cremes*), 2 pieces, .9 oz.	19.0	0
mint/creme (*Oreo* Double Delight), 1 oz.	20.0	1.0
mint or orange (*Pepperidge Farm Milano*), 2 pieces, .9 oz.	16.0	<1.0
rainbow crème (*Austin Snackerz*), 7 pieces, 1 oz.	20.0	<1.0
raspberry (*Pepperidge Farm Milano*), 2 pieces, .9 oz.	16.0	<1.0
vanilla crème (*Health Valley* Bars), 1.7-oz. piece	32.0	1.0
cinnamon:		
(*Roscas*), 3 pieces, 1 oz.	22.0	1.0
(*Stella D'oro* Viennese Breakfast Treats), .8-oz. piece	16.0	0
raisin (*Stella D'oro* Toast), 2 pieces, .9 oz.	20.0	0
coconut:		
(*Arcoiris*), 1 pkg., 6 pieces	44.0	1.0
(*Gamesa* Barras de Coco), 5 pieces, 1 oz.	21.0	<1.0

Food and Measure	carb. (gms)	fiber (gms)
(*Hawaianas*), 3 pieces, 1 oz.	22.0	<1.0
filled (*Almond Joy*), 2 pieces, 1 oz.	17.0	<1.0
crème sandwich (*Country Choice* Organic Duplex), 2 pieces, 1 oz.	19.0	0
crème-filled stick, 2 pieces, .9 oz.:		
chocolate hazelnut (*Pepperidge Farm Pirouette*)	10.0	<1.0
mint chocolate (*Pepperidge Farm Pirouette*)	19.0	0
vanilla (*Pepperidge Farm Pirouette*)	18.0	0
devil's food:		
(*Tree of Life* Monster Fat Free), ¼ piece	20.0	2.0
cake (*SnackWell's*), .6-oz. piece	12.0	0
chocolate (*Tree of Life* Fat Free), .8-oz. piece	15.0	1.0
egg biscuits (*Stella D'oro* Jumbo), 2 pieces, 1.2 oz.	26.0	0
egg biscuits (*Stella D'oro* Roman), 1.2-oz. piece	21.0	0
fig filled/bar:		
(*Barbara's*), .7-oz. piece	14.0	0
(*Barbara's* Wheat Free/Whole Wheat), .7-oz. piece	13.0	1.0
(*Newtons*), 2 pieces, 1.1 oz.	22.0	1.0
(*Newtons*), 2-oz. pkg.	40.0	3.0
(*Tofutti Tofiggy*), 1.1-oz. piece	21.0	0
apple cinnamon or raspberry (*Barbara's*), .7-oz. piece	14.0	1.0
blueberry (*Barbara's*), .7-oz. piece	15.0	0
fortune (*Port Arthur*), 3 pieces	23.0	0
fruit slices (*Stella D'oro*), 1.2 oz.	20.0	1.0
fudge:		
(*Stella D'oro* Swiss), 2 pieces, 1.2 oz.	22.0	1.0
double (*Murray* Sugar Free), 3 pieces, 1.2 oz.	23.0	2.0
sticks (*Keebler Fudge Shoppe*), 3 pieces, 1 oz.	19.0	0
sticks (*Keebler Fudge Shoppe* Fudge Lovers), 3 pieces, 1 oz.	17.0	<1.0
stripe (*Keebler Fudge Shoppe*), 3 pieces, 1.1 oz.	20.0	<1.0
stripe (*Keebler Fudge Shoppe* Sugar Free), 3 pieces, 1 oz.	18.0	1.0
stripe, mini (*Keebler Fudge Shoppe*), 14 pieces, 1.1 oz.	20.0	<1.0
fudge sandwich:		
(*Keebler E.L. Fudge Butterfinger* Blasted), 2 pieces, 1.2 oz.	23.0	<1.0
(*Keebler E.L. Fudge* S'mores Blasted), 2 pieces, 1.2 oz.	23.0	0

Food and Measure	carb. (gms)	fiber (gms)
double stuffed (*Keebler E.L. Fudge*), 2 pieces, 1.2 oz. ...	23.0	0
fudge cookies (*Keebler E.L. Fudge*), 2 pieces, .9 oz. ...	18.0	<1.0
mini (*Keebler E.L. Fudge*), 7 pieces, 1 oz.	21.0	0
ginger:		
(*Country Choice*), .8-oz. piece	17.0	<1.0
(*Pepperidge Farm* Gingerman), 4 pieces, .9 oz.	21.0	<1.0
snaps (*Country Choice*), 5 pieces	19.0	2.0
snaps (*Murray* Sugar Free), 7 pieces, 1.1 oz.	23.0	0
snaps (*Nabisco*), 4 pieces, 1 oz.	22.0	0
ginger-lemon sandwich (*Carr's*), 2 pieces, 1 oz.	19.0	<1.0
ginger-lemon sandwich (*Country Choice* Cremes), 2 pieces, 1 oz.	19.0	0
graham cracker:		
amaranth or oat bran (*Health Valley Graham Crackers*), 6 pieces, 1 oz.	22.0	3.0
cinnamon (*Barbara's* Organic Go Go), 8 pieces, 1.1 oz.	23.0	<1.0
cinnamon (*Honey Maid*), 1.1 oz.	25.0	1.0
cinnamon (*Honey Maid* Low Fat), 1.1 oz.	26.0	1.0
cinnamon (*New Morning*), 2 pieces, 1.1 oz.	24.0	<1.0
cinnamon (*Ricanelas*), 8 pieces, 1.1 oz.	24.0	2.0
cinnamon (*Teddy Grahams*), 1.25-oz. pkg.	27.0	1.0
cinnamon, sticks (*Honey Maid*), 1-oz. pkg.	23.0	1.0
cinnamon or honey (*Teddy Grahams*), 24 pieces, 1.1 oz.	23.0	1.0
honey (*Honey Maid*), 1.1 oz.	24.0	1.0
honey (*Honey Maid* Low Fat/Sticks), 1.1 oz.	25.0	1.0
honey (*New Morning*), 2 pieces, 1.1 oz.	24.0	1.0
honey (*New Morning* Bites), 22 pieces, 1 oz.	18.0	0
honey (*Teddy Grahams*), 1.25-oz. pkg.	26.0	1.0
honey or lemon ginger (*Barbara's* Organic Go Go), 8 pieces, 1.1 oz.	22.0	<1.0
graham, chocolate:		
(*Barbara's* Organic Go Go), 8 pieces, 1.1 oz.	23.0	1.0
(*Honey Maid/Honey Maid* Sticks), 1.1 oz.	24.0	1.0
(*New Morning* Bites), 22 pieces, 1 oz.	19.0	0
(*Teddy Grahams*), 1.25-oz. pkg.	26.0	1.0
or chocolate chip (*Teddy Grahams*), 1.1 oz.	22.0	1.0

Food and Measure	carb. (gms)	fiber (gms)
graham, fudge coated:		
(*Keebler Fudge Shoppe*), 3 pieces, 1 oz.	19.0	<1.0
mini (*Keebler Fudge Shoppe*), 10 pieces, 1.2 oz.	22.0	<1.0
graham sandwich:		
chocolate, crème (*Teddy Grahams Bearwiches*),		
1.1-oz. piece	21.0	1.0
chocolate or honey, butter (*New Morning*),		
2 pieces, 1 oz.	18.0	0
honey, crème (*Teddy Grahams Bearwiches*),		
1-oz. piece	21.0	0
honey, vanilla (*New Morning*), 2 pieces, 1 oz.	19.0	0
s'mores (*Austin*), 7 pieces, 1 oz.	21.0	0
s'mores (*Ritz Bits*), 1.1 oz.	22.0	1.0
granola (*Tree of Life* Monster), ⅕ piece	19.0	1.0
hazelnut créme sandwich (*Bahlsen*), 3 pieces, 1.1 oz.	19.0	0
lemon nut (*Pepperidge Farm*), 3 pieces, 1.1 oz.	19.0	2.0
lemon wafers (*Murray* Sugar Free), 4 pieces, 1 oz.	19.0	0
lemon sandwich:		
(*Austin Lemon Ohs!*), 1 pkg.	37.0	<1.0
(*Emperador*), 1 pkg., 6 pieces	45.0	1.0
(*Murray* Sugar Free), 3 pieces, 1 oz.	19.0	<1.0
(*SnackWell's* Sugar Free), 3 pieces, 1.1 oz.	24.0	0
lemon tartlets (*Bonne Maman*), .6-oz. piece	11.0	0
macadamia nut crunch (*Mauna Loa*), 2 pieces, .9 oz.	15.0	1.0
macaroon:		
coconut (*Streit's*), 2 pieces, 1 oz.	12.0	2.0
honey (*Tree of Life* Monster), ⅕ piece	17.0	1.0
oatmeal (*Famous Amos*), 3 pieces, 1.2 oz.	23.0	<1.0
maple pecan (*Tree of Life* Monster Fat Free), ¼ piece	21.0	2.0
marshmallow, chocolate:		
(*Arcoiris*), 2 pieces, 1 oz.	18.0	<1.0
(*Mallomars*), 2 pieces, .9 oz.	17.0	1.0
fudge (*Twirls*), 1.1 oz.	20.0	0
marshmallow sandwich (*Arcoiris*), 1 pkg., 6 pieces	43.0	1.0
mint, chocolate coated:		
(*Keebler Fudge Shoppe Grasshopper*), 4 piece, 1 oz.	19.0	<1.0
(*York*), 2 pieces, 1 oz.	17.0	1.0
mint sandwich (*Country Choice* Cremes), 2 pieces, 1 oz.	19.0	0

Food and Measure	carb. (gms)	fiber (gms)
oatmeal:		
(*Barbara's*), .6-oz. piece	8.0	<1.0
(*Country Choice* Old Fashioned), .8-oz. piece	16.0	1.0
(*Murray* Sugar Free), 3 pieces, 1.1 oz.	21.0	1.0
(*SnackWell's* Sugar Free), .8 oz.	17.0	1.0
(*Tree of Life* Wheat Free Americana), .8-oz. piece	11.0	1.0
peanut crunch (*Health Valley*), .8-oz. piece	14.0	1.0
oatmeal raisin:		
(*Country Choice*), .8-oz. piece	16.0	1.0
(*Famous Amos*), 4 pieces, 1 oz.	21.0	<1.0
(*Grandma's* Homestyle), 1.4-oz. piece	30.0	1.0
(*Health Valley*), .8-oz. piece	14.0	1.0
(*Health Valley Cafe Creations*), .8-oz. piece	15.0	1.0
(*Pepperidge Farm Santa Cruz*), .9-oz. piece	23.0	2.0
golden (*Tree of Life* Fat Free), .8-oz. piece	16.0	1.0
orange (*Morelianas*), .9 oz.	19.0	0
peanut butter:		
(*Chips Ahoy!*), .5-oz. piece	9.0	0
(*Country Choice*), .8-oz. piece	13.0	<1.0
(*Grandma's* Homestyle), 1.4-oz. piece	24.0	1.0
(*Health Valley* Mini), 4 pieces, 1 oz.	16.0	0
(*Murray* Sugar Free), 3 pieces, 1.1 oz.	17.0	1.0
(*Tofutti*), 1.1-oz. piece	18.0	0
(*Tree of Life* Monster), ⅕ piece	17.0	1.0
(*Tree of Life* Wheat Free Georgia), .8-oz. piece	8.0	1.0
cup (*Keebler Chips Deluxe*), .6-oz. piece	10.0	0
filled (*Reese's*), 2 pieces, 1 oz.	17.0	<1.0
fudge sticks (*Keebler Fudge Shoppe*), 3 pieces, 1 oz.	18.0	<1.0
swirl (*Health Valley* Bars), 1.7-oz. piece	33.0	1.0
peanut butter sandwich:		
(*Nutter Butter*), 1 oz.	18.0	1.0
(*Nutter Butter* Bites), 10 pieces, 1.1 oz.	20.0	1.0
(*Nutter Butter* Bites), 1.25-oz. pkg.	23.0	1.0
crèmes (*Grandma's*), 5 pieces, 1.2 oz.	28.0	1.0
double stuffed (*Keebler E.L. Fudge*), 2 pieces, 1.2 oz.	21.0	<1.0
pecan, wheat free (*Foods by George*), 3.25-oz. piece	50.0	1.0
rainbow chips sandwich crèmes (*Keebler Chips Deluxe*), .6-oz. piece	11.0	0

Food and Measure	carb. (gms)	fiber (gms)
raspberry (*Pepperidge Farm Chantilly*), 2 pieces, .9 oz.	23.0	<1.0
raspberry bar (*Newtons*), 2 pieces, 1 oz.	21.0	1.0
shortbread:		
(*Barbara's*), .6-oz. piece	9.0	<1.0
(*Lorna Doone*), 4 pieces, 1 oz.	19.0	0
(*Murray* Sugar Free), 8 pieces, 1.1 oz.	22.0	1.0
(*Pepperidge Farm*), 2 pieces, .9 oz.	16.0	<1.0
(*Sandies* Simply Shortbread), .6-oz. piece	10.0	0
(*SnackWell's* Sugar Free), 3 pieces, 1.1 oz.	22.0	1.0
fudge dipped (*Murray* Sugar Free), 5 pieces, 1 oz.	20.0	<1.0
fudge stripe (*SnackWell's*), .8 oz.	16.0	1.0
pecan (*Murray* Sugar Free), 3 pieces, 1.1 oz.	18.0	<1.0
pecan, caramel or chocolate chip, or cinnamon swirl (*Sandies*), .6-oz. piece	9.0	0
strawberry filled (*Health Valley Bars*), 1.7-oz. piece	33.0	1.0
spice (*Stella D'oro* Pfeffernusse), .9 oz.	18.0	0
strawberry:		
(*Newtons*), 2 pieces, 1 oz.	20.0	1.0
(*Pepperidge Farm Verona*), 3 pieces, .9 oz.	22.0	<1.0
cheesecake (*Sandies* Fruit Delights), .6-oz. piece	11.0	<1.0
yogurt bar (*Newtons*), 2 pieces, 1.3 oz.	26.0	1.0
strawberry sandwich (*Emperador*), 2 pieces, .9 oz.	19.0	<1.0
sugar (*Pepperidge Farm*), 3 pieces, 1.1 oz.	20.0	<1.0
sugar wafer:		
(*Biscos*), 8 pieces, 1 oz.	21.0	0
(*Gamesa*), 3 pieces, 1.2 oz.	23.0	0
strawberry (*Gamesa*), 3 pieces, 1.2 oz.	24.0	0
vanilla (*Gamesa*), 3 pieces, 1.2 oz.	25.0	0
vanilla (*Murray* Sugar Free), 4 pieces, 1 oz.	19.0	0
vanilla sandwich:		
(*Austin* Cremes), 1 pkg.	37.0	<1.0
(*Country Choice* Cremes), 2 pieces, 1 oz.	19.0	0
(*Emperador*), 2 pieces, .9 oz.	19.0	0
(*Grandma's* Mini Bites), 9 pieces, 1.1 oz.	22.0	<1.0
(*Grandma's* Sandwich Cremes), 5 pieces, 1.5 oz.	30.0	<1.0
(*Health Valley Cookie Cremes*), 2 pieces, .9 oz.	19.0	0
(*Murray* Sugar Free Cremes), 3 pieces, 1 oz.	19.0	<1.0

Food and Measure	carb. (gms)	fiber (gms)
(*SnackWell's*), 2 pieces, .9 oz.	20.0	0
(*SnackWell's*), 1.7-oz. pkg.	38.0	1.0
(*Vienna Fingers*), 2 pieces, 1.1 oz.	21.0	0
rainbow crème (*Austin Snackerz*), 7 pieces, 1 oz.	21.0	0
vanilla wafer:		
(*Country Choice*), 7 pieces	19.0	2.0
(*Keebler* Reduced Fat), 8 pieces, 1.1 oz.	25.0	<1.0
(*Murray* Sugar Free), 9 pieces, 1 oz.	22.0	<1.0
(*Murray* Sugar Free Reduced Fat), 8 pieces, 1.1 oz.	25.0	<1.0
(*Nilla*), 8 pieces, 1.1 oz.	21.0	0
(*Nilla* Reduced Fat), 8 pieces, 1 oz.	24.0	0
fudge dipped (*Murray* Sugar Free), 4 pieces, 1.1 oz.	19.0	<1.0
mini, golden (*Murray* Sugar Free), 18 pieces, 1.1 oz.	21.0	<1.0
Cookie, frozen or refrigerated, ready-to-bake, 1 piece, except as noted:		
chocolate candy, with chips (*Pillsbury*)	16.0	0
chocolate chip:		
(*Kineret*)	17.0	0
(*Pillsbury* Family Size), 1 oz., 1½'' ball	17.0	<1.0
(*Pillsbury* Reduced Fat), 1 oz., 1½'' ball	19.0	<1.0
(*Pillsbury Big Deluxe Classics*)	25.0	<1.0
(*Pillsbury Ready To Bake*)	15.0	<1.0
(*Pillsbury Ready To Bake* Sugar Free)	16.0	3.0
with caramel, pecans (*Pillsbury Big Deluxe Classics* Turtle Supreme)	25.0	<1.0
chips and chunks (*Pillsbury Ready To Bake*)	15.0	<1.0
double, chips and chunks (*Pillsbury*), 1 oz., 1½'' ball	17.0	<1.0
mini (*Pillsbury Ready To Bake* Bites), 4 pieces	15.0	1.0
walnut (*Pillsbury*), 1 oz., 1½'' ball	16.0	<1.0
walnut (*Pillsbury Ready To Bake*)	14.0	0
chocolate chunk (*Pillsbury*), 1 oz., 1½'' ball	17.0	<1.0
gingerbread (*Pillsbury*), 1 cutout piece	12.0	0
oatmeal chocolate chip (*Pillsbury*), 1 oz., 1½'' ball	17.0	<1.0
oatmeal raisin (*Pillsbury Big Deluxe Classics*)	26.0	1.0
peanut butter:		
(*Pillsbury*), 1 oz., 1½'' ball	17.0	0
(*Pillsbury Ready To Bake* Reese's Pieces)	15.0	0
cup (*Pillsbury Big Deluxe Classics*)	24.0	<1.0

Food and Measure	carb. (gms)	fiber (gms)
sugar:		
(*Pillsbury*), 2 slices, ¼"	19.0	0
(*Pillsbury Ready To Bake*)	15.0	0
Christmas or Easter with images (*Pillsbury*)	18.0	0
shapes, all varieties (*Pillsbury*), 2 pieces	17.0	0
white chunk macadamia (*Pillsbury Big Deluxe Classics*) ..	24.0	<1.0
Cookie, mix, 2 pieces*:		
chocolate chip/chunk, double (*Betty Crocker*)	21.0	0
chocolate peanut butter chip (*Betty Crocker*)	30.0	0
oatmeal chocolate chip (*Betty Crocker*)	21.0	0
peanut butter (*Betty Crocker*)	20.0	0
rainbow chocolate candy or sugar (*Betty Crocker*)	22.0	0
Cookie crumbs:		
(*Oreo*), 2 tbsp.	13.0	1.0
(*Oreo* Crunchies), 2 tbsp.	8.0	0
Cookie pie crust, see "Pie crust"		
Coquito nuts (*Frieda's*), 11 pieces, 1 oz.	5.0	3.0
Coriander, fresh, ¼ cup	.1	.1
Coriander, dried:		
leaf, 1 tsp.	.3	.1
seed, 1 tsp.	1.0	.5
Corn, fresh:		
baby, .28-oz. ear	2.0	.2
golden or white, raw, 5-oz. ear	27.2	3.9
golden or white, kernels, boiled, drained, ½ cup	20.6	2.3
white, boiled, drained, 2.72-oz. ear	19.3	2.1
Corn, canned, ½ cup, except as noted:		
baby, whole, stir-fry (*Port Arthur*)	3.0	4.0
kernel, golden:		
(*Del Monte*)	18.0	3.0
(*Del Monte* Supersweet/Supersweet No Salt)	11.0	3.0
(*Del Monte* Supersweet Vac Pac/Vac Pac No Salt)	13.0	3.0
(*Freshlike*)	17.0	2.0
(*Green Giant*)	18.0	2.0
(*Green Giant* 50% Less Sodium)	17.0	2.0
(*Green Giant Niblets* Extra Sweet), ⅓ cup	10.0	2.0
(*Green Giant Niblets* No Salt), ⅓ cup	13.0	2.0

Food and Measure	carb. (gms)	fiber (gms)
(*Green Giant Niblets* Vac Pac), ⅓ cup	16.0	<1.0
(*S&W*)	11.0	3.0
(*S&W* Vac Pac)	13.0	3.0
(*Veg-All*)	16.0	2.0
(*Westbrae Natural* Organic)	14.0	2.0
kernel, golden/white, (*Del Monte* Supersweet)	18.0	2.0
kernel, golden/white, (*Green Giant* Vac Pac), ⅓ cup	11.0	1.0
kernel, white:		
(*Del Monte*)	11.0	3.0
(*Green Giant* Shoepeg Vac Pac), ⅓ cup	16.0	1.0
(*Westbrae Natural* Organic)	20.0	1.0
cream style:		
(*Del Monte/Del Monte* No Salt)	20.0	2.0
(*Del Monte* Supersweet/Supersweet No Salt)	14.0	2.0
(*Freshlike/Veg-All*), ⅓ cup	21.0	2.0
(*Green Giant*)	19.0	1.0
(*S&W*)	14.0	2.0
seasoned (*Glory* Skillet Corn)	22.0	2.0
white (*Del Monte*)	21.0	2.0
in butter sauce (*Del Monte Savory Sides*)	14.0	<1.0
with diced pepper (*Freshlike* Selects)	16.0	1.0
with diced pepper (*Green Giant Mexicorn*), ⅓ cup	14.0	1.0
seasoned (*Del Monte* Fiesta Supersweet)	12.0	2.0
with tomato and black beans (*Del Monte Savory Sides* Santa Fe)	16.0	1.0
Corn, dried (*John Cope's*), ¼ cup	15.0	1.0
Corn, freeze-dried, ½ cup:		
(*AlpineAire*)	16.0	3.0
(*Mountain House*)	16.0	2.0
Corn, frozen:		
on cob (*Green Giant*), 4.4-oz. ear	22.0	3.0
on cob (*Green Giant* Nibbers Halves), ½ ear, 2.2 oz.	14.0	1.0
kernel, golden:		
(*Birds Eye* Sweet), ⅔ cup	21.0	1.0
(*Birds Eye* Super Sweet), ⅔ cup	14.0	2.0
(*Cascadian Farm* Super Sweet), ¾ cup	16.0	2.0
(*Cascadian Farm* Sweet), ¾ cup	18.0	2.0

Food and Measure	carb. (gms)	fiber (gms)
(*C&W/C&W Early Harvest*/Organic/Petite), ⅔ cup	19.0	1.0
(*Green Giant Niblets*), ⅓ cup cooked	17.0	2.0
(*Green Giant Niblets* Extra Sweet), ⅓ cup cooked	13.0	2.0
(*McKenzie's* Southern), ½ cup	19.0	1.0
(*Dr. Praeger's*), ⅔ cup	21.0	1.0
(*Tree of Life*), ⅔ cup	19.0	1.0
kernel, golden/white:		
(*C&W* Petite), ⅔ cup	19.0	1.0
(*Green Giant Select*), ¾ cup	14.0	2.0
baby (*Birds Eye*), ⅔ cup	20.0	2.0
kernel, white:		
(*C&W* Petite), ⅔ cup	19.0	1.0
(*Green Giant* Shoepeg), ½ cup	14.0	2.0
(*Green Giant Select* Shoepeg), ¾ cup	20.0	3.0
baby (*Birds Eye*), ⅔ cup	18.0	3.0
in butter sauce:		
(*Birds Eye*, 9 oz.), ½ cup	28.0	2.0
(*Birds Eye*, 24 oz.), ¾ cup	22.0	1.0
(*Cascadian Farm*), ½ cup	19.0	2.0
(*Green Giant Niblets*), ½ cup, cooked	19.0	2.0
(*Green Giant Niblets* Boil-in-Bag), ⅔ cup	22.0	2.0
white (*Green Giant* Shoepeg), ¾ cup	21.0	3.0
cream style (*Green Giant*), ½ cup	23.0	2.0
fried (*Glory* Savory Accents), ½ cup	24.0	2.0
Corn, whole-grain:		
1 oz.	21.1	2.1
1 cup	123.3	12.2
Corn bran, crude, 1 cup	65.1	64.3
Corn bread, see "Bread mix, sweet"		
Corn bread and bean entree, frozen, red beans		
(*Moosewood*), 10-oz. pkg.	62.0	9.0
Corn cake mix, sweet, dry (*Chi-Chi's*), ½ cup	22.0	0
Corn combinations, frozen:		
baby carrots, sugar snap peas (*C&W*), ⅔ cup	10.0	2.0
baby corn and green beans, peas (*Birds Eye*), ¾ cup	13.0	2.0
baby corn and vegetable blend (*Birds Eye*), ⅔ cup	9.0	3.0
black beans, tomatoes (*C&W Corn Salsa*), 1 cup	18.0	3.0
broccoli florets, red peppers (*C&W*), ⅔ cup	14.0	1.0

Food and Measure	carb. (gms)	fiber (gms)
and peas, herb butter sauce (*Green Giant*), ¾ cup	14.0	3.0
red peppers, roasted, Southwestern (*Green Giant*), ¾ cup	17.0	2.0
Corn crisps/chips (see also "Snack chips"), 1 oz., except as noted:		
(*Corn Nuts* Original)	20.0	2.0
(*Dipsy Doodles*)	16.0	1.0
(*Fritos*)	15.0	1.0
(*Fritos* King Size/*Fritos Scoops!*)	16.0	1.0
(*O-Ke-Doke* Puffs), 2½ cups	18.0	<1.0
(*Sun Chips* Original)	19.0	2.0
(*Wise/Moore's*)	16.0	1.0
barbecue:		
(*Bugles* Smokin'), 1.1 oz.	18.0	0
(*Corn Nuts*)	20.0	4.0
(*Dipsy Doodles/Moore's*)	16.0	1.0
(*Fritos*)	16.0	1.0
honey (*Fritos Flavor Twists*)	16.0	1.0
butter flavor (*Chester's* Puffcorn)	12.0	<1.0
butter flavor (*Hain PureSnax Zoinks*), 1.1 oz.	23.0	<1.0
cheese:		
(*Barbara's* Puff Bakes)	13.0	0
(*Barbara's* Puffs)	16.0	0
(*Bugles*), 1.1 oz.	18.0	<1.0
(*Cheese Doodles* Crunchy)	20.0	0
(*Cheese Doodles* Puffed)	13.0	0
(*Cheetos* Crunchy)	15.0	<1.0
(*Cheetos* Crunchy Baked!)	19.0	0
(*Cheetos* Puffs/Twisted)	13.0	0
(*Cheetos Asteroids*)	15.0	1.0
(*Cheetos Edge* Puffs)	7.0	<1.0
(*Chester's* Puffcorn)	12.0	0
(*Snyder's* Twist)	15.0	<1.0
chili (*Bugles*), 1.1 oz.	18.0	0
hot (*Cheetos Asteroids Flamin' Hot*)	13.0	<1.0
hot (*Cheetos Flamin' Hot*)	14.0	<1.0
hot (*Cheetos Flamin' Hot* Limón)	15.0	<1.0
hot (*Chester's Flamin' Hot* Fries)	17.0	<1.0
jalapeño (*Barbara's* Puffs)	16.0	0

Food and Measure	carb. (gms)	fiber (gms)
nacho (*Bugles*), 1.1 oz.	18.0	<1.0
nacho (*Corn Nuts*)	19.0	2.0
nacho (*Doodle Twisters*)	16.0	1.0
cheese, cheddar:		
(*Shiloh Farms* Curls)	13.0	0
(*Sun Chips* Harvest)	19.0	2.0
ranch (*Fritos Flavor Twists*)	17.0	1.0
with rice (*Snyder's CheddAirs* Puffs)	20.0	n.a.
white (*Barbara's* Puff Bakes)	13.0	0
white (*Cheetos* Puffs)	16.0	<1.0
white (*Hain PureSnax Zoinks*), 1.1 oz.	22.0	1.0
chili cheese (*Fritos*)	15.0	1.0
chili lime (*Sabritones*)	13.0	1.0
chili picante (*Corn Nuts*)	19.0	2.0
hot (*Fritos Flamin' Hot*)	15.0	1.0
mac and cheese (*Cheese Doodles*)	12.0	0
onion:		
(*Funyuns* Rings)	18.0	<1.0
(*Funyuns* Rings Mini), 1 pkg.	30.0	1.0
French (*Sun Chips*)	18.0	2.0
rings (*Wise*), .5 oz.	10.0	1.0
ranch (*Corn Nuts*)	19.0	2.0
salsa (*Corn Nuts* Jalisco)	20.0	2.0
tortilla:		
(*Cape Cod* Whole Earth)	19.0	2.0
(*Cape Cod* Whole Earth Reduced Carb)	11.0	2.0
(*Doritos* Ranchero!)	17.0	1.0
(*Doritos* Toasted Corn)	18.0	1.0
(*D.L. Jardine's* Texaditas)	19.0	2.0
(*Garden of Eatin'* White Chips/Mini Strips/Rounds)	19.0	2.0
(*Guiltless Gourmet* White Corn)	22.0	2.0
(*Santitas*)	19.0	1.0
(*Snyder's*)	23.0	1.0
(*Tostitos* Bite Size)	17.0	1.0
(*Tostitos* Bite Size Baked!)	24.0	2.0
(*Tostitos* Light)	20.0	1.0
(*Tostitos* Restaurant Style)	19.0	1.0
(*Tostitos* Rounds/*Tostitos Scoops!*)	18.0	1.0

Food and Measure	carb. (gms)	fiber (gms)
(*Tostitos Edge*)	9.0	3.0
(*Tostitos Gold*)	19.0	1.0
black pepper jack (*Doritos*)	18.0	1.0
cheese (*Doritos* Spicier Nacho!)	18.0	1.0
cheese (*Doritos Nacho Cheesier*)	17.0	1.0
cheese (*Doritos Nacho Cheesier* Baked!)	21.0	2.0
cheese (*Doritos Nacho Cheesier* Light)	18.0	1.0
cheese (*Guiltless Gourmet* Mucho Nacho)	20.0	3.0
cheese, four (*Doritos*)	17.0	1.0
cheese, nacho (*Snyder's*)	16.0	1.0
cheese, nacho (*Wise Bravos!*)	17.0	1.0
cheese, white nacho (*Doritos* Natural)	17.0	1.0
chili (*Kettle Fire Roasted Chili* Organic)	18.0	2.0
chili lime (*Garden of Eatin'*)	18.0	2.0
chili lime (*Guiltless Gourmet*)	22.0	2.0
garlic herb (*Cape Cod* Whole Earth)	19.0	2.0
guacamole (*Doritos*)	16.0	1.0
guacamole (*Garden of Eatin'*)	19.0	2.0
lime, hint of (*Tostitos*)	19.0	1.0
with mixed grains (*Garden of Eatin' Garden Grains*)	18.0	2.0
multigrain, black bean, garlic, onion (*Kettle* Organic)	16.0	2.0
multigrain, 5 grain (*Kettle* Organic)	18.0	2.0
pico de gallo (*Garden of Eatin'*)	18.0	3.0
ranch (*Doritos Cooler Ranch* Baked!)	21.0	2.0
ranch (*Doritos Cooler Ranch*/Cool Natural)	18.0	1.0
ranch (*Doritos Edge*)	9.0	3.0
ranch (*Doritos Rollitos Cooler Ranch*)	17.0	1.0
salsa (*Doritos*)	17.0	1.0
salsa verde (*Doritos*)	19.0	1.0
sesame rye, with caraway (*Kettle* Organic)	17.0	2.0
taco (*Doritos*)	18.0	1.0
taco (*Doritos Rollitos* Zesty)	17.0	1.0
tamari (*Garden of Eatin'*)	18.0	3.0
veggie (*Cape Cod* Whole Earth)	18.0	1.0
tortilla, blue corn:		
(*Garden of Eatin'*/*Garden of Eatin' Red Hot Blues*)	18.0	2.0
(*Garden of Eatin' Little Soy Blue/Sunny Blues*)	17.0	2.0
(*Garden of Eatin' Sesame Blues*)	16.0	2.0

Food and Measure	carb. (gms)	fiber (gms)
(*Guiltless Gourmet*)	22.0	2.0
(*Kettle* Organic)	18.0	2.0
(*Snyder's* Organic/Organic Sesame)	17.0	n.a.
(*Tostitos* Natural)	19.0	1.0
black bean, spicy (*Guiltless Gourmet*)	22.0	2.0
sesame (*Cape Cod* Whole Earth)	19.0	2.0
sesame (*Kettle* Blue Moons Organic)	19.0	2.0
tortilla, red corn:		
(*Garden of Eatin'*)	18.0	1.0
(*Guiltless Gourmet*)	22.0	2.0
salsa (*Garden of Eatin'*)	18.0	3.0
tortilla, yellow corn:		
(*Garden of Eatin'*/*Garden of Eatin'* Mini Rounds)	18.0	2.0
(*Guiltless Gourmet*/*Guiltless Gourmet* Unsalted)	22.0	2.0
(*Kettle Little Dippers* Organic)	19.0	2.0
(*Santitas*)	19.0	1.0
(*Snyder's*)	23.0	1.0
(*Tostitos* Natural)	19.0	1.0
(*Tostitos* Santa Fe)	20.0	1.0
black bean (*Garden of Eatin'*)	18.0	4.0
black bean chili (*Garden of Eatin'*)	17.0	4.0
cheese, nacho (*Garden of Eatin'*)	18.0	2.0
chili verde or chipotle (*Guiltless Gourmet*)	22.0	2.0
Corn dogs, see "Frankfurter, wrapped"		
Corn flour:		
(*Shiloh Farms*), ¼ cup	27.0	5.0
whole-grain, 1 oz.	21.8	3.8
whole-grain, 1 cup	89.9	15.7
masa, 1 oz.	21.6	2.7
masa, 1 cup	87.0	10.9
Corn fritters, frozen (*Delta Pride*), 3 pieces	19.0	0
Corn grits, ¼ cup:		
(*Quaker* Quick)	29.0	2.0
white (*Arrowhead Mills*)	33.0	1.0
yellow (*Arrowhead Mills*)	30.0	1.0
Corn relish (*Mrs. Renfro's*), 1 tbsp.	4.0	0
Corn soufflé, frozen (*Stouffer's*), ½ cup	21.0	1.0

Food and Measure	carb. (gms)	fiber (gms)
Corn syrup, dark or light, 2 tbsp.	31.0	0
Cornflake crumbs (*Kellogg's*), 2 tbsp.	9.0	0
Cornichon, see "Pickle"		
Cornish hen, meat only, without added ingredients	0	0
Cornmeal (see also "Corn flour" and "Polenta"):		
(*Goya* Fine), 3 tbsp.	23.0	1.0
blue (*Arrowhead Mills*), ⅓ cup	25.0	5.0
white, stone ground (*Hodgson Mill*), <¼ cup	22.0	3.0
yellow:		
(*Arrowhead Mills*), ⅓ cup	27.0	3.0
(*Hodgson Mill*), <¼ cup	22.0	3.0
(*Shiloh Farms*), ¼ cup	27.0	3.0
self-rising (*Hodgson Mill*), <¼ cup	21.0	3.0
whole grain, ½ cup	46.9	4.5
Cornstarch (*Argo*), 1 tbsp.	7.0	0
Cottonseed flour, partially defatted, 1 cup	38.1	2.8
Cottonseed kernels, roasted, 1 tbsp.	2.2	.6
Cottonseed meal, partially defatted, 1 oz.	10.9	<1.0
Couscous, dry, except as noted:		
(*Fantastic*), ¼ cup	43.0	2.0
(*Hodgson Mill*), ⅓ cup	47.0	5.0
(*Marrakesh Express*), 1 cup*	45.0	1.0
(*Near East*), ⅓ cup or 1 cup*	46.0	2.0
(*Shiloh Farms*), ¼ cup	43.0	7.0
whole wheat (*Fantastic*), ¼ cup	45.0	7.0
whole wheat (*Shiloh Farms*), ¼ cup	34.0	8.0
whole wheat, with flax seed and soy, ⅓ cup:		
(*Hodgson Mill*)	48.0	6.0
garlic basil or Parmesan (*Hodgson Mill*)	50.0	6.0
Couscous, freeze-dried, precooked (*AlpineAire*), 1 oz. . .	20.0	1.0
Couscous dish, mix, dry:		
basil pesto (*Fantastic*), ⅓ cup	41.0	3.0
broccoli and cheese (*Near East*), 2 oz.	41.0	3.0
broccoli and cheese (*Near East*), 1 cup*	42.0	3.0
chicken, herb (*Near East*), 2 oz. or 1 cup*	42.0	3.0
chicken vegetable or curry (*Marrakesh Express*), 1 cup* .	39.0	2.0
curry (*Near East* Mediterranean), 2 oz. or 1 cup*	42.0	3.0

Food and Measure	carb. (gms)	fiber (gms)
garlic, roasted:		
olive oil (*Fantastic*), ⅓ cup	43.0	3.0
olive oil (*Near East*), 2 oz. or 1 cup*	41.0	2.0
red pepper (*Fantastic*), ⅓ cup	41.0	3.0
mango salsa (*Marrakesh Express*), 1 cup*	38.0	1.0
Moroccan pasta (*Marrakesh Express*), 1 cup*	45.0	1.0
mushroom, wild (*Marrakesh Express*), 1 cup*	39.0	1.0
mushroom, wild, herb (*Near East*), 2 oz. or 1 cup*	42.0	3.0
Parmesan (*Marrakesh Express*), 1 cup*	38.0	2.0
Parmesan (*Near East*), 2 oz. or 1 cup*	41.0	2.0
pine nut, Parmesan (*Fantastic*), ⅓ cup	41.0	3.0
pine nut, toasted (*Near East*), 2 oz. or 1 cup*	40.0	2.0
sun-dried tomato (*Marrakesh Express*), 1 cup*	39.0	2.0
tomato lentil (*Near East*), 2 oz. or 1 cup*	42.0	3.0
Couscous entree, frozen, stew, with vegetables (*Moosewood* Moroccan), 10-oz. pkg.	32.0	5.0
Cousins Subs:		
subs, 7½''':		
BLT	45.0	1.0
cappacola and cheese	48.0	1.0
cheese steak, regular or double	46.0	1.0
cheese steak, Philly	49.0	1.0
chicken breast or chicken cheddar deluxe	46.0	1.0
club	48.0	2.0
Genoa and cappacola or provolone	48.0	1.0
gyro	55.0	2.0
ham and provolone	47.0	2.0
Italian, regular or special	48.0	1.0
meatball and provolone	50.0	2.0
pepperoni melt	47.0	2.0
pizza sub	50.0	2.0
pork, barbecue, slow-roasted	63.0	1.0
provolone	46.0	2.0
roast beef	46.0	1.0
seafood with crab	53.0	1.0
tuna	46.0	2.0
turkey breast	48.0	1.0
veggie, garden or hot	49.0	2.0

Food and Measure	carb. (gms)	fiber (gms)
sub, lower fat, 7½"		
BLT	45.0	1.0
chicken breast	46.0	1.0
club	48.0	2.0
ham	47.0	2.0
roast beef or steak	46.0	1.0
turkey breast	48.0	1.0
veggie, garden	49.0	2.0
veggie, hot	49.0	1.0
sub, mini, 4"		
ham, lower fat, or ham and provolone	30.0	1.0
Italian, special	31.0	1.0
meatballs and provolone	32.0	1.0
provolone	30.0	1.0
seafood with crab	33.0	1.0
tuna	30.0	1.0
turkey breast, regular or lower fat	31.0	1.0
ciabatta sandwich:		
chicken, Sedona	36.0	4.0
club, Tuscan	33.0	2.0
pork, Cubano	38.0	1.0
fries:		
large	72.0	1.0
medium	55.0	1.0
small	38.0	1.0
salad:		
chef	15.0	3.0
chicken, Oriental sesame	20.0	4.0
chicken Sedona	14.0	5.0
garden	14.0	3.0
garden, with chicken or Italian	15.0	3.0
seafood	19.0	3.0
side	7.0	1.0
tuna	14.0	3.0
soup, 8 oz. regular:		
broccoli cheese	15.0	3.0
cheese	18.0	2.0
chicken dumpling	19.0	3.0

Food and Measure	carb. (gms)	fiber (gms)
chicken noodle	18.0	1.0
chicken rice	21.0	2.0
chili	26.0	14.0
clam chowder	19.0	3.0
potato, cream of	24.0	3.0
tomato basil ravioli	22.0	1.0
vegetable beef	13.0	2.0
breads:		
ciabatta	47.0	1.0
Italian or Parmesan-asiago, 15"	84.0	0
wheat, 15"	84.0	6.0
wrap, low-carb	19.0	12.0
chocolate chip cookie	25.0	1.0
Cowpeas (see also "Black-eyed peas"), fresh, ½ cup:		
raw:		
immature seeds	13.7	3.6
leafy tips, chopped	.9	n.a.
pods, with seeds	4.5	n.a.
boiled, drained:		
immature seeds	16.8	4.1
leafy tips, chopped	.7	n.a.
pods, with seeds	3.3	n.a.
Cowpeas, canned or frozen, see "Black-eye peas"		
Cowpeas, catjang, see "Catjang"		
Crab, meat only, 4 oz.:		
Alaska king, raw or boiled, poached, or steamed	0	0
blue, raw	.1	0
blue, boiled, poached, or steamed	0	0
Dungeness, raw	.8	0
Dungeness, boiled, poached, or steamed	1.1	0
queen, raw or boiled, poached, or steamed	0	0
Crab, canned, 2 oz., except as noted:		
with leg meat or lump (*Brunswick*)	1.0	0
lump, regular, or leg meat (*Yankee Clipper*)	2.0	0
lump, jumbo, or claw (*Orleans*)	0	0
pink or white lump (*Bumble Bee*)	0	0
white lump (*Crown Prince*)	1.0	0

Food and Measure	carb. (gms)	fiber (gms)
"Crab," imitation, frozen, ½ cup, 3 oz., except as noted:		
chunk, flake, or leg style (*Louis Kemp Crab Delights*)	11.0	0
shredded (*Louis Kemp Crab Delights* Easy Shreds)	13.0	0
from surimi, 1 oz.	3.0	0
Crab apple, fresh:		
(*Frieda's*), 5 oz.	28.0	.0
1 oz.	5.7	.3
sliced, ½ cup	11.0	.6
Crab apple, spiced, in jars (*Lucky Leaf/Musselman's*),		
1 piece	8.0	1.0
Crab cake, frozen:		
(*Nancy's Seafood*), 6 pieces, 3 oz.	16.0	1.0
deviled, breaded (*Mrs.Paul's*), 2.9-oz. piece	12.0	3.0
Maryland style:		
(*Mrs. Friday's*), 2.25-oz. piece	7.0	0
(*Phillips*), 3-oz. piece	7.0	<1.0
mini (*Yankee Trader*), 6 pieces, 2.5 oz.	8.0	1.0
Crab cake seasoning (*Old Bay* Classic), ⅙ pkg.	2.0	0
Crab spread, with jalapeños (*Sau•Sea*), 2 tbsp.	1.0	0
Cracker (see also "Snack chips"):		
(*Barbara's* Rite Lite Rounds Original), 5 pieces, .5 oz.	11.0	0
(*Bremner* Cracker), 7 pieces, .5 oz.	10.0	0
(*Bremner* Wafer), 7 pieces, .5 oz.	11.0	0
(*Goldfish* Original), 55 pieces, 1.1 oz.	20.0	<1.0
(*Lavosh-Hawaii* Classic/Bite Size), 1 oz.	19.0	1.0
(*Munch'ems* Original), 41 pieces, 1.1 oz.	21.0	1.0
(*Sabrosas*), 11 pieces, 1.1 oz.	20.0	0
bacon (*Nabisco* Baked), 1.1 oz.	19.0	2.0
bruschetta vegetable (*Health Valley*), 6 pieces, .5 oz.	10.0	1.0
butter/butter flavor:		
(*Keebler Club* Low Salt/Original), 4 pieces, .5 oz.	9.0	0
(*Keebler Club* Reduced Fat), 5 pieces, .6 oz.	12.0	0
(*Ritz* Low Sodium/ Original), 5 pieces, .6 oz.	10.0	0
(*Ritz* Reduced Fat), 5 pieces, .5 oz.	11.0	0
(*Ritz* Sticks), 1.1 oz.	19.0	1.0
(*Ritz* Top'ems), .5 oz.	10.0	0
(*Sara Lee* Country), 7 pieces, 1.1 oz.	20.0	<1.0

Food and Measure	carb. (gms)	fiber (gms)
(*Toasteds* Buttercrisp), 5 pieces, .6 oz.	10.0	0
(*Town House* Low Salt), 5 pieces, .6 oz.	10.0	<1.0
(*Town House* Original), 5 pieces, .6 oz.	9.0	<1.0
(*Town House* Reduced Fat), 6 pieces, .5 oz.	11.0	<1.0
(*Tree of Life* Golden Classic), 5 pieces, .5 oz.	12.0	0
garlic (*Ritz*), .6 oz.	10.0	0
thins (*Pepperidge Farm*), 4 pieces, .5 oz.	10.0	0
wheat (*Town House*), 5 pieces, .6 oz.	9.0	<1.0
caraway (*Bremner* Wafer), 7 pieces, .5 oz.	11.0	0
cheese:		
(*Barbara's* Cheese Bites), 22 pieces, 1 oz.	20.0	<1.0
(*Cheese Nips* Big), 1 oz.	18.0	1.0
(*Cheez-It* Big), 13 pieces, .1 oz.	18.0	<1.0
(*Cheez-It* Original), 27 pieces, 1.1 oz.	18.0	<1.0
(*Cheez-It* Reduced Fat), 29 pieces, 1.1 oz.	20.0	<1.0
(*Cheez-It Twisterz* Hot Wings Cheesy Blue), 17 pieces, 1.1 oz.	19.0	<1.0
(*Doritos Nacho Cheesier Golden Toast*), 1 pkg.	25.0	1.0
(*Pepperidge Farm* Snack Sticks), 25 pieces, 1.1 oz.	20.0	<1.0
colors (*Goldfish*), 55 pieces, 1.1 oz.	20.0	<1.0
four (*Cheese Nips*), 1.1 oz.	19.0	1.0
four (*Goldfish* Crisps), 37 pieces, 1.1 oz.	18.0	<1.0
hot and spicy (*Cheez-It*), 26 pieces, 1.1 oz.	17.0	<1.0
hot and spicy (*Goldfish* Explosive), 51 pieces, 1.1 oz.	17.0	1.0
jalapeño (*Doritos Golden Toast*), 1 pkg.	26.0	1.0
sour cream and onion (*Cheez-It*), 25 pieces, 1.1 oz.	19.0	0
cheese, cheddar:		
(*Annie's* Bunnies), 1.1 oz., 50 pieces	19.0	1.0
(*Austin Dolphins & Friends*), 60 pieces, 1.1 oz.	20.0	<1.0
(*Better Cheddars*), 22 pieces, 1.1 oz.	18.0	1.0
(*Better Cheddars* Reduced Fat), 24 pieces, 1.1 oz.	20.0	3.0
(*Cheese Nips* Mini Go Pack), 1.1 oz.	19.0	1.0
(*Cheese Nips* Reduced Fat), 31 pieces, 1.1 oz.	21.0	1.0
(*Cheetos Golden Toast*), 1 pkg.	25.0	1.0
(*Cheez-It Twisterz*), 17 pieces,. 1.1 oz.	19.0	<1.0
(*Goldfish*), 55 pieces, 1.1 oz.	20.0	<1.0
(*Goldfish* Baby), 89 pieces, 1.1 oz.	19.0	<1.0
(*Goldfish* Giant), 14 pieces, 1.1 oz.	19.0	1.0

Food and Measure	carb. (gms)	fiber (gms)
(*Munch'ems*), 39 pieces, 1.1 oz.	19.0	1.0
(*TLC* Country), 18 pieces, 1.1 oz.	20.0	<1.0
(*Triscuit*), 1 oz.	19.0	3.0
barbecue (*Annie's* Bunnies), 1.1 oz., 50 pieces	18.0	2.0
barbecue (*Cheez-It*), 25 pieces, 1.1 oz.	17.0	<1.0
extra (*Goldfish*), 51 piece, 1.1 oz.	18.0	1.0
jack (*Cheez-It*), 26 pieces, 1.1 oz.	18.0	0
jalapeño (*Cheese Nips*), 1.1 oz.	19.0	1.0
ranch (*Annie's* Bunnies), 1.1 oz., 50 pieces	17.0	2.0
salsa (*Cheese Nips*), 1.1 oz.	19.0	1.0
white (*Cheez-It*), 26 pieces, 1.1 oz.	18.0	<1.0
whole wheat (*Annie's* Bunnies), 1.1 oz., 50 pieces	17.0	3.0
cheese sandwich:		
(*Austin* Bite Size), 14 pieces, 1.1 oz.	17.0	0
(*Pepperidge Farm* Mini), 1-oz. pkg.	18.0	<1.0
(*Ritz Bits*), 1.1 oz.	18.0	0
(*Ritz Bits*), 1.5-oz. pkg.	25.0	1.0
American/mozzarella (*Ritz Bits*), 1.1 oz.	17.0	0
cheddar on wheat (*Austin*), 1.4-oz. pkg.	24.0	<1.0
cheddar jack or grilled cheese (*Austin*), 1.4-oz. pkg.	23.0	<1.0
jalapeño cheddar (*Ritz Bits*), 1.1 oz.	17.0	0
chicken flavor (*Chicken in a Bisket*), 12 pieces, 1.1 oz.	18.0	1.0
corn bread (*Town House Bistro*), 2 pieces, .6 oz.	11.0	<1.0
corn bread, all varieties (*Health Valley*), 4 pieces, .5 oz.	11.0	1.0
cream cheese–chive wafer sandwich (*Austin*), 1 pkg.	24.0	<1.0
croissant (*Carr's*), 3 pieces, .5 oz.	10.0	0
flatbread, chive garlic (*Margaret's Artisan*), .9-oz. piece	18.0	<1.0
garlic and herb, bite size (*Tree of Life* Fat Free), 12 pieces, .5 oz.	12.0	0
graham cracker, see "Cookie"		
herb, garden (*Health Valley*), 6 pieces, .5 oz.	10.0	1.0
herb and garlic (*Tree of Life*), 10 pieces, 1.1 oz.	22.0	1.0
matzo (*Manischewitz*), 1.1-oz. piece	27.0	1.0
matzo (*Streit's*)	25.0	1.0
multigrain:		
(*Town House Bistro*), 2 pieces, .6 oz.	11.0	<1.0
(*Wheat Thins*), 17 pieces, 1.1 oz.	21.0	2.0

Food and Measure	carb. (gms)	fiber (gms)
5 grain (*Harvest Crisps*), 1.1 oz.	23.0	1.0
7 grain (*TLC*), 15 pieces, 1.1 oz.	22.0	2.0
7 grain (*Wheatables*), 17 pieces, 1.1 oz.	20.0	1.0
10 grain (*Lavosh-Hawaii*), 1 oz.	19.0	3.0
onion:		
(*Toasteds*), 5 pieces, .6 oz.	10.0	0
French (*Health Valley*), 10 pieces, .5 oz.	10.0	1.0
slightly (*Lavosh-Hawaii*), 1 oz.	19.0	1.0
toasted (*Tree of Life*), 10 pieces, 1.1 oz.	22.0	1.0
Parmesan (*Goldfish*), 60 pieces, 1.1. oz.	19.0	<1.0
Parmesan and garlic (*Cheez-It*), 26 pieces, 1.1 oz.	19.0	0
peanut butter sandwich:		
(*Austin* PB & J), 1.4-oz. pkg.	24.0	<1.0
(*Pepperidge Farm* Mini), 1-oz. pkg.	18.0	<1.0
(*Ritz Bits*), 1.25-oz. pkg.	21.0	1.0
(*Ritz Bits,* 9.5 oz.), 1 oz.	16.0	1.0
cheese (*Cheese Nips*), 1.4-oz. pkg.	23.0	1.0
cheese or toast (*Frito Lay*), 1 pkg.	23.0	1.0
toast (*Austin* Toasty), 1.4-oz. pkg.	23.0	1.0
pepper, cracked:		
(*Health Valley*), 5 pieces, .5 oz.	10.0	1.0
(*Tree of Life*), 10 pieces, 1.1 oz.	23.0	<1.0
bite size (*Tree of Life* Fat Free), 12 pieces, .5 oz.	12.0	0
peppercorn (*Lavosh-Hawaii*), 1 oz.	20.0	1.0
pizza (*Goldfish*), 55 pieces, 1.1 oz.	19.0	2.0
pizza (*Goldfish* Explosive), 51 pieces, 1.1 oz.	19.0	1.0
poppy seed, savory (*Barbara's* Rite Lite Rounds), 5 pieces, .5 oz.	11.0	0
pumpernickel (*Pepperidge Farm* Snack Sticks), 15 pieces, 1 oz.	22.0	2.0
ranch (*Munch'ems*), 39 pieces, 1.1 oz.	20.0	1.0
ranch (*TLC* Natural), 15 pieces, 1.1 oz.	22.0	2.0
rice, brown:		
(*Eden*), 1.1 oz.	22.0	2.0
(*Westbrae Natural* Wafers No Salt), 7 pieces, .5 oz.	11.0	0
nori maki (*Eden*), 15 pieces, 1.1 oz.	24.0	2.0
sesame (*San-J*), 5 pieces, 1 oz.	19.0	1.0
sesame (*Westbrae Natural* Wafers), 7 pieces, .5 oz.	11.0	0

Food and Measure	carb. (gms)	fiber (gms)
sesame, black (*San-J*), 5 pieces, 1 oz.	17.0	1.0
tamari (*San-J*), 6 pieces, 1.1 oz.	26.0	1.0
tamari or 5-spice (*Westbrae Natural* Wafers), 7 pieces, .5 oz.	11.0	0
rice bran (*Health Valley*), 6 pieces, 1 oz.	19.0	3.0
rosemary (*Carr's*), 7 pieces, 1 oz.	19.0	<1.0
rosemary garlic (*Lavosh-Hawaii*), 1 oz.	19.0	1.0
rye:		
(*Town House Bistro*), 2 pieces, .6 oz.	10.0	<1.0
(*Triscuit* Deli Style), 1 oz.	19.0	3.0
caraway (*Lavosh-Hawaii*), 1 oz.	20.0	1.0
saltines, 5 pieces, .5 oz.:		
(*Krispy* Original)	11.0	<1.0
(*Premium* Fat Free)	12.0	0
(*Premium* Gold/Low Sodium/Original 4 oz.)	10.0	0
(*Premium* Original/Unsalted Top)	11.0	0
(*Zesta* Fat Free)	13.0	0
(*Zesta* Original/Reduced Sodium/Unsalted Top)	11.0	0
with multigrain (*Premium*)	10.0	0
whole wheat (*Krispy*)	11.0	<1.0
whole wheat (*Zesta*)	11.0	<1.0
savory (*Sociables*), 7 pieces, .5 oz.	9.0	1.0
sesame:		
(*Bremner* Wafer), 7 pieces, .5 oz.	11.0	0
(*Health Valley*), 5 pieces, .5 oz.	10.0	1.0
(*Pepperidge Farm* Snack Sticks), 12 pieces, 1.1 oz.	20.0	1.0
(*Toasteds*), 5 pieces, .6 oz.	10.0	<1.0
cheese sticks (*Twigs*), 1.1 oz.	18.0	3.0
and flax seed (*Tree of Life*), 10 pieces, 1.1 oz.	23.0	1.0
honey (*TLC*), 15 pieces, 1.1 oz.	22.0	2.0
tamari (*Barbara's* Rite Lite Rounds), 5 pieces, .5 oz.	10.0	0
soda/water:		
(*Carr's Table Water*), 5 pieces, .6 oz.	13.0	<1.0
(*Wellington* Traditional), 4 pieces, .5 oz.	12.0	0
assorted (*Carr's* Biscuits for Cheese), 2 pieces, .4 oz.	8.0	<1.0
cracked pepper (*Carr's Table Water*), 5 pieces, .6 oz.	13.0	<1.0
cracked pepper trio (*Sara Lee*), 7 pieces, 1.1 oz.	22.0	<1.0
garlic, roasted (*Carr's Table Water*), 5 pieces, .6 oz.	12.0	<1.0

Food and Measure	carb. (gms)	fiber (gms)
poppy and sesame (*Carr's*), 4 pieces, .6 oz.	9.0	<1.0
soup/oyster, .5 oz.:		
(*Bremner* Oyster Cracker), 50 pieces	10.0	0
(*Bremner* Soup/Chili Cracker), 50 pieces	11.0	0
(*Krispy*), 17 pieces	12.0	0
(*Premium*), 23 pieces	11.0	0
(*Zesta*), 45 pieces	10.0	0
sour cream and onion (*Goldfish* Crisps),		
37 pieces, 1.1 oz.	17.0	<1.0
sour cream and onion (*Munch 'ems*), 39 pieces, 1.1 oz. ..	20.0	1.0
Swiss cheese (*Nabisco* Baked), 1 oz.	18.0	2.0
tomato (*Garden Savory*), 4 pieces, .5 oz.	9.0	0
vegetable:		
(*Sara Lee* Harvest), 6 pieces, 1 oz.	19.0	<1.0
(*Vegetable Thins* Baked), 14 pieces, 1.1 oz.	19.0	2.0
garden (*Harvest Crisps*), 1.1 oz.	22.0	1.0
garden (*Tree of Life*), 10 pieces, 1.1 oz.	22.0	<1.0
garden, bite size (*Tree of Life* Fat Free),		
12 pieces, .5 oz.	12.0	0
wheat:		
(*Pepperidge Farm* Hearty), 3 pieces, .5 oz.	10.0	1.0
(*Pepperidge Farm* Snack Sticks), 30 pieces, 1.1 oz. ...	22.0	1.0
(*Toasteds*), 5 pieces, .6 oz.	10.0	<1.0
(*Wheat Thins* Big), 11 pieces, 1.1 oz.	21.0	1.0
(*Wheat Thins* Low Sodium/Original), 16 pieces, 1.1 oz.	21.0	1.0
(*Wheatables* Original), 19 pieces, 1.1 oz.	20.0	1.0
(*Wheatables* Reduced Fat), 19 pieces, 1.1 oz.	22.0	2.0
(*Wheatsworth*), 5 pieces, .6 oz.	10.0	1.0
cracked (*Bremner* Wafer), 7 pieces, .5 oz.	11.0	0
golden (*Sara Lee*), 6 pieces, 1 oz.	18.0	1.0
honey (*Wheat Thins*), 1.1 oz.	21.0	1.0
honey (*Wheatables*), 17 pieces, 1.1 oz.	20.0	1.0
ranch (*Wheat Thins*), 1 oz.	19.0	1.0
stoned (*Health Valley* Low Fat), 5 pieces, .5 oz.	10.0	1.0
stoned (*Red Oval Farms/Red Oval Farms* Lower Sodium),		
2 pieces, .5 oz.	10.0	1.0
wheat, whole:		
(*Barbara's Wheatines*), 4 pieces, .5 oz.	11.0	<1.0

Food and Measure	carb. (gms)	fiber (gms)
(*Carr's*), 2 pieces, .6 oz.	11.0	1.0
(*Health Valley*), 6 pieces, .5 oz.	10.0	2.0
(*Ritz*), 5 pieces, .5 oz.	11.0	1.0
(*Triscuit* Original/Low Sodium), 1 oz.	19.0	3.0
(*Triscuit* Reduced Fat), 1 oz.	21.0	3.0
(*Triscuit* Thin Crisps), 15 pieces, 1.1 oz.	21.0	3.0
cracked pepper (*Barbara's Wheatines*), 4 pieces, .5 oz.	11.0	1.0
garlic, roasted or herb, garden (*Triscuit*), 1 oz.	20.0	3.0
zwieback (*Nabisco*), .3-oz. piece	6.0	0
Cracker meal, ¼ cup:		
(*Golden Dipt* Fry Easy)	23.0	0
(*Nabisco*)	22.0	1.0
matzo meal (*Manischewitz*)	23.0	1.0
matzo meal (*Streit's*)	24.0	1.0
Cranberry, fresh, ½ cup:		
(*Dole*)	7.0	2.0
(*Ocean Spray*)	7.0	2.0
whole	6.0	2.0
chopped	7.0	2.3
Cranberry, canned, see "Cranberry fruit blend" and "Cranberry sauce"		
Cranberry, dried, ⅓ cup, 1.4 oz.:		
(*Craisins*)	33.0	2.0
(*Frieda's*)	28.0	2.0
(*Shiloh Farms*)	33.0	1.0
(*Tree of Life*)	35.0	3.5
cherry flavor (*Craisins*)	33.0	2.0
orange flavor (*Craisins*)	34.0	2.0
Cranberry beans:		
boiled, ½ cup	21.5	3.0
canned, ½ cup	19.7	n.a.
Cranberry drink, 8 fl. oz.:		
(*Langers* Caribbean)	34.0	0
(*Langers* Diet)	8.0	0
(*Ocean Spray*)	32.0	0
(*R.W. Knudsen* Concentrate)	13.0	0
(*Walnut Acres*)	26.0	0

Food and Measure	carb. (gms)	fiber (gms)
cocktail:		
(*Langers*)	35.0	0
(*Langers* Diet)	8.0	0
(*Nantucket Nectars*)	34.0	0
(*Ocean Spray*)	33.0	0
(*Ocean Spray* Calcium)	37.0	0
(*Ocean Spray* Light)	10.0	0
(*Ocean Spray* Reduced Calorie)	13.0	0
nectar (*Santa Cruz Organic*)	27.0	0
white:		
(*Langers*)	28.0	0
(*Ocean Spray*)	29.0	0
(*Ocean Spray* Light)	10.0	0
Cranberry drink blend, 8 fl. oz., except as noted:		
all varieties (*Langers* Diet/Low Carb)	8.0	0
apple:		
(*Langers* Fuji)	39.0	0
(*Minute Maid*), 11.5-fl.-oz. can	60.0	0
(*Cranapple*)	40.0	0
white cranberry (*Ocean Spray*)	30.0	0
apple raspberry (*Minute Maid*)	33.0	0
apple raspberry (*Minute Maid*), 11.5-fl.-oz. can	46.0	0
berry (*Langers*)	34.0	0
cherry (*Cran•Cherry*)	39.0	0
cherry (*Cran•Grape* Light)	10.0	0
grape:		
(*Cran•Grape*)	40.0	0
(*Langers*)	41.0	0
(*Minute Maid*), 11.5-fl.-oz. can	39.0	0
(*Ocean Spray*)	41.0	0
grapefruit (*SoBe Elixer 3C*)	28.0	0
mango (*Cran•Mango*)	35.0	0
orange (*Langers*)	33.0	0
orange (*Nantucket Nectars* Organic)	31.0	0
peach, white cranberry (*Ocean Spray*)	30.0	0
raspberry:		
(*Cran•Raspberry*)	34.0	0
(*Cran•Raspberry* Light)	10.0	0

Food and Measure	carb. (gms)	fiber (gms)
(*Langers*)	36.0	0
(*R.W. Knudsen*)	31.0	0
(*Snapple*)	29.0	0
white cranberry (*Langers*)	28.0	0
strawberry (*Cran•Strawberry*)	37.0	0
tangerine (*Cran•Tangerine*)	35.0	0
white cranberry (*Ocean Spray*)	31.0	0
wildberry (*Ocean Spray Cravin' Less Sugar*)	20.0	0
Cranberry fruit blend, orange or raspberry		
(*Cran•Fruit*), ¼ cup	29.0	1.0
Cranberry juice, 8 fl. oz.:		
(*After the Fall* Cape Cod)	30.0	0
(*L&A* Delight)	34.0	0
(*L&A* 100)	35.0	0
(*Langers*)	35.0	0
(*Northland*)	35.0	0
(*R.W. Knudsen* Just Cranberry)	14.0	0
(*R.W. Knudsen* Nectar)	34.0	0
frozen* (*Cascadian Farm*)	29.0	0
white cranberry (*L&A* 100)	40.0	0
white cranberry (*Langers*)	40.0	0
Cranberry juice blend, 8 fl. oz.:		
(*Ocean Spray*)	35.0	0
apple, red delicious (*Ocean Spray*)	32.0	0
berry, mixed (*Langers*)	34.0	0
berry, mixed (*Ocean Spray*)	38.0	0
blueberry (*Walnut Acres*)	29.0	0
grape (*Langers*)	38.0	0
grape (*Ocean Spray* Concord)	37.0	0
kiwi (*Ceres*)	28.0	0
peach (*Ocean Spray* Georgia)	34.0	0
raspberry:		
(*After the Fall*)	32.0	0
(*Langers*)	36.0	0
(*Ocean Spray* Pacific)	34.0	0
(*Walnut Acres*)	27.0	<1.0
raspberry grape (*Nantucket Nectars*)	38.0	0
Cranberry juice cocktail, see "Cranberry drink"		

Food and Measure	carb. (gms)	fiber (gms)
Cranberry juice concentrate (*Tree of Life*), 8 tsp.	28.0	0
Cranberry sauce, can or jar, ¼ cup, except as noted:		
(*R.W. Knudsen*), 1 tbsp.	6.0	0
jellied (*Ocean Spray*)	25.0	1.0
whole (*Ocean Spray*)	27.0	1.0
whole or jellied (*Harvest Moon*)	26.0	1.0
whole or jellied (*S&W*)	26.0	1.0
Cranberry twist drink mixer (*Rose's* Cocktail Infusions),		
1.5 fl. oz.	15.0	0
Crayfish, without added ingredients	0	0
Cream:		
half and half:		
(*Darigold*), 2 tbsp.	1.0	0
(*Organic Valley*)	1.0	0
(*Simply Smart* Fat Free), 2 tbsp.	2.0	0
1 cup	10.4	0
1 tbsp.	.6	0
light, coffee or table:		
(*Hood*), 1 tbsp.	<1.0	0
1 cup	8.8	0
1 tbsp.	.6	0
medium (25% fat), 1 cup	8.3	0
medium (25% fat), 1 tbsp.	.5	0
sour, see "Cream, sour"		
whipped topping, see "Cream topping"		
whipping[1], light:		
(*Darigold*), 1 tbsp.	1.0	0
(*Hood*), 1 tbsp.	<1.0	0
1 cup	7.1	0
1 tbsp.	.4	0
whipping[1], heavy:		
(*Darigold*), 1 tbsp.	1.0	0
(*Hood*), 1 tbsp.	0	0
(*Organic Valley*)	0	0
1 cup	6.6	0
1 tbsp.	.4	0

[1]Unwhipped; volume approximately doubled when whipped.

Food and Measure	carb. (gms)	fiber (gms)
Cream, clotted (*The Devon Cream Company*), 2 tbsp.	<1.0	0
Cream, sour, 2 tbsp., except as noted:		
(*Breakstone's*)	1.0	0
(*Darigold*)	2.0	0
(*Knudsen Hampshire*)	1.0	0
(*Organic Valley*)	1.0	0
1 cup	9.8	0
light (low fat):		
(*Breakstone's*)	2.0	0
(*Darigold*)	3.0	0
(*Knudsen* Light/*Knudsen* Light 16 oz.)	2.0	0
(*Organic Valley*)	1.0	0
nonfat:		
(*Breakstone's* 8 oz.)	5.0	0
(*Breakstone's* 16 oz.)	6.0	0
(*Darigold*)	4.0	0
(*Knudsen Free*)	5.0	0
Cream, sour, powder (*AlpineAire*), 2 oz.	20.0	0
"Cream," sour, nondairy (*Tofutti Better Than Sour Cream/Sour Supreme*), 2 tbsp.	9.0	0
Cream puffs, frozen:		
chocolate, mini:		
(*Delizza*), 7 pieces, 3.5 oz.	33.5	.1
(*Ritch & Famous* Dreamy), 4 pieces, 1.7 oz.	13.0	1.0
vanilla, French, mini (*Ritch & Famous*), .4-oz. piece	3.0	0
Cream of tartar, 1 tsp.	1.9	0
Cream topping, 2 tbsp.:		
(*Cool Whip/Cool Whip* Extra Creme)	2.0	0
(*Cool Whip* Free/*Cool Whip* Lite)	3.0	0
(*Hood* Instant)	<1.0	0
(*Hood* Instant Light)	1.0	0
(*Reddi Wip* Extra Creamy/Original)	<1.0	0
(*Reddi Wip* Fat Free/Chocolate)	1.0	0
Creamer, 2 tbsp.:		
half and half:		
(*Coffee-mate*)	1.0	0
hazelnut (*Coffee-mate*)	8.0	0
vanilla (*Coffee-mate*)	4.0	0

Food and Measure	carb. (gms)	fiber (gms)
powder (*Coffee-mate* Latte Creations Classic)	12.0	0
powder, mocha or vanilla (*Coffee-mate* Latte Creations) ..	14.0	0
Creamer, nondairy:		
fluid, 1 tbsp.:		
(*Coffee-mate/Coffee-mate* Fat Free)	2.0	0
(*Coffee-mate* Low Fat)	1.0	0
(*Country Creamer*)	2.0	0
(*Silk*)	1.0	0
powder, 1 tsp.		
(*Coffee-mate* Low Fat)	1.0	0
(*Coffee-mate* Lite)	2.0	0
(*Cremora*)	<1.0	0
(*Cremora* Fat Free)	2.0	0
(*Cremora* Lite & Creamy/Royal)	1.0	0
(*Cremora* No Carb)	0	0
Creamer, nondairy, flavored:		
fluid, 1 tbsp.:		
all varieties (*Coffee-mate*)	5.0	0
café mocha or Irish creme (*Coffee-mate* Fat Free)	5.0	0
hazelnut or French vanilla (*Silk*)	3.0	0
vanilla, French (*Coffee-Mate* Fat Free)	2.0	0
powder, 4 tsp.:		
all varieties (*Coffee-Mate* Fat Free)	11.0	0
all varieties, except vanilla nut (*Coffee-mate*)	9.0	0
dulce de leche (*Cremora*)	9.0	0
hazelnut (*Cremora Nutty for Hazelnut*)	<1.0	0
vanilla (*Cremora* Ooh-la-la)	<1.0	0
vanilla nut (*Coffee-mate*)	8.0	0
Crème fraîche:		
(*Santé*), 2 tbsp.	<1.0	0
(*Vermont Butter & Cheese*), 1 oz.	1.0	0
Crepe, 1 piece:		
(*A&B Famous*), 1.4 oz.	9.0	0
(*Frieda's*), .4 oz.	5.0	0
Cress, garden: raw, ½ cup	1.4	.3
boiled, drained, ½ cup	2.6	.5
Cress, water, see "Watercress"		
Croaker, Atlantic, without added ingredients	0	0

Food and Measure	carb. (gms)	fiber (gms)
Croissant:		
butter, 1-oz. piece	13.0	.7
apple, 2-oz. piece	21.0	1.4
cheese, 1.5-oz. piece	19.7	1.1
Croissant, frozen, French style:		
(*Sara Lee* Original), 1.5-oz. piece	20.0	1.0
petite (*Sara Lee*), 2 pieces, 2 oz.	26.0	1.0
Crookneck squash:		
(*Frieda's* Baby), ⅔ cup, 2 oz.	3.0	1.0
sliced, raw, ends trimmed, ½ cup	2.6	.7
sliced, boiled, drained, ½ cup	3.9	1.3
Crookneck squash, canned, cut, drained, ½ cup	3.2	1.1
Crookneck squash, frozen, boiled, sliced, ½ cup	5.3	1.2
Croutons (see also "Salad toppers"):		
Caesar salad:		
(*Mrs. Cubbison's*), 5 pieces	4.0	0
(*Pepperidge Farm* Generous Cut Classic), 6 pieces	4.0	0
(*Pepperidge Farm* Generous Cut Fat Free), 6 pieces	5.0	0
cheese, sourdough (*Pepperidge Farm* Generous Cut), 6 pieces	4.0	0
cheese and garlic (*Mrs. Cubbison's*), 5 pieces	4.0	0
garlic and butter or onion (*Mrs. Cubbison's*), 5 pieces	5.0	0
garlic and cheese or onion (*Pepperidge Farm* Classic Cut), 11 pieces	5.0	0
herb (*Mrs. Cubbison's* Fat Free), 5 pieces	5.0	0
Italian, zesty (*Pepperidge Farm* Generous Cut), 6 pieces	4.0	0
pepper, cracked, and Parmesan (*Pepperidge Farm* Generous Cut), 6 pieces	4.0	0
ranch:		
buttermilk (*Pepperidge Farm* Generous Cut), 6 pieces	5.0	0
cool herb (*Mrs. Cubbison's*), 5 pieces	5.0	0
seasoned (*Mrs. Cubbison's*), 5 pieces	4.0	0
seasoned (*Pepperidge Farm* Classic Cut), 11 pieces	5.0	0
Crowder peas, see "Peas, crowder"		
Cucumber, with peel:		
(*Chiquita*), ⅓ medium, 3.5 oz.	3.0	1.0
(*Frieda's* Hothouse/Japanese), ⅔ cup, 3 oz.	2.0	1.0

Food and Measure	carb. (gms)	fiber (gms)
1 medium, 8¼" long	8.3	2.4
sliced, ½ cup	1.4	.4
Cucumber, pickled, see "Pickles"		
Cucuzza squash (*Frieda's*), ¾ cup, 3 oz.	3.0	0
Cumin seeds, ground, 1 tsp.	.9	.2
Cupcake, see "Cake, snack"		
Curacao, blue (*Angostura*), 1 fl. oz.	19.0	0
Currants:		
fresh, black, Europe, ½ cup	8.6	3.0
fresh, red or white, ½ cup	7.7	2.4
dried, Zante, ½ cup	53.3	4.9
Curry paste (see also "Curry sauce base"):		
green (*Thai Kitchen*), 1 tbsp.	2.0	0
hot:		
(*Patak's/Patak's* Vindaloo), 2 tbsp.	4.0	0
(*Patak's* Garam Masala), 2 tsp.	4.0	0
(*Patak's* Kashmiri Masala), 1 tsp.	<1.0	0
hot, vindaloo (*Neera's*), 2 tsp.	3.0	1.0
medium, 2 tbsp.:		
(*Patak's* Balti)	6.0	<1.0
(*Patak's* Biryani Paste)	3.0	0
(*Patak's* Tikka Masala)	5.0	<1.0
mild (*Patak's*), 2 tbsp.	8.0	4.0
red (*Thai Kitchen*), 1 tbsp.	2.0	0
tandoori (*Neera's* Grilling), 2 tsp.	3.0	1.0
tandoori (*Patak's*), 2 tbsp.	3.0	2.0
Curry powder:		
1 tbsp.	3.7	1.0
1 tsp.	1.2	.3
Masala (*Neera's*), 2 tsp.	3.0	1.0
Masala (*Neera's* Garam), ¼ tsp.	0	0
Curry sauce, cooking (see also "Thai sauce"), ½ cup:		
chile, hot, with coriander or cumin (*Patak's* Vindaloo)	15.0	1.0
coconut, rich creamy, mild (*Patak's* Korma 10 oz.)	11.0	2.0
coriander and lemon, tangy, medium (*Patak's* Tikka Masala 10 oz.)	13.0	2.0
sweet peppers and coconut, hot (*Patak's* Jalfrezi)	12.0	2.0

Food and Measure	carb. (gms)	fiber (gms)
tomato, rich, mild (*Patak's* Dopiaza)	13.0	1.0
tomato, spicy, and cardamom (*Patak's* Rogan Josh)	12.0	1.0
Curry sauce base (see also "Curry paste"), 1 tsp.:		
green, yellow, or red (*A Taste of Thai*)	1.0	1.0
Panang (*A Taste of Thai*)	2.0	0
Cusk, without added ingredients	0	0
Custard apple, trimmed, 1 oz.	7.1	1.0
Custard marrow, see "Chayote"		
Cuttlefish, meat only:		
raw, 4 oz.	.9	0
boiled or steamed, 4 oz.	1.9	0
Cuttlefish, canned, in ink (*Goya*), ¼ cup	2.0	0

D

Food and Measure	carb. (gms)	fiber (gms)
Dahl/Dal, see "Lentil dish, mix"		
Daikon, fresh or dried, see "Radish, Oriental"		
Daikon, pickled (*Eden*), 2 slices, .5 oz.	1.0	0
Daiquiri drink mixer:		
(*Trader Vic's* Hawaiian), 4 fl. oz.	42.0	0
banana, frozen (*Bacardi*), 2 fl. oz.	36.0	0
peach, frozen (*Bacardi*), 2 fl. oz.	32.0	0
strawberry:		
(*Bacardi*), 4 fl. oz.	46.0	0
(*Mr & Mrs T*), 3.5 fl. oz.	34.0	0
frozen (*Bacardi*), 2 fl. oz.	32.0	0
Daiquiri/Margarita drink mixer, 4 fl. oz.:		
lime, mango, or strawberry (*Daiq-or-Rita*)	55.0	1.0
peach (*Daiq-or-Rita*)	41.0	1.0
strawberry (*Holland House*)	46.0	0
Dairy Queen/Brazier, 1 serving:		
burgers:		
DQ Homestyle burger or cheeseburger	29.0	2.0
DQ Homestyle double cheeseburger	30.0	2.0
DQ Homestyle double cheeseburger, with bacon	31.0	2.0
DQ Ultimate	29.0	2.0
Flame Thrower	27.0	2.0
Grillburger, bacon cheese	40.0	1.0
Grillburger, California or mushroom Swiss	37.0	1.0
Grillburger, classic or ½ lb., with or without cheese ...	41.0	2.0
chicken sandwich, crispy	50.0	4.5
chicken sandwich, grilled	26.0	2.0
Chicken Strip Basket, 4-piece	92.0	7.0
Chicken Strip Basket, 6-piece	102.0	9.0

Food and Measure	carb. (gms)	fiber (gms)
hot dog, regular	19.0	1.0
hot dog, chili 'n cheese	22.0	2.0
popcorn shrimp basket	88.0	7.0
fries:		
large	72.0	5.0
medium	56.0	4.0
small	45.0	3.0
onion rings	45.0	3.0
salad, without dressing:		
crispy chicken	21.0	6.0
grilled chicken	12.0	4.0
side salad	6.0	2.0
salad dressing:		
DQ blue cheese	4.0	0
DQ honey mustard	18.0	0
DQ ranch	3.0	0
honey mustard or ranch, nonfat	13.0	0
Italian, nonfat	3.0	0
ranch, buttermilk, nonfat	6.0	0
red French, nonfat	10.0	0
Thousand Island, nonfat	16.0	0
Blizzard:		
banana split, large	134.0	2.0
banana split, medium	97.0	1.0
banana split, small	73.0	<1.0
chocolate chip cookie, large	193.0	0
chocolate chip cookie, medium	150.0	0
chocolate chip cookie, small	105.0	0
Oreo cookie, large	148.0	2.0
Oreo cookie, medium	103.0	1.0
Oreo cookie, small	83.0	<1.0
Reese's Cup, large	152.0	0
Reese's Cup, medium	114.0	0
Reese's Cup, small	87.0	0
Blizzard CheeseQuake:		
blueberry, large	148.0	1.0
blueberry, medium	108.0	1.0
blueberry, small	78.0	0

Food and Measure	carb. (gms)	fiber (gms)
raspberry, large	165.0	1.0
raspberry, medium	119.0	1.0
raspberry, small	84.0	1.0
strawberry, large	136.0	1.0
strawberry, medium	97.0	1.0
strawberry, small	71.0	0
cones:		
DQ soft serve, chocolate or vanilla, ½ cup	22.0	0
chocolate, medium	53.0	0
chocolate, small	37.0	0
dipped, large	85.0	0
dipped, medium	59.0	1.0
dipped, small	42.0	1.0
vanilla, large	76.0	0
vanilla, medium	53.0	0
vanilla, small	38.0	0
DQ round cake, ⅛ cake	56.0	<1.0
malt, chocolate, large	222.0	2.0
malt, chocolate, medium	153.0	2.0
malt, chocolate, small	111.0	1.0
Misty slush, medium	74.0	0
Misty slush, small	56.0	0
MooLatte:		
caramel, 16 oz.	96.0	0
caramel, 24 oz.	139.0	0
cappuccino, 16 oz.	68.0	0
cappuccino, 24 oz.	102.0	0
mocha, 16 oz.	80.0	1.0
mocha, 24 oz.	118.0	1.0
vanilla, 16 oz.	87.0	0
vanilla, 24 oz.	127.0	0
novelties:		
Buster Bar	45.0	2.0
Chocolate Dilly bar	25.0	0
DQ fudge bar	13.0	0
DQ sandwich	31.0	1.0
DQ vanilla orange bar	17.0	0

Food and Measure	carb. (gms)	fiber (gms)
lemon *DQ Freez'r*	20.0	0
Starkiss	21.0	0
Royal Treats:		
banana split	96.0	3.0
Brownie Earthquake	112.0	0
Peanut Buster parfait	99.0	2.0
Triple Chocolate Utopia	96.0	5.0
strawberry shortcake	70.0	1.0
shake, chocolate:		
large	186.0	2.0
medium	129.0	2.0
small	93.0	1.0
sundae, chocolate:		
large	100.0	1.0
medium	71.0	0
small	49.0	0
sundae, strawberry:		
large	83.0	<1.0
medium	58.0	<1.0
small	40.0	0
Dandelion greens:		
raw (*Frieda's*), 2 cups, 3 oz.	8.0	3.0
raw, ½ cup chopped, 1 oz.	2.6	1.0
boiled, drained, chopped, ½ cup	3.3	1.5
Danish, 1 piece:		
cheese (*Entenmann's*), 3.5 oz.	60.0	<1.0
pineapple cheese (*Entenmann's*), 4 oz.	45.0	1.0
Dasheen, see "Taro"		
Date, dried:		
(*Dole*), 1.4 oz.	33.0	3.0
(*Frieda's* Medjool), 2–3 pieces, 1.4 oz.	31.0	3.0
(*Shiloh Farms* Deglet Noor), 5–6 pieces, 1.4 oz.	31.0	3.0
(*Sunsweet*), 5–6 pieces or ¼ cup chopped, 1.4 oz.	32.0	3.0
(*Tree of Life* Deglet Noor), 5 pieces, 1.5 oz.	31.0	3.0
10 pieces, 2.9 oz.	61.0	6.2
pitted, ½ cup	65.4	6.7
Date, Indian, see "Tamarindo"		

Food and Measure	carb. (gms)	fiber (gms)
Date-nut rolls, with coconut, almonds		
(*Shiloh Farms*), 1½ pieces, 1.4 oz.	30.0	4.0
Del Taco, 1 serving:		
breakfast:		
burrito, breakfast	24.0	1.0
burrito, egg and cheese	39.0	3.0
burrito, steak and egg	41.0	3.0
hash brown sticks, 5 pieces	20.0	0
hash brown sticks, 8 pieces	32.0	0
Macho Bacon & Egg Burrito	82.0	6.0
quesadilla, bacon and egg	40.0	2.0
burgers:		
bun taco	37.0	4.0
cheeseburger or hamburger	37.0	3.0
Del Cheeseburger/Double Del Cheeseburger/		
Bacon Double Del Cheeseburger	35.0	4.0
burrito:		
bean and cheese, green or red	38.0	6.0
carnitas	41.0	3.0
chicken, spicy	66.0	8.0
chicken works	57.0	4.0
Del Beef	42.0	3.0
Del Classic Chicken	41.0	3.0
Del Combo	61.0	11.0
Deluxe Combo	64.0	12.0
Deluxe Del Beef	45.0	4.0
half pound green	59.0	13.0
half pound red	65.0	13.0
Macho Beef	89.0	7.0
Macho Chicken	111.0	16.0
Macho Combo	113.0	17.0
steak works	58.0	5.0
veggie works	69.0	9.0
quesadilla:		
cheddar	39.0	2.0
chicken cheddar	41.0	2.0
chicken spicy jack	40.0	2.0
spicy jack	38.0	2.0

Food and Measure	carb. (gms)	fiber (gms)
taco:		
Big Fat	39.0	3.0
Big Fat Chicken/Steak	38.0	3.0
carnitas	18.0	2.0
chicken, soft	16.0	1.0
chicken or steak del carbon	19.0	2.0
fish, crispy	30.0	2.0
taco	11.0	1.0
taco, soft	16.0	1.0
ultimate	13.0	2.0
salad:		
chicken, deluxe	77.0	15.0
Deluxe Taco Salad	76.0	14.0
taco salad	10.0	2.0
nachos/sides:		
beans/cheese cup	44.0	16.0
chips/salsa, medium	43.0	3.0
fries:		
chili cheese	51.0	5.0
Deluxe Chili Cheese	53.0	6.0
macho	68.0	6.0
medium	47.0	5.0
small	34.0	3.0
Macho Nachos	113.0	15.0
nachos	40.0	2.0
rice cup	27.0	1.0
shakes:		
chocolate	117.0	1.0
strawberry	100.0	1.0
vanilla	97.0	0
Delicata squash (*Frieda's*), ¾ cup, 3 oz.	7.0	1.0
Denny's, 1 serving:		
breakfast menu, without bread or syrup:		
All-American Slam	3.0	1.0
Belgian waffle platter	28.0	0
corned beef hash slam	11.0	1.0
country-fried steak and eggs	13.0	6.0
country scramble	79.0	4.0

Food and Measure	carb. (gms)	fiber (gms)
Denver scramble	75.0	4.0
French Slam	74.0	3.0
French toast platter	110.0	3.0
Grand Slam	33.0	2.0
Grand Slam Slugger	74.0	3.0
grits, 4 oz.	18.0	0
ham-cheddar omelet	5.0	0
hash browns	20.0	2.0
hash browns, with cheddar cheese	21.0	2.0
hash browns, with onion, cheese, gravy	54.0	3.0
heartland scramble	79.0	8.0
Lumberjack Slam, with hash browns	73.0	3.0
meat lover's	72.0	3.0
meat lover's scramble	82.0	8.0
meat lover's skillet	27.0	10.0
Moons Over My Hammy	42.0	2.0
pancakes, 3, or pancake platter	47.0	2.0
potatoes, country fried	23.0	10.0
sirloin steak and eggs	1.0	1.0
Slim Slam	39.0	1.0
T-bone steak/eggs	1.0	1.0
Ultimate Omelette	8.0	1.0
veggie-cheese omelet	11.0	2.0
breakfast items:		
bacon, 4 strips	1.0	0
bagel, dry	46.0	0
biscuit, dry	22.0	0
cinnamon apple filling	21.0	1.0
cream cheese	1.0	0
egg, 1	>1.0	0
eggs, 2, and hash browns	20.0	2.0
English muffin, dry	24.0	1.0
ham, grilled slice	6.0	0
oatmeal, *Quaker*	18.0	3.0
sausage, 4 links	0	0
syrup, maple	36.0	0
syrup, maple, sugar free	9.0	0
toast, 1 piece, dry	17.0	1.0

Food and Measure	carb. (gms)	fiber (gms)
toppings, 3 oz.:		
blueberry	26.0	0
cherry	21.0	0
strawberry	26.0	1.0
whipped cream	2.0	0
sandwiches, without fries:		
bacon, lettuce, and tomato	50.0	2.0
Boca Burger	64.0	9.0
burger, classic	56.0	4.0
burger, classic, with cheese	57.0	4.0
burger, mushroom Swiss	63.0	5.0
chicken, barbecued	86.0	5.0
chicken, grilled, without dressing	56.0	4.0
chicken melt, Italian	68.0	7.0
chicken melt hoagie	43.0	2.0
chicken ranch melt	57.0	3.0
club	45.0	2.0
fish	30.0	3.0
Philly melt hoagie	58.0	5.0
The Super Bird	32.0	2.0
soup, 8 oz.:		
broccoli cheddar	41.0	2.0
chicken noodle	14.0	1.0
clam chowder	55.0	4.0
vegetable beef	11.0	2.0
appetizers, without condiments:		
Buffalo strips	43.0	0
Buffalo wings	11.0	2.0
chicken strips	55.0	0
mozzarella sticks	49.0	6.0
nacho	117.0	11.0
Sampler	124.0	4.0
smothered cheese fries	69.0	0
entrees, without sides:		
burgers, mini, 6 pieces, with onion rings	179.0	10.0
chicken, grilled	15.0	1.0
chicken strips	55.0	0
country fried steak	30.0	11.0

Food and Measure	carb. (gms)	fiber (gms)
fish and chips	83.0	6.0
shrimp, fried	18.0	1.0
shrimp, fried and scampi	15.0	1.0
shrimp scampi skillet	3.0	.3
sirloin steak	1.0	1.0
steak and shrimp	31.0	2.0
T-bone steak	0	0
turkey, roast, with stuffing, gravy	62.0	2.0
sides/condiments:		
applesauce	15.0	1.0
barbecue sauce	11.0	0
bread stuffing	19.0	1.0
brown gravy	2.0	0
coleslaw	14.0	2.0
corn	23.0	3.0
cottage cheese or country gravy	2.0	0
fries, without salt	57.0	0
fries, seasoned	35.0	0
garlic dinner bread, 2 pieces	15.0	1.0
green beans	8.0	3.0
marinara sauce	7.0	1.0
onion rings	38.0	1.0
pico de gallo	5.0	1.0
potato, baked	51.0	5.0
potato, mashed	23.0	2.0
sour cream	2.0	0
tartar sauce	3.0	0
tomato, 3 slices	3.0	1.0
turkey gravy	29.0	0
salad, without dressing, except as noted:		
Caesar, side, with dressing	20.0	2.0
chef's	14.0	4.0
chicken breast, grilled	10.0	4.0
chicken strip, fried	26.0	4.0
garden, side	6.0	2.0
taco	57.0	8.0
salad croutons	12.0	1.0

Food and Measure	carb. (gms)	fiber (gms)
salad dressing:		
blue cheese, Caesar, or ranch	1.0	0
French or low cal Italian	3.0	0
honey mustard	20.0	0
ranch, fat free	6.0	0
Thousand Island	5.0	0
dessert/shakes:		
apple crisp à la mode	133.0	6.0
banana split	121.0	6.0
carrot cake	99.0	2.0
cheesecake	51.0	0
float, cola or root beer	47.0	0
hot fudge brownie à la mode	147.0	6.0
milkshake	76.0	<1.0
milkshake, malted	82.0	<1.0
Oreo Blender Blaster	112.0	2.0
pie, without topping:		
apple	64.0	1.0
blueberry	90.0	5.0
chocolate peanut butter	64.0	3.0
coconut cream	63.0	3.0
French silk	54.0	4.0
sundae, single scoop	14.0	0
sundae, double scoop	29.0	0
toppings, 2 oz.:		
blueberry	17.0	0
cherry	14.0	0
chocolate	34.0	1.0
fudge	30.0	1.0
strawberry	17.0	1.0
whipped cream	2.0	0
Dessert, freeze-dried, 1 serving:		
apple almond crisp (*AlpineAire*)	57.0	4.0
apple blueberry cobbler (*AlpineAire*)	38.0	4.0
bananas Foster (*AlpineAire*)	47.0	2.0
cheesecake, blackberry (*AlpineAire* Mountain)	134.0	1.0
cheesecake, blueberry (*Mountain House*), ¼ pouch, ½ cup	37.0	<1.0

Food and Measure	carb. (gms)	fiber (gms)
chocolate hazelnut Bavarian cream (*AlpineAire*)	36.0	4.0
ice cream, Neapolitan (*Mountain House*)	15.0	0
ice cream, Neapolitan, sandwich (*Mountain House*)	25.0	1.0
peach crumble, deep dish (*AlpineAire*)	48.0	1.0
raspberry crumble (*Mountain House*), ¼ pouch, ½ cup ..	31.0	3.0
Dill dip (*Litehouse Dilly*), 2 tbsp.	2.0	0
Dill see, 1 tsp.	1.2	.4
Dill weed, fresh:		
5 sprigs	.1	<.1
1 cup	.6	.2
Dill weed, dried, 1 tsp.	.6	.1
Dip, see specific listings		
Dipping sauce, see specific listings		
Dock:		
raw, chopped, 1 cup	4.3	3.9
boiled, drained, 4 oz.	3.3	<1.0
Dolphin fish, without added ingredients	0	0
Domino's Pizza:		
deep dish, 12", ⅛ pie:		
America's Favorite Feast/Deluxe Feast	29.0	2.0
Bacon Cheeseburger Feast	28.0	2.0
Barbecue Feast	32.0	2.0
beef, cheese, ham, or pepperoni	28.0	2.0
ExtravaganZZa Feast	30.0	2.0
green pepper, onion, and mushroom	30.0	2.0
Hawaiian Feast, or ham and pineapple	30.0	2.0
MeatZZa Feast/Pepperoni Feast	29.0	2.0
pepperoni and sausage, or sausage	29.0	2.0
Vegi Feast	30.0	2.0
deep dish, 14", ⅛ pie:		
America's Favorite Feast/Deluxe Feast	42.0	3.0
Bacon Cheeseburger Feast	41.0	3.0
Barbecue Feast	46.0	2.0
beef, cheese, ham, or pepperoni	41.0	2.0
ExtravaganZZa Feast	43.0	3.0
green pepper, onion, and mushroom	42.0	3.0
ham and pineapple	42.0	2.0
Hawaiian Feast	43.0	3.0

Food and Measure	carb. (gms)	fiber (gms)
MeatZZa Feast	40.0	3.0
Pepperoni Feast	42.0	3.0
pepperoni and sausage	41.0	3.0
sausage	42.0	3.0
Vegi Feast	43.0	3.0
hand-tossed, 12", ⅛ pie:		
America's Favorite Feast/Deluxe Feast	29.0	2.0
Bacon Cheeseburger Feast	28.0	2.0
Barbecue Feast	31.0	1.0
beef, cheese, ham, or pepperoni	28.0	2.0
ExtravaganZZa Feast	30.0	2.0
green pepper, onion, and mushroom	29.0	2.0
ham and pineapple	29.0	2.0
Hawaiian Feast	30.0	2.0
MeatZZa Feast	29.0	2.0
Pepperoni Feast	28.0	2.0
pepperoni and sausage or sausage	28.0	2.0
Vegi Feast	29.0	2.0
hand-tossed, 14", ⅛ pie:		
America's Favorite Feast/Deluxe Feast	39.0	2.0
Bacon Cheeseburger Feast	38.0	2.0
Barbecue Feast	43.0	2.0
beef, cheese, ham, or pepperoni	38.0	2.0
ExtravaganZZa Feast	40.0	3.0
green pepper, onion, and mushroom	39.0	2.0
ham and pineapple	40.0	2.0
Hawaiian Feast	41.0	2.0
MeatZZa Feast	39.0	2.0
Pepperoni Feast	39.0	2.0
pepperoni and sausage or sausage	39.0	2.0
Vegi Feast	40.0	3.0
thin crust, 12", ⅛ pie:		
America's Favorite Feast/Deluxe Feast	15.0	1.0
Bacon Cheeseburger Feast	14.0	1.0
Barbecue Feast	17.0	1.0
beef, cheese, ham, or pepperoni	14.0	1.0
ExtravaganZZa Feast	16.0	1.0
green pepper, onion, and mushroom	15.0	1.0

Food and Measure	carb. (gms)	fiber (gms)
ham and pineapple	15.0	1.0
Hawaiian Feast	16.0	1.0
MeatZZa Feast	15.0	1.0
Pepperoni Feast	14.0	1.0
pepperoni and sausage or sausage	14.0	1.0
Vegi Feast	15.0	1.0
thin crust, 14'', ⅛ pie:		
America's Favorite Feast/Deluxe Feast	20.0	2.0
Bacon Cheeseburger Feast	19.0	1.0
Barbecue Feast	24.0	1.0
beef, cheese, ham, or pepperoni	19.0	1.0
ExtravaganZZa Feast	21.0	2.0
green pepper, onion, and mushroom	21.0	2.0
ham and pineapple	21.0	1.0
Hawaiian Feast	21.0	2.0
MeatZZa Feast	20.0	2.0
Pepperoni Feast	20.0	1.0
pepperoni and sausage	19.0	2.0
sausage	20.0	2.0
Vegi Feast	21.0	2.0
salad, *Amazin' Greens,* garden fresh, ½ cont.	4.5	1.6
salad, *Amazin' Greens,* grilled chicken Caesar, ½ cont.	4.2	1.3
sides, 1 piece or cont.:		
bread stick	12.0	0
Buffalo Chicken Kickers	3.0	0
Buffalo wings, barbecue	2.0	0
Buffalo wings, hot	1.0	0
cheesy bread	13.0	0
Cinna Stix	15.0	1.0
icing, sweet	57.0	0
sauce, dipping:		
blue cheese or ranch	2.0	0
garlic	0	0
hot	4.0	0
marinara	5.0	0
Donuts, 1 piece, except as noted:		
plain (*Awrey's*), 2 pieces, 2.8 oz.	38.0	0
plain (*Entenmann's Softee*), 1.7 oz.	24.0	<1.0

Food and Measure	carb. (gms)	fiber (gms)
chocolate coated, mini (*Hostess Donettes*), 3 pieces, 1.5 oz.	21.0	0
chocolate frosted (*Entenmann's*), 2 oz.	28.0	1.0
crumb, mini (*Hostess Donettes*), 3 pieces, 2 oz.	31.0	0
crumb topped (*Entenmann's*), 2.1 oz.	35.0	<1.0
glazed (*Entenmann's*), 1.8 oz.	25.0	<1.0
Dough, sweet (*Rhodes*), 1.8 oz.	24.0	1.0
Dow gok, see "Yardlong bean"		
Drum, freshwater, without added ingredients	0	0
Duck, domesticated or wild, without added ingredients	0	0
Duck fat, 2 tbsp.	0	0
Duck sauce, see "Sweet and sour sauce"		
Dulce de leche topping, see "Caramel topping"		
Dulse flakes, see "Seaweed"		
Dumpling squash, see "Sweet dumpling squash"		
Dumplings, frozen:		
chicken, see "Chicken entree, frozen"		
meatless, (*Health is Wealth* Potstickers), 1.6 oz., 2 pieces	11.0	1.0
steamed (*Health is Wealth*), 1.6 oz., 2 pieces	12.0	1.0
Dunkin' Donuts, 1 serving:		
breakfast sandwich:		
bacon, egg, and cheese:		
bagel	69.0	2.0
croissant	39.0	0
English muffin	34.0	1.0
egg and cheese:		
bagel	71.0	2.0
biscuit	32.0	1.0
croissant	39.0	0
English muffin	34.0	1.0
ham, egg, and cheese:		
bagel	71.0	2.0
croissant	38.0	0
English muffin	34.0	1.0
sausage, egg, and cheese:		
bagel	72.0	2.0
biscuit	32.0	1.0

Food and Measure	carb. (gms)	fiber (gms)
croissant	39.0	0
English muffin	35.0	1.0
steak, egg, and cheese bagel	66.0	2.0
steak, mushroom, and Swiss bagel	67.0	2.0
bagel:		
plain	62.0	2.0
blueberry	66.0	2.0
cinnamon raisin	65.0	3.0
everything	67.0	3.0
harvest	61.0	7.0
multigrain	68.0	5.0
onion	61.0	3.0
poppy seed	65.0	3.0
reduced carb	45.0	14.0
salsa	60.0	2.0
salt	62.0	2.0
sesame	64.0	3.0
sourdough	71.0	2.0
wheat	62.0	4.0
biscuit	29.0	1.0
croissant, plain	37.0	0
croissant, reduced carb	19.0	2.0
cream cheese, 2 oz.:		
plain	4.0	0
plain, lite	6.0	0
chive	4.0	2.0
salmon	2.0	0
strawberry	9.0	0
vegetable, garden	4.0	0
Shedd's buttermatch, 1 tbsp.	0	0
panini, chicken fajita	57.0	3.0
panini, meatball or steak	56.0	3.0
cookies, 2 pieces:		
chocolate chunk, regular or white chocolate	28.0	1.0
chocolate chunk with walnuts	27.0	1.0
oatmeal raisin pecan	29.0	1.0
donuts:		
apple crumb	34.0	1.0

Food and Measure	carb. (gms)	fiber (gms)
apple crumb cake	41.0	1.0
apple n'spice	29.0	1.0
Bavarian kreme	30.0	1.0
black raspberry	32.0	1.0
blueberry cake	35.0	1.0
blueberry crumb or Boston kreme	36.0	1.0
chocolate coconut	31.0	1.0
chocolate frosted	29.0	1.0
chocolate frosted cake	40.0	1.0
chocolate-glazed cake	33.0	1.0
chocolate kreme filled	35.0	1.0
cinnamon cake	34.0	1.0
crueller, French	17.0	1.0
double chocolate cake	37.0	2.0
gingerbread, glazed	35.0	1.0
glazed	25.0	1.0
glazed cake	41.0	1.0
jelly filled	32.0	1.0
lemon burst	35.0	3.0
lemon cake	28.0	0
maple frosted	29.0	1.0
old-fashioned cake	28.0	1.0
powdered cake	36.0	1.0
strawberry	32.0	1.0
strawberry frosted	30.0	1.0
sugar raised	22.0	1.0
vanilla kreme filled	36.0	1.0
whole wheat glazed	32.0	2.0
donut fancies:		
apple fritter	41.0	1.0
chocolate iced Bismark	50.0	1.0
bow tie donut	34.0	1.0
coffee roll	33.0	1.0
coffee roll, frosted	36.0	1.0
eclair	39.0	1.0
glazed fritter	31.0	1.0
donut *Munchkins:*		
cinnamon, 4 pieces	31.0	1.0

Food and Measure	carb. (gms)	fiber (gms)
cake, 4 pieces	27.0	1.0
cake, glazed, 3 pieces	38.0	1.0
cake, powdered, 4 pieces	31.0	1.0
chocolate cake, glazed, 3 pieces	26.0	1.0
glazed, 5 pieces	27.0	1.0
jelly filled, 5 pieces	30.0	1.0
lemon filled, 4 pieces	23.0	0
sugar raised, 7 pieces	26.0	1.0
donut sticks, cake:		
plain	35.0	1.0
chocolate, glazed	49.0	2.0
cinnamon	42.0	1.0
glazed	51.0	1.0
jelly	61.0	1.0
powdered	42.0	1.0
muffins:		
banana walnut	69.0	3.0
blueberry	73.0	2.0
blueberry, reduced fat	75.0	2.0
chocolate chip	89.0	2.0
coffee cake muffin	78.0	1.0
corn	77.0	1.0
cranberry orange	66.0	3.0
English	32.0	1.0
honey bran	79.0	5.0
pumpkin	83.0	3.0
pastry and pie:		
apple Danish	36.0	0
apple pie	82.0	4.0
apple pie à la mode	107.0	4.0
cheese Danish	32.0	0
cinnamon stick	60.0	2.0
s'mores	20.0	1.0
strawberry cheese Danish	33.0	0
Coolatta:		
coffee, with cream	40.0	0
coffee, with milk	42.0	0
coffee, with 2% milk or skim milk	41.0	0

Food and Measure	carb. (gms)	fiber (gms)
lemonade	49.0	0
orange mango	66.0	2.0
strawberry fruit	72.0	1.0
vanilla bean	70.0	1.0
espresso drinks, hot:		
cappuccino, with milk	7.0	0
with milk and sugar	21.0	0
with soy milk	6.0	1.0
with soy milk and sugar	20.0	1.0
latte, with milk	10.0	0
with milk and sugar	22.0	0
with soy milk	8.0	1.0
with soy milk and sugar	22.0	1.0
caramel swirl	36.0	0
caramel swirl, soy	34.0	1.0
mocha swirl	37.0	1.0
mocha swirl, soy	35.0	1.0
peppermint mocha	51.0	1.0
white chocolate raspberry	42.0	0
latte, iced:		
with milk	11.0	0
with milk and sugar	23.0	0
with soy milk	8.0	1.0
with soy milk and sugar	20.0	1.0
caramel swirl, with milk	37.0	0
caramel swirl, with soy milk	34.0	1.0
mocha swirl, with milk	38.0	1.0
mocha swirl, with soy milk	35.0	2.0
drinks, other:		
Dunkaccino	35.0	0
hot chocolate	38.0	2.0
vanilla chai	40.0	0
Durian, fresh:		
½ of 1.3-lb. fruit	81.5	11.4
chopped, ½ cup	32.9	4.6
Dutch brand loaf, see "Lunch meat"		

E

Food and Measure	carb. (gms)	fiber (gms)
Eclair, chocolate, frozen:		
(*Smart Ones*), 2.1-oz. piece	25.0	1.0
mini (*Delizza* Belgian), 7 pieces, 3.5 oz.	32.2	.9
mini (*Ritch & Famous*), 1 piece, .6 oz.	5.0	0
Edamame (see also "Soybean"), fresh (*Frieda's*),		
½ cup in pod or 1 cup shelled, 2.6 oz.	10.0	3.0
Edamame, frozen:		
in pod, ½ cup (*C&W*)	8.0	5.0
in pod, ½ cup (*Dr. Praeger's*)	6.0	7.5
shelled (*Cascadian Farm*), ⅔ cup	9.0	4.0
shelled (*Dr. Praeger's*), ½ cup	8.0	5.0
Eel, without added ingredients	0	0
Egg, chicken:		
raw, 1 large:		
whole	.6	0
white only	.3	0
yolk, with small portion of white	.3	0
cooked, hard-boiled, chopped, 1 cup	1.5	0
cooked, boiled, poached, or scrambled, 1 large	.6	0
Egg, chicken, dried:		
whole, 1 oz.	1.4	0
whole, stabilized, 1 oz.	.7	0
white, flakes, 1 oz.	1.2	0
yolk, 1 oz.	.1	0
Egg, duck, 1 egg	1.0	0
Egg, goose, 1 egg	1.9	0
Egg, quail, 1 egg	<.1	0
Egg, substitute, ¼ cup:		
(*Egg Beaters*)	1.0	0

Food and Measure	carb. (gms)	fiber (gms)
(*Kineret* Light'n Tasty)	1.0	0
(*Morningstar Farms Better'n Eggs*)	0	0
(*Morningstar Farms Scramblers*)	2.0	0
(*Tofutti Egg Watchers*)	1.0	0
cheese and chive, garden vegetable, or Southwestern (*Egg Beaters*)	1.0	0
Egg, turkey, 1 egg	.9	0
Egg breakfast, freeze-dried, 1 serving:		
with bacon (*Mountain House* Can), ⅔ cup	7.0	0
with bacon (*Mountain House* Pouch)	12.0	<1.0
with ham and peppers (*Mountain House* Can), ⅔ cup	6.0	<1.0
with ham and peppers (*Mountain House* Pouch)	14.0	1.0
omelet, ranch with beef (*AlpineAire*)	17.0	1.0
scrambled (*AlpineAire*)	2.0	0
scrambled (*Mountain House*)	14.0	0
scrambling/omelet mix (*AlpineAire*)	3.0	0
Egg breakfast, frozen (see also "Breakfast pocket/sandwich" and specific listings):		
omelet:		
cheese, three (*Jimmy Dean*), 4.3 oz.	5.0	<1.0
ham and cheese, with home fries (*Aunt Jemima Great Starts*), 5.2-oz. pkg.	19.0	1.0
Western style (*Jimmy Dean*), 4.3 oz.	6.0	<1.0
scrambled, with hash browns, 1 pkg.:		
with bacon (*Aunt Jemima Great Starts*), 5.25 oz.	16.0	<1.0
with sausage (*Aunt Jemima Great Starts*), 6.25 oz. ...	18.0	2.0
Egg roll (see also "Spring roll"), frozen or refrigerated, 1 roll, except as noted:		
broccoli (*Health is Wealth*), 3 oz.	23.0	2.0
pizza (*Health is Wealth*), 3 oz.	23.0	3.0
seafood or shrimp, with sauce (*Chung's*), 3.1 oz.	24.0	2.0
spinach (*Health is Wealth*), 3 oz.	20.0	3.0
vegetable:		
(*Empire*), 3 oz.	15.0	3.0
(*Health is Wealth* Oriental), 3 oz.	23.0	2.0
(*Kahiki*), 3 oz.	23.0	2.0
mini (*Barney's*), 3 pieces, 2.4 oz.	22.0	1.0

Food and Measure	carb. (gms)	fiber (gms)
with sauce (*Chung's*), 3.1 oz.	25.0	2.0
vegetable/vegetarian (*Health is Wealth*), 3 oz.	21.0	2.0
Egg roll entree, frozen, vegetable (*Lean Cuisine*		
Everyday Favorites), 9-oz. pkg.	60.0	3.0
Egg roll sauce (see also "Sweet and sour sauce") orange		
(*Port Arthur*), 2 tbsp.	13.0	0
Egg roll wrapper (see also "Wrappers")		
(*Frieda's*), 2 pieces	28.0	1.0
Eggnog, dairy, ½ cup:		
(*Darigold*)	22.0	0
(*Darigold* Light)	20.0	0
(*Hood* Fat Free)	18.0	0
(*Hood* Golden/Light/Vanilla)	22.0	0
(*Hood Carb Countdown* Reduced Sugar)	9.0	0
(*Organic Valley*)	15.0	0
(*Turkey Hill*)	23.0	0
(*Turkey Hill CarbIQ*)	11.0	2.0
Eggnog, canned (*Borden*), ½ cup	17.0	0
"Eggnog," nondairy (*Silk* Nog), ½ cup	15.0	0
Eggplant, fresh:		
raw (*Frieda's* Chinese/Japanese), ⅔ cup, 3 oz.	5.0	2.0
raw, 1'' pieces, ½ cup	2.5	1.0
boiled, drained, 1'' cubes, ½ cup	3.2	1.2
Eggplant appetizer:		
babaghanoush (*Cedar's*), 2 tbsp.	5.0	3.0
caponata (*Alessi*), ⅓ cup	7.0	4.0
spread (*Peloponnese*), 2 tbsp.	3.0	0
Eggplant dip (*Victoria*), 2 tbsp.	2.0	1.0
Eggplant entree, frozen:		
bhartha (*Ethnic Gourmet*), 12-oz. pkg.	46.0	8.0
cutlets, breaded (*Dominex*), 3-oz. piece	18.0	1.0
Parmesan (*Cedarlane*), 5 oz.	16.0	3.0
Parmesan (*Cedarlane Carb Buster*), 9.5 oz.	15.0	4.0
parmigiana, with sauce (*Celentano*), ½ of 14-oz. pkg. . . .	13.0	3.0
rollettes (*Celentano*), 10 oz.	20.0	4.0
Eggplant entree, pkg. (*Tasty Bite* Punjab),		
½ of 10-oz. pkg.	13.0	2.0

Food and Measure	carb. (gms)	fiber (gms)
Eggplant relish, Indian (*Patak's* Brinjal), 1 tbsp.	5.0	0
Eggplant spread, see "Eggplant appetizer"		
Eight ball squash (*Frieda's*), 1 cup, 4.4 oz.	4.0	1.0
El Pollo Loco, 1 serving:		
chicken, all cuts, flame-grilled	0	0
tortilla, corn, 6", 3 pieces	42.0	3.0
tortilla, flour, 6.5", 3 pieces	48.0	3.0
burritos:		
BRC	79.0	6.0
chicken, spicy	64.0	6.0
Chicken Lover's Burrito	55.0	2.0
Classic Chicken Burrito	81.0	6.0
Grilled Fiesta Burrito	91.0	5.0
Twice Grilled Burrito	62.0	2.0
Ultimate Chicken Burrito	84.0	6.0
favorites:		
chicken nachos	90.0	12.0
chicken quesadilla	53.0	2.0
cheese quesadilla	51.0	2.0
chicken taquito, 2 pieces	43.0	3.0
chicken soft taco	18.0	1.0
taco al carbon	18.0	1.0
bowl, chicken Caesar	47.0	5.0
bowl, Pollo	84.0	12.0
salad:		
Caesar	17.0	4.0
Caesar, without dressing	15.0	4.0
fiesta	29.0	5.0
fiesta, without dressing	26.0	4.0
Monterray Pollo Salad	17.0	3.0
Monterray Pollo Salad, without dressing	12.0	3.0
tostada	83.0	11.0
tostada, without shell	42.0	7.0
salad dressing:		
chipotle	3.0	1.0
cilantro	1.0	0
cilantro, lite	5.0	0

Food and Measure	carb. (gms)	fiber (gms)
Italian, lite	2.0	0
ranch, buttermilk	2.0	0
Thousand Island	7.0	0
sides:		
black beans	35.0	5.0
coleslaw	12.0	2.0
corn cobbette	10.0	1.0
fries	61.0	0
garden salad	8.0	2.0
gravy	2.0	0
macaroni and cheese	25.0	2.0
pinto beans	24.0	9.0
mashed potatoes	23.0	2.0
Spanish rice	33.0	1.0
vegetables, fresh	6.0	4.0
condiments:		
guacamole	5.0	0
jalapeño hot sauce	0	0
salsa, avocado or house	1.0	0
salsa, pico de gallo, or spicy chipotle	1.0	0
tortilla chips	34.0	3.0
sour cream	2.0	0
Serrano pepper, fried	3.0	0
dessert:		
churro	24.0	1.0
caramel flan	43.0	0
Foster's Freeze, without cone	30.0	0
Elderberries, ½ cup	13.3	5.1
Elderberry nectar (*R.W. Knudsen*), 8 fl. oz.	29.0	0
Elk, meat only, without added ingredients	0	0
Empanada, frozen, 2 pieces, 4.75 oz.:		
beef (*Goya*)	58.0	2.0
cheese (*Goya*)	44.0	2.0
pizza (*Goya*)	56.0	40
Emu, meat only, without added ingredients	0	0
Enchilada, frozen, 1 piece:		
beef, with sauce (*El Monterey*), 4 oz.	16.0	2.0
beef, with sauce (*El Monterey*), 5 oz.	18.0	2.0

Food and Measure	carb. (gms)	fiber (gms)
cheese (*Cedarlane*), 4.8 oz.	19.0	2.0
cheese, with sauce (*El Monterey*), 4 oz.	15.0	1.0
cheese, with sauce (*El Monterey*), 5 oz.	16.0	1.0
chicken, with Suiza sauce (*El Monterey*), 5 oz.	19.0	1.0
Enchilada dinner, frozen, 1 pkg.:		
black bean (*Amy's* Whole Meal), 10 oz.	55.0	9.0
cheese (*Amy's* Whole Meal), 9 oz.	38.0	6.0
Enchilada entree, frozen, 1 pkg., except as noted:		
(*Amy's* Bowls Santa Fe), 10 oz.	47.0	10.0
black bean vegetable (*Amy's*), ½ of 9.5-oz. pkg. or ⅟₇ of 35-oz. pkg.	26.0	3.0
cheese:		
(*Amy's*), ½ of 9-oz. pkg.	18.0	2.0
(*Amy's* Family Size), ⅟₇ of 35-oz. pkg.	19.0	2.0
(*Linda McCartney*), 5-oz. piece	23.0	2.0
chicken:		
(*Healthy Choice*), 9 oz.	46.0	6.0
(*Healthy Choice*), 11.3 oz.	59.0	8.0
(*Lean Cuisine Everyday Favorites*), 9 oz.	49.0	3.0
(*Stouffer's* Family Style Recipes), ⅛ of 57-oz. pkg.	33.0	2.0
Suiza (*Smart Ones*), 9 oz.	38.0	3.0
pie, 3-layer (*Cedarlane*), ½ of 11-oz. pkg.	27.0	3.0
spinach feta (*Cedarlane Carb Buster*), 9 oz.	11.0	4.0
vegetable, garden (*Cedarlane*), ½ of 9-oz. pkg.	20.0	3.0
Enchilada sauce, ¼ cup:		
(*La Victoria* Traditional)	2.0	0
(*Pace*)	5.0	1.0
all varieties (*Old El Paso*)	3.0	0
green chili (*La Victoria*)	3.0	1.0
green chili (*Las Palmas*)	3.0	0
hot (*Las Palmas*)	2.0	0
medium or mild (*Las Palmas*)	2.0	1.0
red chili (*La Victoria*)	2.0	0
tomato (*Las Palmas*)	5.0	<1.0
Enchilada sauce mix:		
(*Lawry's*), 2 tsp.	4.0	<1.0
(*McCormick*), 2 tsp.	3.0	0
Endive, chopped, ½ cup	.8	.8

Food and Measure	carb. (gms)	fiber (gms)
Endive, Belgian, see "Chicory, witloof"		
Epazote, raw, 2 sprigs	.3	.2
Eppaw, raw, ½ cup	15.8	n.a.
Escarole, see "Endive"		
European soldier bean, canned (*Westbrae Natural*		
Organic Heirloom Beans), ½ cup	16.0	5.0

F

Food and Measure	carb. (gms)	fiber (gms)
Fajita, frozen or refrigerated:		
beef or chicken (*Tyson* Meal Kit), 3.8-oz. piece*	17.0	2.0
chicken (*Birds Eye Voila!*), 1 cup*	13.0	3.0
chicken (*Smart Ones Bistro Selections*), 9.25-oz. pkg.	33.0	3.0
Fajita kit, pkg.:		
(*Old El Paso* No-Fuss Dinner Kit) ⅕ pkg. mix	33.0	1.0
(*Old El Paso* No-Fuss Dinner Kit), 2 fajitas*	36.0	2.0
(*Taco Bell* Dinner Home Originals), ⅕ pkg. mix	38.0	3.0
Fajita marinade/sauce, see "Marinade"		
Fajita seasoning (*McCormick*), ¼ tsp.	0	0
Fajita seasoning mix:		
(*Chi-Chi's*), ¼ pkg.	7.0	0
(*D.L. Jardine's*), 1 tsp.	1.0	0
(*Lawry's*), 2 tsp.	3.0	0
marinade (*McCormick*), 2 tsp.	2.0	0
Falafel mix:		
(*Fantastic*), ¼ cup	21.0	6.0
(*Near East*), ¼ cup or about 2½ patties*	18.0	5.0
Farfalle pasta entree, frozen, spinach pesto sauce		
(*Moosewood*), 10-oz. pkg.	57.0	6.0
Farina, whole-grain:		
dry, 1 oz.	22.1	.8
cooked, 1 cup	24.6	3.3
Farro, see "Spelt"		
Fava bean, see "Broad bean, mature"		
Feijoa, raw:		
(*Frieda's*), 5 oz.	15.0	0
with skin, 1 medium, 2.3 oz.	5.3	0
pureed, ½ cup	12.9	0

223

Food and Measure	carb. (gms)	fiber (gms)
Fennel, bulb:		
(*Andy Boy*), 1 medium bulb	17.0	7.3
(*Frieda's*), ¾ cup, 3 oz.	6.0	0
8.3-oz. bulb	17.1	7.3
sliced, 1 cup	6.3	2.7
Fennel seed, 1 tsp.	1.1	<1.0
Fenugreek seed, 1 tsp.	2.2	<1.0
Fettuccine:		
dry, see "Pasta"		
refrigerated:		
(*DiGirono*), 2.5 oz.	39.0	2.0
(*Monterey Carb Smart* Egg Recipe), 3.5 oz.	27.0	5.0
plain or spinach (*Buitoni*), 1¼ cups	45.0	2.0
Fettuccine dish, freeze-dried (*AlpineAire*		
Leonardo da Fettuccine), 1 serving	44.0	1.0
Fettuccine dish, mix, 1 cup*		
Alfredo (*Annie's* Organic)	43.0	2.0
curly, cheddar, broccoli sauce (*Annie's* Natural)	51.0	1.0
Fettuccine entree, frozen, 1 pkg.:		
Alfredo:		
(*Healthy Choice*), 8 oz.	36.0	4.0
(*Lean Cuisine Everyday Favorites*), 9.25 oz.	44.0	2.0
(*Linda McCartney*), 10 oz.	35.0	4.0
(*Michelina's* Authentico), 9 oz.	46.0	3.0
(*Michelina's Lean Gourmet*), 9 oz.	41.0	2.0
(*Smart Ones*), 9.25 oz.	39.0	3.0
(*Stouffer's*), 11.5 oz.	49.0	3.0
with chicken, see "Chicken entree, frozen"		
Fettuccine entree, pkg., Alfredo (*Kraft It's Pasta Anytime*),		
11.5-oz. pkg.	74.0	4.0
Fiddlehead fern, fresh, 4 oz.	6.3	n.a.
Fig, fresh:		
1 large, 2.3 oz.	12.3	2.1
1 medium, 1.8 oz.	9.6	1.7
Fig, canned:		
in light syrup, ½ cup	22.6	2.3
in heavy syrup, ½ cup	29.7	2.8

Food and Measure	carb. (gms)	fiber (gms)
Fig, dried:		
(*Shiloh Farms* Adriatic/Black Mission), ⅓ cup	26.0	5.0
(*Shiloh Farms* Calimyrna), 2 figs, 1.6 oz.	30.0	4.0
10 figs, 6.6 oz.	122.2	17.4
Filberts, see "Hazelnuts"		
Filo dough, frozen:		
(*Athens* Twin Pack), 5 sheets, 9'' × 14'', 2 oz.	37.0	1.0
(*Athens/Apollo*), about 2½ sheets, 14'' × 18'', 2 oz.	37.0	1.0
extra thick (*Apollo* Country Style), 2-oz. sheet	33.0	<1.0
shells, mini (*Athens*), 2 shells	4.0	0
shredded (*Athens/Apollo*), ⅛ of 12-oz. pkg.	22.0	<1.0
Fireweed, leaves, fresh, 1 cup	4.4	2.4
Fish, see specific listings		
Fish cake, see "Fish entree" and specific fish listings		
Fish coating mix (see also "Batter and breading mix" and "Seafood coating mix"), seasoned:		
(*Don's Chuck Wagon*), ¼ cup	21.0	1.0
(*Golden Dipt* Fish Fry), 1⅓ tbsp.	6.0	0
(*Oven Fry*), ⅛ pkg.	9.0	0
Cajun (*Golden Dipt* Fry Easy), 1⅓ tbsp.	6.0	0
fish and chips mix (*Don's Chuck Wagon*), ¼ cup	21.0	1.0
fish and chips mix, batter (*Golden Dipt* Fry Easy), ¼ cup .	20.0	0
Fish dinner, frozen, 1 pkg.:		
herb baked (*Healthy Choice*), 10.9 oz.	55.0	5.0
lemon pepper (*Healthy Choice*), 10.7 oz.	49.0	5.0
Fish entree, frozen (see also specific fish listings):		
cake, breaded (*Kineret*), 2 pieces, 4 oz.	23.0	1.0
cake, breaded (*Dr. Praeger's*), 1 piece, 2.9 oz.	14.0	<1.0
fillet, baked, lemon pepper (*Lean Cuisine* Cafe Classics), 9-oz. pkg.	20.0	7.0
fillet, beer batter (*Gorton's*), 2 pieces, 3.6 oz.	18.0	0
fillet, beer batter (*Mrs. Paul's* Tenders), 4 pieces, 4 oz. . . .	22.0	1.0
fillet, breaded:		
(*Dr. Praeger's*), 2.1-oz. piece	11.0	<1.0
(*Ian's* Natural), 3.5-oz. piece	32.0	2.0
crunchy (*Mrs. Paul's*), 2 pieces, 3.7 oz.	22.0	0
sandwich (*Dr. Praeger's*), 4 oz.	19.0	<1.0

fillet, grilled:

	carb. (gms)	fiber (gms)
Alfredo, with broccoli (*Gorton's* Meal), 10-oz. pkg.	14.0	5.0
Caesar Parmesan, Cajun, Italian herb, char-grilled, or garlic butter (*Gorton's*), 3.8-oz. piece	1.0	0
garlic butter (*Mrs. Paul's* Meals), 11-oz. pkg.	34.0	3.0
lemon butter or pepper (*Gorton's*), 3.8-oz. piece	1.0	0
lemon pepper, with rice and vegetables (*Gorton's* Meal), 10-oz. pkg.	34.0	3.0
fillet, with macaroni and cheese (*Stouffer's* Homestyle), 9-oz. pkg.	47.0	2.0
nuggets (*Dr. Praeger's* Fishies), 4 pieces, 1.6 oz.	9.0	<1.0
portions, breaded:		
crunchy (*Kineret* 11.4 oz.), 2 pieces, 3.8 oz.	27.0	<1.0
crunchy (*Kineret* 20 oz.), 2 pieces, 4 oz.	29.0	<1.0
with shrimp, crab and vegetables (*Oven Poppers*), 4.5-oz. piece	13.0	0
with spinach and cheese (*Oven Poppers*), 4.5-oz. piece ..	8.0	0
sticks, breaded:		
(*Dr. Praeger's*), 3 pieces, 2.8 oz.	14.0	<1.0
(*Ian's* Natural), 5 pieces, 3.3 oz.	24.0	1.0
(*Kineret*), 5 pieces, 3.8 oz.	30.0	<1.0
(*Mrs. Paul's*), 6 pieces, 3.4 oz.	21.0	1.0
(*Van de Kamp's*), 6 pieces, 4 oz.	23.0	0
crunchy (*Kineret* 10.8 oz.), 6 pieces, 3.6 oz.	28.0	<1.0
crunchy (*Kineret* 25 oz.), 6 pieces, 3.1 oz.	29.0	1.0
with macaroni and cheese (*Stouffer's Maxaroni*), 7.75-oz. pkg.	35.0	1.0
Fish oil, all varieties, 2 tbsp.	0	0
Fish sauce, Thai, see "Thai sauce"		
Fish seasoning, see specific listings		
Fish seasoning mix, see "Fish coating mix"		
Flatfish, without added ingredients	0	0
Flavor enhancer, see "Monosodium glutamate"		
Flax seeds:		
(*Arrowhead Mills*), 3 tbsp.	9.0	7.0
(*Hodgson Mill*), 2 tbsp.	4.0	4.0
(*Tree of Life/Tree of Life* Organic Golden), 3 tbsp.	11.0	6.0
brown (*Shiloh Farms*), 3 tbsp.	11.0	6.0

Food and Measure	carb. (gms)	fiber (gms)
golden (*Arrowhead Mills*), 3 tbsp.	10.0	9.0
golden (*Shiloh Farms*), 1 tbsp.	3.0	3.0
Flounder, without added ingredients	0	0
Flounder entree, frozen, 5-oz. piece:		
au gratin (*Oven Poppers*)	5.0	1.0
stuffed:		
with broccoli, cheese (*Oven Poppers*)	4.0	1.0
with crab (*Oven Poppers*)	15.0	0
with garlic, shrimp, and almonds (*Oven Poppers*)	16.0	0
Flour, see "Wheat flour" and specific listings		
Flour, mixed grains (*Arrowhead Mills Perfect Harvest*),		
¼ cup	24.0	4.0
Focaccia, mix, see "Bread, mix"		
Foo qua, see "Balsam pear"		
Frankfurter, 1 link, except as noted:		
(*Ball Park* Bun Size/Franks), 2 oz.	3.0	0
(*Ball Park* Fat Free), 1.8 oz.	6.0	0
(*Ball Park* Lite), 1.8 oz.	3.0	0
(*Ball Park* Single), 1.6 oz.	3.0	0
(*Hatfield*), 2 oz.	1.0	0
(*Hatfield* Original), 1.6 oz.	0	0
(*Hatfield* Reduced Sodium/*Phillies*), 2 oz.	1.0	0
(*Healthy Choice*), 1.75 oz.	6.0	0
(*Hormel* Fat Free), 1.8 oz.	5.0	0
(*Dietz & Watson* Gourmet Lite), 2 oz.	3.0	0
(*Oscar Mayer* Wieners Light), 1.6 oz.	1.0	0
beef:		
(*Ball Park* Bun Size/Franks), 2 oz.	3.0	0
(*Ball Park* Fat Free), 1.8 oz.	7.0	0
(*Ball Park* Grillmaster/Grillmaster Deli), 2.9 oz.	3.0	0
(*Ball Park* Lite), 1.8 oz.	3.0	0
(*Ball Park* Single), 1.6 oz.	2.0	0
(*Boar's Head* Lite/Skinless), 1.6 oz.	0	0
(*Boar's Head* Natural Casing), 2 oz.	1.0	0
(*Dietz & Watson* Fat Free), 2 oz.	4.0	0
(*Dietz & Watson* Gourmet Lite), 2 oz.	3.0	0
(*Hatfield*), 2 oz.	1.0	0
(*Healthy Choice*), 1.75 oz.	7.0	0

Food and Measure	carb. (gms)	fiber (gms)
(*Hebrew National*), 1.7 oz.	1.0	0
(*Hebrew National* Family/Party Pack), 2 oz.	1.0	0
(*Hebrew National* 97% Fat Free), 1.7 oz.	3.0	0
(*Hebrew National* Reduced Fat), 1.7 oz.	0	0
(*Hormel*), 2 oz.	0	0
(*Hormel* Fat Free), 1.8 oz.	5.0	0
(*Nathan's* Casing), 2 oz.	1.0	1.0
(*Nathan's* Skinless), 2 oz.	1.0	0
(*Oscar Mayer XXL* Deli Style/Premium), 2.7 oz.	1.0	0
(*Shiloh Farms*) 2 oz.	0	0
(*Wranglers*), 2 oz.	1.0	0
dinner (*Hebrew National*), 4 oz.	1.0	0
uncured (*Organic Valley*), 2 oz.	1.0	0
cheese:		
(*Ball Park* Single), 1.6 oz.	2.0	0
(*Hatfield*), 2 oz.	1.0	0
(*Wranglers*), 2 oz.	1.0	0
chicken (*Organic Valley*), 2 oz.	1.0	0
cocktail:		
beef (*Boar's Head*), 5 pieces, 2 oz.	0	0
beef (*Hormel* Smokies), 6 pieces, 2 oz.	2.0	0
regular or cheese (*Hormel* Smokies), 6 pieces, 2 oz.	1.0	0
hot and spicy (*Ball Park Grillmaster*), 2.9 oz.	4.0	0
hot and spicy (*Oscar Mayer XXL*), 2.7 oz.	1.0	0
jalapeño (*Wranglers*), 2 oz.	7.0	0
pork and beef (*Boar's Head*), 2 oz.	0	0
salmon (*A&B Famous*), 2 pieces, 2.6 oz.	4.0	0
smoked:		
(*Ball Park* Bun Size Smokies), 2 oz.	2.0	0
(*Ball Park Grillmaster* Smokehouse), 2.9 oz.	3.0	0
(*Johnsonville* Natural Casing Wieners), 1.75 oz.	1.0	0
(*Oscar Mayer XXL* Original), 2.7 oz.	1.0	0
(*Wranglers*), 2 oz.	1.0	0
regular or cheese (*Hormel* Smokies), 1 oz.	0	0
turkey:		
(*Louis Rich/Oscar Mayer*), 1.6 oz.	2.0	0
(*Louis Rich/Oscar Mayer* Bun Length), 2 oz.	3.0	0
cheese (*Louis Rich/Oscar Mayer*), 1.6 oz.	2.0	0

Food and Measure	carb. (gms)	fiber (gms)
smoked, white (*Ball Park* Bun Size), 1.8 oz.	5.0	0
uncured (*Health is Wealth*), 1.5 oz.	1.0	0
"Frankfurter," vegetarian, 1 piece, except as noted:		
canned (*Loma Linda* Big Franks/Low Fat), 1.8 oz.	3.0	2.0
frozen/refrigerated:		
(*Morningstar Farms Veggie Dogs*), 2 oz.	6.0	1.0
(*Quorn* Dogs), 1.5 oz.	3.0	2.0
(*Worthington Leanies*), 1.4 oz.	2.0	1.0
(*Yves* The Good Dog), 1.8 oz.	2.0	0
(*Yves* Tofu Dogs), 1.3 oz.	2.0	0
(*Yves* Veggie Dogs), 1.6 oz.	1.0	1.0
(*Yves* Veggie Dogs Jumbo), 2.7 oz.	7.0	2.0
hot and spicy (*Yves* Chili Dogs), 1.8 oz.	3.0	2.0
wrapped:		
(*Morningstar Farms* Corn Dogs), 2.5 oz.	22.0	3.0
(*Loma Linda* Corn Dogs), 2.5 oz.	22.0	3.0
mini (*Morningstar Farms* Corn Dogs), 4 pieces, 2.7 oz.	21.0	1.0
Frankfurter, wrapped:		
(*Hebrew National* Franks in a Blanket), 5 pieces, 2.9 oz.	8.0	1.0
corn dogs (*Oscar Mayer*), 3.2-oz. piece	25.0	1.0
Franks and beans, see "Beans and franks"		
French toast, frozen:		
(*Aunt Jemima* Homestyle), 2 pieces	39.0	2.0
(*Pepperidge Farm* Homestyle), 1 piece	23.0	1.0
cinnamon:		
(*Aunt Jemima*), 3 pieces	34.0	2.0
sticks (*Aunt Jemima*), 5 pieces	50.0	2.0
swirl (*Pepperidge Farm*), 1 piece	24.0	2.0
sticks (*Pillsbury* Original), 6 pieces with syrup	68.0	1.0
sticks, cinnamon (*Pillsbury*), 6 pieces with syrup	69.0	1.0
sticks, toaster, 2 pieces:		
(*Eggo* French Toaster Sticks Original)	36.0	1.0
cinnamon (*Eggo* French Toaster Sticks)	37.0	1.0
Frog's legs, without added ingredients	0	0
Frosting, ready-to-spread, 2 tbsp.:		
butter cream:		
(*Betty Crocker* Rich & Creamy)	20.0	0

Food and Measure	carb. (gms)	fiber (gms)
(*Betty Crocker* Whipped)	14.0	0
(*Duncan Hines*)	22.0	0
caramel or cherry (*Betty Crocker* Rich & Creamy)	20.0	0
chocolate:		
(*Betty Crocker* Pour & Frost)	18.0	1.0
(*Betty Crocker* Rich & Creamy)	18.0	0
(*Betty Crocker* Whipped)	13.0	1.0
(*Duncan Hines* Classic)	22.0	0
almond or milk (*Betty Crocker* Rich & Creamy)	18.0	0
dark (*Betty Crocker* Rich & Creamy)	17.0	0
dark, fudge (*Duncan Hines*)	20.0	0
milk (*Betty Crocker* Pour & Frost)	18.0	0
milk (*Betty Crocker* Whipped)	14.0	0
milk (*Duncan Hines*)	22.0	0
chocolate chip:		
triple fudge (*Betty Crocker* Rich & Creamy)	22.0	1.0
vanilla (*Betty Crocker* Rich & Creamy)	23.0	0
coconut (*Duncan Hines* Supreme)	24.0	0
coconut pecan (*Betty Crocker* Rich & Creamy)	17.0	0
cream cheese (*Betty Crocker* Whipped)	14.0	0
cream cheese, plain or strawberry (*Betty Crocker* Rich & Creamy)	20.0	0
lemon:		
(*Betty Crocker* Rich & Creamy)	20.0	0
(*Betty Crocker* Whipped)	14.0	0
(*Duncan Hines* Supreme)	24.0	0
rainbow chip (*Betty Crocker* Rich & Creamy)	20.0	0
sour cream, chocolate (*Betty Crocker* Rich & Creamy)	18.0	0
sour cream, white (*Betty Crocker* Rich & Creamy)	20.0	0
strawberry (*Betty Crocker* Whipped)	14.0	0
vanilla:		
(*Betty Crocker* Pour & Frost or Rich & Creamy)	20.0	0
(*Betty Crocker* Whipped)	14.0	0
(*Duncan Hines* Classic)	24.0	0
with rainbow sprinkles (*Betty Crocker* Toppers)	21.0	0
vanilla, French:		
(*Betty Crocker* Rich & Creamy)	23.0	0

Food and Measure	carb. (gms)	fiber (gms)
(*Betty Crocker* Whipped)	14.0	0
(*Duncan Hines*)	24.0	0
white, fluffy (*Betty Crocker* Whipped)	14.0	0
Frosting mix:		
fudge ("*Jiffy*"), ¼ cup	28.0	<1.0
white ("*Jiffy*"), ¼ cup	27.0	0
white, fluffy (*Betty Crocker* Homestyle), 3 tbsp.	24.0	0
Frozen desserts, see "Ice cream" and specific listings		
Fructose:		
(*Estee*), 1 tsp.	4.0	0
(*Tree of Life*), 1 tbsp.	1.0	0
Fruit, see specific listings		
Fruit, mixed, can or jar (see also "Fruit cocktail"), ½ cup, except as noted:		
(*Dole Fruit Bowls*), 4 oz.	22.0	1.0
in juice:		
(*Del Monte*), 4-oz. cup	13.0	<1.0
(*Del Monte Fruit Naturals Fruit Cup*), 4.5 oz.	13.0	<1.0
(*Del Monte Orchard Select*)	19.0	<1.0
chunky (*Del Monte*)	15.0	1.0
chunky (*S&W* Natural Style)	19.0	3.0
tropical (*Del Monte*), 4-oz. cup	18.0	<1.0
tropical (*Del Monte Fruit Naturals*)	18.0	<1.0
in extra light syrup:		
(*Del Monte Fruit Cup* Lite), 4.5 oz.	13.0	<1.0
Ambrosia (*Del Monte Sunfresh*)	16.0	2.0
chunky (*Del Monte*)	15.0	1.0
citrus (*Del Monte Sunfresh*)	20.0	0
in gelatin, cherry (*Del Monte*), 4.5-oz. cup	23.0	0
in light syrup:		
(*Del Monte*), 4-oz. cup	18.0	<1.0
cherry (*Del Monte*)	22.0	<1.0
cherry (*Del Monte*), 4-oz. cup	18.0	<1.0
cherry (*Del Monte* Very Cherry)	22.0	<1.0
citrus (*Del Monte*)	20.0	0
tropical (*Del Monte Sunfresh*)	20.0	0
tropical (*Dole*)	20.0	1.0
tropical, with passion fruit juice (*Del Monte Sunfresh*)	21.0	1.0

Food and Measure	carb. (gms)	fiber (gms)
in heavy syrup (*Del Monte Fruit Cups*), 4.5 oz.	20.0	<1.0
in heavy syrup, chunky (*Del Monte*)	24.0	1.0
tropical (*Dole Fruit Bowls*), 4 oz.	16.0	2.0
Fruit, mixed, candied, 1 oz.	23.4	.5
Fruit, mixed, dried, ¼ cup, 1.4 oz.:		
(*Express*).	24.0	3.0
(*SunRidge Farms* Tropical Mix)	30.0	1.0
(*Sunsweet* Morsels)	28.0	2.0
(*Sunsweet* Tropical Mix)	32.0	2.0
(*Sunsweet* Orchard Mix)	25.0	3.0
Fruit, mixed, frozen (*McKenzie's*), ⅓ of 16-oz. pkg.	13.0	2.0
Fruit bar, frozen (see also "Ice bar," "Iced confection bar," and "Sorbet bar"), 1 piece, except as noted:		
all varieties:		
(*Breyer's* Bars No Sugar)	5.0	0
(*Breyer's* Swirl)	13.0	0
(*Minute Maid* Juice Bars)	15.0	0
(*Popsicle* All Natural)	12.0	0
(*Popsicle* Fantastic Fruity)	13.0	0
(*Popsicle* Mini Bars)	19.0	0
(*Popsicle Scribblers* Juice Pops), 2 pieces	16.0	0
(*Welch's* No Sugar Variety Pack)	6.0	0
except orange (*Tropicana* Real Fruit Variety Pack)	12.0	0
except orange (*Tropicana* Real Fruit Variety Pack No Sugar)	6.0	0
except tropical (*Welch's* Variety Pack)	11.0	0
banana, creamy:		
(*FrozFruit* Cream)	20.0	<1.0
(*Fruit-a-Freeze*)	18.0	<1.0
(*Fruit-a-Freeze* Single)	24.0	<1.0
chocolate dipped (*FrozFruit*)	22.0	1.0
chocolate dipped (*Fruit-a-Freeze*)	21.0	1.0
berry, wild (*Whole Fruit*)	20.0	0
cantaloupe (*FrozFruit*)	15.0	0
cantaloupe (*Fruit-a-Freeze*)	14.0	0
cappuccino (*Fruit-a-Freeze*)	19.0	0
cherry (*FrozFruit*)	16.0	<1.0

Food and Measure	carb. (gms)	fiber (gms)
coconut, creamy:		
(*FrozFruit* Cream)	18.0	2.0
(*Fruit-a-Freeze*)	19.0	<1.0
(*Fruit-a-Freeze* Single)	26.0	<1.0
(*Tropicana* Chunks of Fruit)	16.0	0
(*Whole Fruit*)	21.0	0
chocolate dipped (*FrozFruit*)	24.0	8.0
chocolate dipped (*Fruit-a-Freeze*)	22.0	1.0
grape (*Welch's*)	19.0	0
grape (*Whole Fruit*)	20.0	0
lemon:		
(*Dr. Praeger's* Sensible Treats)	24.0	0
(*FrozFruit*)	19.0	0
(*Fruit-a-Freeze* Single)	21.0	0
lemonade:		
(*Tropicana* Cooler)	18.0	0
(*Whole Fruit*)	20.0	0
soft (*Minute Maid* Tubes)	25.0	0
lime:		
(*FrozFruit*)	22.0	0
(*Fruit-a-Freeze*)	15.0	0
(*Fruit-a-Freeze* Single)	21.0	0
(*Whole Fruit*)	20.0	0
key, creamy (*Fruit-a-Freeze*)	20.0	0
mango (*FrozFruit*)	26.0	<1.0
mango (*Fruit-a-Freeze* Single)	26.0	0
mango pineapple (*Fruit-a-Freeze*)	15.0	0
orange:		
(*Tropicana* Real Fruit)	16.0	0
(*Tropicana* Real Fruit Variety Pack)	13.0	0
(*Tropicana* Real Fruit Variety Pack No Sugar)	7.0	0
with light ice cream (*Whole Fruit* Orange & Cream)	16.0	0
peach:		
(*Dr. Praeger's* Sensible Treats)	25.0	<1.0
(*FrozFruit Smoothie.Yum* Give Peach a Chance)	21.0	0
(*Whole Fruit*)	23.0	0
piña colada (*FrozFruit* Cream)	22.0	1.0

Food and Measure	carb. (gms)	fiber (gms)
pineapple (*FrozFruit*)	20.0	0
pineapple (*Fruit-a-Freeze* Single)	21.0	0
strawberry:		
(*Breyer's*), 1.75 fl. oz.	12.0	0
(*Breyer's*), 3.75 fl. oz.	30.0	<1.0
(*Dr. Praeger's* Sensible Treats)	16.0	<1.0
(*FrozFruit*)	23.0	<1.0
(*Fruit-a-Freeze*)	15.0	0
(*Fruit-a-Freeze* Single)	20.0	0
(*Tropicana* Chunks of Fruit)	14.0	<1.0
(*Whole Fruit*)	21.0	0
strawberry, chocolate coated (*Dr. Praeger's* Sensible Treats)	31.0	<1.0
strawberry, creamy:		
(*FrozFruit* Cream)	22.0	<1.0
(*Fruit-a-Freeze*)	18.0	0
chocolate dipped (*Fruit-a-Freeze*)	21.0	<1.0
chocolate dipped (*FrozFruit*)	18.0	1.0
strawberry banana (*FrozFruit* Smoothie. Yum Yumtonic)	34.0	1.0
tangerine (*Whole Fruit*)	20.0	0
tropical:		
(*Breyer's*)	20.0	0
(*FrozFruit*)	21.0	<1.0
(*Welch's Tropical Coolers* Variety Pack)	11.0	0
(*Whole Fruit*)	26.0	0
watermelon (*FrozFruit*)	17.0	0
watermelon (*Fruit-a-Freeze*)	14.0	0
Fruit cocktail, can or jar, ½ cup:		
(*Del Monte Carb Clever*)	11.0	<1.0
in juice:		
(*Del Monte Fruit Naturals*)	15.0	1.0
(*S&W* Natural Style)	20.0	2.0
with liquid	14.1	1.2
in extra light syrup (*Del Monte Lite*)	15.0	1.0
in light syrup (*S&W*)	18.0	1.0
in light syrup, with liquid	18.8	1.4
in heavy syrup:		
(*Del Monte*)	24.0	1.0

Food and Measure	carb. (gms)	fiber (gms)
(*S&W*)	23.0	1.0
with liquid	23.4	1.2
Fruit dip, 2 tbsp.:		
caramel:		
(*Litehouse* Lowfat)	28.0	0
(*Litehouse* Original)	25.0	0
(*Litehouse* Premium Dip Sleeve)	20.0	0
chocolate (*Litehouse*)	24.0	0
toffee (*Litehouse*)	27.0	0
chocolate:		
(*Litehouse*)	19.0	0
milk (*Baker's* Dipping Real)	9.0	0
semisweet, dark (*Baker's* Dipping Real)	9.0	1.0
strawberry or vanilla crème (*Litehouse*)	9.0	0
Fruit drink blend (see also "Citrus drink" and specific listings), 8 fl. oz., except as noted:		
(*Capri Sun* Splash Cooler), 6.75 fl. oz.	27.0	0
(*R.W. Knudsen* Razzleberry)	33.0	0
(*R.W. Knudsen* Razzleberry Box)	28.0	0
(*Simply Nutritious* Mega Antioxidant)	29.0	0
(*Simply Nutritious* Mega C or Morning Blend)	31.0	0
(*Simply Nutritious* Mega Green)	30.0	0
(*Simply Nutritious* Vita Juice)	29.0	0
(*V8 Splash* Medley)	28.0	0
lemon ginger enchinacea (*Simply Nutritious*)	29.0	0
punch:		
(*Hood*)	32.0	0
(*Langers* Cocktail)	30.0	0
(*Lincoln*)	34.0	0
(*Minute Maid* Carton/Jug)	31.0	0
(*Minute Maid Coolers*), 6.75-fl.-oz. pouch	26.0	0
(*Minute Maid* Plastic)	28.0	0
(*Nantucket Nectars*)	32.0	0
(*Ocean Spray*)	32.0	0
(*Snapple*)	29.0	0
canned	29.5	.3
frozen* (*Minute Maid*)	30.0	0
frozen*	28.9	.4

Food and Measure	carb. (gms)	fiber (gms)
herbal (*AriZona* Rx Power)	26.0	0
tropical:		
(*Ocean Spray Cravin' Less Sugar*)	20.0	0
(*Santa Cruz Organic* Box)	31.0	0
(*Snapple-a-Day*), 11.5 fl. oz.	43.0	5.0
(*SoBe* Lizard Lightning)	33.0	0
(*V8 Splash*)	27.0	0
colada (*V8 Splash* Smoothies)	30.0	1.0
tropical punch:		
(*Capri Sun*), 6.75 fl. oz.	25.0	0
(*Minute Maid*)	30.0	0
(*Minute Maid Coolers*), 6.75-fl.-oz. pouch	26.0	0
(*R.W. Knudsen* Box)	29.0	0
frozen* (*Minute Maid*)	28.0	0
Fruit glaze, see specific fruit listings		
Fruit juice blend (see also specific listings), 8 fl. oz.,		
except as noted:		
(*Bolthouse Farms* Green Goddess)	33.0	1.0
(*Ceres* Medley)	31.0	2.0
(*Langers* Autumn/Spring/Winter Blend)	30.0	0
(*Langers* Summer Blend)	31.0	0
(*Minute Maid* Medley), 11.5-fl.-oz. can	42.0	0
(*Minute Maid* Medley), 12-fl.-oz. bottle	43.0	0
punch (*Juicy Juice*)	29.0	0
punch (*Minute Maid*), 6.75-fl.-oz. box	24.0	0
tropical (*Santa Cruz Organic*)	33.0	0
Fruit pectin (*Sure•Jell*), ⅛ tsp.	0	0
Fruit protector (*Sure•Jell Ever Fresh*), ⅛ tsp.	<1.0	0
Fruit sauce, Asian, four (*Heaven and Earth*), 1 tbsp.	5.0	0
Fruit snack (see also specific listings),		
all fruits:		
(*Animal Planet*), .8-oz. pouch	17.0	0
(*Fruit by the Foot*), ¾-oz. roll	17.0	0
(*Fruit Gushers*), .8-oz. pouch	20.0	0
(*Fruit Rippers*), .6-oz. pouch	11.0	0
(*Fruit Roll-Ups*), .5-oz. roll	12.0	0
except apricot, blackberry, mango, strawberry, and tropical		
(*Stretch Island* Fruit Leather), .5-oz. bar	12.0	1.0

Food and Measure	carb. (gms)	fiber (gms)
all shapes/characters (*Betty Crocker* Fruit Snacks), .8-oz. pouch	21.0	0
apricot, mango, strawberry, or tropical (*Stretch Island* Fruit Leather), .5-oz. bar	11.0	1.0
blackberry (*Stretch Island* Fruit Leather), .5-oz. bar	12.0	2.0
Fruit spread (see also "Jam and preserves" and specific listings), all fruits, 1 tbsp.:		
(*Cascadian Farm*)	10.0	0
(*Harvest Moon*)	8.0	0
(*Smucker's Simply 100% Fruit*)	10.0	0
Fruit-nut mix, see "Trail mix"		
Fudge, see "Candy"		
Fudge topping, see "Chocolate topping"		
Fuki, see "Butterbur"		
Furikake, see "Sesame seed condiment"		
Fuzzy navel, drink mixer, frozen (*Bacardi*), 2 fl. oz.	29.0	0

G

Food and Measure	carb. (gms)	fiber (gms)
Gai choy, see "Cabbage, mustard"		
Gai lan, see "Kale, Chinese"		
Galanga, raw (*Frieda's*), ⅔ cup, 3 oz.	13.0	2.0
Garbanzo beans:		
dry (*Arrowhead Mills*), ¼ cup	27.0	8.0
dry (*Shiloh Farms*), ¼ cup	29.0	6.0
boiled, ½ cup	22.5	2.9
pre-soaked (*Frieda's*), ⅓ cup	23.0	22.0
Garbanzo beans, canned, ½ cup:		
(*Allens/East Texas Fair* Chick Peas)	19.0	8.0
(*Bush's*)	22.0	9.0
(*Eden* Organic)	19.0	5.0
(*Old El Paso*)	16.0	4.0
(*Progresso* Chick Peas)	20.0	5.0
(*S&W/S&W* 50% Less Salt)	19.0	5.0
(*Westbrae Natural* Organic)	18.0	5.0
(*Zapata*)	20.0	8.0
Garlic, fresh:		
(*Frieda's* Elephant), chopped, 1 tbsp.	1.0	0
trimmed, 1 oz.	9.4	.6
1 clove, .1 oz.	1.0	.1
granulated or minced, 1 tsp.	2.9	0
Garlic, in jars:		
crushed (*Christopher Ranch*), 1 tsp.	1.0	0
crushed (*McCormick* California Style), 1 tsp.	0	0
marinated (*Frieda's*), 1 oz.	7.0	0
minced (*McCormick* California Style), 1 tsp.	1.0	0
Garlic bread, see "Bread, frozen"		
Garlic bread sprinkle (*McCormick*), ¼ tsp.	0	0

Food and Measure	carb. (gms)	fiber (gms)
Garlic and herb sauce mix (*Golden Dipt Bag 'n Season*), 1 tbsp.	3.0	0
Garlic juice (*McCormick*), ¼ tsp.	0	0
Garlic oil (*Watkins* Liquid Spice), 1 tsp.	0	0
Garlic paste (*Italia in Tavola*), 1 tbsp.	3.0	0
Garlic pepper:		
(*Lawry's*), ¼ tsp.	0	0
(*McCormick* California Style/Grinder), ¼ tsp.	0	0
1 tsp.	1.8	.3
Garlic powder:		
1 tsp.	2.3	0
with parsley (*Lawry's*), ¼ tsp.	<1.0	0
Garlic relish, Indian, medium (*Patak's*), 1 tbsp.	3.0	0
Garlic salt, ¼ tsp.:		
(*Lawry's*)	0	0
(*McCormick*/California Style/Parsley/*Season-All*)	0	0
Garlic seasoning:		
herb (*McCormick 1 Step*), ¾ tsp.	1.0	0
roasted, and bell pepper (*McCormick 1 Step*), 1 tsp.	2.0	0
Garlic spread:		
(*Lawry's*), 1 tbsp.	2.0	0
(*Lawry's* Concentrate), 2 tsp.	1.0	0
(*McCormick*/McCormick Herb), ½ tbsp.	1.0	0
Garlic sprouts, fresh (*Jonathan's*), 1 cup	14.0	3.0
Garlic-herb dip mix (*Fantastic* Soup/Dip), 2¼ tsp.	5.0	0
Gefilte fish, in jars, without gel:		
(*Manischewitz*), 2.3-oz. piece	1.0	<1.0
(*Manischewitz* Fishlets), 7 pieces, 2 oz.	2.0	<1.0
(*Rokeach*), 2-oz. piece	2.0	1.0
sweet, 2-oz. piece	4.1	0
whitefish/pike (*Manischewitz*), 2.3-oz. piece	3.0	<1.0
whitefish/pike (*Rokeach* Old Vienna), 2-oz. piece	4.0	1.0
Gefilte fish, frozen, cooked (*A&B Famous*), 2 oz.	9.0	1.0
Gefilte fish, frozen, uncooked:		
(*BenZ's*), 3 oz.	19.0	0
(*Dr. Praeger's*), 1.8 oz.	6.0	0
(*Ungar's*), 1.8 oz.	4.5	0
(*Ungar's* Lite), 2.4 oz.	5.0	2.0

Food and Measure	carb. (gms)	fiber (gms)
gluten free (*A&B Famous*), 2 oz.	7.0	1.0
low cholesterol (*A&B Famous*), 2 oz.	8.0	1.0
salmon (*A&B Famous*), 2 oz.	4.0	1.0
salmon (*Ungar's*), 1.8 oz.	6.0	0
sugar free:		
(*A&B Famous*), 2 oz.	4.0	1.0
(*A&B Famous* Gourmet), 2 oz.	2.0	<1.0
(*Ungar's*), 1.8 oz.	3.0	0
sweet (*A&B Famous*), 2 oz.	7.0	<1.0
sweet and savory (*A&B Famous* Hungarian Style), 2 oz.	9.0	1.0
Gelatin, unflavored (*Knox*), ¼ pkt.	0	0
Gelatin dessert, ready-to-eat, 3.5 oz.:		
all fruit flavors:		
(*Hunt's Snack Packs Juicy Gels*)	24.0	0
(*Jell-O*)	17.0	0
(*Jell-O* Sugar Free)	0	0
cherry and blue raspberry (*Jell-O X-Treme*)	17.0	0
with fruit, see specific fruit listings		
watermelon and green apple (*Jell-O X-Treme*)	24.0	0
Gelatin dessert mix, ½ cup*:		
all fruit flavors (*Jell-O*)	17.0	0
all fruit flavors (*Jell-O* Sugar Free)	0	0
Gelatin sticks, all flavors (*Jell-O X-Treme*), 1 piece	16.0	0
Gemelli pasta dish, mix, with roasted garlic,		
Parmesan sauce (*Annie's*), 1 cup*	50.0	1.0
Ginger, trimmed root:		
1 oz.	4.3	.6
sliced, ¼ cup	3.6	.5
Ginger, candied or crystallized:		
(*Frieda's*), 9 pieces, 1.1 oz.	26.0	0
(*Tree of Life*), 7 pieces, 1.4 oz.	37.0	1.0
Ginger, ground, 1 tsp.	1.3	.2
Ginger, pickled:		
Japanese, 1 oz.	2.1	0
with shiso leaves (*Eden*), 1 tbsp., .5 oz.	3.0	1.0
Ginger, Thai, see "Galanga"		
Ginger-garlic oil (*Watkins* Liquid Spice), 1 tsp.	0	0

Food and Measure	carb. (gms)	fiber (gms)
Ginkgo nut, shelled:		
raw, 1 oz.	10.7	<1.0
canned, drained, 1 oz.	6.3	2.6
dried, 1 oz.	20.6	n.a.
Glace, cake, see "Fruit, mixed, candied"		
Glaze, see "Ham glaze" and specific fruit listings		
Glaze sauce, see "Grilling sauce" and "Marinade"		
Gluten, see "Wheat gluten"		
Gnocchi, potato:		
pkg. (*Bellino*), 1 cup	46.0	3.0
pkg., with spinach (*Bellino*), ¾ cup	41.0	2.0
refrigerated (*Rienzi*), 1½ cups	30.0	2.0
refrigerated, with cheese (*Rienzi*), 1½ cups	30.0	0
Goat, meat only, without added ingredients	0	0
Gobo root, see "Burdock root"		
Godfather's Pizza:		
original, medium, ⅛ pie:		
all meat combo or bacon cheeseburger	35.0	2.0
cheese	34.0	1.0
combo	36.0	3.0
combo, super	37.0	3.0
Hawaiian	37.0	2.0
Hawaiian, super	36.0	2.0
hot stuff	35.0	2.0
humble pie	34.0	2.0
pepperoni	34.0	1.0
taco or veggie	36.0	2.0
taco, super	36.0	3.0
original, large, ¹⁄₁₀ pie:		
all meat combo	38.0	2.0
bacon cheeseburger or combo	37.0	2.0
cheese	36.0	1.0
combo, super	39.0	3.0
Hawaiian	39.0	2.0
Hawaiian, super	38.0	2.0
hot stuff	37.0	2.0
humble pie	38.0	2.0

Food and Measure	carb. (gms)	fiber (gms)
pepperoni	36.0	1.0
taco	38.0	2.0
taco, super	39.0	3.0
veggie	45.0	3.0
golden, medium, ⅛ pie:		
all meat combo	27.0	1.0
cheese or bacon cheeseburger	26.0	1.0
combo	27.0	2.0
combo, super	28.0	2.0
Hawaiian	28.0	1.0
Hawaiian, super	27.0	1.0
hot stuff or humble pie	27.0	1.0
pepperoni	26.0	1.0
taco or veggie	27.0	2.0
taco, super	28.0	2.0
golden, large, ⅒ pie:		
all meat combo	29.0	2.0
bacon cheeseburger	29.0	1.0
cheese	28.0	1.0
combo	30.0	2.0
combo, super	31.0	2.0
Hawaiian or super Hawaiian	30.0	1.0
hot stuff or humble pie	29.0	1.0
pepperoni	28.0	1.0
taco, super taco, or veggie	30.0	2.0
thin, medium, ⅛ pie:		
all meat combo	20.0	1.0
bacon cheeseburger	19.0	1.0
cheese	19.0	>1.0
combo or combo, super	21.0	2.0
Hawaiian or super Hawaiian	21.0	1.0
hot stuff	20.0	0
humble pie	20.0	1.0
pepperoni	19.0	>1.0
taco or veggie	20.0	1.0
taco, super	21.0	2.0
thin, large, ⅒ pie:		
all meat combo or bacon cheeseburger	20.0	1.0

Food and Measure	carb. (gms)	fiber (gms)
cheese	19.0	>1.0
combo	21.0	2.0
combo, super	22.0	2.0
Hawaiian	22.0	1.0
Hawaiian, super	21.0	1.0
hot stuff or humble pie	20.0	1.0
pepperoni	19.0	>1.0
taco or veggie	21.0	1.0
taco, super	21.0	2.0
extras:		
bread stick, 1 piece	14.0	1.0
cheese sticks	18.0	1.0
potato wedges, 4 oz.	24.0	4.0
apple dessert:		
alum. pan, ⅙	28.0	1.0
small, ⅙	37.0	1.0
medium, ⅛	39.0	1.0
large, ⅒	42.0	1.0
cherry dessert:		
alum. pan, ⅙	29.0	1.0
small, ⅙	38.0	1.0
medium, ⅛	40.0	1.0
large, ⅒	44.0	1.0
chocolate chip cookie, alum. pan, ⅙	30.0	0
cinnamon streusel:		
alum. pan, ⅙	30.0	1.0
small, ⅙	39.0	1.0
medium, ⅛	40.0	1.0
large, ⅒	45.0	1.0
M&M's streusel:		
alum. pan, ⅙	31.0	1.0
small, ⅙	42.0	1.0
medium, ⅛	45.0	1.0
large, ⅒	51.0	1.0
Golden nugget squash (*Frieda's*), ¾ cup, 3 oz.	7.0	1.0
Goose, meat only, without added ingredients	0	0
Goose fat, 2 tbsp.	0	0
Goose liver, see "Liver" and "Pâté"		

Food and Measure	carb. (gms)	fiber (gms)
Gooseberries, fresh, ½ cup	7.6	3.2
Gordita entree kit:		
with ranch sauce (*Old El Paso* Dinner Kit), ¼ pkg.*	34.0	1.0
with red sauce (*Old El Paso* Dinner Kit), ¼ pkg.*	36.0	1.0
Gourd, boiled, ½ cup:		
dishcloth, 1" slices	12.8	<1.0
white-flower, 1" cubes	2.7	<1.0
Gourd, dried, see "Kanpo"		
Grain salad, see "Tabouli" and specific listings		
Grains, mixed, dish, mix (see also specific listings):		
brown rice and wheat:		
barley, chicken herb (*Near East*), 2 oz. or 1 cup*	51.0	6.0
bulgur, roasted garlic (*Near East*), 2 oz. or 1 cup*	41.0	5.0
pecan and garlic (*Near East*), 2 oz. or 1 cup*	37.0	4.0
white rice and pearled wheat, creamy Parmesan:		
(*Near East*), 2 oz. or 1 cup*	48.0	3.0
Granadilla, see "Passion fruit"		
Granola, see "Cereal, ready-to-eat"		
Granola/cereal bar, 1 bar, except as noted:		
(*Cascadian Farm* Harvest Berry Granola)	27.0	1.0
(*Froot Loops*)	16.0	<1.0
(*Frosted Flakes*)	19.0	<1.0
all varieties:		
(*Health Valley* Cobbler Cereal/ Low Fat Cobbler Cereal) .	27.0	1.0
(*Health Valley* Fat Free Granola)	35.0	3.0
(*Health Valley* Fat Free Bakes)	19.0	3.0
(*Health Valley* Low Fat Tarts/Creme Sandwich)	28.0	1.0
(*Nature Valley* Chewy Granola)	26.0	1.0
(*Nutri-Grain* Cereal)	27.0	1.0
(*Nutri-Grain* Minis), 1 pouch	32.0	<1.0
except dipped varieties (*PowerBar Harvest*)	45.0	4.0
almond, roasted (*Nature Valley* Crunchy Granola), 2 bars .	28.0	2.0
apple:		
cobbler (*Nutri-Grain Twists*)	27.0	1.0
crisp (*Nature Valley* Crunchy Granola), 2 bars	29.0	2.0
Dutch (*Health Valley* Moist & Chewy Granola)	22.0	2.0
apple berry (*Uncle Sam* Cereal)	28.0	3.0

Food and Measure	carb. (gms)	fiber (gms)
apple cinnamon (*Nature Valley* Chewy Trail Mix)	25.0	1.0
apple cinnamon or banana (*PowerBar*)	45.0	3.0
banana (*Nutri-Grain* Muffin)	30.0	1.0
banana nut:		
(*Nature Valley* Crunchy Granola), 2 bars	28.0	2.0
(*PowerBar Harvest* Dipped)	45.0	4.0
chocolate (*Save the Forest* Trail Mix)	19.0	1.0
berry:		
mixed (*Nature Valley* Chewy Trail Mix)	26.0	1.0
wild (*Health Valley* Moist & Chewy Granola)	22.0	2.0
wild (*PowerBar*)	45.0	3.0
blueberry:		
(*Honey Maid* Soft Baked)	27.0	1.0
(*Nutri-Grain* Muffin)	31.0	<1.0
and yogurt (*Barbara's Puffins* Cereal & Milk)	24.0	3.0
brown sugar cinnamon (*All-Bran* Cereal)	27.0	5.0
cappuccino and cream (*Nutri-Grain Twists*)	28.0	1.0
caramel nut crunch (*Nutri-Grain* Chewy Granola Bites),		
1 pouch	18.0	1.0
carob chip (*Barbara's Nature's Choice* Granola)	15.0	<1.0
carrot cake (*PowerBar Harvest* Dipped)	45.0	3.0
chocolate:		
(*PowerBar*)	45.0	3.0
almond toffee (*GoLean* Cereal)	45.0	6.0
caramel (*GoLean* Crunchy! Cereal Karma)	26.0	5.0
cinnamon (*Cafe Creations* Danish)	27.0	2.0
cookie, double (*PowerBar Pria*)	16.0	0
crème (*Hershey's SnackBarz*)	17.0	0
double (*PowerBar Harvest* Dipped)	45.0	3.0
espresso (*Cafe Creations*)	27.0	2.0
fudge brownie (*PowerBar Protein Plus*)	36.0	2.0
honey graham (*PowerBar Pria*)	16.0	0
peanut (*GoLean* Crunchy! Cereal Bliss)	30.0	5.0
peanut butter (*PowerBar*)	45.0	3.0
peanut butter (*PowerBar Protein Plus*)	38.0	1.0
peanut crunch (*PowerBar Pria*)	16.0	0
raspberry (*Cafe Creations*)	27.0	2.0

Food and Measure	carb. (gms)	fiber (gms)
chocolate chip/chunk:		
(*Nutri-Grain* Chewy Granola)	18.0	<1.0
(*Nutri-Grain* Chewy Granola Bites), 1 pouch	20.0	1.0
cinnamon:		
(*Nature Valley* Crunchy Granola), 2 bars	29.0	2.0
raisin (*Barbara's Nature's Choice* Granola)	14.0	<1.0
(*Nutri-Grain* Muffin)	32.0	1.0
raisin (*Save the Forest* Cereal)	19.0	2.0
roll (*PowerBar Harvest* Dipped)	45.0	3.0
cocoa (*Rice Krispies*)	17.0	<1.0
cookies and cream:		
(*GoLean* Cereal)	50.0	6.0
(*PowerBar*)	45.0	2.0
(*PowerBar Protein Plus*)	38.0	1.0
cranberry crunch (*Save the Forest* Trail Mix)	14.0	2.0
crème caramel crisp (*PowerBar Pria*)	17.0	0
French toast (*Barbara's Puffins* Cereal & Milk)	25.0	3.0
fruit and nut (*Cascadian Farm* Granola)	24.0	1.0
fruit and nut (*Nature Valley* Chewy Trail Mix)	25.0	2.0
honey oat (*All-Bran* Cereal)	27.0	5.0
honey oat raisin (*Nutri-Grain* Chewy Granola)	18.0	1.0
honey vanilla yogurt (*GoLean* Cereal)	49.0	6.0
lemon lime (*GoLean* Crunchy! Cereal)	32.0	5.0
malt nut (*PowerBar*)	45.0	3.0
malted chocolate crisp (*GoLean* Cereal)	49.0	6.0
maple brown sugar (*Nature Valley* Crunchy Granola), 2 bars	29.0	2.0
marshmallow crème (*Hershey's SnackBarz* S'Mores)	18.0	0
mint chocolate cookie (*PowerBar Pria*)	16.0	1.0
mocha java (*GoLean* Cereal)	50.0	6.0
multigrain (*Cascadian Farm* Granola)	27.0	1.0
multigrain, all fruit varieties (*Barbara's Nature's Choice* Cereal)	25.0	2.0
nut, triple (*Skippy* Trail Mix)	19.0	2.0
nutty s'mores (*Skippy* Trail Mix)	23.0	1.0
oatmeal (*Honey Maid*)	24.0	1.0
oatmeal raisin:		
(*GoLean* Cereal)	49.0	6.0

Food and Measure	carb. (gms)	fiber (gms)
(*Honey Maid* Soft Baked)	27.0	1.0
(*PowerBar*)	45.0	3.0
(*Uncle Sam* Cereal)	28.0	3.0
iced (*PowerBar Harvest* Dipped)	45.0	3.0
oats and honey (*Barbara's Nature's Choice* Granola)	14.0	<1.0
oats and honey (*Nature Valley* Crunchy Granola), 2 bars	29.0	2.0
peanut butter:		
(*Barbara's Nature's Choice* Granola)	13.0	<1.0
(*Hershey's SnackBarz*)	16.0	<1.0
(*Nature Valley* Crunchy Granola), 2 bars	30.0	2.0
(*PowerBar*)	45.0	3.0
(*Skippy* Snack Bar Granola)	18.0	1.0
all varieties (*Health Valley* Peanut Butter Bars)	26.0	1.0
chocolate (*GoLean* Cereal)	48.0	6.0
chocolate chip (*Barbara's Puffins* Cereal & Milk)	22.0	3.0
and fudge (*Skippy* Snack Bar Granola)	18.0	1.0
and strawberry (*Skippy* Snack Bar Granola)	14.0	1.0
peanut crunch (*Health Valley* Moist & Chewy Granola)	19.0	2.0
raspberry (*Save the Forest* Cereal)	19.0	2.0
raspberry crème stripe (*PowerBar*)	45.0	2.0
spice cake, frosted (*GoLean* Cereal)	49.0	6.0
strawberry cheesecake (*Nutri-Grain Twists*)	26.0	<1.0
strawberry shortcake (*PowerBar Pria*)	17.0	0
toffee chocolate chip (*PowerBar Harvest* Dipped)	45.0	4.0
vanilla crisp (*PowerBar*)	45.0	3.0
vanilla crisp French (*PowerBar Pria*)	16.0	0
yogurt:		
strawberry (*Barbara's Puffins* Cereal & Milk)	24.0	3.0
strawberry/vanilla (*Nutri-Grain*)	27.0	1.0
strawberry vanilla (*GoLean* Cereal)	50.0	6.0
vanilla (*PowerBar Protein Plus*)	37.0	1.0
Grape, fresh:		
(*Del Monte*), 1½ cups	24.0	1.0
(*Dole* Green), 1½ cups	24.0	1.0
(*Frieda's* Champagne), ½ cup, 3 oz.	15.0	1.0
American type (slip-skin), 10 medium	4.1	.3
American type (slip-skin), peeled and seeded, ½ cup	7.9	.6

Food and Measure	carb. (gms)	fiber (gms)
European type (adherent skin):		
seeded, 1 lb.	72.0	2.7
seedless, 10 medium	8.9	.3
seedless or seeded, ½ cup	14.2	.5
Grape, canned, seedless, in heavy syrup, with liquid,		
½ cup	25.1	.5
Grape drink, 8 fl. oz.:		
(*Nantucket Nectars* Organic Concord)	31.0	0
(*Newman's Own* Gorilla Grape)	34.0	0
(*Ocean Spray Cravin' Less Sugar*)	22.0	0
(*R.W. Knudsen* Box)	38.0	0
(*Santa Cruz Organic* Box)	24.0	0
(*SoBe Grape Grog*)	30.0	0
canned	28.8	0
cocktail, frozen* (*Minute Maid*)	33.0	0
grapeade:		
(*AriZona*)	31.0	0
(*Nantucket Nectars*)	33.0	0
(*Snapple*)	29.0	0
punch (*Minute Maid*)	32.0	0
Grape drink mix (*Lincoln*), 8 fl. oz.*	32.0	0
Grape juice, 8 fl. oz., except as noted:		
(*Juicy Juice*)	34.0	0
(*L&A* Plus)	40.0	0
(*Langers* Cocktail/Plus)	40.0	0
(*Nantucket Nectars*)	39.0	0
(*R.W. Knudsen*)	37.0	0
(*R.W. Knudsen* Concord)	40.0	0
(*R.W. Knudsen* Organic)	39.0	0
(*Santa Cruz Organic* Concord)	40.0	0
(*Walnut Acres* Concord)	31.0	0
blend:		
(*Minute Maid*), 6.75-fl.-oz. box	26.0	0
(*Minute Maid*), 11.5-fl.-oz. can	45.0	0
(*Minute Maid*), 12-fl.-oz. bottle	47.0	0
canned or bottled	37.9	.3
frozen* (*Cascadian Farm* Concord)	32.0	0
frozen* sweetened	31.9	.3

Food and Measure	carb. (gms)	fiber (gms)
white grape:		
(*Ceres* Hanport)	30.0	0
(*Juicy Juice*)	38.0	0
(*Langers* Plus)	40.0	0
(*Santa Cruz Organic*)	39.0	0
Grape juice concentrate, Concord (*Tree of Life*),		
9 tsp.	40.0	0
Grape leaves, fresh:		
1 cup	2.4	1.5
1 medium leaf	.5	.3
Grape leaves, in jar:		
(*Fanci Food*), 2 leaves	0	0
(*Krinos*), 1 leaf	0	1.0
Grape leaves, stuffed:		
(*Cedar's*), 6 pieces, 4.9 oz.	22.0	.0
(*Peloponnese*), 6 pieces, 4.9 oz.	27.0	.0
Grapefruit, fresh:		
(*Dole*), ½ medium	16.0	6.0
(*Sunkist*), ½ medium, 5.4 oz.	16.0	6.0
all areas/varieties, ½ large, 4.7 oz.	13.4	1.8
all areas/varieties, sections, 1 cup	18.6	2.5
all areas, pink/red, ½ medium, 3¾''	9.5	n.a.
all areas, pink/red, sections, 1 cup	17.7	n.a.
all areas, white, ½ medium, 3¾''	9.9	1.3
all areas, white, sections, 1 cup	17.7	2.5
California/Arizona:		
pink/red, ½ medium, 3¾''	11.9	1.4
pink/red, sections with juice, 1 cup	22.3	2.6
white, ½ medium, 3¾''	10.7	1.3
white, sections, with juice, 1 cup	20.9	2.6
Florida:		
pink/red, ½ medium, 3¾''	9.2	1.4
pink/red, sections with juice, 1 cup	17.3	2.5
white, ½ medium, 3¾''	9.7	.2
white, sections with juice, 1 cup	18.8	.4
Grapefruit, can or jar, ½ cup, except as noted:		
in juice:		
(*Fanci Food*), ⅔ cup	14.0	0

Food and Measure	carb. (gms)	fiber (gms)
white (*Del Monte Sunfresh*)	9.0	2.0
with liquid	11.4	.5
in extra light syrup, red (*Del Monte Fruit Naturals*)	16.0	<1.0
in extra light syrup, red (*Del Monte Sunfresh*)	14.0	<1.0
in light syrup, red (*Del Monte Sunfresh*)	19.0	2.0
in light syrup, with liquid	19.6	.5
Grapefruit, Chinese, see "Pummelo"		
Grapefruit drink, ruby red, 8 fl. oz.:		
(*Hood Carb Countdown*)	5.0	0
(*Langers*)	33.0	0
(*Langers* Diet)	10.0	0
(*Langers* Low Carb)	8.0	0
(*Minute Maid*)	34.0	0
(*Ocean Spray/Ocean Spray* Cocktail)	30.0	0
(*Ocean Spray Light Ruby*)	10.0	0
Grapefruit drink blend, ruby red, 8 fl. oz.:		
lemonade, strawberry, or tangerine (*Ocean Spray Ruby*)	31.0	0
mango (*Ocean Spray Ruby•Mango*)	30.0	0
tropical (*Langers*)	34.0	0
Grapefruit juice, 8 fl. oz.:		
(*Nantucket Nectars*)	23.0	0
(*Ocean Spray* Premium)	24.0	0
(*S&W*)	25.0	0
pink:		
(*Ocean Spray* Premium)	28.0	0
(*Organic Valley*)	21.0	0
(*Tree Ripe*)	24.0	0
ruby red (*Ocean Spray* Premium)	32.0	0
ruby red (*R.W. Knudsen* Rio Red)	35.0	0
canned, unsweetened	22.1	.3
fresh, pink or white	22.7	.3
frozen*, (*Minute Maid* with Calcium)	25.0	0
frozen*, unsweetened	24.0	.3
Gravlax, see "Salmon, marinated"		
Gravy, see specific listings		
Gravy, country, in jars, cream or sausage (*Campbell's*), ¼ cup	3.0	0

Food and Measure	carb. (gms)	fiber (gms)
Gravy mix (see also specific listings), ¼ cup*:		
country style (*McCormick* Lowfat)	5.0	0
country style, regular or sausage flavor (*McCormick*)	4.0	0
golden or savory (*Road's End Organics*)	5.0	0
home style (*McCormick*)	4.0	0
Gravy seasoning, see "Browning sauce"		
Great northern beans:		
dry (*Shiloh Farms*), ¼ cup	29.0	8.0
boiled, ½ cup	18.6	6.2
Great northern beans, canned, ½ cup:		
(*Allens*)	19.0	7.0
(*Bush's*)	18.0	7.0
(*Eden* Organic)	20.0	8.0
(*Westbrae Natural* Organic)	19.0	6.0
with sausage (*Trappey's*)	18.0	7.0
seasoned (*Glory*)	15.0	3.0
Green beans (see also "Snap beans"), fresh:		
raw, cut (*Glory*), 2 cups	5.0	3.0
raw, ½ cup	3.9	1.9
boiled, drained, ½ cup	4.9	2.0
Green beans, can or jar, ½ cup:		
all styles, except Italian cut (*Del Monte*)	4.0	2.0
whole (*Allens*)	6.0	3.0
whole (*Freshlike* Selects)	7.0	3.0
whole or cut (*S&W*)	4.0	2.0
cut:		
(*Allens* No Salt)	3.0	2.0
(*Allens/Sunshine*)	6.0	3.0
(*Freshlike*)	7.0	3.0
(*Freshlike* No Salt)	4.0	2.0
(*Freshlike* Selects)	5.0	2.0
(*Green Giant/Green Giant* Kitchen Sliced/Low Sodium) .	4.0	1.0
(*Veg-All*)	4.0	2.0
(*Westbrae Natural* Organic)	4.0	1.0
dilled (*S&W*)	5.0	1.0
with liquid	4.2	1.8
cut or French (*Del Monte* No Salt)	4.0	2.0

Food and Measure	carb. (gms)	fiber (gms)
French style:		
(*Allens/Sunshine*)	4.0	2.0
(*Freshlike*)	3.0	3.0
(*Freshlike* No Salt)	4.0	2.0
(*Green Giant*)	4.0	1.0
(*Veg-All*)	4.0	2.0
(*Westbrae Natural* Organic)	4.0	1.0
seasoned (*Del Monte*)	4.0	2.0
Italian cut:		
(*Allens* Shellouts)	9.0	3.0
(*Allens/Sunshine*)	7.0	3.0
(*Del Monte*)	6.0	3.0
seasoned (*Allens/Sunshine*)	8.0	3.0
seasoned (*Glory* Pole Beans)	9.0	2.0
seasoned (*Glory* String Beans)	6.0	2.0
Green beans, freeze-dried, l serving:		
(*Mountain House*)	6.0	2.0
almondine (*AlpineAire*)	13.0	5.0
Green beans, frozen:		
whole:		
(*Birds Eye*), 1 cup	5.0	2.0
(*Cascadian Farm* Petite), 1 cup	5.0	2.0
(*C&W* Haricots Verts/Petite), ¾ cup	4.0	2.0
(*Green Giant Select*), 1 cup	4.0	2.0
cut:		
(*Birds Eye*), ⅔ cup	5.0	2.0
(*Cascadian Farm*), ¾ cup	6.0	2.0
(*Green Giant*), ½ cup cooked	4.0	2.0
(*McKenzie's* Pole Beans), ½ cup	4.0	2.0
(*Dr. Praeger's*), ⅔ cup	5.0	2.0
(*Tree of Life*), ⅔ cup	4.0	2.0
French (*C&W*), ⅔ cup	4.0	2.0
Italian cut (*Birds Eye*), ¾ cup	5.0	2.0
Italian cut (*C&W*), ¾ cup	4.0	2.0
boiled, drained, ½ cup	4.4	2.0
in garlic butter (*Green Giant*), ½ cup cooked	6.0	2.0
Green beans, pickled, in jars, hot (*Tillen Farms*), ¼ cup	3.0	0

Food and Measure	carb. (gms)	fiber (gms)
Green beans combinations, canned, ½ cup:		
casserole:		
(*Allens*)	6.0	1.0
(*Del Monte Savory Sides*)	11.0	2.0
(*Glory*)	9.0	2.0
and potatoes:		
(*Allens/Sunshine*)	10.0	2.0
(*Glory* String Beans)	10.0	2.0
with ham flavor (*Del Monte*)	6.0	1.0
Green beans combinations, frozen:		
with almonds:		
(*Cascadian Farm* Bag), ¾ cup	10.0	4.0
(*Cascadian Farm* Box), ⅔ cup	8.0	2.0
(*C&W*), 1 cup	9.0	3.0
(*Green Giant*), ½ cup cooked	4.0	2.0
toasted (*Birds Eye* Medley), 1 cup	10.0	5.0
toasted, lightly (*Birds Eye*), ¾ cup	8.0	3.0
baby, mixed, with carrots (*Birds Eye*), 1 cup	6.0	2.0
casserole (*Green Giant*), ⅔ cup	7.0	2.0
and spaetzle, in sauce (*Birds Eye* Bavarian), 1 cup	16.0	3.0
stir-fry (*Birds Eye* Crisp), 1 cup cooked	19.0	2.0
Green peas, see "Peas, green"		
Greens, see specific listings		
Greens, mixed, salad, see "Salad blend"		
Greens, mixed, canned, ½ cup:		
(*Allens* No Salt)	8.0	4.0
all varieties (*Bush's*)	3.0	2.0
seasoned (*Allens/Sunshine*)	6.0	1.0
seasoned (*Glory*)	7.0	3.0
Grenadine syrup:		
(*Angostura*), 1 tsp.	4.0	0
(*Giroux*), 2 tbsp.	26.0	0
(*Trader Vic's*), 2 tbsp.	23.0	0
Grilling sauce (see also "Barbecue sauce," "Marinade," and specific listings), 2 tbsp., except as noted:		
garlic, roasted, and herb (*McCormick Grill Mates*)	7.0	0
hickory barbecue (*McCormick Grill Mates*)	17.0	0

Food and Measure	carb. (gms)	fiber (gms)
honey mustard (*McCormick Grill Mates*)	15.0	0
Hunan (*House of Tsang* Hibachi Smokehut), 1 tbsp.	8.0	0
Italian grill (*World Harbors*)	4.0	0
lemon butter dill (*Golden Dipt*)	4.0	0
lemon butter dill (*Golden Dipt* Fat Free)	7.0	0
mesquite (*McCormick Grill Mates*)	12.0	0
peanut, Thai (*House of Tsang* Hibachi), 1 tbsp.	4.0	0
pepper, cracked (*San-J*)	5.0	<1.0
sesame, sweet ginger (*House of Tsang* Hibachi), 1 tbsp.	8.0	0
steak, kobe (*House of Tsang* Hibachi), 1 tbsp.	2.0	0
steak, Montreal (*McCormick Grill Mates*)	7.0	0
sweet and hot chili (*San-J*)	6.0	<1.0
teriyaki (*House of Tsang* Hibachi), 1 tbsp.	10.0	0
teriyaki (*McCormick Grill Mates*)	12.0	0
Grilling seasoning (*Watkins*), ¼ tsp.	0	0
Grits, see "Corn grits" and "Barley grits"		
Grog mixer, see "Navy grog drink mixer"		
Ground cherry, ½ cup	7.8	2.0
Grouper, without added ingredients	0	0
Guacamole, frozen or refrigerated:		
(*Calavo* Fiesta), 2 tbsp.	2.0	2.0
(*Calvao* Homestyle/Spicy), 2 tbsp.	3.0	2.0
(*Calavo* Original), 2 tbsp.	3.0	0
(*Kraft*), 2 tbsp.	3.0	0
(*Tofutti Sour Supreme*), 2 tbsp.	1.0	0
Mexican or Western (*Calavo*), 2 tbsp.	3.0	0
mild (*Calavo*), 2 tbsp.	4.0	2.0
with salsa (*San Pedro's* Holy Guacamole!), 1 oz.	3.0	0
spicy (*Goya*), 2 tbsp.	3.0	2.0
Guacamole seasoning (*Lawry's*), ½ tsp.	1.0	0
Guava (see also "Feijoas"):		
(*Frieda's*), 3-oz. piece	10.0	5.0
1 medium, 4 oz.	10.7	4.9
½ cup	9.8	4.5
strawberry, ½ cup	21.2	7.8
Guava, in jars, whole in syrup (*Herdez*), 4 pieces, 4.5 oz.	32.0	5.0

Food and Measure	carb. (gms)	fiber (gms)
Guava drink blend, 8 fl. oz.:		
(*Nantucket Nectars*)	33.0	0
passion fruit (*V8 Splash*)	27.0	0
strawberry (*R.W. Knudsen*)	27.0	0
Guava juice (*Ceres*), 8 fl. oz.	29.0	0
Guava nectar (*Goya*), 12 fl. oz.	59.0	2.0
Guava sauce, ½ cup	11.3	4.3
Guavadilla, see "Passion fruit"		
Guinea hen, meat only, without added ingredients	0	0
Gyros mix, dry (*Casbah*), .65 oz.	12.0	0

H

Food and Measure	carb. (gms)	fiber (gms)
Habas, see "Broad beans, mature"		
Haddock, fresh or smoked, without added ingredients ...	0	0
Haddock entree, frozen:		
fillet, battered (*Van de Kamp's*), 2 pieces, 3.7 oz.	20.0	0
fillet, breaded (*Mrs. Paul's*), 4-oz. piece	17.0	0
with shrimp, crab, vegetables (*Oven Poppers*), 5-oz. piece	12.0	1.0
Hake, see "Whiting"		
Halibut, Atlantic/Pacific, without added ingredients	0	0
Halvah, chocolate, vanilla, or marble (*Joyva*), 2 oz.	18.0	2.0
Ham, fresh, without added ingredients	0	0
Ham, cured, whole leg:		
whole leg, unheated, 4 oz. or 1 cup	.1	0
whole leg, roasted, 4 oz. or 1 cup chopped or diced	0	0
boneless:		
13% fat, unheated, 4 oz.	0	0
13% fat, roasted, 4 oz.	.5	0
extra lean, 4% fat, unheated, 4 oz.	0	0
extra lean, 4% fat, roasted, 4 oz.	.6	0
extra lean, 4% fat, roasted, chopped, or diced, 1 cup ..	.7	0
Ham, deviled, see "Ham spread"		
Ham, refrigerated or canned, 3 oz., except as noted:		
(*Black Label* Refrigerator Can)	1.0	0
(*Bilinski* Champagne Ham)	1.0	0
(*Cure 81*)	0	0
(*Curemaster*)	0	0
(*Spiral Cure 81*)	1.0	0
chunk (*Hormel*), 2 oz.	0	0
extra lean, 4% fat:		
unheated, 4 oz. or 1 cup chopped or diced	0	0

Food and Measure	carb. (gms)	fiber (gms)
roasted, 4 oz.	.6	0
roasted, 1 cup	.7	0
smoked (*Organic Valley*)	1.0	0
steak, cooked:		
(*Hatfield* Traditional)	3.0	0
honey (*Hatfield*)	5.0	0
maple (*Hatfield*)	6.0	0
"Ham," vegetarian, slices (*Yves*), 2.2 oz.	6.0	1.0
Ham and cheese loaf:		
(*Hansel 'n Gretel*), 2 oz.	3.0	0
(*Oscar Mayer*), 1 oz.	1.0	0
Ham and cheese pocket/sandwich, frozen, 1 piece:		
(*Hot Pockets*), 4.5 oz.	33.0	3.0
(*Lean Pockets* Ultra), 4.5 oz.	19.0	7.0
cheddar, 4.5 oz.:		
(*Croissant Pockets*)	36.0	3.0
(*Lean Pockets*)	40.0	3.0
(*Smart Ones Smartwich*)	38.0	1.0
sub (*Michelina's Hot Subs*), 2.1 oz.	32.0	1.0
Ham entree, frozen, sausage Jambalaya:		
(*Glory* Savory Singles), 11-oz. pkg.	42.0	2.0
(*Glory* Savory Singles Family Size), 1 cup	38.0	2.0
Ham entree mix, and au gratin potatoes		
(*Betty Crocker Complete Meals*), 1/5 pkg.	37.0	2.0
Ham glaze:		
(*Boar's Head* Sugar & Spice), 2 tbsp.	30.0	0
(*Crosse & Blackwell*), 1 tbsp.	8.0	0
(*Reese's*), 1 tbsp.	5.0	0
Ham lunch meat (see also "Proscuitto"), 2 oz., except as noted:		
(*Boar's Head* Deluxe/Deluxe 42% Lower Sodium)	2.0	0
(*Deli Delight*)	2.0	0
(*Dietz & Watson* Gourmet Lite/Tiffany)	1.0	0
(*Hansel 'n Gretel* Deluxe)	1.0	0
(*Hatfield Deli Choice* Ham Off the Bone)	2.0	0
(*Healthy Deli* Zero Carb Deluxe/Less Sodium Fat Free)	0	0
(*Williams* Old Fashion)	1.0	0

Food and Measure	carb. (gms)	fiber (gms)
baked:		
(*Healthy Choice* Hearty Slices), 1 oz.	1.0	0
(*Healthy Choice* Tub), 2 slices, 2 oz.	1.0	0
(*Healthy Choice* Deli Thin), 6 slices, 2 oz.	1.0	0
(*Sara Lee* Homestyle)	2.0	0
(*Williams* Home)	2.0	0
brown sugar:		
(*Oscar Mayer* Deli Style Shaved), 1.8 oz.	3.0	0
(*Oscar Mayer* Deli Style Thin Sliced)	4.0	0
(*Sara Lee*)	5.0	0
(*Sara Lee* Sliced), 2 slices, 1.6 oz.	4.0	0
(*Tyson* Bag), .9-oz. slice	1.0	0
Black Forest:		
(*Boar's Head*)	2.0	0
(*Dietz & Watson*)	2.0	0
(*Healthy Deli*)	1.0	0
(*Hormel*)	0	0
(*Sara Lee*)	1.0	0
(*Tyson*), 1-oz. slice	0	0
boiled (*Oscar Mayer* 96% Fat Free), 2.2 oz.	1.0	0
capicola/cappy:		
(*Black Bear* Capocollo), 1 oz.	<1.0	0
(*Boar's Head* Cappy)	3.0	0
(*Hansel 'n Gretel*)	2.0	0
(*Healthy Deli*)	2.0	0
Italian (*Boar's Head* Capocollo), 1 oz.	0	0
chopped (*Hormel Black Label*)	3.0	0
chopped (*Oscar Mayer*), 1 oz.	1.0	0
cinnamon apple (*Healthy Deli*)	4.0	0
cooked:		
(*Alpine Lace* 97% Fat Free)	2.0	0
(*Hatfield Deli Choice* Imported)	1.0	0
(*Hatfield Deli Choice* Premium)	2.0	0
(*Healthy Choice*)	1.0	0
(*Healthy Choice* Hearty Slices), 1 oz.	1.0	0
(*Healthy Choice* Deli Thin), 4 slices, 1.8 oz.	2.0	0
(*Hormel*)	0	0
(*Oscar Mayer* 96% Fat Free), 2.2 oz.	1.0	0

Food and Measure	carb. (gms)	fiber (gms)
(*Sara Lee* Old Fashioned)	1.0	0
(*Tyson* Bag), 2 slices, 1.6 oz.	0	0
(*Tyson* Box), 5 slices, 1.8 oz.	0	0
fresh, seasoned (*Boar's Head*)	0	0
glazed (*Hansel 'n Gretel*)	2.0	0
glazed (*Healthy Deli* Deluxe)	2.0	0
honey/honey cured:		
(*Alpine Lace* 97% Fat Free)	2.0	0
(*Healthy Choice*)	2.0	0
(*Healthy Choice* Hearty Slices), 1 oz.	1.0	0
(*Healthy Choice* Tub), 5 slices, 1.9 oz.	2.0	0
(*Healthy Choice* Deli Thin), 4 slices, 1.8 oz.	2.0	0
(*Healthy Deli*)	2.0	0
(*Hormel*)	3.0	0
(*Louis Rich Carving Board* 97% Fat Free), 2.1 oz.	2.0	0
(*Oscar Mayer*), 2.2 oz.	2.0	0
(*Sara Lee* Sliced), 2 slices, 1.6 oz.	1.0	0
(*Sara Lee/Sara Lee* Bavarian)	2.0	0
(*Tyson* Bag), 2 slices, 1.6 oz.	1.0	0
(*Tyson* Box), 5 slices, 1.8 oz.	1.0	0
chopped (*Oscar Mayer* 96% Fat Free), 1 oz.	4.0	0
cured (*Tyson*), .9-oz. slice	2.0	0
honey maple (*Healthy Choice* Hearty Slices), 1 oz.	1.0	0
honey maple (*Healthy Choice* Deli Thin), 4 slices, 1.8 oz.	1.0	0
honey mustard (*Healthy Choice* Deli Thin), 4 slices, 1.8 oz.	3.0	0
jalapeño (*Healthy Deli*)	3.0	0
loaf (*Deli Delight*)	3.0	0
maple:		
(*Healthy Choice*)	3.0	0
(*Healthy Deli* Vermont)	3.0	0
(*Williams* Buffet)	1.0	0
glazed (*Boar's Head Honey Coat*)	3.0	0
honey (*Sara Lee*)	4.0	0
peppered:		
(*Boar's Head* Gourmet)	2.0	0
(*Dietz & Watson*)	0	0
(*Hatfield Deli Choice*)	2.0	0

Food and Measure	carb. (gms)	fiber (gms)
(*Healthy Deli*)	2.0	0
(*Sara Lee*)	2.0	0
spiced, see "Lunch meat"		
pesto Parmesan, oven-roasted (*Boar's Head*)	0	0
rosemary sun-dried tomato (*Boar's Head*)	2.0	0
smoked:		
(*Boar's Head Sweet Slice*)	1.0	0
(*Healthy Choice*)	2.0	0
(*Sara Lee* Smokehouse)	1.0	0
(*Oscar Mayer* Deli Style Thin Sliced)	0	0
(*Oscar Mayer* 96% Fat Free Wallet Pack), 2.2 oz.	0	0
double (*Healthy Deli*)	1.0	0
double (*Hormel*)	0	0
maple glaze (*Dietz & Watson*)	2.0	0
tavern:		
(*Boar's Head*)	2.0	0
(*Dietz & Watson* Gourmet Lite)	1.0	0
(*Hatfield Deli Choice*), 3 oz.	3.0	0
(*Healthy Deli*)	1.0	0
honey (*Sara Lee*)	2.0	0
Virginia:		
(*Boar's Head*)	2.0	0
(*Deli Delight*)	3.0	0
(*Dietz & Watson* Gourmet Lite)	2.0	0
(*Hansel 'n Gretel*)	2.0	0
(*Hatfield Deli Choice*)	4.0	0
(*Healthy Choice*)	2.0	0
(*Healthy Deli* Zero Carb)	0	0
(*Sara Lee* Sliced), 2 slices, 1.6 oz.	2.0	0
(*Tyson*), .9-oz. slice	0	0
oven baked (*Healthy Deli*)	3.0	0
smoked (*Healthy Choice*), 2 slices, 2 oz.	2.0	0
smoked (*Healthy Choice Deli Thin*), 4 slices, 1.8 oz.	2.0	0
smoked (*Healthy Deli*)	2.0	0
Ham patties:		
(*Hormel*), 2-oz. patty	1.0	0
and cheese (*Hormel*), 2-oz. patty	0	0

Food and Measure	carb. (gms)	fiber (gms)
Ham spread, deviled:		
(*Hormel Cure 81*), 4 tbsp.	2.0	0
(*Underwood*), ¼ cup	0	0
Hamburger, see "Beef pocket/sandwich"		
"Hamburger," vegetarian, see "Burger, vegetarian"		
Hamburger entree mix, 1 cup*, except as noted:		
cheddar melt (*Hamburger Helper*)	28.0	1.0
cheese, three (*Hamburger Helper*)	30.0	1.0
cheeseburger:		
bacon (*Hamburger Helper*)	33.0	1.0
macaroni (*Annie's* Organic Skillet Meal)	27.0	1.0
macaroni (*Hamburger Helper*)	34.0	1.0
chili macaroni (*Hamburger Helper*)	28.0	1.0
enchilada, cheesy (*Hamburger Helper*)	38.0	<1.0
fettuccine Alfredo (*Hamburger Helper*)	24.0	1.0
hash browns, cheesy (*Hamburger Helper*)	38.0	2.0
Italian, zesty (*Hamburger Helper*)	30.0	1.0
lasagna:		
(*Betty Crocker Complete Meals* Pasta Bake), ⅕ pkg.	35.0	2.0
(*Hamburger Helper Oven Favorites*), ⅙ pkg.*	29.0	1.0
cheesy (*Annie's* Organic Skillet Meal)	26.0	1.0
four cheese (*Hamburger Helper*)	27.0	1.0
meat loaf, mashed potato (*Hamburger Helper Oven Favorites*), ⅙ pkg.*	30.0	2.0
Parmesan, Italian (*Hamburger Helper*)	29.0	1.0
pasta (*Hamburger Helper*)	25.0	1.0
penne, tomato basil (*Hamburger Helper*)	30.0	1.0
Philly cheesesteak (*Hamburger Helper*)	24.0	1.0
pizza, double cheese (*Hamburger Helper*)	33.0	1.0
potato, cheesy baked or garlic (*Hamburger Helper*)	27.0	1.0
quesadilla, double cheese (*Hamburger Helper*)	37.0	1.0
ravioli and cheese (*Hamburger Helper*)	32.0	1.0
rice Oriental (*Hamburger Helper*)	31.0	0
Romanoff or spaghetti (*Hamburger Helper*)	26.0	1.0
Salisbury (*Hamburger Helper*)	24.0	1.0
shells, cheesy (*Hamburger Helper*)	29.0	1.0
Stroganoff:		
(*Annie's* Organic Skillet Meal)	24.0	1.0

Food and Measure	carb. (gms)	fiber (gms)
(*Hamburger Helper*)	26.0	1.0
creamy, with pasta (*Campbell's Supper Bakes*), ⅙ pkg. mix	31.0	1.0
potatoes (*Hamburger Helper*)	23.0	1.0
taco:		
(*Hamburger Helper*)	28.0	1.0
crunchy (*Hamburger Helper*)	32.0	1.0
soft, bake (*Hamburger Helper Oven Favorites*), ⅙ pkg.*	32.0	0
Hard sauce (*Crosse & Blackwell*), 2 tbsp.	24.0	0
Hardee's, 1 serving:		
breakfast:		
big country platter, without syrup or butter:		
bacon or ham	90.0	3.0
chicken	104.0	4.0
sausage	91.0	4.0
steak, country	98.0	4.0
biscuit:		
bacon	35.0	0
bacon or ham, egg, and cheese	37.0	0
chicken fillet	50.0	1.0
ham, country	36.0	0
omelet, loaded	37.0	0
sausage or sausage and egg	36.0	0
sausage, smoked	37.0	0
steak, country	44.0	0
biscuit, *Made From Scratch*	35.0	0
Biscuit 'N' Gravy	47.0	0
Biscuit 'N' Gravy bowl, loaded	49.0	0
breakfast bowl, low carb	6.0	2.0
burrito, loaded	38.4	n.a.
croissant, sunrise, bacon or ham	28.0	0
croissant, sunrise, sausage	29.0	0
Frisco sandwich	39.0	2.0
pancakes, 3 pieces	55.0	2.0
tortilla scrambler	18.0	0
breakfast sides:		
biscuit gravy	12.0	0
butter blend pkt.	0	0

Food and Measure	carb. (gms)	fiber (gms)
Cinnamon 'N' Raisin biscuit	40.0	0
Cinnamon 'N' Raisin biscuit, apple	42.0	0
croissant	26.0	0
grits	16.0	0
Hash Rounds, large	45.0	2.0
Hash Rounds, medium	34.0	1.0
Hash Rounds, small	25.0	1.0
pancake syrup	21.0	0
burgers:		
cheeseburger, ⅓ lb.	52.0	2.0
six dollar burger, ½ lb.	60.0	3.0
slammer	19.0	0
slammer, with cheese	20.0	0
Thickburger:		
⅓ lb.	54.0	3.0
⅓ lb. bacon cheese	50.0	3.0
⅓ lb. chili cheese	55.0	4.0
⅓ lb. low carb	5.0	2.0
⅓ lb. mushroom 'N' Swiss	48.0	2.0
⅓ lb. Western bacon	69.6	3.0
½ lb. grilled sourdough	49.0	3.0
⅔ lb. double	53.0	3.0
⅔ lb. double bacon cheese	51.0	3.0
⅔ lb. monster	48.7	n.a.
sandwiches:		
beef, roast	29.0	2.0
Big Roast Beef	38.0	2.0
chicken, big fillet	73.0	4.0
chicken, charbroiled	53.0	4.0
barbecued	45.0	2.0
low carb club	11.0	2.0
chicken, spicy	46.0	2.0
hot dog	22.0	1.0
Hot Ham 'N' Cheese	30.0	2.0
Hot Ham 'N' Cheese, big	40.0	2.0
chicken:		
fried, breast	29.0	0
fried, leg	15.0	0

Food and Measure	carb. (gms)	fiber (gms)
fried, thigh	30.0	0
fried, wing	23.0	0
strips, 3 pieces	27.0	1.0
strips, 5 pieces	45.0	2.0
sides:		
chili cheese fries	67.0	7.0
coleslaw, small	20.0	2.0
Crispy Curls, large	60.0	5.0
Crispy Curls, medium	52.0	4.0
Crispy Curls, small	43.0	4.0
fries, large	78.0	6.0
fries, medium	67.0	5.0
fries, small	51.0	4.0
gravy, chicken	3.0	0
potatoes, mashed, small	17.0	0
sauce/condiments:		
dipping sauce, 1 oz.:		
barbecue	10.0	0
honey mustard	6.0	0
ranch	2.0	0
sweet and sour	11.0	0
horseradish or mayo pkt.	1.0	0
hot sauce pkt.	0	0
ketchup pkt.	2.0	0
shakes, 16 fl. oz.:		
chocolate, hand-dipped	61.0	0
chocolate, soft serve	137.0	0
strawberry, hand-dipped	58.0	0
strawberry, soft serve	128.0	0
vanilla, hand-dipped	52.0	0
vanilla, soft serve	98.0	0
desserts:		
apple turnover	36.0	1.0
chocolate chip cookie	44.0	0
twist cone	34.0	0
Hash, see "Beef hash"		
Hazelnut, shelled:		
raw (*Shiloh Farms*), ¼ cup	5.0	4.0

Food and Measure	carb. (gms)	fiber (gms)
raw (*Tree of Life*), ¼ cup	5.0	3.0
chopped (*Planters*), 2-oz. pkg.	9.0	5.0
dried, 1 oz.	4.4	1.7
dried, chopped, 1 cup	17.6	7.0
dry-roasted, salted, 1 oz.	5.1	<2.0
oil-roasted, salted, 1 oz.	5.4	1.8
Hazelnut spread:		
(*Nutella*), 2 tbsp.	19.0	0
butter (*Kettle Roaster Fresh* Unsalted), 1 oz.	5.0	0
Hazelnut syrup (*Ferrara*), 2 oz.	32.0	0
Head cheese:		
(*Hansel 'n Gretel*), 2 oz.	2.0	0
pork, 2 oz.	0	0
Heart, braised or simmered, 4 oz.:		
beef	.5	0
chicken, broiler-fryer	.1	0
lamb	2.2	0
pork	.5	0
turkey	2.3	0
veal	.1	0
Herbs, see specific listings		
Herbs, mixed, seasoning (*Lawry's* Pinch of Herbs), ¼ tsp.	0	0
Herring, fresh, kippered, or smoked, without added ingredients	0	0
Herring, canned (see also "Sardine"):		
in hot sauce (*Beach Cliff/Brunswick* Louisiana), 3.75-oz. can	2.0	0
lemon/cracked pepper, drained (*Brunswick* Seafood Snacks 3.5 oz.), 3.2 oz.	0	0
mustard sauce (*Beach Cliff/Brunswick* Fish Steaks), 3.75-oz. can	2.0	0
smoked, golden (*Brunswick* Seafood Snacks), 3.25-oz. can	0	0
in soybean oil with chili, jalapeño, or hot pepper, drained (*Beach Cliff/Brunswick* Fish Steaks), 3.4 oz.	1.0	0
teriyaki sauce (*Brunswick* Seafood Snacks), 3.5-oz. can	5.0	0

Food and Measure	carb. (gms)	fiber (gms)
tomato basil sauce (*Brunswick* Seafood Snacks), 3.5-oz. can	2.0	0
in water, drained (*Brunswick* Fish Steaks 3.75 oz.), 3.3 oz.	0	0
Herring, kippered, see "Herring"		
Herring, pickled, in jars:		
in cream or wine sauce (*Acme*), 5 pieces, 2 oz.	7.0	1.0
in wine sauce (*Nathan's*), ¼ cup	7.0	0
in wine sauce, tidbits (*Skansen*), 5 pieces, 2 oz.	7.0	<1.0
Herring oil, 2 tbsp.	0	0
Hibiscus cooler (*Santa Cruz Organic*), 8 fl. oz.	24.0	0
Hickory nut, dried, shelled, 1 oz.	5.2	1.8
Hiziki, see "Seaweed"		
Hoisin sauce:		
(*House of Tsang*), 1 tsp.	4.0	0
(*Ka•Me*), 2 tbsp.	15.0	0
(*Kikkoman*), 2 tbsp.	17.0	0
1 tbsp.	7.1	.4
Hollandaise sauce, in jars (*Reese*), 2 tbsp.	1.0	0
Hollandaise sauce mix:		
(*McCormick*), 1 tsp.	1.0	0
(*Produce Partners*), 2 tsp.	2.0	0
Hominy, dry, white (*Goya*), ¼ cup	39.0	0
Hominy, canned, ½ cup:		
golden (*Allens/Allens* Pepi-Hominy)	27.0	4.0
golden (*Bush's*)	13.0	3.0
white (*Allens*)	22.0	4.0
white (*Bush's*)	14.0	4.0
Hominy grits, see "Corn grits"		
Hommus, see "Hummus"		
Honey, 1 tbsp.:		
(*Aunt Sue's/Grandma's/Sue Bee*)	17.0	0
raw, all varieties (*Tree of Life*)	17.0	0
Honey bun, see "Bun, sweet"		
Honey butter, see "Butter, flavored"		
Honey mustard, see "Mustard blend" and "Pretzel dip"		
Honey pepper sauce (*Neera's* Barbados), 2 tsp.	5.0	0
Honey roll sausage, beef, 1 oz.	.6	0

Food and Measure	carb. (gms)	fiber (gms)
Honeycomb (*Frieda's*), ½ cup, 3 oz.	70.0	0
Honeydew melon:		
(*Del Monte*), ¹⁄₁₀ melon, 4.7 oz.	13.0	1.0
(*Dole*), ¹⁄₁₀ melon	13.0	1.0
¹⁄₁₀ melon, 7" x 2"	11.8	.8
cubed, 1 cup	15.6	1.0
Horned melon (*Frieda's*), 3.5-oz. melon	3.0	1.0
Horseradish, fresh, ½ cup:		
leafy tips, raw, chopped	.8	.2
leafy tips, boiled, drained, chopped	2.3	.4
pods, raw, sliced	4.3	1.6
pods, boiled, drained, sliced	4.8	2.5
Horseradish, prepared, 1 tsp.:		
(*Boar's Head*)	0	0
extra hot (*Silver Spring*)	0	0
Horseradish mustard, see "Mustard blend"		
Horseradish sauce, 1 tsp.:		
(*Boar's Head* Pub Style)	1.0	0
(*Heinz*)	1.0	0
(*Kraft*)	1.0	0
(*Sara Lee*)	0	0
Hot dog, see "Frankfurter"		
Hot dog sauce, see "Chili sauce"		
Hot fudge sauce, see "Chocolate topping"		
Hot sauce, 1 tsp., except as noted:		
(*Bufalo* Especial/Picante Clasica)	0	0
(*Cajun Bayou* Gator Swamp Sauce), 1 tbsp.	1.0	0
(*D.L. Jardine's* Texas Kicker XX)	<1.0	1.0
(*Da'Bomb* The Final Answer), 2 tsp.	2.0	0
(*Frank's* Red Hot Xtra Hot)	0	0
(*Glory*)	0	0
(*Fiesta* Quest for Fire)	1.0	0
(*Tabasco*)	0	0
(*Taco Bell*)	0	0
(*TryMe* Tennessee/Yucatán Sunshine)	0	0
(*TryMe Tiger Sauce* Original)	2.0	0
(*World Harbors*), 2 tbsp.	7.0	0
(*Zapata*)	0	0

Food and Measure	carb. (gms)	fiber (gms)
cayenne (*D.L. Jardine's* Texas Champagne)	0	0
cayenne (*Cajun Bayou*)	1.0	0
chipotle (*Tabasco*)	<1.0	0
chipotle or jalapeño (*Bufalo*)	0	0
garlic or jalapeño (*Tabasco*)	0	0
garlic pepper (*Cajun Bayou*), 1 tbsp.	1.0	0
habañero (*D.L. Jardine's* Blazin' Saddle XXX)	<1.0	<1.0
habañero (*Tabasco*)	1.0	0
jalapeño (*Cajun Bayou*)	1.0	0
jalapeño (*D.L. Jardine's* Texapeppa)	0	0
Hubbard squash:		
raw (*Frieda's* Blue/Orange), ¾ cup, 3 oz.	7.0	2.0
raw, 1 cup	10.1	2.7
baked, cubed, ½ cup	11.0	2.9
boiled, drained, mashed, ½ cup	7.6	3.4
Hummus, 2 tbsp., except as noted:		
(*Guiltless Gourmet* Original)	4.0	1.0
all varieties (*Cedar's*)	5.0	3.0
all varieties, except artichoke garlic and roasted garlic		
(*Athenos*)	5.0	1.0
artichoke garlic (*Athenos*)	4.0	1.0
garlic, roasted (*Athenos*)	6.0	<.10
garlic, roasted (*Guiltless Gourmet*)	4.0	1.0
Hummus, mix, dry, original or spinach Parmesan (*Fantastic*),		
2 tbsp.	11.0	1.0
Hunter sauce mix (*McCormick*), 1 tsp.	4.0	0
Hush puppies, frozen:		
(*Delta Pride*), 3 pieces	21.0	n.a.
(*McKenzie's*), 2 oz.	23.0	2.0
jalapeño (*Delta Pride*), 3 pieces	20.0	n.a.
Hush puppy mix (*Golden Dipt* Fry Easy), ¼ cup	25.0	0
Hyacinth beans, immature, boiled, drained, ½ cup	4.1	n.a.
Hyacinth beans, dried, boiled, ½ cup	20.1	n.a.

I

Food and Measure	carb. (gms)	fiber (gms)
Ice:		
all flavors (*Luigi's* Swirls), 6 fl. oz.	39.0	0
cherry:		
(*Luigi's* Italian), 6 fl. oz.	32.0	<1.0
(*Popsicle Zone*), 12 fl. oz.	62.0	0
slush (*Popsicle Screwball*), 3.75 fl. oz.	27.0	0
chocolate fudge (*Luigi's* Italian), 6 fl. oz.	40.0	<1.0
grape (*Luigi's* Italian), 6 fl. oz.	31.0	<1.0
lemon:		
(*Chill* Soft Serve), 6 fl. oz.	38.0	0
(*Luigi's* Italian), 6 fl. oz.	30.0	<1.0
(*Popsicle Zone*), 12 fl. oz.	60.0	0
lemonade, soft:		
(*Breyer's*), 12 fl. oz.	74.0	0
(*Minute Maid*), 4-oz. tube	25.0	0
(*Minute Maid*), 12 fl. oz.	77.0	0
strawberry (*Minute Maid*), 4-oz. tube	26.0	0
strawberry (*Minute Maid*), 12 fl. oz.	78.0	0
orange (*Chill* Soft Serve), 6 fl. oz.	41.0	0
orange (*Chill Orange Overload*), ¾ of 6-fl.-oz. cup	24.0	0
rainbow (*Popsicle* Snow Cone), 7 fl. oz.	7.0	0
raspberry (*Chill Blue Raspberry Blast*), ¾ of 6-oz. cup . . .	26.0	0
strawberry:		
(*Chill* Soft Serve), 6 fl. oz.	36.0	0
(*Chill Very Strawberry*), ¾ of 6-oz. cup	23.0	0
(*Luigi's* Italian), 6 fl. oz.	31.0	<1.0
Ice bar (see also "Iced confection bar" and "Fruit bar"), 1 piece:		
(*Eskimo Pie* Great American Chilly Pops 12 Pack)	10.0	0

Food and Measure	carb. (gms)	fiber (gms)
(*Eskimo Pie* Great American Jr. Single)	10.0	0
(*Eskimo Pie* Great American Single)	26.0	0
(*Popsicle Big Stick* Big Reds)	17.0	0
(*Popsicle Firecracker*), 4.5 fl. oz.	20.0	0
(*Popsicle Firecracker/Firecracker Jr.*), 1.6 fl. oz.	10.0	0
(*Popsicle Great White*), 1.75 fl. oz.	11.0	0
(*Popsicle Great White*), 3 fl. oz.	18.0	0
(*Popsicle Hyper Stripe*)	19.0	0
all flavors:		
(*Darigold* Super Pops)	23.0	0
(*Hendrie's* Stix)	9.0	0
(*Hoodsie* Pops)	16.0	0
(*LifeSavers* Pops)	10.0	0
(*LifeSavers* Sugar Free Pops)	2.0	0
(*Popsicle* Ice Pops)	11.0	0
(*Popsicle* Sugar Free)	4.0	0
(*Popsicle* Sugar Free), 2 bars	9.0	2.0
(*Popsicle* Swirl Bar)	13.0	0
(*Popsicle Lick-a-Color*), 2 fl. oz.	13.0	0
(*Popsicle Lick-a-Color*), 3.5 fl. oz.	22.0	0
(*Popsicle Rainbow*), 1.75 fl. oz.	11.0	0
(*Popsicle Rainbow*), 3.5 fl. oz.	22.0	0
(*Popsicle* Super Twin)	16.0	0
(*Popsicle* Tingle Twister)	13.0	0
(*Popsicle* Towering Tornado)	21.0	0
cherry:		
(*Eskimo Pie* Red Rocket Single)	10.0	0
(*Popsicle* Red Zone)	19.0	0
(*Popsicle* Torpedo)	8.0	0
cherry pineapple swirl (*Popsicle Big Stick*)	12.0	0
citrus (*Hendrie's* Stix)	10.0	0
citrus, berry (*Hendrie's* No Sugar)	2.0	0
tropical (*Popsicle* Sugar Free)	4.0	0
Ice cream, ½ cup:		
(*Ben & Jerry's Chubby Hubby*)	31.0	1.0
(*Ben & Jerry's Dublin Mudslide*)	28.0	<1.0
(*Ben & Jerry's everything but the…/Fossil Fuel/ In A Crunch*)	30.0	1.0

Food and Measure	carb. (gms)	fiber (gms)
(*Ben & Jerry's Fudge Central*)	31.0	1.0
(*Ben & Jerry's The Gobfather/Marsha Marsha Marshmallow*)	32.0	2.0
(*Ben & Jerry's half baked*)	34.0	<1.0
(*Ben & Jerry's Karamel Sutra*)	32.0	1.0
(*Creamy Commotions Moose Tracks*)	21.0	1.0
(*Dreyer's/Edy's* Grand Turtle Sundae)	18.0	0
(*Dreyer's/Edy's* Grand Light *French Silk*)	19.0	0
(*Healthy Choice* Double Karma)	28.0	<1.0
(*Healthy Choice* Happy Together)	29.0	<1.0
(*Hood* Heavenly Hash)	21.0	0
(*Hood* Heavenly Hash Light)	22.0	0
(*Turkey Hill* Turtle)	21.0	1.0
almond (*Darigold* Avalanche)	17.0	1.0
almond, toasted (*Dreyer's* Grand)	15.0	0
almond hazelnut swirl (*Häagen-Dazs*)	26.0	<1.0
almond praline (*Dreyer's* Grand)	21.0	0
almond praline (*Hood* Delight Light)	23.0	0
apple pie (*Dreamery* Deep Dish)	34.0	0
Bailey's Irish Cream (*Häagen-Dazs*)	23.0	0
banana:		
(*Breyer's Fresa*)	20.0	0
split (*Dreamery*)	31.0	1.0
split (*Häagen-Dazs*)	31.0	0
split (*Turkey Hill*)	19.0	1.0
foster (*Häagen-Dazs*)	28.0	0
banana fudge chunk (*Breyer's*)	21.0	<1.0
banana fudge chunk, walnut (*Ben & Jerry's Chunky Monkey*)	30.0	1.0
berry (*Dreamery* Blue Ribbon Pie)	31.0	<1.0
berry (*Turkey Hill* Berried Treasure)	22.0	0
brownie sundae (*Hood* Light)	23.0	0
brownie sundae, double (*Hood* Fat Free)	27.0	0
butter almond (*Breyer's*)	14.0	<1.0
butter almond (*Turkey Hill* Philadelphia Style)	15.0	0
butter brickle (*Turkey Hill*)	18.0	0
butter crunch, toffee (*Hood* Light)	23.0	0
butter crunch, toffee (*Peak Pleasures*)	21.0	0

Food and Measure	carb. (gms)	fiber (gms)
butter pecan:		
(*Ben & Jerry's*)	20.0	0
(*Breyer's*)	14.0	0
(*Breyer's* Light)	15.0	4.0
(*Creamy Commotions Janas* Sticky Bun)	21.0	0
(*Dreamery* Triple)	30.0	1.0
(*Dreyer's/Edy's* Grand/Light)	16.0	0
(*Dreyer's/Edy's* Homemade Old Fashioned/No Sugar)	15.0	0
(*Dreyer's/Edy's Carb Benefit*)	13.0	6.0
(*Endulge*)	12.0	4.0
(*Green's* Light)	16.0	0
(*Green's* No Sugar)	4.0	0
(*Green's* Southern)	16.0	<1.0
(*Häagen-Dazs*)	21.0	<1.0
(*Healthy Choice*)	20.0	1.0
(*Healthy Choice* No Sugar)	18.0	3.0
(*Turkey Hill*)	15.0	0
(*Turkey Hill CarbIQ*)	11.0	4.0
butterscotch (*Hood* Blast)	20.0	0
with candy (*Breyer's Almond Joy*)	19.0	1.0
with candy (*Breyer's Snickers/Snickers Cruncher*)	20.0	0
cappuccino, see "coffee," below"		
caramel:		
(*Darigold* Killer)	21.0	0
(*Green's* Snapper)	19.0	0
(*Healthy Choice* Crazy for Caramel)	23.0	<1.0
(*Peak Pleasures* Caramel Cup Goldmine)	22.0	0
with chocolate (*Dreyer's/Edy's* Grand *Ultimate Caramel Cup*)	22.0	0
caramel cone (*Häagen-Dazs*)	32.0	0
caramel fudge (*Breyer's*)	20.0	0
caramel fudge brownie (*Healthy Choice*)	21.0	1.0
caramel praline crunch (*Breyer's*)	22.0	0
caramel toffee bar (*Dreamery* Heaven)	32.0	0
cashew praline (*Dreamery*)	30.0	0
cherry (*Green's* Whitehouse)	18.0	0
cherry, black (*Turkey Hill*)	18.0	0

Food and Measure	carb. (gms)	fiber (gms)
cherry chocolate chip:		
(*Ben & Jerry's Cherry Garcia*)	26.0	<1.0
(*Breyer's*)	18.0	0
(*Dreamery ba da Bing*)	33.0	1.0
(*Edy's* Grand)	19.0	0
(*Healthy Choice* Mambo)	21.0	<1.0
cherry fudge, ripple (*Turkey Hill* Fat Free No Sugar)	22.0	4.0
cherry fudge, truffle (*Häagen-Dazs* Light)	37.0	0
cherry vanilla:		
(*Breyer's*)	17.0	0
(*Häagen-Dazs*)	23.0	0
(*Stonyfield* Organic)	24.0	0
sweet (*Turkey Hill* Philadelphia Style)	18.0	0
chocolate:		
(*Ben & Jerry's*)	25.0	2.0
(*Ben & Jerry's* Chocolate Therapy)	30.0	2.0
(*Breyer's*)	17.0	<1.0
(*Breyer's* Extra Creamy)	18.0	<1.0
(*Breyer's* 98% Fat Free)	20.0	4.0
(*Darigold* Totally)	17.0	1.0
(*Dreyer's/Edy's* Grand/Grand Light)	16.0	0
(*Dreyer's/Edy's* Homemade)	19.0	0
(*Dreyer's/Edys* No Sugar)	13.0	0
(*Dreyer's/Edy's Carb Benefit*)	13.0	7.0
(*Endulge*)	13.0	5.0
(*Green's*)	17.0	<1.0
(*Häagen-Dazs*)	22.0	1.0
(*Stonyfield* Organic)	22.0	1.0
(*Turkey Hill* Philadelphia Style)	18.0	0
(*Turkey Hill CarbIQ*)	11.0	4.0
Belgian dark (*Godiva*)	26.0	2.0
brownie (*Healthy Choice* Brownie Bliss)	25.0	1.0
with cake (*Dreyer's/Edy's* Grand *Blue Ribbon Chocolate Cake*)	20.0	0
with chocolate hearts (*Godiva*)	32.0	2.0
Dutch (*Häagen-Dazs* Light)	33.0	<1.0
Dutch (*Turkey Hill*)	18.0	1.0

Food and Measure	carb. (gms)	fiber (gms)
Dutch (*Turkey Hill* Fat Free No Sugar)	20.0	6.0
French (*Breyer's* Light)	20.0	<1.0
milk (*Godiva* Classic)	28.0	1.0
pecan, brownie, caramel (*Healthy Choice* Turtle Fudge Cake)	23.0	<1.0
triple (*Dreyer's/Edy's* Grand *Triple Chocolate Thunder*)	18.0	0
triple (*Dreyer's/Edy's* No Sugar)	16.0	0
truffle (*Dreamery* Explosion)	31.0	1.0
chocolate brownie (*Peak Pleasures*)	23.0	0
chocolate brownie, with candy (*M&M's*)	22.0	0
chocolate brownie, fudge:		
(*Ben & Jerry's*)	32.0	2.0
(*Ben & Jerry's* Organic)	30.0	2.0
(*Breyer's* 98% Fat Free No Sugar)	20.0	4.0
(*Dreamery* Brownie Turtle Sundae)	33.0	2.0
(*Endulge*)	15.0	5.0
(*Healthy Choice* No Sugar)	21.0	1.0
double (*Dreyer's/Edys* No Sugar)	17.0	0
chocolate cake, German (*Turkey Hill*)	22.0	1.0
chocolate caramel:		
(*Breyer's* No Sugar)	18.0	3.0
fudge (*Darigold* Gooey Cluster)	21.0	0
swirl (*Dreyer's/Edy's* Grand)	19.0	0
chocolate cheesecake (*Godiva*)	36.0	1.0
chocolate chip:		
(*Breyer's*)	17.0	0
(*Dreyer's/Edy's* Grand)	18.0	0
(*Dreyer's/Edy's* Grand Light)	17.0	0
(*Dreyer's/Edy's Carb Benefit*)	14.0	6.0
(*Peak Pleasures*)	20.0	0
chocolate (*Häagen-Dazs*)	26.0	2.0
chocolate chip cookie dough:		
(*Ben & Jerry's*)	32.0	0
(*Breyer's*)	20.0	0
(*Dreamery* Grandma's)	32.0	0
(*Dreyer's/Edy's* Grand)	21.0	0
(*Dreyer's/Edy's* Grand Light)	19.0	0
(*Dreyer's/Edys* No Sugar)	16.0	0

Food and Measure	carb. (gms)	fiber (gms)
(*Green's*)	21.0	0
(*Häagen-Dazs*)	29.0	0
(*Turkey Hill*)	20.0	0
swirl (*Dreyer's/Edy's* Grand *Nestle Toll House*)	21.0	0
chocolate chunk, chocolate (*Healthy Choice*)	21.0	1.0
chocolate chunk, milk (*Dreyer's/Edy's* Homemade)	18.0	0
chocolate fudge:		
(*Breyer's Fudgsicle*)	17.0	1.0
(*Dreyer's/Edy's* Fat/Sugar Free)	22.0	0
chunks with nuts (*Ben & Jerry's New York Super Fudge Chunk*)	29.0	2.0
mousse (*Edy's* Grand)	19.0	0
sundae (*Edy's* Grand)	20.0	0
chocolate malt (*Creamy Commotions* Choco Malt Chip)	22.0	0
chocolate malt, nuts (*Dreamery* Nuts About Malt)	29.0	1.0
chocolate marshmallow:		
(*Turkey Hill*)	23.0	1.0
caramel fudge (*Ben & Jerry's Phish Food*)	37.0	1.0
swirl (*Green's*)	21.0	<1.0
chocolate mocha silk (*Healthy Choice*)	24.0	1.0
chocolate peanut butter:		
(*Dreyer's/Edy's* Grand)	17.0	0
(*Häagen-Dazs*)	27.0	2.0
(*Peak Pleasures*)	21.0	0
swirl (*Endulge*)	14.0	5.0
chocolate pretzel (*Creamy Commotions Snyder's*)	22.0	0
chocolate pretzel (*Turkey Hill*)	21.0	1.0
chocolate rainbow (*Breyer's*)	16.0	0
chocolate raspberry:		
(*Stonyfield* Organic)	25.0	1.0
truffle (*Godiva*)	32.0	2.0
truffle, white (*Häagen-Dazs*)	32.0	1.0
white (*Godiva*)	32.0	0
coconut creme pie (*Turkey Hill*)	21.0	1.0
coffee:		
(*Ben & Jerry's*)	21.0	0
(*Breyer's*)	15.0	0
(*Dreyer's/Edy's* Grand)	15.0	0

Food and Measure	carb. (gms)	fiber (gms)
(*Häagen-Dazs*)	21.0	0
(*Häagen-Dazs* Light)	32.0	0
(*Hood Caribbean Coffee Royale* Light)	18.0	0
(*Starbucks* Classic)	26.0	0
(*Stonyfield* Organic Decaf)	21.0	0
(*Turkey Hill* Philadelphia Style)	16.0	0
almond fudge (*Healthy Choice* Jumpin' Java)	25.0	<1.0
almond fudge (*Healthy Choice* No Sugar)	20.0	1.0
almond fudge (*Starbucks*)	29.0	1.0
caramel, espresso chips (*Creamy Commotions* Alpine Espresso)	20.0	0
caramel cappuccino swirl (*Starbucks*)	30.0	0
cappuccino chocolate chunk (*Healthy Choice*)	20.0	<1.0
chocolate chip (*Peak Pleasures* Java Chip Trails)	19.0	0
chocolate chip (*Starbucks* Java Chip)	29.0	0
Colombian (*Turkey Hill*)	16.0	0
espresso chip (*Edy's* Grand)	17.0	0
fudge swirl (*Dreamery* Mudslide)	28.0	1.0
latte (*Starbucks* Low Fat)	30.0	0
latte, white chocolate (*Starbucks*)	31.0	0
toffee (*Ben & Jerry's Heath* Crunch)	29.0	0
cookie dough, see "chocolate chip cookie dough," above		
with cookies (*Breyer's Oreo*)	20.0	0
with cookies (*Breyer's Twix*)	21.0	0
cookies and cream:		
(*Ben & Jerry's* Sweet Cream Organic)	24.0	0
(*Breyer's*)	18.0	<1.0
(*Darigold*)	18.0	0
(*Dreyer's/Edy's* Grand)	19.0	0
(*Dreyer's/Edy's* Grand Light)	18.0	0
(*Green's*)	18.0	0
(*Häagen-Dazs*)	23.0	0
(*Healthy Choice*)	21.0	<1.0
(*Turkey Hill*)	19.0	0
chocolate covered (*Godiva*)	32.0	<1.0
cookie sandwich (*Peak Pleasures*)	21.0	0
crème brûlée (*Häagen-Dazs*)	23.0	0
crème caramel (*Stonyfield* Organic)	26.0	0

Food and Measure	carb. (gms)	fiber (gms)
dulce de leche:		
(*Breyer's*)	20.0	0
(*Häagen-Dazs*)	28.0	0
(*Häagen-Dazs* Light)	33.0	0
eggnog (*Hood* Holiday)	16.0	0
eggnog (*Turkey Hill*)	17.0	0
espresso, see "coffee," above		
fudge:		
(*Peak Pleasures* River Rapids)	20.0	0
double (*Dreyer's/Edy's* Grand)	19.0	0
hot, sundae (*Dreamery*)	29.0	<1.0
ripple (*Turkey Hill*)	20.0	0
latte, see "coffee," above		
lemon pie (*Turkey Hill* Southern)	22.0	0
macadamia brittle (*Häagen-Dazs*)	25.0	0
maple walnut (*Hood*)	17.0	0
mango (*Häagen-Dazs*)	28.0	<1.0
mint:		
with candy (*Breyer's M&M's*)	19.0	0
with candy (*M&M's*)	20.0	0
with cookies (*Breyer's Oreo*)	23.0	0
with cookies (*Peak Pleasures* Cookie Caverns)	21.0	0
mint chocolate chip:		
(*Breyer's*)	17.0	0
(*Breyer's* Light)	19.0	0
(*Darigold* Cool)	17.0	0
(*Dreyer's/Edy's* Grand)	18.0	0
(*Dreyer's/Edy's* Grand Light)	17.0	0
(*Dreyer's/Edy's* No Sugar)	13.0	0
(*Dryer's/Edy's* Carb Benefit)	14.0	6.0
(*Endulge*)	14.0	4.0
(*Green's*)	17.0	0
(*Häagen-Dazs*)	26.0	<1.0
(*Häagen-Dazs* Light)	34.0	0
(*Healthy Choice*)	20.0	<1.0
(*Healthy Choice* No Sugar)	18.0	1.0
(*Turkey Hill* Premium)	17.0	1.0
(*Turkey Hill* Philadelphia Style)	18.0	0

Food and Measure	carb. (gms)	fiber (gms)
(*Turkey Hill CarbIQ*)	14.0	4.0
fudge swirl (*Dreyer's/Edy's* Grand *Andes Cool Mint*) . . .	19.0	0
mint chocolate cookie (*Ben & Jerry's*)	26.0	0
mocha almond fudge:		
(*Breyer's*)	18.0	2.0
(*Darigold*)	18.0	1.0
(*Dreyer's* Grand)	17.0	0
(*Dreyer's* Grand Light)	16.0	0
(*Häagen-Dazs*)	28.0	<1.0
mud pie (*Darigold*)	21.0	1.0
mud pie (*Starbucks*)	32.0	1.0
Neapolitan:		
(*Darigold*)	16.0	0
(*Dreyer's/Edy's* Grand)	16.0	0
(*Dreyer's/Edy's* Grand Light)	15.0	0
(*Dreyer's/Edy's* No Sugar)	13.0	0
(*Green's* Metropolitan)	17.0	0
(*Turkey Hill/Turkey Hill* Philadelphia Style)	17.0	0
oatmeal cookie chunk (*Ben & Jerry's*)	31.0	<1.0
peach:		
(*Breyer's*)	17.0	0
(*Dreyer's/Edy's* Homemade Grovestand)	17.0	0
(*Green's* Just Peachy!)	17.0	0
and cream (*Häagen-Dazs*)	29.0	0
and cream (*Turkey Hill*)	17.0	0
peanut brittle (*Turkey Hill* Light No Sugar)	19.0	5.0
peanut butter:		
(*Breyer's Twix*)	18.0	<1.0
(*Turkey Hill* Mania)	20.0	0
(*Turkey Hill CarbIQ* Paradise)	13.0	4.0
chunk, chocolate (*Dreamery*)	29.0	2.0
fudge (*Breyer's*)	17.0	<1.0
ripple (*Turkey Hill*)	16.0	1.0
twirl (*Green's*)	16.0	<1.0
peanut butter cup:		
(*Ben & Jerry's*)	27.0	1.0
(*Breyer's Reese's Peanut Butter Cups*)	22.0	0
(*Dreyer's/Edy's* Grand)	19.0	0

Food and Measure	carb. (gms)	fiber (gms)
(*Healthy Choice*)	21.0	<1.0
chocolate (*Turkey Hill*)	18.0	1.0
fudge (*Dreyer's/Edy's* Grand/Grand Light Fudge Tracks)	18.0	0
peppermint stick (*Turkey Hill*)	19.0	0
pineapple coconut (*Häagen-Dazs*)	25.0	0
pineapple upside-down cake (*Turkey Hill*)	21.0	0
pistachio (*Ben & Jerry's*)	21.0	<1.0
pistachio (*Häagen-Dazs*)	22.0	<1.0
praline and caramel (*Healthy Choice*)	23.0	<1.0
raspberry:		
black (*Dreamery* Avalanche)	27.0	1.0
black (*Green's* Blast)	20.0	0
black (*Turkey Hill*)	18.0	0
black, ripple (*Peak Pleasures*)	20.0	0
raspberry brownie (*Dreamery A la Mode*)	27.0	1.0
raspberry cheesecake (*Turkey Hill CarbIQ*)	16.0	4.0
raspberry vanilla swirl (*Dreyer's/Edy's* Fat/Sugar Free)	19.0	0
rocky road:		
(*Breyer's*)	20.0	<1.0
(*Darigold*)	19.0	<1.0
(*Dreyer's/Edy's* Grand/Grand Light)	17.0	0
(*Green's*)	19.0	1.0
(*Häagen-Dazs*)	29.0	1.0
(*Healthy Choice*)	25.0	<1.0
(*Turkey Hill*)	22.0	1.0
rum raisin (*Häagen-Dazs*)	22.0	0
rum raisin (*Turkey Hill*)	19.0	0
s'mores (*Dreamery*)	39.0	1.0
s'mores (*Häagen-Dazs* Light)	42.0	<1.0
spumoni (*Dreyer's/Edy's* Grand)	16.0	0
strawberry:		
(*Ben & Jerry's*)	26.0	0
(*Ben & Jerry's* Organic)	21.0	0
(*Breyer's*)	15.0	0
(*Darigold* Summer)	16.0	0
(*Dreamery Strawberry Fields*)	26.0	1.0
(*Dreyer's/Edy's* Grand Light)	17.0	0
(*Dreyer's/Edy's* Grand Real)	16.0	0

Food and Measure	carb. (gms)	fiber (gms)
(*Dreyer's/Edy's* No Sugar)	13.0	0
(*Green's*)	17.0	0
(*Häagen-Dazs*)	23.0	<1.0
and cream (*Dreyer's/Edy's* Homemade)	17.0	0
and cream (*Turkey Hill*)	16.0	1.0
strawberry cheesecake:		
(*Dreamery* New York)	27.0	0
(*Häagen-Dazs*)	28.0	0
(*Creamy Commotions Janas*)	22.0	0
graham swirl (*Ben & Jerry's* Primary Berry Graham)	29.0	1.0
strawberry shortcake (*Breyer's*)	23.0	0
tin roof sundae:		
(*Darigold*)	19.0	0
(*Healthy Choice*)	21.0	1.0
(*Turkey Hill*)	19.0	0
tiramisu (*Dreamery*)	31.0	0
toffee bar (*Breyer's Heath*)	22.0	0
toffee bar (*Dreyer's/Edy's* Grand Crunch)	19.0	0
vanilla:		
(*Ben & Jerry's*)	21.0	0
(*Ben & Jerry's* Organic)	18.0	0
(*Breyer's*)	15.0	0
(*Breyer's* Calcium Rich/Lactose Free)	14.0	0
(*Breyer's* Extra Creamy/Light All Natural)	17.0	0
(*Breyer's* Homemade)	16.0	0
(*Breyer's* Light)	18.0	0
(*Breyer's* 98% Fat Free)	20.0	4.0
(*Breyer's* No Sugar)	15.0	3.0
(*Darigold* Very)	16.0	0
(*Dreamery*)	25.0	0
(*Dreamery* Fortunate)	33.0	1.0
(*Dreyer's/Edy's* Fat/Sugar Free)	20.0	0
(*Dreyer's* Grand)	14.0	0
(*Dreyer's/Edy's* Grand Light/Homemade)	15.0	0
(*Dreyer's/Edy's* No Sugar)	14.0	0
(*Edy's* Grand)	15.0	0
(*Endulge*)	13.0	4.0
(*Green's/Green's* Light)	17.0	0

Food and Measure	carb. (gms)	fiber (gms)
(*Green's* No Sugar)	3.0	0
(*Häagen-Dazs*)	21.0	0
(*Healthy Choice*)	19.0	<1.0
(*Healthy Choice* No Sugar)	17.0	1.0
(*Peak Pleasures* Snowdrift)	17.0	0
(*Stonyfield* Organic)	20.0	0
(*Turkey Hill* Original)	16.0	0
bean (*Dreyer's/Edy's* Grand)	15.0	0
bean (*Dreyer's/Edy's* Carb Benefit)	13.0	6.0
bean (*Green's* Philly)	17.0	0
bean (*Häagen-Dazs* Light)	29.0	0
bean (*Healthy Choice* In the Beginning)	21.0	<1.0
bean (*Turkey Hill/Turkey Hill* Philadelphia Style)	16.0	0
bean (*Turkey Hill* Fat Free No Sugar)	19.0	5.0
bean (*Turkey Hill* CarbIQ)	11.0	4.0
French (*Breyer's*)	15.0	0
French (*Breyer's* Light)	18.0	0
French (*Breyer's* No Sugar)	14.0	3.0
French (*Darigold*)	17.0	0
French (*Dreyer's/Edy's* Grand)	17.0	0
French (*Dreyer's/Edy's* Grand Light)	15.0	0
French (*Green's*)	18.0	0
French (*Peak Pleasures* Summit)	18.0	0
French (*Turkey Hill*)	16.0	0
vanilla, with candy (*M&M's*)	22.0	0
vanilla, with chocolate caramel hearts (*Godiva*)	32.0	1.0
vanilla, with chocolate dip cone (*Dreamery* Coney Island Waffle Cone)	32.0	1.0
vanilla, with chocolate wafers (*Edy's* Grand Ice Cream Sandwich)	19.0	0
vanilla, with raspberry, brownie swirl (*Ben & Jerry's* Dave Matthews Band Magic Brownies)	29.0	0
vanilla caramel, fudge (*Ben & Jerry's*)	31.0	0
vanilla caramel, pecan (*Godiva*)	33.0	0
vanilla and chocolate:		
(*Breyer's* Light)	18.0	0
(*Breyer's* No Sugar)	15.0	3.0
(*Breyer's* Take Two)	16.0	0

Food and Measure	carb. (gms)	fiber (gms)
(*Dreyer's/Edy's* Grand)	16.0	0
(*Green's*)	17.0	0
(*Peak Pleasures* Twin Peaks)	16.0	0
(*Turkey Hill*)	17.0	0
swirl (*Dreyer's/Edy's* Fat/Sugar Free)	20.0	0
vanilla, chocolate, and strawberry (*Breyer's*)	16.0	0
vanilla chocolate chip (*Häagen-Dazs*)	26.0	<1.0
vanilla custard (*Dreyer's/Edy's* Homemade)	17.0	0
vanilla fudge:		
(*Breyer's* Checks)	19.0	0
(*Dreyer's/Edy's* Grand *French Vanilla Fudge Pie*)	20.0	0
(*Häagen-Dazs*)	26.0	0
brownie (*Breyer's*)	19.0	<1.0
brownie (*Stonyfield* Organic)	28.0	0
with candy (*Breyer's M&M's*)	20.0	0
swirl (*Endulge*)	14.0	4.0
swirl (*Green's*)	21.0	0
twirl (*Breyer's*)	18.0	<1.0
twirl (*Breyer's* No Sugar)	19.0	3.0
vanilla peanut butter fudge (*Green's* Pocono Paws)	21.0	0
vanilla Swiss almond (*Endulge*)	14.0	5.0
vanilla Swiss almond (*Häagen-Dazs*)	24.0	<1.0
vanilla toffee (*Ben & Jerry's Heath*)	29.0	0
"Ice cream," nondairy, ½ cup:		
(*Purely Decadent Soy Delicious* Turtle Tracks)	31.0	5.0
almond pecan (*It's Soy Delicious*)	24.0	1.0
banana, with chocolate (*Purely Decadent Soy Delicious* Swinging Anna)	31.0	5.0
"butter" pecan (*Organic Soy Delicious*)	22.0	1.0
"butter" pecan (*Tofutti* Better Pecan)	22.0	0
cappuccino (*RiceDream*)	23.0	1.0
carob, plain or almond (*RiceDream*)	24.0	2.0
carob, peppermint (*It's Soy Delicious*)	24.0	1.0
chai (*It's Soy Delicious* Tiger)	24.0	2.0
cheesecake, blueberry, chocolate, or strawberry (*Tofutti* Cheesecake Supreme)	20.0	0
cherry (*Purely Decadent Soy Delicious* Nirvana)	32.0	5.0

Food and Measure	carb. (gms)	fiber (gms)
chocolate:		
(*It's Soy Delicious* Awesome)	24.0	1.0
(*Organic Soy Delicious* Velvet)	23.0	2.0
(*Purely Decadent Soy Delicious* Obsession)	36.0	5.0
(*Sweet Nothings*)	27.0	3.0
(*Tofutti* No Sugar)	12.0	0
(*Tofutti* Super Soy Supreme New York, New York)	22.0	0
(*Tofutti* Supreme)	18.0	0
Swiss (*Dr. Preager's* Sensible Treats)	21.0	3.0
chocolate almond (*It's Soy Delicious*)	24.0	2.0
chocolate brownie almond (*Purely Decadent Soy Delicious*)	34.0	6.0
chocolate coffee (*It's Soy Delicious* Mexican)	22.0	1.0
chocolate cookie crunch (*Tofutti*)	26.0	0
chocolate fudge (*Tofutti* Low Fat)	25.0	0
chocolate peanut butter (*It's Soy Delicious*)	25.0	1.0
chocolate peanut butter (*Organic Soy Delicious*)	23.0	1.0
cocoa marble fudge (*RiceDream*)	25.0	2.0
coffee marshmallow swirl (*Tofutti* Low Fat)	24.0	0
cookie:		
(*Purely Decadent Soy Delicious* Avalanche)	32.0	5.0
(*RiceDream* Cookies n' Dream)	26.0	1.0
and "cream" (*Organic Soy Delicious*)	25.0	4.0
dulce de leche (*Organic Soy Delicious*)	25.0	4.0
espresso (*It's Soy Delicious*)	25.0	1.0
green tea (*It's Soy Delicious*)	24.0	2.0
mango raspberry (*It's Soy Delicious*)	25.0	2.0
mango raspberry (*Sweet Nothings*)	29.0	2.0
mint, chunky, with chocolate (*Purely Decadent Soy Delicious* Madness)	35.0	6.0
mint chocolate chip (*Tofutti*)	21.0	0
mint chocolate chip or carob chip (*RiceDream*)	26.0	1.0
mint fudge (*Sweet Nothings*)	30.0	3.0
mint fudge, marble (*Organic Soy Delicious*)	25.0	1.0
mocha fudge:		
(*Dr. Preager's* Sensible Treats)	21.0	1.0
(*Organic Soy Delicious*)	27.0	1.0

Food and Measure	carb. (gms)	fiber (gms)
(*Sweet Nothings*)	30.0	3.0
almond (*Purely Decadent Soy Delicious*)	32.0	6.0
Neapolitan (*Organic Soy Delicious*)	23.0	1.0
Neapolitan (*RiceDream*)	24.0	2.0
orange vanilla swirl (*RiceDream*)	24.0	1.0
peanut butter (*Purely Decadent Soy Delicious Zig Zag*)	32.0	5.0
pistachio almond (*It's Soy Delicious*)	23.0	3.0
praline (*RiceDream* Supreme Pralines n' Dream)	24.0	1.0
praline, pecan (*Purely Decadent Soy Delicious*)	33.0	5.0
raspberry (*It's Soy Delicious*)	25.0	1.0
raspberry à la mode (*Purely Decadent Soy Delicious*)	34.0	5.0
rocky road (*Purely Decadent Soy Delicious*)	31.0	5.0
strawberry:		
(*Dr. Preager's* Sensible Treats)	20.0	<1.0
(*Organic Soy Delicious*)	23.0	1.0
(*RiceDream*)	24.0	1.0
(*Sweet Nothings* Cool)	30.0	2.0
(*Tofutti* No Sugar)	12.0	0
vanilla:		
(*Dr. Preager's* Sensible Treats)	25.0	2.0
(*It's Soy Delicious*)	25.0	1.0
(*Organic Soy Delicious* Old Fashioned)	24.0	5.0
(*Purely Decadent Soy Delicious* Purely)	29.0	6.0
(*RiceDream*)	23.0	1.0
(*SoyDream*)	17.0	1.0
(*Sweet Nothings*)	28.0	3.0
(*Tofutti*/Super Soy Supreme Bella)	20.0	0
creamy (*Organic Soy Delicious*)	23.0	1.0
vanilla almond:		
bark (*Tofutti*)	21.0	0
Swiss (*Purely Decadent Soy Delicious*)	31.0	6.0
Swiss (*RiceDream*)	25.0	1.0
vanilla fudge:		
(*It's Soy Delicious*)	25.0	2.0
(*Sweet Nothings*)	30.0	3.0
(*Tofutti*)	25.0	0
(*Tofutti* Low Fat)	24.0	0

Food and Measure	carb. (gms)	fiber (gms)
vanilla orange (*Organic Soy Delicious* Twisted)	24.0	4.0
wildberry (*Tofutti* Supreme)	24.0	0
Ice cream bar (see also "Iced confection bar"), 1 piece, except as noted:		
(*Ben & Jerry's half baked*)	46.0	2.0
(*Scribblers* Ice Cream Pops), 2 pieces	17.0	0
almond, toasted:		
(*Eskimo Pie*/Premium Single)	27.0	0
(*Eskimo Pie* King Size)	21.0	0
(*Good Humor*), 3 fl. oz.	22.0	<1.0
(*Good Humor*), 4 fl. oz.	30.0	<1.0
butter pecan (*Endulge* Single)	11.0	3.0
candy center, with chocolate, crisps:		
(*Eskimo Pie* Crunch Bar)	21.0	0
(*Good Humor* Crunch Bar)	24.0	<1.0
caramel fudge swirl (*Endulge* Caramel Turtle Sundae)	12.0	4.0
caramel and peanuts, with chocolate:		
(*Klondike Planters*)	28.0	1.0
(*Klondike Planters* Single)	25.0	<1.0
caramel crunch (*Klondike*)	26.0	0
cherry, with chocolate (*Ben & Jerry's Cherry Garcia*)	29.0	2.0
chocolate, with chocolate:		
(*Dove* Original 4-Pack)	27.0	3.0
(*Dove* Original Single)	32.0	3.0
(*Klondike*)	23.0	<1.0
dark (*Häagen-Dazs*)	24.0	<1.0
chocolate eclair:		
(*Eskimo Pie*)	26.0	<1.0
(*Eskimo Pie* King Size)	31.0	1.0
(*Eskimo Pie* Premium King Size Single)	26.0	<1.0
(*Good Humor*), 3 fl. oz.	20.0	<1.0
(*Good Humor*), 4 fl. oz.	30.0	<1.0
(*Hood*)	14.0	0
(*No Pudge*)	23.0	4.0
(*Popsicle Col. Crunch*)	20.0	<1.0
chocolate fudge swirl (*Endulge/Endulge* Single)	12.0	4.0
coffee, with chocolate (*Klondike* Cappuccino Bar)	24.0	0
coffee almond crunch (*Häagen-Dazs*)	23.0	<1.0

Food and Measure	carb. (gms)	fiber (gms)
cookies and cream:		
(*Eskimo Pie* No Sugar)	15.0	3.0
(*Good Humor*)	21.0	<1.0
(*No Pudge*)	21.0	6.0
cookie coated (*Good Humor Oreo*)	28.0	<1.0
dulce de leche (*Häagen-Dazs*)	28.0	0
fudge, with chocolate (*Darigold* Fudge & Cream)	17.0	0
mint, with chocolate:		
(*Eskimo Pie* Peppermint Pattie)	24.0	1.0
(*Eskimo Pie* Thin Mint)	23.0	1.0
(*Klondike York* Peppermint Pattie)	24.0	<1.0
Neapolitan, with chocolate (*Klondike*)	24.0	<1.0
peanut butter:		
(*Darigold* Cup)	13.0	0
(*Good Humor Reese's*)	27.0	<1.0
with chocolate (*Butterfinger*)	17.0	0
swirl (*Endulge*)	12.0	4.0
strawberry shortcake:		
(*Eskimo Pie*)	26.0	0
(*Eskimo Pie* King Size)	30.0	<1.0
(*Eskimo Pie* Premium Single)	26.0	0
(*Eskimo Pie* Reduced Fat)	15.0	3.0
(*Good Humor*), 3 fl. oz.	21.0	0
(*Good Humor*), 4 fl. oz.	30.0	<1.0
(*No Pudge*)	23.0	4.0
(*Popsicle Col. Crunch*)	21.0	0
toffee with chocolate (*Klondike Heath*)	26.0	0
vanilla with chocolate:		
(*Darigold*)	14.0	0
(*Good Humor*), 2.75 fl. oz.	19.0	<1.0
(*Good Humor*), 4 fl. oz.	23.0	<1.0
(*Klondike* Original)	24.0	0
(*Klondike* Slim-a-Bear No Sugar Reduced Fat)	21.0	4.0
(*Popsicle*)	15.0	1.0
(*Popsicle Sprinklers*), 2.1 fl. oz.	18.0	0
(*Popsicle Sprinklers*), 3 fl. oz.	26.0	0
almond (*Klondike Hershey*)	20.0	<1.0

Food and Measure	carb. (gms)	fiber (gms)
chocolate stripe (*Good Humor Number 1 Bar*)	21.0	<1.0
crisps (*Eskimo Pie* No Sugar)	13.0	0
crisps (*Klondike Krunch*), 4 fl. oz.	24.0	0
crisps (*Klondike Krunch*), 5 fl. oz.	25.0	0
dark (*Dove* Original 4-Pack)	26.0	2.0
dark (*Dove* Original Single)	32.0	2.0
dark (*Endulge*)	11.0	3.0
dark (*Eskimo Pie*)	15.0	0
dark (*Eskimo Pie* Giant King Size Single)	35.0	2.0
dark (*Eskimo Pie* King Size)	21.0	<1.0
dark (*Eskimo Pie* No Sugar)	13.0	0
dark (*Good Humor*)	15.0	<1.0
dark (*Häagen-Dazs*)	23.0	<1.0
dark (*Klondike*)	24.0	<1.0
dark, miniatures (*Dove* Original), 5 pieces	32.0	2.0
milk (*Dove* 4-Pack)	25.0	1.0
milk (*Dove* Single)	31.0	1.0
milk (*Endulge*)	12.0	4.0
milk (*Endulge* Single)	12.0	5.0
milk (*Eskimo Pie*)	14.0	0
milk (*Eskimo Pie*) King Size/Premium)	21.0	0
milk (*Eskimo Pie* King Size Single)	23.0	0
milk (*Good Humor*)	15.0	0
milk (*Häagen-Dazs*)	22.0	0
milk, with almonds (*Dove* 4-Pack)	23.0	1.0
milk, with almonds (*Dove* Single)	28.0	1.0
milk, caramel toffee crunch (*Dove* 4-Pack)	29.0	1.0
milk, caramel toffee crunch (*Dove* Single)	35.0	1.0
milk, with crunchy cookies (*Dove* 4-Pack)	27.0	1.0
milk, miniatures (*Dove* Original), 5 pieces	30.0	1.0
mini (*Klondike* Snack Size), 2 pieces	15.0	0
mini (*Klondike Movie Bites*), 4.48-fl.-oz. pkg.	26.0	0
mini (*Popsicle*), 2 pieces	18.0	0
vanilla cookie (*Popsicle WWE*)	23.0	1.0
vanilla almond (*Ben & Jerry's*)	30.0	2.0
vanilla with chocolate ice cream (*Endulge* Fudge & Cream)	7.0	2.0
vanilla fudge swirl (*Endulge*)	12.0	4.0

Food and Measure	carb. (gms)	fiber (gms)
"Ice cream" bar, nondairy, 1 bar:		
chocolate (*RiceDream*)	32.0	2.0
chocolate with nuts (*RiceDream* Nutty Bar)	23.0	2.0
chocolate fudge (*Tofutti* Coffee Break/Treats)	6.0	0
chocolate fudge (*Tofutti* Totally Fudge)	19.0	0
chocolate center:		
peanut butter, dark chocolate (*Tofutti* Monkey Bars)	22.0	0
vanilla, dark chocolate (*Tofutti* Hooray Hooray		
No Sugar)	10.0	0
vanilla:		
(*RiceDream*)	33.0	1.0
with dark chocolate (*Toffuti* Marry Me)	22.0	0
with fruit ice coating (*Tofutti* Kid Sticks)	15.0	0
with nuts (*RiceDream* Nutty Bar)	23.0	2.0
vanilla, chocolate, or strawberry, with dark chocolate		
(*Tofutti* Delights)	7.0	0
Ice cream cone, filled, 1 piece:		
(*Choco Taco*)	35.0	1.0
chocolate, with chocolate (*Klondike* Slim-a-Bear 96%		
Fat Free)	36.0	3.0
chocolate, with nuts (*Drumstick* Sundae)	33.0	<1.0
chocolate, with nuts (*Klondike*)	29.0	1.0
cookies and cream (*Eskimo Pie*)	28.0	5.0
cookies and cream (*No Pudge*)	29.0	3.0
mint, with nuts (*Drumstick* Sundae)	38.0	<1.0
vanilla, with chocolate:		
(*Klondike* Slim-a-Bear 96% Fat Free)	35.0	3.0
and brownie (*No Pudge* Fudgy Brownie Cones)	32.0	4.0
and candy (*M&M's*)	32.0	1.0
vanilla, with chocolate, nuts:		
(*Drumstick* Sundae)	33.0	<1.0
(*Endulge*)	19.0	7.0
(*Eskimo Pie* Giant Sundae)	30.0	1.0
(*Eskimo Pie* No Sugar)	24.0	<1.0
(*Good Humor* Sundae), 4 fl. oz.	31.0	1.0
(*Good Humor* Sundae), 4.3 fl. oz.	29.0	<1.0
(*Good Humor Giant King Cone*)	44.0	1.0
(*Good Humor King Cone*)	30.0	<1.0

Food and Measure	carb. (gms)	fiber (gms)
(*Hood Nutty Royale*)	26.0	<1.0
(*Klondike*)	29.0	<1.0
(*Klondike Big Bear* Sundae)	31.0	<1.0
(*No Pudge* Sundae)	22.0	5.0
with caramel (*Drumstick* Sundae)	36.0	<1.0
with caramel or fudge (*Klondike*)	34.0	<1.0
with caramel (*Klondike Big Bear* Sundae)	35.0	<1.0
with fudge (*Klondike Big Bear* Sundae)	36.0	<1.0
vanilla fudge (*Turkey Hill* Sundae)	33.0	2.0
ice cream cone/cup, unfilled, 1 piece:		
bowl (*Keebler*)	10.0	0
cone:		
chocolate (*Oreo*)	12.0	0
sugar (*Comet*)	12.0	0
sugar or waffle (*Keebler*)	10.0	0
cup:		
(*Comet*)	4.0	0
(*Keebler*)	4.0	0
fudge dipped (*Keebler Fudge Shoppe*)	6.0	0
rainbow (*Comet*)	4.0	0
ice cream cup, filled, 1 cup:		
sundae (*Hoodsie*), 3 fl. oz.	19.0	0
sundae (*Klondike*), 6 fl. oz.	26.0	<1.0
vanilla (*Hoodsie*), 3 fl. oz.	12.0	0
vanilla, with chocolate strawberry swirl (*Good Humor Swirland*), 6 fl. oz.	31.0	0
vanilla, with root beer (*Barq's Floatz*), 4 fl. oz.	22.0	0
ice cream dessert:		
brownie à la mode (*Smart Ones*), 3.1 oz.	33.0	2.0
brownie parfait, double fudge (*Smart Ones*), 3.8 oz.	43.0	1.0
chocolate chip cookie dough sundae (*Smart Ones*), 2.6 oz.	35.0	1.0
ice cream pie, see "Ice cream sandwich"		
ice cream sandwich, with chocolate wafers, except as noted, 1 piece:		
chocolate (*Endulge*)	16.0	5.0
chocolate chip:		
malt (*Turkey Hill*)	32.0	1.0
mint (*Turkey Hill* No Sugar)	31.0	5.0

Food and Measure	carb. (gms)	fiber (gms)
vanilla:		
(*Chipwich*)	37.0	0
(*Chipwich* King)	45.0	<1.0
(*Chipwich* No Sugar)	36.0	3.0
vanilla fudge (*Chipwich*)	36.0	2.0
cookies and cream (*Eskimo Pie*)	34.0	1.0
cookies and cream, sugar cookies (*Chilly Bears*)	24.0	<1.0
mint (*Klondike* Slim-a-Bear 98% Fat Free)	28.0	3.0
mint chocolate chip (*Hood*)	15.0	0
Neapolitan:		
(*Darigold*)	28.0	0
(*Good Humor* Giant)	37.0	<1.0
(*Klondike Big Bear*), 4.23 fl. oz.	28.0	<1.0
(*Klondike Big Bear*), 7 fl. oz.	42.0	1.0
peanut butter ripple (*Turkey Hill*)	28.0	1.0
vanilla:		
(*Darigold*)	28.0	0
(*Endulge*)	15.0	4.0
(*Eskimo Pie* Giant King Size)	36.0	0
(*Eskimo Pie* No Sugar)	27.0	<1.0
(*Eskimo Pie* Slender Pie Clamshell No Sugar)	28.0	4.0
(*Good Humor*), 3 fl. oz.	25.0	<1.0
(*Good Humor*), 3.5 fl. oz.	25.0	0
(*Good Humor* Giant), 6 fl. oz.	36.0	0
(*Healthy Choice*)	24.0	<1.0
(*Klondike* Slim-a-Bear 98% Fat Free)	28.0	3.0
(*Klondike* Slim-a-Bear No Sugar)	25.0	2.0
(*Klondike Big Bear*), 4.23 fl. oz.	28.0	0
(*Klondike Big Bear*), 7 fl. oz.	42.0	<1.0
(*Popsicle* Mini)	15.0	0
(*Turkey Hill*)	26.0	0
(*Turkey Hill* Double Decker)	29.0	1.0
brownie, with candy (*M&M's*)	28.0	0
brownie batter swirl (*No Pudge*)	30.0	3.0
brownie chunk (*No Pudge*)	30.0	4.0
chocolate chip cookie (*Good Humor*)	41.0	1.0
chocolate chip cookie (*Klondike Big Bear*)	38.0	1.0
chocolate chip cookie, giant (*Klondike Hershey*)	66.0	2.0

Food and Measure	carb. (gms)	fiber (gms)
gingerbread cookie (*Eskimo Pie* Gingerbread Men)	26.0	<1.0
peanut butter candy (*Klondike Reese's Pieces*)	37.0	1.0
vanilla cookie, with candy (*M&M's*)	29.0	1.0
vanilla, with cookie pieces (*Klondike Oreo* Cookie)	34.0	2.0
vanilla caramel swirl, vanilla cookie (*Healthy Choice*)	27.0	<1.0
vanilla fudge (*Eskimo Pie* Slender Pie Clamshell No Sugar)	28.0	4.0
vanilla fudge swirl (*Healthy Choice*)	27.0	<1.0
vanilla fudge chip, with fudge swirl cookie (*Ben & Jerry's* 'Wich)	45.0	1.0
vanilla strawberry chocolate (*Eskimo Pie* Giant King Size).	37.0	1.0
"Ice cream" sandwich, nondairy, 1 piece:		
blueberry swirl, mini (*Tofutti Cuties*)	20.0	0
chocolate:		
(*RiceDream* Pie)	39.0	2.0
(*Soy Delicious Li'l Buddies*)	28.0	3.0
mini (*Tofutti Cuties*)	16.0	0
swirl, mini (*Tofutti Cuties* Wave)	20.0	0
chocolate chip, chocolate chip wafers (*Tofutti Too Too's*) .	30.0	0
coffee, mini (*Tofutti Cuties* Coffee Break)	16.0	0
cookies and cream, mini (*Tofutti Cuties*)	17.0	0
mint (*RiceDream* Pie)	39.0	2.0
mint chocolate chip, mini (*Tofutti Cuties*)	19.0	0
mocha (*RiceDream* Pie)	40.0	1.0
peanut butter, mini (*Tofutti Cuties*)	20.0	0
strawberry swirl, mini (*Tofutti Cuties* Wave)	20.0	0
vanilla:		
(*RiceDream* Pie)	40.0	1.0
(*Soy Delicious Li'l Buddies*)	28.0	3.0
mini (*Tofutti Cuties*)	17.0	0
mini (*Tofutti Cuties* No Sugar)	11.0	0
with vanilla wafer, mini (*Tofutti Cuties*)	16.0	0
wildberry, mini (*Tofutti Cuties*)	17.0	0
Ice cream and sherbet or sorbet, see "Sherbet" and "Sorbet"		
Iced confection bar, dairy (see also "Ice bar" and "Fruit bar"), 1 piece, except as noted:		
all varieties:		
(*CarbSmart Creamsicle*)	5.0	1.0

Food and Measure	carb. (gms)	fiber (gms)
(*Hawaiian Punch Arctic Surfer Pops*)	12.0	0
(*Popsicle* Rainbow Floats/*Sherbet Cyclone*)	11.0	0
coffee:		
(*Frappuccino*)	20.0	9.0
fudge (*Frappuccino Java Fudge*)	25.0	4.0
fudge (*Hood* Java Smoothie)	17.0	0
fudge:		
(*Darigold* Super Fudge)	30.0	1.0
(*Eskimo Pie* No Sugar)	11.0	0
(*Fudgsicle*), 1.75 fl. oz.	11.0	<1.0
(*Fudgsicle*), 2.5 fl. oz.	18.0	1.0
(*Fudgsicle*), 2.7 fl. oz.	17.0	<1.0
(*Fudgsicle* Fat Free)	14.0	<1.0
(*Fudgsicle* Mini), 2 bars	16.0	<1.0
(*Fudgsicle* No Sugar 12 Pack), 2 bars	12.0	0
(*Fudgsicle* No Sugar 20 Pack), 2 bars	18.0	4.0
(*Fudgsicle* Sugar Free), 2 bars	9.0	2.0
(*Healthy Choice*)	13.0	0
(*Hendrie's* Fat Free Stix)	15.0	1.0
(*Klondike* Slim-a-Bear)	22.0	4.0
(*Simply Slender*), 1.75 fl. oz.	9.0	0
(*Simply Slender*), 2.5 fl. oz.	21.0	1.0
chocolate (*Endulge*)	12.0	5.0
double (*Supersicle Firecracker*)	29.0	1.0
mocha (*Frappuccino*)	22.0	3.0
orange sherbet (*Popsicle Pop-Ups*)	19.0	0
orange sherbet/vanilla ice cream:		
(*Creamsicle*), 1.75 fl. oz.	13.0	0
(*Creamsicle*), 2.5 fl. oz.	18.0	0
(*Creamsicle*), 2.7 fl. oz.	20.0	0
(*Creamsicle* No Sugar)	5.0	1.0
(*Creamsicle* Sugar Free), 2 bars	10.0	6.0
(*Hood* Orange Cream)	18.0	0
(*Minute Maid* Swirl Bars), 3-oz. tube	16.0	0
rainbow (*Popsicle Pop-Ups*)	19.0	0
Icing, cake, see "Frosting"		
Irish cream syrup (*Ferrara*), 2 oz.	32.0	0

J

Food and Measure	carb. (gms)	fiber (gms)
Jack in the Box, 1 serving:		
breakfast:		
biscuit, sausage	41.0	2.0
biscuit, sausage, egg, and cheese	50.0	2.0
burrito	32.0	22.0
burrito, with salsa	34.0	22.0
burrito, meaty	29.0	2.0
burrito, meaty, with salsa	30.0	2.0
Breakfast Jack	34.0	0
croissant, sausage	42.0	1.0
croissant, supreme	41.0	1.0
hash browns	13.0	2.0
sausage sandwich, extreme	37.0	0
sourdough sandwich	37.0	2.0
ultimate sandwich	58.0	2.0
burgers:		
cheeseburger, bacon	50.0	2.0
cheeseburger, junior bacon	32.0	0
cheeseburger, ultimate	52.0	2.0
cheeseburger, ultimate, bacon	53.0	2.0
hamburger	30.0	0
hamburger, with cheese	31.0	0
hamburger deluxe	32.0	0
hamburger deluxe, with cheese	34.0	0
Jumbo Jack	52.0	2.0
Jumbo Jack, with cheese	55.0	2.0
Sourdough Jack	36.0	2.0
chicken/fish:		
chicken breast strips	39.0	3.0

Food and Measure	carb. (gms)	fiber (gms)
chicken ciabatta, bruschetta, or classic	69.0	4.0
chicken fajita pita	33.0	0
chicken sandwich	39.0	1.0
chicken sandwich, with bacon	39.0	2.0
chicken sandwich, with cheese	40.0	1.0
chicken sandwich Cordon Bleu	33.0	2.0
fish & chips	69.0	4.0
Jack's Spicy Chicken	62.0	3.0
Jack's Spicy Chicken, with cheese	63.0	3.0
sourdough grilled chicken club	35.0	2.0
Southwest pita	35.0	4.0
sandwiches:		
Pannido, deli trio	53.0	2.0
Pannido, ham and turkey	54.0	2.0
Pannido, zesty turkey	51.0	2.0
ultimate club	52.0	2.0
tacos/snacks:		
bacon cheddar potato wedges	45.0	5.0
egg roll, 1 piece	26.0	2.0
egg roll, 3 pieces	55.0	6.0
jalapeños, stuffed, 3 pieces	22.0	2.0
jalapeños, stuffed, 7 pieces	51.0	4.0
taco	15.0	2.0
taco, monster	20.0	3.0
fries:		
natural, large	69.0	5.0
natural, medium	47.0	4.0
natural, small	35.0	3.0
seasoned curly, large	60.0	6.0
seasoned curly, medium	45.0	5.0
seasoned curly, small	30.0	3.0
onion rings	51.0	3.0
salad:		
chicken, Asian	58.0	8.0
chicken, Southwest	56.0	7.0
chicken Caesar	10.0	3.0
chicken club	34.0	5.0
side salad	16.0	0

Food and Measure	carb. (gms)	fiber (gms)
sauces/dressing:		
dipping sauce:		
barbecue	11.0	0
buttermilk house	3.0	0
Frank's Red Hot Buffalo or tartar	2.0	0
sweet and sour	11.0	0
dressing:		
balsamic, low fat or creamy Caesar	6.0	0
ranch	4.0	0
ranch, lite	3.0	0
herb mayo, reduced fat	1.0	0
mayo onion sauce or soy sauce	1.0	0
taco sauce	0	0
shakes, ice cream:		
caramel, creamy, large	173.0	1.0
caramel, creamy, medium	109.0	0
caramel, creamy, small	87.0	0
chocolate, large	178.0	2.0
chocolate, medium	111.0	1.0
chocolate, small	89.0	1.0
Oreo cookie, large	161.0	2.0
Oreo cookie, medium	103.0	1.0
Oreo cookie, small	81.0	1.0
strawberry, large	167.0	0
strawberry, medium	106.0	0
strawberry, small	84.0	0
strawberry banana, large	199.0	0
strawberry banana, medium	122.0	0
strawberry banana, small	100.0	0
vanilla, large	129.0	0
vanilla, medium	85.0	0
vanilla, small	65.0	0
dessert, cheesecake	34.0	0
dessert, double fudge cake	49.0	4.0
Jackfruit, fresh, trimmed, 1 oz.	6.8	.5
Jackfruit, canned, in syrup, ½ cup	21.3	.8
Jackson wonder beans, canned (*Westbrae Natural Organic Heirloom Beans*), ½ cup	19.0	5.0

Jalapeño, see "Pepper, jalapeño"
Jalapeño sauce, see "Hot sauce" and specific listings
Jam and preserves (see also "Fruit spreads"), 1 tbsp.:
all fruits:

	carb. (gms)	fiber (gms)
(*Smucker's*)	13.0	0
(*Smucker's* Low Sugar)	6.0	0
(*Smucker's* Sugar Free)	5.0	0
grapefruit marmalade, pink (*Bellisimo*)	12.0	0
orange marmalade (*Cascadian Farm*)	11.0	0
orange marmalade (*Dundee*)	14.0	0

Java plum:

3 medium, .4 oz.	1.4	<1.0
seeded, ½ cup	10.5	<1.0

Jelly, fruit, 1 tbsp.:

all fruits (*Smucker's*)	13.0	0
apple mint (*Great Expectations*)	13.0	0
guava (*Goya*)	14.0	0
Jelly, hot pepper (*Reese*), 1 tbsp.	13.0	0

Jerk sauce, see "Barbecue sauce" and "Marinade"
Jerk seasoning:

(*McCormick* Caribbean), ¼ tsp.	0	0
dry rub (*Neera's* Jamaican), 1 tsp.	2.0	0
spice paste (*Neera's* Jamaican), 2 tsp.	4.0	1.0

Jerusalem artichoke:

(*Frieda's Sunchoke*), ½ cup, 3 oz.	14.0	1.0
sliced, ½ cup	13.1	1.2

Jew's ear, see "Pepeao"
Jicama, see "Yam beans"
Jujube:

raw, seeded, 1 oz.	5.7	n.a.
dried, 1 oz.	20.1	n.a.

Jute, potherb, ½ cup:

raw	.8	n.a.
boiled, drained	3.1	.9

K

Food and Measure	carb. (gms)	fiber (gms)
Kabocha squash (*Frieda's*), ¾ cup, 3 oz.	7.0	1.0
Kahn choy, see "Celery, Chinese"		
Kale, fresh:		
raw (*Glory*), 2.8 oz.	8.0	2.0
raw, chopped, ½ cup	3.4	.7
boiled, drained, chopped, ½ cup	3.7	3.6
Kale, canned, ½ cup:		
(*Allens* No Salt)	3.0	2.0
(*Bush's*)	4.0	2.0
seasoned (*Allens/Sunshine*)	5.0	1.0
seasoned (*Glory*)	6.0	3.0
Kale, frozen, boiled, drained, chopped, ½ cup	3.4	1.3
Kale, Chinese, fresh:		
(*Frieda's* Chinese Broccoli), 1 cup, 3 oz.	3.0	0
cooked, 1 cup	3.3	2.2
Kale, Scotch, ½ cup:		
raw, chopped	2.8	.6
boiled, drained, chopped	3.7	.8
Kamranga, see "Carambola"		
Kamut, grain (*Shiloh Farms*), ¼ cup	35.0	9.0
Kamut flakes, see "Cereal, ready-to-eat"		
Kamut flour (*Arrowhead Mills*), ⅓ cup	25.0	4.0
Kanpo, dried:		
.2-oz. strip	4.1	n.a.
½ cup	15.6	n.a.
Kasha, see "Buckwheat groats"		
Kefir, 8 fl. oz.:		
plain:		
(*Lifeway* Original)	12.0	0

Food and Measure	carb. (gms)	fiber (gms)
(*Lifeway Organic/Lifeway* Nonfat/Lowfat)	8.0	0
(*Lifeway Slim6*)	3.0	2.0
flavored, all varieties:		
(*Lifeway* Nonfat)	28.0	0
(*Lifeway Organic/Lifeway* Lowfat)	21.0	0
(*Lifeway Slim6*)	8.0	2.0
soy blend, see "Soy beverage"		
Ketchup, 1 tbsp.:		
(*Annie's Naturals* Organic)	3.0	0
(*Del Monte*)	4.0	0
(*Heinz*)	4.0	0
(*Hunt's/Hunt's* No Salt)	4.0	0
(*Muir Glen*)	4.0	0
(*Red Gold*)	5.0	0
(*Red Pack*)	4.0	0
(*S&W*)	4.0	0
(*Tree of Life*)	3.0	0
fruit sweetened (*Westbrae Natural*/No Salt)	3.0	0
fruit sweetened (*Westbrae Natural* Squeeze)	4.0	0
garlic, zesty (*Heinz*)	5.0	0
hot and spicy (*Heinz Kick'rs*)	4.0	0
jalapeño, smoked, spicy (*Fiesta*)	3.0	0
unsweetened (*Westbrae Natural* UnKetchup)	1.0	0
KFC, 1 serving:		
chicken:		
Extra Crispy:		
breast	19.0	0
drumstick	5.0	0
thigh	12.0	0
whole wing	10.0	0
hot and spicy:		
breast	20.0	0
drumstick	4.0	0
thigh	14.0	0
whole wing	9.0	0
Original Recipe:		
breast	11.0	0
drumstick	4.0	0

Food and Measure	carb. (gms)	fiber (gms)
thigh	12.0	0
whole wing	5.0	0
chicken, popcorn:		
family	173.0	1.0
individual	23.0	0
large	34.0	1.0
chicken pot pie	70.0	5.0
chicken strips, 3 pieces	17.0	0
chicken wings, honey barbecue–sauced, 6 pieces	12.0	1.0
chicken wings, *Hot Wings,* 6 pieces	8.0	1.0
meal, strips, oven-roasted, with green beans, rice	50.0	6.0
meal, *Tender* Roast fillet, with green beans, rice	41.0	4.0
sides, individual:		
baked beans	46.0	7.0
biscuit, 2 oz.	23.0	0
coleslaw	22.0	3.0
corn on cob, 3"	13.0	3.0
corn on cob, 5.5"	26.0	7.0
green beans	7.0	2.0
macaroni and cheese	30.0	4.0
potato salad	22.0	1.0
potato wedges	30.0	3.0
potatoes, mashed	16.0	1.0
potatoes, mashed, with gravy	18.0	1.0
rice, seasoned	32.0	2.0
sandwiches:		
crunch, double	42.0	3.0
crunch, triple	49.0	3.0
honey barbecue	41.0	1.0
KFC snacker	31.0	2.0
KFC snacker, honey barbecue	32.0	2.0
Tender Roast	24.0	1.0
Tender Roast, without sauce	23.0	1.0
Twister, crispy	55.0	3.0
Twister, oven roast	50.0	4.0
salad, without dressing or croutons:		
BLT, crispy	21.0	4.0
BLT, roasted	8.0	4.0

Food and Measure	carb. (gms)	fiber (gms)
Caesar, crispy	20.0	3.0
Caesar, roasted	6.0	3.0
salad croutons, 1 pkt.	9.0	0
salad dressing, 1 pkt.:		
Caesar, Parmesan	4.0	0
Italian, light	8.0	0
ranch	3.0	0
ranch, fat free	8.0	0
dessert:		
apple pie, mini, 3 pieces	46.0	2.0
applesauce	24.0	1.0
cake, double chocolate chip	31.0	2.0
Lil' Bucket:		
chocolate cream	37.0	2.0
fudge brownie	44.0	1.0
lemon crème	65.0	2.0
strawberry shortcake	34.0	0
pie, 1 slice:		
apple	44.0	2.0
lemon meringue	40.0	1.0
pecan	68.0	2.0
sweet potato	44.0	1.0
Kidney beans:		
dry, dark (*Shiloh Farms*), ¼ cup	29.0	10.0
boiled, ½ cup	20.1	6.5
Kidney beans, canned, ½ cup:		
red:		
(*Eden* Organic)	18.0	10.0
(*Progresso*)	20.0	8.0
(*S&W*)	23.0	6.0
(*S&W* 50% Less Salt)	21.0	6.0
(*Westbrae Natural* Organic)	18.0	5.0
red, dark:		
(*Allens*)	22.0	8.0
(*Bush's*)	21.0	7.0
(*Progresso*)	20.0	6.0
(*Trappey's*)	28.0	5.0

Food and Measure	carb. (gms)	fiber (gms)
red, light:		
(*Allens/Trappey's*)	22.0	8.0
(*Bush's*)	20.0	7.0
with bacon (*Trappey's*)	23.0	7.0
with chili (*Trappey's*)	20.0	7.0
with jalapeño (*Trappey's*)	19.0	6.0
white, cannellini:		
(*Bush's*)	18.0	6.0
(*Eden* Organic)	17.0	5.0
(*Goya*)	18.0	7.0
(*Progresso*)	16.0	5.0
Kidney beans, sprouted, raw, ½ cup	3.8	<1.0
Kidneys, braised:		
beef or lamb, 4 oz.	1.1	0
pork or veal, 4 oz. or 1 cup chopped	0	0
Kielbasa, 2 oz.:		
(*Boar's Head*)	0	0
(*Healthy Choice* Polska)	6.0	0
turkey (*Louis Rich* Polska)	2.0	0
Kim chee (*Frieda's*), ¼ cup, 2 oz.	2.0	1.0
Kippers, see "Herring"		
Kiwi, fresh:		
(*Del Monte*), 2 medium, 5.2 oz.	24.0	4.0
(*Dole*), 2 medium, 5.2 oz.	24.0	4.0
(*Frieda's/Frieda's* Baby/Gold), 5 oz.	21.0	5.0
1 large, 3.7 oz.	13.5	3.1
1 medium, 3.1 oz.	11.3	2.6
Kiwi drink blend, 8 fl. oz.:		
berry (*Nantucket Nectars*)	30.0	0
raspberry or strawberry (*Langers* Juice Cocktail)	29.0	0
strawberry:		
(*ArIZona*)	29.0	0
(*Ocean Spray*)	31.0	0
(*Ocean Spray Cravin' Less Sugar*)	19.0	0
(*R.W. Knudsen*)	30.0	0
(*Snapple*)	28.0	0
(*Snapple* Diet)	5.0	0

Food and Measure	carb. (gms)	fiber (gms)
Kiwi-strawberry juice (*Juicy Juice*), 8 fl. oz. . . . . , . .	29.0	0
Knockwurst, 1 link:		
(*Karl Ehmer*), 4 oz.	1.0	0
(*Schaller & Weber* Knackwurst), 2 oz.	2.0	0
beef (*Boar's Head*), 4 oz.	1.0	0
beef (*Hebrew National*), 3 oz.	1.0	0
Kohlrabi:		
raw (*Frieda's*), ⅔ cup or ½ cup sliced	4.3	2.5
boiled, drained, sliced, ½ cup	5.5	.9
Krispy Kreme:		
donuts, 1 piece:		
blueberry, glazed	43.0	<1.0
blueberry filled, powdered	33.0	<1.0
cake, powdered	37.0	<1.0
cake, traditional	25.0	<1.0
caramel kreme crunch	43.0	<1.0
cheesecake, New York	35.0	<1.0
chocolate, glazed, cake	41.0	2.0
chocolate, glazed, cruller	37.0	<1.0
chocolate, iced:		
cake	37.0	<1.0
custard filled	35.0	<1.0
glazed	33.0	<1.0
kreme filled or with sprinkles	38.0	<1.0
chocolate brownie deluxe	33.0	2.0
cinnamon, glazed	24.0	<1.0
cinnamon apple filled	32.0	<1.0
cinnamon bun	28.0	<1.0
cinnamon twist	33.0	1.0
cruller, glazed	26.0	<1.0
dulce de leche	30.0	<1.0
key lime pie	40.0	<1.0
kreme filled, glazed	38.0	<1.0
lemon filled, glazed	35.0	<1.0
maple iced glazed	32.0	<1.0
pumpkin spice cake	42.0	<1.0
raspberry filled, glazed	39.0	<1.0
sour cream, glazed	42.0	<1.0

Food and Measure	carb. (gms)	fiber (gms)
strawberry filled, powdered	33.0	<1.0
sugar	21.0	0
frozen blends, without whipped cream:		
chocolate, double, with or without coffee:		
12 oz.	69.0	0
16 oz.	93.0	0
20 oz.	116.0	0
latte:		
12 oz.	69.0	0
16 oz.	92.0	0
20 oz.	114.0	0
original, with or without coffee:		
12 oz.	70.0	0
16 oz.	95.0	0
20 oz.	117.0	0
raspberry:		
12 oz.	74.0	0
16 oz.	99.0	0
20 oz.	123.0	0
Kumquat:		
(*Frieda's*), 5 oz.	23.0	9.0
1 medium, 7 oz.	3.1	1.3
seeded, 1 oz.	4.7	1.9
Kuri squash, see "Red kuri squash"		
Kuzu root (*Eden* Organic), .3 oz.	8.0	0

L

Food and Measure	carb. (gms)	fiber (gms)
Lamb, meat only, without added ingredients	0	0
Lamb's quarters, boiled, drained, chopped, ½ cup	4.5	1.9
Lard:		
(*Goya* Achiotina), 1 tbsp.	0	0
pork, 1 tbsp.	0	0
Lasagna entree, freeze-dried, 1 serving:		
meat sauce:		
(*Mountain House* Can/Four), 1 cup	29.0	2.0
(*Mountain House* Double), ½ pouch	36.0	2.0
(*Mountain House* Single)	45.0	3.0
vegetable (*Mountain House*), ½ pouch	35.0	3.0
Lasagna entree, frozen, 1 pkg., except as noted:		
Alfredo (*Michelina's* Authentico), 9 oz.	38.0	2.0
bake, (*Healthy Choice*), 9 oz.	36.0	5.0
bake, (*Stouffer's*), 11.5 oz.	47.0	4.0
Bolognese (*Smart Ones*), 9 oz.	43.0	4.0
cheese:		
(*Amy's*), 10.3 oz.	35.0	4.0
(*Ian's* Natural Low Carb), ½ of 12-oz. pkg.	9.0	3.0
five (*Lean Cuisine Everyday Favorites* Classic), 11.5 oz.	48.0	4.0
five (*Michelina's Lean Gourmet*), 8.5 oz.	38.0	5.0
five (*Stouffer's*), 10.75 oz.	39.0	4.0
five (*Stouffer's* Family Style Recipes),		
⅟₁₁ of 96-oz. pkg.	32.0	3.0
four (*Michelina's* Authentico), 8 oz.	43.0	3.0
four (*Uncle Ben's* Pasta Bowl), 12 oz.	41.0	7.0
four, layered (*Michelina's* Authentico), 8 oz.	30.0	1.0
with chicken (*Lean Cuisine* Cafe Classics), 10 oz.	36.0	4.0
with meatless ground round (*Cedarlane*), 10 oz.	45.0	3.0

Food and Measure	carb. (gms)	fiber (gms)
chicken:		
(*Stouffer's* Family Style Recipes), ⅕ of 39-oz. pkg.	29.0	2.0
(*Stouffer's* Family Style Recipes), ¹⁄₁₁ of 96-oz. pkg. ...	34.0	3.0
Florentine (*Lean Cuisine Everyday Favorites*), 10 oz. ...	35.0	3.0
Florentine (*Smart Ones*), 10.5 oz.	36.0	5.0
Florentine, bake (*Lean Cuisine* Cafe Classics), 10 oz.	35.0	3.0
meat sauce:		
(*Lean Cuisine Everyday Favorites*), 10.5 oz.	43.0	4.0
(*Smart Ones* Traditional), 10.5 oz.	38.0	3.0
(*Stouffer's*), 10.5 oz.	37.0	3.0
(*Stouffer's*), ⅓ of 21-oz. pkg.	27.0	2.0
(*Stouffer's* Family Style Recipes), ⅕ of 40-oz. pkg.	28.0	2.0
(*Stouffer's* Family Style Recipes), ⅐ of 57-oz. pkg.	31.0	2.0
(*Stouffer's* Family Style Recipes), ¹⁄₁₂ of 96-oz. pkg. ...	27.0	2.0
four cheese (*Michelina's* Authentico), 9 oz.	40.0	3.0
layered (*Michelina's Lean Gourmet*), 8 oz.	34.0	5.0
meatless (*Boca*), 10.5 oz.	41.0	5.0
mozzarella (*Michelina's* Zap'ems), 8 oz.	39.0	3.0
primavera (*Michelina's* Zap'ems), 8 oz.	35.0	3.0
seafood (*Contessa* Minute Meal Bowl), 10 oz.	35.0	3.0
tomato sauce, sausage (*Stouffer's*), 10⅞ oz.	41.0	4.0
vegetable:		
(*Amy's*), 9.5 oz.	35.0	5.0
(*Amy's* Family Size), ⅐ of 45-oz. pkg.	25.0	4.0
(*Cedarlane Carb Buster*), 9.5 oz.	19.0	9.0
(*Stouffer's*), 10.5 oz.	43.0	5.0
(*Stouffer's* Family Style Recipes), ¹⁄₁₂ of 96-oz. pkg. ...	36.0	3.0
(*Yves* Veggie), 10.5 oz.	51.0	4.0
garden (*Amy's*), 10.25 oz.	41.0	5.0
garden (*Cedarlane* Low Fat), ½ of 10-oz. pkg.	26.0	2.0
tofu (*Amy's*), 9.5 oz.	41.0	6.0
Lasagna entree mix, see "Hamburger entree mix"		
Lecithin granules:		
(*Shiloh Farms*), 2 tbsp.	1.0	0
(*Tree of Life*), 1 tbsp.	1.0	0
Leek, with lower leaf portion, fresh:		
raw:		
(*Frieda's*), 1 cup, 3 oz.	12.0	2.0

Food and Measure	carb. (gms)	fiber (gms)
9.9-oz. leek	17.6	2.2
chopped, ½ cup	7.4	.9
boiled, drained, 4.4-oz. leek	9.5	1.2
boiled, drained, chopped, ½ cup	4.0	.5
Leek, freeze-dried, 1 tbsp.	.2	<1.0
Lemon, fresh:		
(*Dole*), 2-oz. fruit	5.0	1.0
(*Del Monte*), 2-oz. fruit	5.0	1.0
(*Sunkist*), 2-oz. fruit	5.0	<1.0
2⅛" lemon, 3.8 oz.	11.6	n.a.
1 wedge, ¼ medium	2.9	n.a.
peeled, 2⅛" lemon	5.4	1.6
Lemon butter dill sauce, see "Grilling sauce"		
Lemon curd, 1 tbsp.:		
(*Crosse & Blackwell*)	13.0	0
(*Dickenson's*)	14.0	0
(*Grant's*)	10.0	0
(*Laird's Larder*)	15.0	0
Lemon dill sauce mix (*Golden Dipt Bag 'n Season*),		
1 tbsp.	6.0	0
Lemon drink (see also "Lemonade") (*Santa Cruz*		
Organic Box), 8 fl. oz.	28.0	0
Lemon drink blend, ginger echinacea (*Santa Cruz*		
Organic), 8 fl. oz.	25.0	0
Lemon garlic herb sauce (*Litehouse*), 2 tbsp.	8.0	0
Lemon grass, fresh:		
1 tbsp.	1.2	n.a.
1 cup	16.9	n.a.
Lemon grass sauce, see "Marinade"		
Lemon herb seasoning (*McCormick 1 Step*), 1 tsp.	1.0	0
Lemon juice:		
fresh, ½ cup	10.5	.5
fresh, 1 tbsp.	1.3	.1
bottled (*Santa Cruz Organic*), 1 tsp.	0	0
Lemon peel, fresh, 1 tbsp.	1.0	.6
Lemon pepper, ¼ tsp., except as noted:		
(*Lawry's*)	0	0
(*McCormick* California Style)	0	0

Food and Measure	carb. (gms)	fiber (gms)
1 tsp.	1.5	.3
and lime seasoning rub (*Ducks Unlimited*)	0	0
salt (*McCormick*)	0	0
Lemonade, 8 fl. oz., except as noted:		
(*AriZona*)	27.0	0
(*Minute Maid* Carton/Jug)	31.0	0
(*Nantucket Nectars* Squeezed)	32.0	0
(*R.W. Knudsen* Juice Box)	28.0	0
(*Santa Cruz Organic*)	24.0	0
(*Snapple* Super Sour)	33.0	0
(*SoBe MacLizard's* Special Recipe)	30.0	0
(*Tropicana*)	27.0	0
(*Turkey Hill*)	29.0	0
pink:		
(*Hi-C Blast*)	32.0	0
(*Minute Maid* Carton/Jug)	30.0	0
(*Minute Maid* Cooler), 6.75-fl.-oz. box	25.0	0
(*Nantucket Nectars* Squeezed)	29.0	0
pink or white:		
(*Minute Maid*), 12-fl.-oz. cont.	42.0	0
(*Minute Maid*), 6.75-fl.-oz. box	25.0	0
(*Minute Maid* Plastic/Can)	28.0	0
(*Newman's Own/Newman's Own* Virgin)	27.0	0
(*Snapple*)	28.0	0
(*Walnut Acres*)	29.0	0
frozen*:		
(*Cascadian Farm*)	28.0	0
(*Minute Maid*)	29.0	0
pink	25.9	0
white	26.0	.3
sparkling (*Santa Cruz Organic*), 12 fl. oz.	26.0	0
tea, see "Tea, iced"		
Lemonade fruit blend, 8 fl. oz.:		
cranberry (*Nantucket Nectars* Squeezed)	30.0	0
cranberry, white (*Langers*)	30.0	0
limeade (*Nantucket Nectars*)	29.0	0
mango (*Bolthouse Farms*)	30.0	<1.0
peach (*Nantucket Nectars* Squeezed)	35.0	0

Food and Measure	carb. (gms)	fiber (gms)
peach (*V8 Splash*)	27.0	0
raspberry:		
(*Langers*)	29.0	0
(*Minute Maid* Carton)	32.0	0
(*Minute Maid* Plastic)	28.0	0
(*Santa Cruz Organic*)	23.0	0
(*Turkey Hill*)	29.0	0
(*V8 Splash*)	27.0	0
frozen* (*Minute Maid*)	29.0	0
strawberry (*Santa Cruz Organic*)	24.0	0
strawberry kiwi (*Turkey Hill*)	29.0	0
watermelon (*Nantucket Nectars*)	30.0	0
Lemonade, mix*, 8 fl. oz.:		
(*Country Time*)	16.0	0
(*Country Time* Sugar Free)	0	0
raspberry (*Country Time*)	19.0	0
raspberry, strawberry (*Country Time*)	20.0	0
Lentil:		
dry, ¼ cup:		
black Beluga (*Shiloh Farms*)	34.0	9.0
French (*Shiloh Farms*)	30.0	3.0
green (*Arrowhead Mills*)	27.0	7.0
green or split red (*Shiloh Farms*)	27.0	7.0
red (*Arrowhead Mills*)	28.0	7.0
cooked, ½ cup	19.9	7.8
Lentil, canned, ½ cup:		
(*Goya*)	16.0	4.0
(*Westbrae Natural* Organic)	17.0	9.0
black Beluga (*Westbrae Natural* Organic Heirloom)	16.0	4.0
with onion and bay leaf (*Eden* Organic)	13.0	4.0
Lentil, sprouted, raw, ½ cup	8.4	n.a.
Lentil dish, mix:		
(*Neera's* Dal and Seasoning), 1 cup*	23.0	12.0
(*Neera's* Urad and Channa Dal), 1 cup*	18.0	9.0
pilaf, with rice (*Near East*), 2 oz. or 1 cup*	36.0	8.0
Lentil entree, frozen, garlic stew (*Ethnic Gourmet* Dal Bahaar), 12 oz.	53.0	4.0

Food and Measure	carb. (gms)	fiber (gms)
Lentil entree, pkg.:		
(*Tasty Bite* Bengal), ½ of 10-oz. pkg.	16.0	8.0
(*Tasty Bite* Jodhpur), ½ of 10-oz. pkg.	12.0	7.0
(*Tasty Bite* Madras), ½ of 10-oz. pkg.	14.0	5.0
with rice, 9.25-oz. pkg:		
chili (*Tamarind Tree* Dal Makhani)	55.0	14.0
vegetables (*Tamarind Tree* Channa Dal Masala)	62.0	10.0
Lettuce (see also "Salad blend" and "Salad kit"):		
bibb or Boston, 1 head, 5'' diam.	3.8	1.6
bibb or Boston, 2 inner leaves	.4	.5
butterhead (*Frieda's* Limestone), ⅔ cup, 3 oz.	2.0	1.0
iceberg:		
(*Dole*), ⅙ medium	3.0	1.0
1 head, 6'' diam.	11.3	7.5
1 leaf, .7 oz.	.4	.3
shredded (*Dole*), 3 oz.	3.0	1.0
shredded (*Fresh Express Shreds!*), 1½ cups, 3 oz.	3.0	1.0
shredded, 1 cup	1.2	.8
leaf/looseleaf, shredded (*Dole*), 1½ cups, 3 oz.	4.0	2.0
leaf/looseleaf, shredded, ½ cup	1.0	.5
romaine or cos:		
(*Dole*), 6 leaves, 3 oz.	3.0	1.0
(*Ready Pac* Bella), 1½ cups, 3 oz.	2.0	1.0
(*Ready Pac* Caesar), 2½ cups, 2.9 oz.	3.0	1.0
(*Ready Pac* Caesar Organic), 2¾ cups, 3 oz.	2.0	<1.0
hearts (*Fresh Express*), 3 oz.	2.0	1.0
1 inner leaf	.2	.2
shredded, ½ cup	.7	.5
romaine hearts, (*Andy Boy*), 6 leaves, 3 oz.	3.0	1.0
romaine hearts (*Dole/Dole* Organic), 3 oz.	3.0	1.0
Lima beans:		
immature, ½ cup, raw, trimmed	15.7	3.8
immature, ½ cup, boiled, drained	20.1	4.5
mature, dry:		
baby (*Goya*), ¼ cup	23.0	15.0
baby (*Shiloh Farms*), ¼ cup	23.0	15.0
baby, boiled, ½ cup	21.2	7.0

Food and Measure	carb. (gms)	fiber (gms)
large (*Shiloh Farms*), ¼ cup	22.0	12.0
boiled, ½ cup	19.6	6.6
Lima beans, canned (see also "Butter beans"), ½ cup:		
baby (*Eden* Organic)	17.0	4.0
baby, seasoned (*Glory*)	24.0	7.0
green:		
(*Allens/East Texas Fair*)	23.0	8.0
(*Del Monte*)	15.0	4.0
baby (*Freshlike/Freshlike* Selects)	26.0	7.0
baby (*Veg-All*)	15.0	3.0
with bacon (*Trappey's*)	22.0	6.0
green and white (*Allens*)	20.0	9.0
white, with bacon (*Trappey's*)	21.0	6.0
Lima beans, frozen:		
baby, ½ cup:		
(*Birds Eye*)	20.0	5.0
(*C&W/C&W* Petite)	15.0	5.0
(*Green Giant*)	16.0	3.0
(*McKenzie's*)	22.0	5.0
baby, in butter sauce (*Green Giant*), ⅔ cup	20.0	4.0
Fordhook (*Birds Eye*), ½ cup	18.0	4.0
Lime, fresh:		
(*Del Monte*), lime, 2.4-oz.	7.0	2.0
(*Frieda's* Key Lime), 3-oz. lime	9.0	2.0
2"-diam. lime	7.1	1.9
peeled, seeded, 1 oz.	3.0	.8
Lime curd, 1 tbsp.:		
(*Crosse & Blackwell*)	13.0	0
(*Dickenson's*)	14.0	0
Lime drink, see "Limeade"		
Lime juice:		
fresh, ½ cup	11.1	.5
fresh, 1 tbsp.	1.4	.1
bottled (*Angostura*), 1 tsp.	1.0	0
bottled (*Santa Cruz Organic*), 1 tsp.	0	0
sweetened (*Rose's*), 1 tsp.	2.0	0
unsweetened (*Rose's*), 2 tbsp.	2.0	0
unsweetened, 2 tbsp.	2.0	.1

Food and Measure	carb. (gms)	fiber (gms)
Lime relish, Indian, 1 tbsp.:		
hot (*Patak's*)	.5	<1.0
mild (*Patak's*)	0	0
Limeade, 8 fl. oz., except as noted:		
(*Nantucket Nectars* Squeezed)	28.0	0
(*Santa Cruz Organic*)	26.0	0
(*Walnut Acres*)	27.0	0
cherry (*Minute Maid*)	34.0	0
sparkling (*Santa Cruz Organic*), 12 fl. oz.	26.0	0
Ling, without added ingredients	0	0
Ling cod, without added ingredients	0	0
Linguica sausage (*Caspar's*), 2 oz.	1.0	0
Linguine:		
dry, see "Pasta"		
refrigerated (*Buitoni*), 1¼ cups	45.0	2.0
refrigerated (*Monterey Carb Smart* Egg Recipe), 3.5 oz.	27.0	5.0
Linguine entree, frozen, with clams (*Michelina's* Authentico), 8.5-oz. pkg.	50.0	2.0
Liquor¹, all proofs, 1 fl. oz.:	0	0
Litchi, see "Lychee"		
Little Caesars:		
⅛ of 12'' pizza:		
cheese only or pepperoni	23.0	1.0
add toppings:		
bacon	.1	0
beef	.4	.2
extra cheese	.2	0
green pepper	.4	.1
ham	.5	0
hot peppers	0	0
mushrooms	.5	.2
olives, black	.2	.2
onions	.1	.1
pepperoni	.1	0

¹Includes all pure distilled liquors: bourbon, brandy, gin, rum, Scotch, tequila, vodka, etc.

Food and Measure	carb. (gms)	fiber (gms)
pineapple	1.7	.1
sausage, Italian	.1	0
tomato	.4	.1
1/10 of 14" pizza:		
cheese only or pepperoni	25.0	1.0
meatsa	26.0	2.0
supreme	31.0	3.0
veggie	32.0	3.0
add toppings:		
bacon	.1	.1
beef	.4	.2
extra cheese	.2	0
green pepper	.4	.1
ham	.1	0
hot peppers	0	0
mushrooms	.4	.2
olives, black	.2	.2
onions	.6	.1
pepperoni	.1	0
pineapple	1.7	0
sausage, Italian	.2	.1
tomato	.5	.1
deep dish, 1/8 pie:		
large, cheese	37.0	2.0
large, pepperoni	38.0	2.0
medium, cheese or pepperoni	27.0	1.0
slice, 1/6 of 14" pie, cheese or pepperoni	42.0	2.0
deli sandwiches:		
ham and cheese or Italian	66.0	3.0
veggie	67.0	3.0
other items, 1 piece, except as noted:		
Baby Pan!Pan!	34.0	2.0
cheese bread, Italian	13.0	0
chicken wing	0	0
Crazy Bread	15.0	0
Crazy Bread, cinnamon, 2 pieces	19.0	0
Crazy Sauce, 4 oz.	9.0	3.0

Food and Measure	carb. (gms)	fiber (gms)
salad:		
antipasto	6.0	2.0
Caesar	12.0	3.0
Greek	11.0	3.0
tossed	15.0	3.0
salad dressing:		
Caesar	1.0	0
Greek	0	0
Italian or ranch	2.0	0
Italian, fat free	5.0	0
Liver:		
beef, pan-fried, 4 oz.	8.9	0
calves (veal), braised, 4 oz.	4.3	0
calves (veal), pan-fried, 4 oz.	5.1	0
chicken, simmered, 4 oz.	1.0	0
chicken, simmered, chopped, 1 cup	1.2	0
chicken, pan-fried, 4 oz.	1.3	0
duck, raw, 1 oz.	1.0	0
goose, raw, 1 oz.	1.8	0
lamb, braised, 4 oz.	2.9	0
lamb, pan-fried, 4 oz.	4.3	0
pork, braised, 4 oz.	4.3	0
turkey, simmered, 4 oz.	3.9	0
turkey, simmered, chopped, 1 cup	4.8	0
Liver cheese:		
(*Oscar Mayer*), 1.3 oz.	1.0	0
pork, 2 oz.	1.8	0
Liver pâté, see "Pâté"		
Liver sausage, see "Braunschweiger" and "Liverwurst"		
Liver steak, beef, organic (*Organic Valley*), 2 oz.	3.0	0
Liverwurst (see also "Braunschweiger" and "Pâté"), 2 oz.:		
(*Boar's Head* Strassburger)	1.0	0
(*Dietz & Watson*)	0	0
(*Hansel 'n Gretel*)	4.0	0
(*Hatfield Deli Choice*)	3.0	0
onion or smoked (*Boar's Head*)	1.0	0
Liverwurst spread, ¼ cup, 2 oz.	3.2	.4

Food and Measure	carb. (gms)	fiber (gms)
Lo bok, see "Radish, Oriental"		
Lobster, northern, meat only:		
raw, 4 oz.	.6	0
boiled or steamed, 4 oz.	.5	0
boiled or steamed, 1 cup, 5.1 oz.	1.9	0
"Lobster," imitation, chunk or salad style (*Louis Kemp Lobster Delights*), ½ cup, 3 oz.	12.0	0
Lobster, spiny, see "Spiny lobster"		
Lobster sauce, canned (*Progresso*), ½ cup	6.0	2.0
Loganberries, fresh, 1 cup	21.5	n.a.
Loganberries, frozen, ½ cup	9.6	3.6
Long beans, see "Yardlong beans"		
Long John Silver's:		
fish and seafood:		
cod, baked, 1 piece	1.0	0
clams, breaded, 3 oz.	22.0	1.0
fish, battered, 1 piece	17.0	<1.0
shrimp, battered, 1 piece	3.0	0
shrimp, crunchy, basket, 21 pieces	4.0	2.0
shrimp, giant, 1 piece	5.0	0
Chicken Plank, 1 piece	9.0	<1.0
dipping sauce, cocktail, 1 oz.	6.0	0
dipping sauce, tartar, 1 oz.	4.0	0
sandwich, chicken	41.0	3.0
sandwich, fish or *Ultimate Fish*	48.0	3.0
salad, chicken club, without dressing	35.0	5.0
salad, shrimp and seafood, without dressing	22.0	4.0
salad dressing, 1 pkt.:		
French, fat free	12.0	<1.0
Italian, lite	3.0	0
ranch, garden	2.0	0
Thousand Island	7.0	0
sides/starters:		
clam chowder, bowl	23.0	0
coleslaw, 4 oz.	15.0	3.0
cheese sticks, 3 pieces	12.0	1.0
corn cobbette, 1 piece	14.0	3.0
Crumblies, 1 oz.	14.0	1.0

Food and Measure	carb. (gms)	fiber (gms)
fries, large	56.0	5.0
fries, regular	34.0	3.0
hush puppies, 1 piece	9.0	1.0
lobster stuffed crab cake, 1 piece	16.0	1.0
rice, 4 oz.	34.0	3.0
dessert pie:		
chocolate cream	24.0	1.0
pecan	55.0	2.0
pineapple cream	39.0	1.0
Longan, fresh, seeded, 1 oz.	4.3	.3
Longan, dried, 1 oz.	21.0	<1.0
Loquat:		
(*Frieda's*), 5 oz.	17.0	2.0
1 large, .7 oz.	2.4	.3
cubed, 1 cup	18.1	2.5
peeled, seeded, 1 oz.	3.4	.5
Lotus root:		
raw:		
(*Frieda's*), 1 cup, 3 oz.	15.0	4.0
10 slices	14.0	4.0
trimmed, 1 oz.	4.9	1.4
boiled, drained, ½ cup	9.6	1.9
Lotus root, sun-dried (*Eden*), .4 oz.	8.0	2.0
Lotus seeds:		
raw, 1 oz.	4.9	n.a.
dried, 1 oz.	18.3	n.a.
fried, 1 cup	20.6	n.a.
Lox, see "Salmon, smoked"		
Lunch meat, loaf (see also specific listings), 2 oz., except as noted:		
(*Hatfield Deli Choice* Original)	4.0	0
barbecue (*Deli Delight*)	6.0	0
deluxe (*Deli Delight*)	7.0	0
Dutch brand:		
(*Boar's Head*)	2.0	0
(*Deli Delight*)	4.0	0
pepper (*Hatfield Deli Choice*)	3.0	0
Italian (*Deli Delight*)	5.0	0

Food and Measure	carb. (gms)	fiber (gms)
jalapeño (*Hansel 'n Gretel*)	6.0	0
macaroni and cheese (*Hansel 'n Gretel*)	8.0	0
olive:		
(*Boar's Head*)	<1.0	0
(*Hansel 'n Gretel*)	7.0	0
(*Hatfield Deli Choice*)	6.0	0
(*Oscar Mayer*), 1 oz.	2.0	0
(*Tyson* Bag), .9-oz. slice	3.0	0
pepper (*Deli Delight*)	5.0	0
pickle (*Deli Delight*)	7.0	0
pickle (*Tyson* Bag), .9-oz. slice	5.0	0
pickle and pepper (*Boar's Head*)	2.0	0
pickle and pimento (*Hatfield Deli Choice*)	2.0	0
pickle and pimento (*Oscar Mayer*), 1 oz.	2.0	0
spiced (*Hansel 'n Gretel*)	6.0	0
spiced (*Oscar Mayer* Luncheon), 1 oz.	2.0	0
spiced ham (*Boar's Head*)	1.0	0
spiced ham (*Hormel*)	1.0	0
Lunch meat, canned, 2 oz.:		
(*Spam* Classic/Less Salt/Lite)	1.0	0
barbecue (*Spam*)	4.0	0
with cheese (*Spam*)	2.0	0
garlic (*Spam*)	1.0	0
hot and spicy, smoked, or turkey (*Spam*)	2.0	0
Lunch "meat," vegetarian, frozen (*Worthington Wham*), 3 slices, 2 oz.	3.0	0
Lupin, boiled, ½ cup	8.2	2.3
Lychee, fresh:		
(*Frieda's*), 6–8 pieces, 3.5 oz.	14.0	1.0
1 fruit, .3 oz.	1.6	.1
shelled, 1 cup	31.4	2.5
shelled, 1 oz.	4.7	.4
Lychee, dried, 10 fruits, .7 oz.	17.7	1.2
Lychee juice (*Ceres*), 8 fl. oz.	30.0	0

M

Food and Measure	carb. (gms)	fiber (gms)
Macadamia nuts:		
(*Planters*), 1 oz.	4.0	3.0
raw, whole or halves:		
(*Tree of Life*), ¼ cup	5.0	2.0
1 oz.	3.9	2.4
¼ cup	4.6	2.9
chopped (*Planters*), 2-oz. pkg.	8.0	5.0
dried, shelled, 1 oz.	3.9	2.6
dried, shelled, ¼ cup	4.6	3.1
dry-roasted:		
(*Mauna Loa/Mauna Loa* Unsalted), 1 oz.	4.0	2.0
1 oz.	3.8	2.3
whole or halves, ¼ cup	4.5	2.7
oil-roasted, 1 oz.	3.7	n.a.
Macadamia nuts, flavored (see also "Candy"), 1 oz.:		
coated (*Beer Nuts*)	24.0	1.0
coffee glazed (*Mauna Loa* Kona)	10.0	1.0
honey roasted (*Mauna Loa*)	6.0	2.0
onion garlic (*Mauna Loa*)	4.0	2.0
Macaroni (see also "Pasta"):		
uncooked:		
2 oz.	42.4	1.4
elbow, 1 cup	78.4	2.5
enriched, 2 oz.	38.3	1.4
whole wheat, 2 oz.	42.8	4.7
cooked, 1 cup:		
enriched, elbows	39.7	1.8
enriched, spirals	38.0	1.7
small shells	32.6	1.8

Food and Measure	carb. (gms)	fiber (gms)
vegetable, enriched, spirals	35.7	5.8
whole wheat, elbows	37.2	3.9
Macaroni entree, can or pkg., 1 cup, except as noted:		
and beef (*Kid's Kitchen* Beefy Macaroni)	24.0	2.0
and beef (*Kid's Kitchen* Cheezy)	34.0	1.0
and cheese:		
(*Bowl Appétit!*), 1 cont.	56.0	1.0
(*Kid's Kitchen* Cheezy)	32.0	1.0
(*Hormel*), 7.5-oz. can	32.0	1.0
with ham (*Hormel Cure 81* Bowl), 10 oz.	32.0	1.0
and franks (*Kid's Kitchen* Cheezy)	26.0	1.0
Macaroni entree, freeze-dried, and cheese:		
(*Mountain House* Can), 1 cup	33.0	<1.0
(*Mountain House* Double), ½ pouch	45.0	1.0
with beef (*Mountain House* Double), 1 cup	32.0	3.0
with veggies (*AlpineAire* Forever Young), 1 serving	55.0	2.0
Macaroni entree, frozen, 1 pkg., except as noted:		
and beef:		
(*Lean Cuisine Everyday Favorites*), 9.5 oz.	39.0	3.0
(*Michelina's* Zap'ems), 8 oz.	36.0	2.0
(*Stouffer's*), 11.5 oz.	39.0	4.0
and cheese:		
(*Amy's*), 9 oz.	47.0	3.0
(*Amy's* Large Size), 8 oz.	41.0	3.0
(*Glory* Savory Singles), 11 oz.	47.0	1.0
(*Glory* Savory Singles Family Size), 1 cup	38.0	<1.0
(*Healthy Choice*), 9 oz.	40.0	3.0
(*Lean Cuisine Everyday Favorites*), 10 oz.	43.0	1.0
(*Linda McCartney*), 10 oz.	32.0	3.0
(*Michelina's* Authentico/Zap'ems), 8 oz.	41.0	2.0
(*Michelina's Lean Gourmet*), 10 oz.	51.0	3.0
(*Smart Ones*), 10 oz.	45.0	3.0
(*Stouffer's*), ½ of 12-oz. pkg.	32.0	2.0
(*Stouffer's* Family Style Recipes), ⅕ of 40-oz. pkg. ...	37.0	2.0
(*Stouffer's* Family Style Recipes), ⅑ of 76-oz. pkg. ...	38.0	2.0
(*Stouffer's Maxaroni*), 9 oz.	36.0	2.0
with broccoli (*Stouffer's*), 10.5 oz.	39.0	4.0
cheddar, sharp (*Michelina's* Authentico), 10 oz.	50.0	3.0

Food and Measure	carb. (gms)	fiber (gms)
with dessert (*Ian's* Natural Kids Meal), 9 oz.	118.0	3.0
with ham (*Michelina's* Authentico), 8 oz.	34.0	2.0
with rice pasta (*Amy's* Rice Mac & Cheese), 9 oz.	47.0	3.0
and cheese, three (*Moosewood*), 10 oz.	44.0	1.0
and cheese, three (*Smart Ones*), 9 oz.	45.0	2.0
and chili, see "Chili entree"		
and meat sauce (*Organic Classics*), 10 oz.	49.0	3.0
vegetarian, soy cheese (*Amy's*), 9 oz.	42.0	4.0
vegetarian, soy cheese (*Yves* The Good Bowl), 10.5 oz. ..	52.0	3.0
Macaroni entree mix (see also "Shells, pasta, mix"):		
Alfredo, cheesy (*Kraft*), ⅓ of 7.25-oz. pkg.	44.0	2.0
Alfredo, nondairy (*Road's End Organics Mac & Chreese*),		
½ cup mix	50.0	6.0
and cheddar:		
(*Kraft* Deluxe), ¼ of 14-oz. pkg.	44.0	2.0
(*Kraft* Deluxe 2% Milk), ¼ of 14-oz. pkg.	49.0	1.0
sharp (*Kraft* Deluxe), ¼ of 14-oz. pkg.	45.0	1.0
white (*Kraft*), 2 oz.	48.0	2.0
and cheese:		
(*Annie's* Mac & Cheese Single Serve), ¾ cup*	40.0	<1.0
(*DeBoles* Homestyle), ⅓ pkg.	53.0	5.0
(*Kraft* The Cheesiest), 2 oz.	47.0	1.0
(*Kraft* Deluxe Family Size), 3.5 oz.	44.0	2.0
(*Kraft* Thick 'n Creamy), 2 oz.	48.0	2.0
3 cheese (*Kraft*), 2 oz.	48.0	2.0
4 cheese (*Annie's* Creamy Deluxe), 1 cup*	45.0	2.0
4 cheese (*Kraft* Deluxe), ¼ of 14-oz. pkg.	44.0	1.0
rice pasta (*DeBoles*), ¼ pkg.	19.0	0
whole wheat pasta (*DeBoles* Organic), ⅓ pkg.	47.0	8.0
whole wheat pasta (*Hodgson Mill*), 2 oz.	45.0	6.0
and "cheese," nondairy, whole wheat pasta (*Road's End*		
Organics Mac & Chreese), ½ cup	42.0	5.0
Macaroni and cheese, see "Macaroni dish" and		
"Macaroni entree"		
Macaroni salad, refrigerated:		
(*Blue Ridge Farm*), 4 oz. ....,	25.0	1.0
(*Hellmann's* Classic), 4.9 oz.	59.0	3.0
(*Reser's*), ¾ cup	28.0	2.0

Food and Measure	carb. (gms)	fiber (gms)
Mace, ground, 1 tsp.	.9	.1
Mackerel, fresh, canned, or smoked, without added ingredients	0	0
Mahi mahi, see "Dolphin fish"		
Mai Tai drink mixer (*Trader Vic's*), 4 fl. oz.	32.0	0
Malanga, fresh:		
(*Frieda's*), ⅔ cup, 3 oz.	23.0	2.0
sliced, ½ cup	16.0	1.0
Malt cooler (*Bartles & Jaymes*), 12 fl. oz.:		
berry, exotic	33.0	0
blackberry, luscious	39.0	0
blue Hawaiian	28.0	0
cherry, black	32.0	0
classic original	29.0	0
fuzzy navel, kiwi strawberry, or hard lemonade	39.0	0
margarita	46.0	0
melon splash or orange sunset	38.0	0
peach, juicy	33.0	0
piña colada	48.0	0
raspberry or strawberry daiquiri	36.0	0
strawberry cosmopolitan or tropical burst	37.0	0
Malt syrup, see "Barley malt syrup"		
Malted milk powder:		
natural (*Carnation*), 3 tbsp.	15.0	<1.0
chocolate (*Carnation*), 3 tbsp.	18.0	<1.0
Mammy apple:		
½ of 25-oz. fruit	52.9	12.7
peeled, seeded, 1 oz.	3.5	.9
Mandarin orange, see "Tangerine"		
Mango, fresh:		
(*Dole*), ½ medium	17.0	1.0
(*Del Monte*), ½ medium, 4.9 oz.	17.0	1.0
10.6-oz. fruit, 7.3 oz. trimmed	35.2	3.7
sliced, 1 cup	28.1	3.0
Mango, in jars:		
in light syrup (*Del Monte Sunfresh*), ½ cup	19.0	<1.0
in syrup, sliced (*Herdez*), 2 pieces	30.0	5.0

Food and Measure	carb. (gms)	fiber (gms)
Mango, dried:		
(*Sunsweet*), ⅓ cup, 1.4 oz.	34.0	1.0
slices, unsweetened (*SunRidge Farms* Organic),		
3 pieces, 1.4 oz.	11.0	<1.0
slices, unsweetened (*Tree of Life*), 1.4 oz.	7.0	1.0
spears (*SunRidge Farms*), 4 pieces, 1.4 oz.	34.0	1.0
Mango, frozen, chunks:		
(*Contessa*), 1 cup	21.0	2.0
(*C&W*), 1 cup	21.0	2.0
Mango drink, 8 fl. oz., except as noted:		
(*AriZona* Mucho Mango)	27.0	0
(*Langers* Mongo)	30.0	0
(*Snapple* Mango Madness)	29.0	0
nectar (*Goya*), 12 fl. oz.	56.0	2.0
nectar (*Walnut Acres*)	29.0	0
Mango drink blend, 8 fl. oz.:		
melon (*SoBe* Nirvana)	31.0	0
orange (*Langers*)	33.0	0
peach (*R.W. Knudsen*)	30.0	0
peach (*V8 Splash*)	27.0	0
Mango juice, 8 fl. oz.:		
(*After the Fall* Montage)	37.0	0
(*Ceres*)	30.0	1.0
Mango nectar, see "Mango drink"		
Mango relish (see also "Chutney"), Indian:		
hot (*Patak's*), 1 tbsp.	1.5	1.0
mild (*Patak's*), 1 tbsp.	1.0	0
Mangosteen, canned, in syrup, ½ cup	6.7	1.8
Manhattan drink mixer (*Holland House*),		
4 fl. oz.	29.0	0
Manicotti entree, frozen, cheese, 1 pkg.:		
(*Michelina's Lean Gourmet*), 8.5 oz.	48.0	3.0
three cheese (*Healthy Choice*), 11 oz.	46.0	3.0
three cheese (*Stouffer's*), 9 oz.	41.0	2.0
Manioc, see "Yuca"		
Maple syrup, pure, ¼ cup:		
(*Cary's/MacDonald's/Maple Orchard's*)	52.0	0

Food and Measure	carb. (gms)	fiber (gms)
(*Great Expectations*)	53.0	0
(*Tree of Life*)	53.0	0
Margarine, regular, all varieties and blends, 2 tbsp.	0	0
Margarine, flavored, spread, 1 tbsp.		
cinnamon (*Shedd's Country Crock*)	3.0	0
strawberry (*Shedd's Country Crock*)	2.0	0
Margarita drink mixer (see also "Daiquiri/Margarita drink mixer"):		
(*Angostura*), 4 fl. oz.	25.0	0
(*Bacardi*), 3.2 fl. oz.	35.0	0
(*D.L. Jardine's* Texarita), 3.5 fl. oz.	30.0	0
frozen (*Bacardi*), 2 fl. oz.	25.0	0
strawberry (*Trader Vic's*), 4 fl. oz.	40.0	0
Marinade (see also "Grilling sauce" and specific listings), 1 tbsp., except as noted:		
(*A.1.* Chicago)	2.0	0
(*A.1.* New York Steakhouse)	5.0	0
(*Annie's Naturals* Organic Paradise), 2 tbsp.	5.0	0
(*Badias* Mojo)	2.5	0
(*Neera's* Kashmiri), 1 tsp.	5.0	0
(*TryMe Dragon Sauce*), 1 tsp.	1.0	0
Cajun:		
(*A.1.* New Orleans)	5.0	0
(*Golden Dipt*)	2.0	0
(*Litehouse*), 2 tbsp.	7.0	0
cherry soy (*World Harbors* Cheriyaki), 2 tbsp.	14.0	0
chimichurri (*World Harbors*), 2 tbsp.	9.0	0
chipotle (*Lawry's* Baja)	4.0	0
citrus (*Lawry's* Citrus Grill)	3.0	0
fajita:		
(*D.L. Jardine's*)	1.0	0
(*Litehouse*), 2 tbsp.	3.0	0
(*S&W* Southwest)	2.0	1.0
(*World Harbors*), 2 tbsp.	10.0	0
medium (*Zapata*)	<1.0	0
garlic herb (*Golden Dipt*)	1.0	0
garlic and lime (*Lawry's*)	2.0	0
ginger, spicy (*Annie's Naturals* Organic), 2 tbsp.	3.0	0

Food and Measure	carb. (gms)	fiber (gms)
ginger, Thai (*Lawry's*)	2.0	0
Hawaiian (*Lawry's*)	5.0	0
herb and garlic (*Lawry's*)	2.0	0
honey mustard:		
(*Golden Dipt*)	4.0	0
Dijon (*Lawry's*)	4.0	0
Dijon (*Litehouse*), 2 tbsp.	6.0	0
honey soy (*Golden Dipt*)	7.0	0
jerk:		
(*Lawry's* Caribbean)	5.0	0
(*Litehouse* Jamaican), 2 tbsp.	1.0	1.0
(*World Harbors*), 2 tbsp.	18.0	0
lemon grass (*Thai Kitchen* Splash)	<1.0	0
lemon grass, herb (*Annie Chun's*)	4.0	0
lemon herb (*Golden Dipt*)	0	0
lemon pepper:		
(*Golden Dipt*)	1.0	0
(*Lawry's*)	2.0	0
and garlic (*World Harbors*), 2 tbsp.	8.0	0
mango (*World Harbors* Island), 2 tbsp.	14.0	0
mesquite:		
(*Golden Dipt*)	1.0	0
(*Lawry's*)	1.0	0
(*S&W*)	3.0	0
grill (*Litehouse*), 2 tbsp.	4.0	0
mojo (*World Harbors*), 2 tbsp.	5.0	0
pepper, red (*Lawry's* Louisiana)	2.0	0
sesame, toasted (*Quick & Easy Marinade*)	7.0	0
sesame ginger (*Lawry's*)	7.0	0
sesame ginger (*World Harbors* Mandarin)	16.0	0
smoky (*Annie's Naturals* Organic Campfire), 2 tbsp.	1.0	0
tequila lime (*Lawry's*)	4.0	0
teriyaki:		
(*A.1.* Steakhouse)	5.0	0
(*Angostura*)	4.0	0
(*Angostura* All Natural)	1.0	0
(*Annie's Naturals* Organic)	6.0	0
(*Kikkoman*)	2.0	0

Food and Measure	carb. (gms)	fiber (gms)
(*Kikkoman* Lite)	3.0	0
(*Kikkoman Quick & Easy Marinade* Gourmet)	7.0	0
(*Lawry's*)	5.0	0
(*Litehouse* Marinade & Sauce), 2 tbsp.	6.0	0
(*S&W/S&W* Lite)	5.0	0
(*World Harbors*), 2 tbsp.	14.0	0
ginger (*Golden Dipt*)	5.0	0
hickory (*Ducks Unlimited*)	3.0	0
honey (*Ducks Unlimited*)	6.0	0
honey mustard (*Kikkoman Quick & Easy Marinade*)	7.0	0
hot (*World Harbors*), 2 tbsp.	17.0	0
roasted garlic (*Kikkoman*)	5.0	0
roasted garlic herb (*Kikkoman Quick & Easy Marinade*)	4.0	0
white wine (*Golden Dipt*)	1.0	0
Marinade seasoning mix, ¾ tsp.:		
(*Adolph's Marinade in Minutes*)	1.0	0
beef, tenderizing (*Lawry's*)	<1.0	0
Marionberry, see "Blackberry, dried"		
Marjoram, dried, 1 tsp.	.4	.1
Marmalade, see "Jam and preserves"		
Marrow squash, raw, trimmed, 1 oz.	1.0	<1.0
Marshmallow topping, 2 tbsp.:		
(*Smucker's*)	29.0	0
plain, raspberry, or strawberry (*Marshmallow Fluff*)	15.0	0
Masa, see "Cornmeal"		
Matai, see "Water chestnut"		
Matzo, see "Cracker"		
Matzo ball, in jars:		
(*Manischewitz*), 1 cup	27.0	3.0
(*Mrs. Adler's*), 1 cup, 3 pieces with liquid	24.0	1.0
Matzo ball mix, dry (*Manischewitz*), 1½ tbsp.	9.0	<1.0
Matzo meal, see "Cracker crumbs/meal"		
Mayonnaise, 1 tbsp.:		
(*Blue Plate*)	0	0
(*Cains*)	0	0
(*Cains* Fat Free/Reduced Fat)	3.0	0
(*Cains* Light)	2.0	0
(*Hain*)	0	0

Food and Measure	carb. (gms)	fiber (gms)
(*Hain* Lite)	2.0	0
(*Hellmann's/Best Foods*)	0	0
(*Hellmann's/Best Foods* Light)	1.0	0
(*Henri's*)	0	0
(*Hollywood* Canola)	0	0
(*Kraft*)	0	0
(*Kraft* Light)	2.0	0
(*Smart Balance Light*)	2.0	0
(*Smart Beat* Fat Free)	3.0	0
(*Vegenaise*)	1.0	0
bacon and tomato (*Hellmann's*)	1.0	0
chipotle, chili, or smoky (*French's GourMayo*)	1.0	0
dressing:		
(*Kraft* Fat Free)	2.0	0
(*Miracle Whip*)	2.0	0
(*Miracle Whip* Fat Free/Light)	3.0	0
hot and spicy (*Miracle Whip*)	2.0	0
fresh, refrigerated (*Delouis Fils/Delouis Fils* Aioli)	0	0
hot and spicy (*Kraft*)	0	0
sun-dried tomato (*French's GourMayo*)	2.0	0
spicy, smoked jalapeño (*Fiesta*)	12.0	0
wasabi horseradish (*French's GourMayo*)	2.0	0
Mayonnaise dressing, see "Mayonnaise"		
McDonald's, 1 serving:		
breakfast:		
Big Breakfast	53.0	3.0
biscuit, plain	31.0	1.0
biscuit, bacon or sausage, egg, and cheese	36.0	1.0
biscuit, sausage	34.0	1.0
burrito, sausage	26.0	1.0
cinnamon roll	57.0	2.0
cinnamon roll deluxe	86.0	4.0
deluxe breakfast	136.0	4.0
eggs, scrambled, 2	5.0	0
hash browns	15.0	2.0
hotcakes, with sausage	104.0	2.0
hotcakes, with syrup and margarine	102.0	2.0
jam or preserves	9.0	0

Food and Measure	carb. (gms)	fiber (gms)
McGriddles, bacon, egg, and cheese	46.0	1.0
McGriddles, sausage	44.0	1.0
McGriddles, sausage, egg, and cheese	48.0	1.0
McMuffin, egg	30.0	2.0
McMuffin, sausage	31.0	2.0
McMuffin, sausage and egg	39.0	2.0
muffin, English	27.0	2.0
sausage patty	2.0	0
sandwiches:		
Big Mac	46.0	3.0
Big N' Tasty	41.0	3.0
Big N' Tasty, with cheese	43.0	3.0
cheeseburger	35.0	1.0
cheeseburger, double	37.0	1.0
chicken, crispy	50.0	3.0
Chicken McGrill	38.0	3.0
Filet-O-Fish	42.0	1.0
hamburger	33.0	1.0
McChicken	41.0	1.0
McChicken, hot and spicy	42.0	1.0
Quarter Pounder	40.0	3.0
Quarter Pounder, with cheese	43.0	3.0
Quarter Pounder, with cheese, double	46.0	3.0
Chicken McNuggets:		
4 pieces	10.0	0
6 pieces	15.0	0
10 pieces	26.0	0
20 pieces	51.0	0
Chicken McNuggets sauce:		
barbecue	11.0	0
honey	12.0	0
hot mustard	9.0	1.0
sweet 'n sour	11.0	0
Chicken Selects, breast:		
3 pieces	28.0	0
5 pieces	46.0	0
10 pieces	92.0	0

Food and Measure	carb. (gms)	fiber (gms)
Chicken Selects sauce:		
barbecue, chipotle	16.0	0
Buffalo, spicy	1.0	<.10
honey mustard	13.0	1.0
ranch, creamy	3.0	0
fries:		
large	70.0	7.0
medium	47.0	5.0
small	30.0	3.0
ketchup, pkt.	3.0	0
salad, without dressing:		
bacon ranch	9.0	3.0
bacon ranch, with crispy chicken	23.0	3.0
bacon ranch, with grilled chicken	12.0	3.0
Caesar or Cobb	8.0	3.0
Caesar or Cobb, with crispy chicken	23.0	3.0
Caesar or Cobb, with grilled chicken	11.0	3.0
side salad	3.0	1.0
butter garlic croutons	10.0	<1.0
salad dressing (*Newman's Own*), 2 fl. oz.:		
balsamic vinaigrette or creamy Caesar	4.0	0
Cobb or ranch	9.0	0
dessert/shakes:		
apple dippers, plain	8.0	0
apple dippers, with caramel dip	22.0	0
apple pie	39.0	2.0
caramel dip	14.0	0
cone, vanilla, reduced fat	24.0	0
cookies:		
chocolate chip	22.0	<1.0
McDonaldland	42.0	<1.0
McDonaldland chocolate chip	39.0	1.0
oatmeal raisin	22.0	1.0
sugar	22.0	0
fruit 'n yogurt parfait	31.0	<1.0
fruit 'n yogurt parfait, without granola	25.0	0
McFlurry, M&M's, 12 fl. oz.	96.0	<1.0

Food and Measure	carb. (gms)	fiber (gms)
McFlurry, Oreo, 12 fl. oz.	88.0	0
sundaes:		
hot caramel	62.0	0
hot fudge	55.0	1.0
strawberry	51.0	0
sundae peanuts	2.0	1.0
Triple Thick shake:		
chocolate, 12 oz.	76.0	1.0
chocolate, 16 oz.	102.0	1.0
chocolate, 21 oz.	134.0	1.0
chocolate, 32 oz.	203.0	2.0
strawberry, 12 oz.	73.0	0
strawberry, 16 oz.	97.0	0
strawberry, 21 oz.	128.0	0
strawberry, 32 oz.	194.0	0
vanilla, 12 oz.	72.0	0
vanilla, 16 oz.	96.0	0
vanilla, 21 oz.	128.0	0
vanilla, 32 oz.	193.0	0
Meat, potted, see "Meat spread"		
Meat loaf, refrigerated:		
(*Hormel*), 5 oz.	13.0	2.0
seasoned (*Tyson*), 5 oz.	16.0	0
Meat loaf dinner, frozen, 1 pkg.:		
(*Healthy Choice*), 12 oz.	36.0	6.0
(*Stouffer's* Homestyle), 17 oz.	46.0	6.0
(*Swanson Hungry-Man*), 16.5 oz.	87.0	6.0
"Meat" loaf dinner, vegetarian, frozen (*Amy's* Veggie Loaf Meal), 10-oz. pkg.	47.0	7.0
Meat loaf entree, frozen, 1 pkg., except as noted:		
(*Michelina's Lean Gourmet*), 8 oz.	22.0	2.0
(*Stouffer's* Homestyle), 9⅞ oz.	23.0	2.0
and gravy:		
(*Stouffer's* Family Style Recipes), ⅙ of 33-oz. pkg.	10.0	1.0
with mashed potato (*Michelina's* Authentico), 8 oz.	20.0	2.0
with vegetable medley (*Organic Classics*), 9.5 oz.	19.0	4.0
with mashed potato (*Boston Market*), 12 oz.	38.0	3.0

Food and Measure	carb. (gms)	fiber (gms)
with mashed potato (*Smart Ones Bistro Selections*), 9.5 oz.	22.0	5.0
with potato and green beans (*Swanson* Angus), 11 oz.	30.0	4.0
and whipped potato (*Lean Cuisine* Cafe Classics), 9⅜ oz.	29.0	3.0
"Meat" loaf entree, vegetarian, frozen:		
(*Amy's* Veggie Loaf Family Size), ¼ of 23-oz. pkg.	32.0	6.0
(*Hain Vegetarian Classics* Homestyle), 10-oz. pkg.	39.0	16.0
Meat loaf seasoning mix, dry:		
(*Adolph's Meal Makers*), 1 tbsp.	5.0	0
(*Lawry's*), 1 tbsp.	7.0	<1.0
(*McCormick*), 1 tsp.	2.0	0
(*McCormick Bag 'n Season*), 2 tsp.	2.0	0
(*Mrs. Cubbison's*), 1 tbsp.	4.0	0
Meat marinade mix (*McCormick*), 1 tsp.	2.0	0
Meat spread (see also specific listings):		
(*Oscar Mayer* Sandwich Spread), 2 oz.	9.0	0
(*Spam* Spread), 4 tbsp.	1.0	0
with crackers (*Spam* Spread), 1 kit	14.0	1.0
potted meat (*Goya*), ¼ cup	0	0
potted meat (*Hormel*), 4 tbsp.	0	0
Meat tenderizer:		
(*Adolph's* Original/Seasoned), ¼ tsp.	0	0
(*McCormick*/Original/Seasoned), ¼ tsp.	0	0
(*Tone's*), 1 tsp.	1.2	tr.
(*Watkins* Meat Magic), 1 tsp.	1.0	0
Meatball, frozen:		
(*Ian's* Natural Italian), 3 pieces, 3 oz.	10.0	1.0
(*Mama Lucia*), 4 pieces, 3.2 oz.	8.0	0
(*On the Go Bistro* Gourmet), 2 pieces, 3 oz.	6.0	0
(*Organic Classics*), 3 pieces, 3 oz.	5.0	1.0
(*Prima Familia*), 4 pieces, 3.2 oz.	6.0	<1.0
"Meatball," vegetarian, frozen (*Quorn*), 4 pieces, 2.4 oz.	7.0	1.0
Meatball entree, canned, stew (*Dinty Moore*), 1 cup	19.0	1.0
Meatball entree, frozen, 1 pkg.:		
and mashed potato (*Michelina's* Authentico), 8.5 oz.	26.0	3.0
pasta and, see "Penne entree" and "Spaghetti entree"		
Swedish:		
(*Lean Cuisine Everyday Favorites*), 9⅛ oz.	33.0	2.0

Food and Measure	carb. (gms)	fiber (gms)
(*Michelina's Lean Gourmet*), 9 oz.	40.0	3.0
(*Smart Ones*), 9 oz.	34.0	3.0
(*Stouffer's*), 11.5 oz.	39.0	2.0
with gravy, pasta (*Michelina's* Authentico), 10 oz.	41.0	3.0
Meatball pocket, frozen, 4.5-oz. piece:		
cheese, three (*Smart Ones Smartwich*)	39.0	2.0
and mozzarella:		
(*Croissant Pockets*)	45.0	3.0
(*Hot Pockets*)	39.0	2.0
(*Lean Pockets*)	44.0	3.0
(*Lean Pockets* Ultra)	19.0	7.0
Meatball seasoning and sauce mix, Swedish		
(*McCormick*), 2 tsp. seasoning, 1 tsp. sauce mix	4.0	0
Melba sauce (*Roland*), 2 tbsp.	25.0	0
Melogold (*Frieda's*), ½ fruit, 5.9 oz.	13.0	2.0
Melon, see specific melon listings		
Melon balls, frozen, cantaloupe and honeydew, ½ cup	6.9	6
Melon drink, see "Watermelon drink"		
Mesclun, see "Salad blend"		
Mexican beans, see "Pinto beans" and specific listings		
Mexican seasoning mix (*Chi-Chi's* Fiesta Restaurante),		
1 tsp.	2.0	0
Mexican squash (*Frieda's*), ½ cup, 3 oz.	9.0	2.0
Mexican entree, frozen, casserole (*Amy's* Bowls),		
9.5-oz. pkg.	70.0	7.0
Mexican sauce (see also specific listings), cooking:		
cilantro lime (*Pace Mexican Creations*), 1 cup	17.0	7.0
onion and garlic, roasted (*Pace Mexican Creations*), 1 cup	15.0	1.0
roasted ranchero (*Pace Mexican Creations*), ¼ cup	6.0	1.0
verde (*Pace Mexican Creations*), 1 cup	14.0	3.0
Mexican snack rolls, frozen (*Health is Wealth Munchees*),		
6 pieces, 3 oz.	32.0	3.0
Milk, 8 fl. oz.:		
buttermilk:		
(*Darigold* Lowfat)	13.0	0
(*Organic Valley* Lowfat)	12.0	0
cultured	11.7	0

Food and Measure	carb. (gms)	fiber (gms)
whole:		
(*Cool Moos*)	12.0	0
(*Darigold*)	12.0	0
(*Organic Valley*)	12.0	0
3.3% fat	11.4	0
reduced fat (2%):		
(*Cool Moos*)	12.0	0
(*Darigold*)	13.0	0
(*Darigold* White)	14.0	0
(*Organic Valley*)	12.0	0
2% fat	11.7	0
2%, protein fortified	13.5	0
low fat (1%):		
(*Cool Moos*)	12.0	0
(*Darigold/Darigold* Acidophilus/Calcium Extra)	13.0	0
(*Organic Valley*)	13.0	0
(*Organic Valley* Lactose Free)	12.0	0
(*Simply Smart*)	13.0	0
1% fat	11.7	0
1%, protein fortified	13.6	0
skim/fat free:		
(*Darigold*)	13.0	0
(*Darigold* Acidophilus/Trim Deluxe)	14.0	0
(*Organic Valley*)	13.0	0
(*Simply Smart*)	13.0	0
8 fl. oz.	11.9	0
Milk, canned, 2 tbsp.:		
condensed, sweetened:		
(*Carnation*)	22.0	0
(*Eagle Brand/Eagle Brand* Lowfat)	23.0	0
(*Eagle Brand* Fat Free)	24.0	0
evaporated:		
(*Carnation/Carnation* Lowfat)	3.0	0
(*Carnation* Fat Free)	4.0	0
(*Pet*)	3.0	0
skim (*Pet*)	4.0	0
Milk, chocolate, see "Milk, flavored"		

Food and Measure	carb. (gms)	fiber (gms)
Milk, dry:		
buttermilk, sweet cream, 1 cup	58.8	0
buttermilk, sweet cream, 1 tbsp.	3.2	0
buttermilk blend (*Organic Valley*), 3 tbsp.	16.0	0
whole, 1 oz.	10.9	0
whole, 1 cup	49.2	0
nonfat:		
(*Organic Valley*), 3 tbsp.	13.0	0
regular, 1 cup	62.4	0
instant, 3.2-oz. pkt.	35.5	0
Milk, flavored, 8 fl. oz.:		
banana, reduced fat (*Nesquik*)	30.0	0
chocolate:		
(*Hershey's* Creamy MilkShake)	43.0	1.0
whole or reduced fat (*Darigold* Extra/Smooth)	33.0	<1.0
reduced fat (*Hershey's*)	31.0	1.0
reduced fat (*Nesquik*)	32.0	<1.0
reduced fat (*Nesquik* Milkshake)	26.0	<1.0
reduced fat (*Organic Valley*)	23.0	<1.0
reduced fat (*Organic Valley* Ultra)	33.0	2.0
low fat (*Cool Moos*)	32.0	0
low fat (*Hershey's* No Sugar)	15.0	1.0
nonfat (*Nesquik*)	32.0	<1.0
chocolate, double, reduced fat (*Nesquik*)	30.0	<1.0
chocolate mint (*Hershey's York* MilkShake)	52.0	<1.0
coffee, low fat (*Hood*)	28.0	0
cookies and cream (*Hershey's* MilkShake)	45.0	0
mocha, reduced fat (*Nesquik*)	32.0	0
strawberry:		
(*Hershey's* MilkShake)	44.0	0
reduced fat (*Darigold*)	33.0	0
reduced fat (*Hershey's*)	30.0	0
reduced fat (*Nesquik*)	33.0	0
reduced fat (*Nesquik* Milkshake)	25.0	<1.0
low fat (*Cool Moos*)	27.0	0
low fat (*Organic Valley*)	30.0	3.0
vanilla:		
(*Darigold*)	33.0	0

Food and Measure	carb. (gms)	fiber (gms)
(*Hershey's* MilkShake)	55.0	0
reduced fat (*Nesquik* Very)	30.0	0
low fat (*Cool Moos*)	26.0	0
low fat (*Organic Valley*)	28.0	2.0
Milk, goat, 8 fl. oz.:		
(*Meyenberg*)	11.0	0
fresh	10.9	0
"Milk," nondairy, see "Rice beverage" and "Soy beverage"		
Milk, human, 8 fl. oz.	16.9	0
Milk, sheep, 8 fl. oz.	13.1	0
Milkfish, without added ingredients	0	0
Millet:		
dry (*Shiloh Farms*), ¼ cup	34.0	3.0
dry, 1 oz.	20.7	2.4
cooked, 4 oz.	26.8	1.5
Millet flour (*Arrowhead Mills*), ⅓ cup	26.0	3.0
Mincemeat, see "Pie filling"		
Mint, fresh:		
peppermint, 2 tbsp.	.5	<.1
spearmint, 2 tbsp.	.9	.7
Mint, dried, spearmint, 1 tbsp.	.8	.5
Mint sauce (*Crosse & Blackwell*), 1 tsp.	1.0	0
Mirin rice wine, see "Wine, cooking"		
Miso, soy paste:		
(*Eden* Organic Hacho), 1 tbsp.	2.0	1.0
(*Eden* Organic Shiro), 1 tbsp.	5.0	1.0
(*Westbrae Natural* Bag), 1 tsp.	0	0
1 oz.	7.9	1.5
½ cup	38.6	7.6
with barley (*Westbrae Natural* Bag), 1 tsp.	2.0	0
with brown rice:		
(*Eden* Organic Genmai), 1 tbsp.	3.0	1.0
(*Westbrae Natural* Bag), 1 tsp.	<1.0	0
(*Westbrae Natural* Organic Mellow), 1 tsp.	2.0	<1.0
red or white (*Westbrae Natural* Organic Mellow), 1 tsp.	2.0	<1.0
with soybean and barley (*Eden* Organic Mugi), 1 tbsp.	3.0	1.0
Miso condiment, see "Tekka"		
Mocha drink (*Yoo-hoo* Dyna-Mocha), 8 fl. oz.	34.0	1.0

Food and Measure	carb. (gms)	fiber (gms)
Mochi, see "Rice snack"		
Molasses, 1 tbsp.:		
(*Brer Rabbit* Full Flavored/Mild)	15.0	0
(*Grandma's*)	12.0	0
blackstrap:		
(*Brer Rabbit*)	13.0	0
(*New Morning*)	13.0	0
(*Tree of Life*)	11.0	0
mild (*Grandma's*)	14.0	0
robust (*Grandma's*)	12.0	0
Mole sauce:		
(*Doña María*), 2 tbsp.	12.0	2.0
(*Doña María* Verde), 2 tbsp.	6.0	2.0
green (*La Costeña*), 1 tbsp.	8.0	<1.0
hot (*La Costeña*), 1 tbsp.	13.0	1.0
Monkfish, without added ingredients	0	0
Monosodium glutamate:		
(*McCormick*), ¼ tsp.	0	0
(*Tone's*), 1 tsp.	0	0
Moose, meat only, without added ingredients	0	0
Mortadella, 2 oz.:		
(*Boar's Head*)	0	0
beef and pork	1.7	0
with pistachios (*Boar's Head*)	2.0	0
Mothbeans, boiled, 4 oz.	23.8	n.a.
MSG, see "Monosodium glutamate"		
Muffin, 1 piece, except as noted:		
banana walnut, mini (*Hostess*), 2-oz. pkg.	24.0	<1.0
blueberry, gluten free (*Foods by George*), 2.8 oz.	34.0	<1.0
blueberry, mini (*Hostess*), 3 pieces, 1.2 oz.	19.0	0
chocolate chip, mini (*Hostess*), 2-oz. pkg.	28.0	0
corn (*Foods by George*), 2.8 oz.	36.0	1.0
corn, 2 oz.	29.0	1.9
English:		
(*Bays* Original), 2 oz.	27.0	1.0
(*Pepperidge Farm*), 2 oz.	25.0	1.0
(*Thomas'* Original), 2 oz.	25.0	1.0
cinnamon raisin (*Thomas'*), 2.2 oz.	31.0	2.0

Food and Measure	carb. (gms)	fiber (gms)
honey wheat (*Thomas'*), 2 oz.	27.0	2.0
multigrain (*Thomas'*), 2 oz.	25.0	1.0
multigrain (*Thomas'* Light), 2 oz.	22.0	8.0
plain, wheat or raisin (*Country Kitchen* Reduced Calorie), 2 oz.	22.0	5.0
sourdough (*Bays*), 2 oz.	26.0	2.0
sourdough (*Thomas'*), 2 oz.	25.0	1.0
whole wheat (*Pepperidge Farm*), 2 oz.	26.0	3.0
whole wheat (*Thomas'*), 2.2 oz.	22.0	3.0
English, gluten free, 3.6 oz.:		
(*Foods by George*)	39.0	1.0
cinnamon currant (*Foods by George*)	42.0	2.0
rye (*Foods by George* No-Rye)	40.0	2.0
oat bran, 2 oz.	27.5	2.6
Muffin, frozen, chocolate chip (*Smart Ones*), 2.5-oz. piece	39.0	4.0
Muffin, toaster, see "Toaster pastry and muffin"		
Muffin mix (see also "Bread mix, sweet"), 1 piece*, except as noted:		
apple cinnamon or banana nut (*Betty Crocker*)	21.0	0
apple cinnamon (*"Jiffy"*), ¼ cup	28.0	1.0
apple streusel (*Betty Crocker*)	33.0	0
banana nut (*"Jiffy"*), ¼ cup	25.0	2.0
berry, triple (*Betty Crocker*)	23.0	0
blueberry:		
(*Betty Crocker*)	30.0	0
(*Betty Crocker Twice the Blueberries*)	25.0	1.0
(*Duncan Hines* Bakery Style)	25.0	1.0
(*"Jiffy"*), ¼ cup	28.0	1.0
wild (*Betty Crocker*)	28.0	<1.0
wild, whole wheat (*Hodgson Mill*), ¼ cup	32.0	4.0
bran, ¼ cup (*Hodgson Mill*)	27.0	3.0
bran, ¼ cup, with dates (*"Jiffy"*)	26.0	3.0
chocolate, double (*Betty Crocker*)	30.0	0
chocolate chip (*Betty Crocker*)	21.0	0
chocolate chip (*Duncan Hines*)	31.0	1.0
corn, ¼ cup:		
(*Glory*)	25.0	<1.0

Food and Measure	carb. (gms)	fiber (gms)
(*Hodgson Mill*)	28.0	3.0
("*Jiffy*")	28.0	1.0
cranberry orange (*Betty Crocker*)	25.0	0
lemon poppy seed (*Betty Crocker*)	22.0	0
lemon poppy seed (*Betty Crocker Sunkist*)	29.0	0
raspberry ("*Jiffy*"), ¼ cup	26.0	<1.0
whole wheat (*Hodgson Mill*), ¼ cup	27.0	3.0
Mulberries, fresh:		
10 berries, ½ oz.	1.5	.3
½ cup	6.9	1.2
Mullet, without added ingredients	0	0
Multigrain chips, see "Snack chips"		
Mung beans:		
dry (*Shiloh Farms*), ¼ cup	28.0	9.0
boiled, ½ cup	19.3	7.7
Mung bean sprouts:		
raw, 1 cup	6.2	1.9
raw, 1 oz.	1.7	.5
boiled, drained, ½ cup	2.6	.5
Mung bean sprouts, canned, drained, 1 cup	2.7	1.0
Mungo beans, boiled, ½ cup	16.5	5.8
Mushroom (see also specific listings), common:		
raw, pieces or slices, ½ cup	1.5	.4
boiled, drained, pieces, ½ cup	4.0	1.7
Mushroom, breaded, frozen (*Empire* Kosher), 7 pieces,		
2.85 oz.	16.0	1.0
Mushroom, can or jar (see also "Mushroom, straw"):		
whole or sliced:		
(*Green Giant*), ½ cup	4.0	2.0
drained, ½ cup	3.9	1.9
with liquid, ½ cup	3.0	<1.0
in butter (*BinB*), 3-oz. can	4.0	1.0
sliced, with garlic (*Green Giant*), ½ cup	4.0	1.0
sliced, with garlic in butter (*BinB*), 3-oz. can	5.0	1.0
sliced, random (*Fanci Food*), ½ cup	3.0	<1.0
stems and pieces (*Green Giant*), ½ cup	4.0	2.0
Mushroom, chanterelle, dried (*Frieda's*), 2 pieces,		
.14 oz.	2.0	1.0

Mushroom, cloud ear, dried:

Food and Measure	carb. (gms)	fiber (gms)
.2-oz. piece	3.3	3.2
½ cup	10.2	9.8
Mushroom, crimini, brown or Italian, raw, .5-oz. piece	.6	<.1
Mushroom, enoki, fresh:		
(*Frieda's*), ¼ pkg., .9 oz.	2.0	1.0
trimmed, 1 oz.	2.0	.7
1 large, 4⅛" long	.4	<1.0
Mushroom, maitake, dried (*Eden*), .4 oz., about		
10 pieces	7.0	4.0
Mushroom, morel, dried (*Frieda's*), 3 pieces, .14 oz.	2.0	0
Mushroom, oyster:		
fresh, 1 large, 5.2 oz.	9.2	3.6
fresh, 1 small, .5 oz.	.9	.4
dried (*Frieda's*), 3 pieces	2.0	0
Mushroom, pickled, cocktail (*Fanci Food*), 1 oz.	0	0
Mushroom, porcini, dried:		
(*Epicurean Specialty*), ⅓ oz.	2.0	0
(*Frieda's*), 5 pieces	2.0	1.0
Mushroom, portobello:		
fresh, 1 oz.	1.4	.4
dried (*Frieda's*), 7 pieces, .14 oz.	1.0	0
Mushroom, shiitake:		
fresh, raw (*Frieda's*), 3.5 oz.	75.0	11.0
fresh, cooked, 4 medium or ½ cup pieces	10.4	1.5
dried:		
(*Frieda's*), ¼ cup, .14 oz.	3.0	0
4 medium, .5 oz.	11.3	1.7
whole or sliced (*Eden*), 6 pieces, .4 oz.	7.0	5.0
Mushroom, straw:		
canned, drained, ½ cup	4.2	2.3
canned, sliced, stir-fry (*Port Arthur*), ½ cup	3.0	2.0
dried (*Frieda's* Padi Straw), 6 pieces	2.0	0
Mushroom, wood ear, dried (*Frieda's*), 3 pieces, .14 oz.	2.0	0
Mushroom batter mix (*Don's Chuck Wagon*), ¼ cup	21.0	1.0
Mushroom gravy, in jars, ¼ cup:		
(*Campbell's*)	3.0	0
(*Pacific Foods*)	4.0	1.0

Food and Measure	carb. (gms)	fiber (gms)
creamy (*Campbell's*)	4.0	0
rich (*Heinz* Home Style)	3.0	0
Mushroom gravy mix, ¼ cup*:		
(*McCormick*)	2.0	0
shiitake (*Road's End Organics*)	5.0	<1.0
Mushroom sauce, shiitake (*Annie Chun's*), 1 tbsp.	3.0	0
Muskrat, meat only, without added ingredients	0	0
Mussels, blue, meat only:		
raw, 4 oz.	4.2	0
raw, 1 cup	3.4	0
boiled or steamed, 4 oz.	8.4	0
Mussels, canned, in red sauce (*Reese*), 4-oz. can drained	4.0	0
Mussels, smoked:		
(*Ducktrap River*), ¼ cup	3.0	0
(*Roland*), ⅓ cup	3.0	0
Mustard, prepared, 1 tsp., except as noted:		
all varieties (*Westbrae Natural*)	0	0
brown:		
(*Eden* Organic/Squeeze)	1.0	0
spicy (*Grey Poupon*)	0	0
spicy (*Gulden's*)	0	0
Chinese, hot (*Port Arthur*)	0	0
Creole (*Luzianne*), 1 tbsp.	2.0	0
deli style:		
(*Boar's Head*)	0	0
(*French's*)	0	0
(*Grey Poupon*)	0	0
(*Hebrew National*)	0	0
Dijon:		
(*Grey Poupon/Grey Poupon* Country)	1.0	0
(*Maille* Original)	0	0
(*Sara Lee* French Country)	0	0
(*Tree of Life*)	0	0
extra hot (*Maille*)	1.0	0
or yellow (*Annie's Naturals* Organic)	0	0
green pepper, strong (*Delouis Fils*)	<1.0	0
stone ground:		
(*Sara Lee* Bavarian)	0	0

Food and Measure	carb. (gms)	fiber (gms)
with herbs (*Tree of Life*)	<1.0	0
or yellow (*Tree of Life* Organic)	0	0
yellow (*Eden* Organic)	0	0
yellow (*French's*)	0	0
Mustard blend (see also "Pretzel dip"), 1 tsp.:		
honey:		
(*Annie's Naturals* Organic)	2.0	0
(*Boar's Head*)	2.0	0
(*French's*)	1.0	0
(*Westbrae Natural* Organic)	1.0	0
or cranberry (*Sara Lee*)	2.0	0
horseradish or raspberry (*Annie's Naturals* Organic)	1.0	0
horseradish (*Watkins*)	1.0	0
onion, sweet (*French's*)	2.0	0
pepper, garden, trio (*Sara Lee*)	1.0	0
Mustard cabbage, see "Cabbage, mustard"		
Mustard greens, fresh:		
raw (*Glory*), 2 cups	4.0	3.0
raw, chopped (*Del Monte*), 2 cups	5.0	1.0
raw, chopped, 1 oz. or ½ cup	1.4	.6
boiled, drained, ½ cup	1.5	1.4
Mustard greens, canned, ½ cup:		
(*Allens* No Salt)	5.0	3.0
(*Bush's*)	3.0	2.0
seasoned (*Allens/Sunshine*)	6.0	1.0
seasoned (*Glory*)	7.0	3.0
Mustard greens, frozen, chopped, boiled, drained, 1 cup	4.7	4.2
Mustard powder, 1 tsp.	.3	<1.0
Mustard seeds, 1 tsp.	1.2	<1.0
Mustard spinach:		
raw, chopped, 1 cup	5.9	4.2
boiled, drained, chopped, 1 cup	5.0	3.6
Mustard tallow, 1 tbsp.	0	0

N

Food and Measure	carb. (gms)	fiber (gms)
Nacho snack, frozen (*Amy's*), 5–6 pieces	26.0	<1.0
Nacho snack kit, with beans, sauce, chips, salsa (*Taco Bell Ultimate Nachos*), ¼ of 18.5-oz. pkg.	29.0	4.0
Name yam (*Frieda's*), ¾ cup, 3 oz.	24.0	3.0
Nathan's Famous, 1 serving:		
burgers:		
bacon cheeseburger	43.3	1.7
¼ lb. burger	42.3	1.7
¼ lb. burger, with cheese	45.4	1.7
super burger	42.2	2.6
fish sandwich	41.7	13.3
cheesesteak, chicken	62.5	4.8
cheesesteak, original	50.3	4.0
cheesesteak supreme	60.8	4.8
chili, *Nathan's,* 9 oz.	32.0	.9
hot dog	22.7	1.3
hot dog nuggets, 6 pieces	20.0	0
fries:		
large	64.8	8.1
regular	46.4	5.8
super	101.0	12.6
rings onion, large	47.7	2.1
rings onion, small	35.8	1.6
sauce, cheese, 2 oz.	6.4	.9
sauerkraut, ½ cup	5.0	3.0
Natto, ½ cup	12.6	4.8
Navy beans:		
dry (*Shiloh Farms*), ¼ cup	32.0	13.0
boiled, ½ cup	24.0	3.3

Food and Measure	carb. (gms)	fiber (gms)
Navy beans, canned, ½ cup:		
(*Allens*)	19.0	6.0
(*Bush's*)	19.0	6.0
(*Eden* Organic)	20.0	7.0
with bacon (*Trappey's*)	18.0	6.0
with bacon and jalapeño (*Trappey's*)	17.0	6.0
sweet (*Glory*)	27.0	7.0
Navy beans, sprouted, ½ cup	6.8	n.a.
Nectarine:		
(*Del Monte*), 1 medium, 4.9 oz.	16.0	2.0
(*Dole*), 1 medium, 4.9 oz.	16.0	2.0
1 medium, 2½'' diam.	16.0	2.2
sliced, ½ cup	8.1	1.1
Noni juice (*Tree of Life*), 2 tbsp.	4.0	0
Noodle, Asian, 2 oz. dry, except as noted:		
cellophane (*Port Arthur* Bean Thread), 1 cup dry	50.0	1.0
cellophane or long rice	48.8	<1.0
chow mein (*Annie Chun's*)	39.0	3.0
chow mein, fresh (*Frieda's*), 4 oz.	70.0	1.0
chow mein, dried, ½ cup	13.0	.9
crispy (*Frieda's*), ½ cup, 1 oz.	17.0	1.0
kuzu (*Eden*)	48.0	2.0
rice:		
(*Annie Chun's* Hunan/Original/Thai Basil)	50.0	0
(*A Taste of Thai* Original/Thin/Wide)	46.0	2.0
(*Thai Kitchen* Stir-fry/Thin/Wide)	46.0	2.0
sticks (*Port Arthur*), 1 cup dry	48.0	1.0
soba:		
(*Annie Chun's*)	39.0	3.0
buckwheat (*Eden*)	43.0	3.0
buckwheat, lotus root, or mugwort (*Eden*)	37.0	2.0
spelt (*Eden* Organic)	37.0	2.0
whole grain, 70% (*Eden* Organic)	38.0	2.0
wild yam (*Eden* Jinenjo)	37.0	2.0
soba, cooked, 1 cup	24.4	n.a.
somen, uncooked	42.2	2.4
somen, whole grain 80% (*Eden* Organic)	38.0	3.0
somen, cooked, 1 cup	48.5	n.a.

Food and Measure	carb. (gms)	fiber (gms)
thin cut, fresh (*Azumaya*), 1 cup	43.0	2.0
udon:		
(*Eden*)	37.0	3.0
brown rice (*Eden*)	38.0	2.0
brown rice or whole grain, 80% (*Eden* Organic)	38.0	3.0
kamut (*Eden* Organic)	37.0	3.0
udon, cooked, 4 oz.	23.0	n.a.
wide cut (*Azumaya*), 1 cup	43.0	2.0
Noodle, egg:		
dry, 2 oz.:		
enriched	40.3	1.5
whole wheat (*Hodgson Mill*)	34.0	4.0
whole wheat, spinach (*Hodgson Mill*)	32.0	5.0
cooked, 1 cup	39.7	1.8
cooked, spinach, 1 cup	38.8	3.7
Noodle, Chinese, Japanese, or Thai, see "Noodle, Asian"		
Noodle entree, frozen, 1 pkg.:		
Asian, stir-fry (*Amy's*), 10 oz.	41.0	4.0
and chicken, see "Chicken entree, frozen"		
with chicken, peas, carrots (*Michelina's* Authentico), 8 oz.	34.0	2.0
lo mein, vegetable, with tofu (*Ethnic Gourmet*), 11 oz.	60.0	6.0
pad Thai, with tofu (*Ethnic Gourmet*), 11 oz.	84.0	4.0
Romanoff, with meatballs (*Michelina's* Authentico), 10 oz.	42.0	2.0
Stroganoff (*Michelina's* Authentico), 8 oz.	35.0	2.0
Noodle entree, pkg.:		
and chicken (*Kid's Kitchen*), 1 cup	18.0	1.0
ginger shiitake (*Fantastic Fast Naturals*), 1 pkg.	58.0	4.0
pad Thai (*Fantastic Fast Naturals*), 1 pkg.	59.0	5.0
pad Thai sauce (*Tasty Bite*), ⅓ pkg.	49.0	2.0
peanut sauce (*Tasty Bite*), ⅓ pkg.	42.0	1.0
stir-fry sauce (*Tasty Bite*), ⅓ pkg.	40.0	2.0
Thai lemon grass (*Fantastic Fast Naturals*), 1 pkg.	48.0	5.0
vegetables and, see "Vegetable entree, pkg." and "Vegetarian entree, pkg."		
Noodle entree mix:		
chow mein, with sauce, ⅓ pkg.:		
black bean or peanut sesame (*Annie Chun's*)	42.0	2.0
garlic scallion (*Annie Chun's*)	39.0	2.0

Food and Measure	carb. (gms)	fiber (gms)
curry stir-fry (*Thai Kitchen* Noodles & Sauce), 1 cup*	59.0	0
garlic, roasted (*Thai Kitchen* Noodle Cart), 1 pkg.	47.0	0
garlic, savory stir-fry (*Thai Kitchen* Noodles & Sauce),		
1 cup*	46.0	<1.0
lemon grass and chili stir-fry (*Thai Kitchen* Noodles & Sauce),		
1 cup*	60.0	0
pad Thai, with sauce:		
(*Annie Chun's*), ⅓ pkg.	48.0	0
(*A Taste of Thai* for Two), ½ pkg.	89.0	3.5
(*Thai Kitchen Noodle* Cart), 1 pkg.	49.0	<1.0
with chili stir-fry (*Thai Kitchen* Noodles & Sauce),		
1 cup*	73.0	<1.0
stir-fry (*Thai Kitchen* Noodles & Sauce), 1 cup*	93.0	<1.0
peanut, Thai (*Thai Kitchen* Noodle Cart), 1 pkg.	47.0	0
peanut, Thai, stir-fry (*Thai Kitchen* Noodles & Sauce),		
1 cup*	55.0	0
sesame, toasted, stir-fry (*Thai Kitchen* Noodles & Sauce),		
1 cup*	54.0	.5
soba, with soy ginger sauce (*Annie Chun's*), ⅓ pkg.	41.0	3.0
Nopales/Nopalitos, see "Cactus pads"		
Nori, see "Seaweed"		
Nut topping, see specific nut listings		
Nutmeg, ground, 1 tsp.	1.1	.1
Nuts, see specific listings		
Nuts, mixed, 1 oz., except as noted:		
(*Fisher* Less Than 50% Peanuts)	5.0	2.0
(*Frito Lay* Deluxe), ¼ cup, 1 oz.	6.0	2.0
(*Planters*/Deluxe/Lightly Salted/Unsalted)	6.0	2.0
(*Tree of Life* Just Nuts Trail Mix), 1.1 oz.	5.0	2.0
cashew mix:		
almonds, macadamias (*Planters*), ¾ oz.	6.0	2.0
almonds, pecans (*Planters*)	7.0	2.0
jumbo, and mixed nuts (*Planters*)	8.0	1.0
glazed (*Beer Nuts*)	4.0	2.0
honey-roasted (*Kettle*)	8.0	2.0
honey-roasted (*Planters*)	9.0	2.0
macadamia mix:		
(*Mauna Loa* Mixed Nuts)	8.0	2.0

Food and Measure	carb. (gms)	fiber (gms)
cashew mix (*Mauna Loa*)	8.0	1.0
cashews, almonds (*Planters*)	6.0	2.0
peanuts, almonds, pecans, hazelnuts, pistachios (*Planters*)	5.0	3.0
peanuts and cashews, honey (*Planters*)	10.0	2.0

O

Food and Measure	carb. (gms)	fiber (gms)
Oat (see also "Cereal"):		
(*Shiloh Farms* Steel Cut), ¼ cup	29.0	5.0
whole grain, 1 oz.	18.8	3.0
rolled or oatmeal:		
dry (*Shiloh Farms* Rolled), ⅓ cup	23.0	4.0
dry, 1 oz.	19.0	2.9
cooked, 1 cup	25.3	4.0
Oat bran, dry:		
(*Shiloh Farms* 1 lb.), ⅓ cup	23.0	7.0
(*Tree of Life*/Organic), ½ cup	31.0	7.0
1 oz.	18.8	4.5
Oat flour:		
(*Arrowhead Mills*), ⅓ cup	21.0	3.0
(*Shiloh Farms*), ⅓ cup	20.0	4.0
bran (*Hodgson Mill*), ¼ cup	23.0	3.0
bran (*Hodgson Mill* Organic), ¼ cup	24.0	3.0
bran blend (*Hodgson Mill*), <¼ cup	24.0	3.0
Oat groats, ¼ cup:		
(*Arrowhead Mills*)	28.0	4.0
(*Shiloh Farms*)	29.0	4.0
Oco (*Frieda's*), ½ cup, 3 oz.	15.0	1.0
Ocean perch, without added ingredients	0	0
Octopus, meat only:		
raw, 4 oz.	2.5	0
boiled or steamed, 4 oz.	5.0	0
Octopus, canned:		
in olive oil (*Goya*), ¼ cup	3.0	0
spiced, in red sauce (*Reese*), 2 oz.	4.0	0

Food and Measure	carb. (gms)	fiber (gms)
Oheloberry, ½ cup	4.8	n.a.
Oil, all varieties	0	0
Okra, fresh:		
raw, sliced, ½ cup	3.8	1.3
boiled, drained, 8 pods, 3" × ⅝"	6.1	2.1
boiled drained, sliced, ½ cup	5.8	2.0
red, raw (*Frieda's*), 3.5 oz.	8.0	3.0
Okra, canned, ½ cup:		
(*Allens/Trappey's*)	6.0	3.0
(*Glory*)	6.0	2.0
Creole gumbo (*Trappey's*)	6.0	3.0
and tomatoes (*Allens/Trappey's*)	5.0	3.0
and tomatoes and corn (*Allens/Trappey's*)	6.0	4.0
Okra, frozen, ½ cup:		
whole or cut (*McKenzie's*)	5.0	3.0
boiled, drained, sliced	7.5	2.6
with tomatoes and onions (*McKenzie's*)	4.0	2.0
Old-fashioned drink mixer (*Holland House*), 4 fl. oz.	39.0	0
Olive, pickled:		
(*D.L. Jardine's* Martini), .5-oz. piece	0	0
black, see "Greek, black" and "ripe," below		
Calamata (*Krinos*), 3 pieces, .5 oz.	2.0	0
Greek, black:		
10 medium	1.7	0
10 extra large	2.3	0
pitted, 1 oz.	2.5	0
green, with pits:		
10 small	.4	.7
10 large	.5	1.0
10 giant	.9	1.7
green, cracked (*Krinos*), 2 pieces, .5 oz.	2.0	0
green, pitted:		
(*Lindsay*), 5 medium, .5 oz.	1.0	0
1 oz.	.4	.7
with pimento, sliced (*Lindsay*), 2 tbsp.	<1.0	0
ripe, pitted (*Lindsay*), 4 large, .5 oz.	1.0	0
ripe, pitted, sliced (*Lindsay*), 2 tbsp.	1.0	0
salad, with pimento (*Pompeian*), 1 tbsp., .5 oz.	1.0	0

Food and Measure	carb. (gms)	fiber (gms)
stuffed, green:		
with almonds or anchovies (*Reese*), 4 pieces, .5 oz. ..	<1.0	0
with anchovies (*Goya*), 4 pieces, .5 oz.	<1.0	0
with jalapeños (*D.L. Jardine's* Texas Caviar), 2 pieces, .5 oz.	0	0
with pimento (*Pompeian*), 6 pieces, .5 oz.	1.0	0
with pimento, Manzanilla (*Lindsay*), 5 pieces, .5 oz. ...	<1.0	0
with pimento, queen (*Goya*), 1 piece	1.0	0
with pimento, queen (*Lindsay*), 2 pieces, .5 oz.	<1.0	0
with sun-dried tomato (*Byzantine*), 5 pieces	1.5	.7
Olive loaf, see "Lunch meat"		
Olive oil, 2 tbsp.	0	0
Olive paste, black (*Roland*), 1 tbsp.	3.0	1.0
Olive sauce, green (*Italia in Tavola*), 2 tbsp.	0	0
Olive spread:		
(*Lindsay Olivada* Taste of Greece), 2 tbsp.	2.0	0
(*Lindsay Olivada* Taste of Sicily/Tuscany), 2 tbsp.	3.0	0
tapenade (*Cantare*), 1 tbsp.	1.0	0
Omelet, see "Egg breakfast"		
Onion, fresh/stored:		
raw:		
(*Del Monte*), 1 medium, 5.2 oz.	16.0	3.0
(*Frieda's* Boiler/Cipolline), 3 pieces, 3 oz.	7.0	2.0
(*Frieda's* Hawaiian Maui), ⅓ cup, 1.1 oz.	3.0	1.0
(*Frieda's* Pearl), ⅔ cup, 3 oz.	7.0	2.0
1 oz.	2.4	.5
chopped, ½ cup	6.9	1.4
chopped, 1 tbsp.	.9	.2
boiled, drained, chopped, ½ cup	10.7	1.5
boiled, drained, chopped, 1 tbsp.	1.5	.2
Onion, can or jar:		
cocktail (*Crosse & Blackwell*), 1 tbsp.	1.0	0
pickled, sour (*London Pub*), ¼ cup, 1.1 oz.	2.0	0
Onion, dried:		
flakes, 1 tbsp.	4.2	.5
minced (*Lawry's*), ¼ tsp.	<1.0	0
minced, 1 tsp.	1.9	.2
Onion, french fried, canned (*French's* Original), 2 tbsp. ...	3.0	0

Food and Measure	carb. (gms)	fiber (gms)
Onion, frozen (see also "Onion rings"):		
whole:		
(*C&W* Petite), ⅔ cup	7.0	1.0
boiled, drained, ½ cup	7.0	1.5
pearl, white (*Birds Eye*), ⅔ cup	6.0	1.0
chopped, boiled, drained, 1 tbsp.	1.0	.2
chopped, with peppers (*McKenzie's* Seasoning Mix),		
1 oz.	2.0	0
Onion, green, raw, trimmed, with top:		
(*Dole*), ¼ cup	2.0	1.0
chopped, ½ cup	3.7	1.3
chopped, 1 tbsp.	.4	.2
Onion, pickled, see "Onion, can or jar"		
Onion, Welsh, 1 oz.	1.8	<1.0
Onion dip:		
(*Litehouse*), 2 tbsp.	2.0	0
French (*Cabot*), 2 tbsp.	1.0	0
French (*Ruffles*), 4 tbsp.	9.0	2.0
French or green (*Kraft*), 2 tbsp.	3.0	0
Onion dip mix, dry:		
(*Fantastic* Soup/Dip), 2½ tsp.	6.0	1.0
French (*McCormick*), ¾ tsp.	0	0
mushroom (*Fantastic* Soup/Dip), 1½ tbsp.	6.0	<1.0
spring (*McCormick*), ½ tsp.	1.0	0
Onion flavor chips, see "Corn chips/crisps"		
Onion gravy mix (*McCormick*), ¼ cup*	3.0	0
Onion nuggets, frozen, with cheese, breaded (*Kineret*),		
3½ pieces, 2.8 oz.	20.0	6.0
Onion oil (*Watkins* Liquid Spice), 1 tsp.	0	0
Onion powder:		
(*Tone's*), ¼ tsp.	1.0	0
1 tsp.	1.7	.1
Onion ring batter mix, ¼ cup:		
(*Don's Chuck Wagon*)	21.0	1.0
(*Golden Dipt* Fry Easy)	20.0	0
(*Hodgson Mill*)	21.0	1.0
(*Produce Partners Zebbie's*)	18.0	0

Food and Measure	carb. (gms)	fiber (gms)
Onion rings, frozen, breaded:		
(*Kineret*), 6 pieces, 3.2 oz.	26.0	2.0
(*McKenzie's*), 3.25 oz.	28.0	6.0
(*Ore-Ida Onion Ringers*), 5 pieces, 2.9 oz.	21.0	2.0
and strings (*Ian's* Natural), 6–8 pieces, 2.5 oz.	16.0	1.0
heated, 10 rings	27.1	2.9
Onion salt (*McCormick* California Style), ¼ tsp.	0	0
Onion sauce (*Boar's Head* Sweet Vidalia), 1 tbsp.	2.0	0
Onion snack chips, see "Snack chips"		
Onion sprouts (*Jonathan's*), 1 cup	5.0	2.0
Opo squash (*Frieda's*), ⅔ cup, 3 oz.	3.0	0
Opossum, meat only, without added ingredients	0	0
Orange, fresh:		
(*Dole*), 5.4-oz. fruit	21.0	7.0
(*Frieda's* Blood Moro/Cara Cara), 5 oz.	16.0	3.0
(*Frieda's* Seville), 3 oz.	10.0	2.0
(*Sunkist*), 5.4-oz. fruit	21.0	7.0
all varieties, 3 1/16'' fruit, 6.5 oz.	21.6	4.4
all varieties, sections, 1 cup	21.2	4.3
California navel, 2⅞'' fruit, 5 oz.	16.3	3.4
California navel, sections, 1 cup	19.2	4.0
California Valencia, 2⅝'' fruit, 4.25 oz.	14.4	3.0
California Valencia, sections, 1 cup	21.4	4.5
Florida, 2 11/16'' fruit, 5 oz.	16.3	3.4
Florida, sections, 1 cup	21.4	4.4
Orange, mandarin, see "Tangerine"		
Orange drink, 8 fl. oz.:		
(*Hi-C Blast*)	31.0	0
(*Hood Carb Countdown*)	5.0	0
(*Minute Maid* Light)	13.0	0
(*Santa Cruz Organic* Box)	25.0	0
(*Tropicana Pure Premium* Essentials Light'n Healthy)	13.0	0
orange flavor (*Bright & Early*)	30.0	0
orange flavor, frozen* (*Bright & Early*)	29.0	0
orangeade:		
(*AriZona*)	27.0	0
(*Snapple*)	29.0	0

Food and Measure	carb. (gms)	fiber (gms)
(*Tropicana*)	28.0	0
(*Turkey Hill*)	30.0	0
Orange drink blend, 8 fl. oz., except as noted:		
apricot (*Lincoln* Breakfast Cocktail)	29.0	0
carrot (*SoBe Elixir 3C*)	24.0	0
crème (*V8 Splash* Smoothies)	29.0	1.0
grapefruit (*Langers* Ruby)	33.0	0
mango:		
(*Nantucket Nectars*)	32.0	0
(*Newman's Own* Tango)	37.0	0
(*R.W. Knudsen*)	30.0	0
(*Santa Cruz Organic*)	31.0	0
pineapple:		
(*Hood Carb Countdown*)	5.0	0
(*Lincoln*)	32.0	0
(*V8 Splash*)	28.0	0
strawberry (*Minute Maid Coolers*), 6.75-fl.-oz. pouch	26.0	0
Orange juice, 8 fl. oz., except as noted:		
(*Bolthouse Farms*)	24.0	>1.0
(*Hood*)	30.0	0
(*Langers* Plus)	29.0	0
(*Minute Maid*), 11.5-fl.-oz. can	38.0	0
(*Nantucket Nectars* Premium)	27.0	0
(*Ocean Spray*)	31.0	0
(*Organic Valley/Organic Valley* Calcium)	26.0	0
(*R.W. Knudsen*)	23.0	0
(*S&W*)	30.0	0
all varieties (*Minute Maid*)	27.0	0
canned	24.5	.5
chilled	25.1	.5
fresh	25.8	.5
frozen* (*Cascadian Farm*)	29.0	0
Orange juice blend, 8 fl. oz., except as noted:		
carrot (*After the Fall* 24 Karrot)	28.0	0
carrot (*Walnut Acres*)	27.0	0
passion fruit (*Minute Maid*)	31.0	0
tangerine (*Minute Maid*)	27.0	0
tangerine (*Tropicana Pure Premium*)	25.0	0

Food and Measure	carb. (gms)	fiber (gms)
tropical (*Minute Maid*), 6.75-fl.-oz. box	27.0	0
tropical (*Minute Maid*), 11.5-fl.-oz. can	46.0	0
Orange peel, fresh, 1 tbsp.	1.5	.2
Oregano, dried, 1 tsp.	.5	.1
Oriental 5-spice (*Tone's*), 1 tsp.	1.9	.5
Ostrich, meat only, without added ingredients	0	0
Oyster, meat only, 4 oz., except as noted:		
Eastern, wild:		
raw, 6 medium, 3 oz.	3.3	0
baked, broiled, or microwaved	5.4	0
steamed or poached	8.9	0
Eastern, farmed, raw	6.3	0
Eastern, farmed, baked, broiled, or microwaved	8.3	0
Pacific:		
raw	5.6	0
raw, steamed, or poached, 1 medium	2.5	0
boiled or steamed	11.2	0
Oyster, canned:		
whole (*Bumble Bee*), 2 oz.	3.0	0
Eastern, wild, with liquid, 4 oz.	4.4	0
Eastern, wild, with liquid, 1 cup	9.7	0
Oyster, smoked, canned, in olive oil:		
(*Crown Prince*), 3-oz. can	11.0	<1.0
drained (*Brunswick*), 2.3 oz.	7.0	1.0
Oyster dish, frozen, breaded (*Hillman*), 7 pieces, 3 oz. ..	20.0	<1.0
Oyster plant, see "Salsify"		
Oyster sauce, Asian:		
(*Ka•Me*), 1 tbsp.	3.0	0
1 tbsp.	2.0	0
Oyster and shrimp sauce (*TryMe* Caribbean Clipper),		
1 tsp.	2.0	0
Oyster stew, see "Soup, condensed"		

P

Food and Measure	carb. (gms)	fiber (gms)
Pad Thai entree, see "Noodle entree"		
Pad Thai sauce, see "Thai sauce"		
Paella, see "Rice entree, frozen"		
Palak paneer, see "Spinach entree"		
Palm, hearts of, can or jar:		
marinated (*Fanci Food*), ½ cup	8.0	4.0
nuggets (*Fanci Food* for Salad), ½ cup	4.0	2.0
sliced or whole (*Island Blaze*), ⅓ cup	4.0	2.0
spears (*Fanci Food* Jar), ½ cup	5.0	3.0
sticks (*Fanci Food* Can), 2 pieces	3.0	<1.0
1.2-oz. piece	1.5	.8
1 cup	6.8	3.5
Pancake, freeze-dried, blueberry (*AlpineAire*), ½ pkg.	52.0	7.0
Pancake, frozen, 3 pieces, except as noted:		
(*Aunt Jemima* Homestyle)	37.0	1.0
(*Aunt Jemima* Low Fat)	35.0	2.0
(*Aunt Jemima* Mini), 5 pieces	46.0	2.0
(*Ian's Natural*), 1 piece	19.0	1.0
(*Pillsbury* Original)	46.0	1.0
blueberry:		
(*Ian's* Natural), 1 piece	19.0	1.0
(*Pillsbury*)	45.0	1.0
mini (*Pillsbury*), 14 pieces, with syrup	89.0	1.0
buttermilk:		
(*Aunt Jemima*)	37.0	0
(*Eggo*)	51.0	1.0
(*Pillsbury*)	51.0	1.0
mini (*Pillsbury*), 14 pieces, with syrup	84.0	1.0

Food and Measure	carb. (gms)	fiber (gms)
Pancake mix, 3 cakes*, except as noted:		
(*Betty Crocker* Original Complete)	39.0	1.0
(*Betty Crocker* Pouch), 3.3 cakes*	39.0	1.0
(*Shake 'n Pour* Original)	39.0	<1.0
blueberry (*Shake 'n Pour*)	40.0	1.0
buckwheat, (*Don's Chuck Wagon*), ⅓ cup	33.0	1.0
buckwheat (*Hodgson Mill*), ⅓ cup	40.0	3.0
buttermilk:		
(*Betty Crocker* Complete)	39.0	1.0
(*Betty Crocker* Complete Pouch), 3.3 cakes*	39.0	1.0
(*"Jiffy"* Complete), ¼ cup	32.0	<1.0
and honey (*Maple Grove Farms*), ⅓ cup	28.0	3.0
multigrain, with flax seed, soy (*Hodgson Mill*), ⅓ cup .	31.0	5.0
whole wheat (*Hodgson Mill*), ⅓ cup	28.0	4.0
Pancake syrup, 4 tbsp. or ¼ cup:		
(*Aunt Jemima*)	52.0	0
(*Aunt Jemima* Lite)	26.0	0
(*Eggo*)	60.0	0
(*Eggo* Butter Flavor)	41.0	0
(*Eggo* Lite)	27.0	0
(*Hungry Jack*)	51.0	0
(*Karo*)	63.0	0
(*Log Cabin*)	53.0	0
(*Log Cabin* Lite)	25.0	0
(*Mrs. Butterworth's*)	55.0	0
(*Mrs. Butterworth's* Lite)	24.0	0
(*Smucker's* No Sugar)	8.0	0
(*Vermont Maid*)	53.0	0
(*Vermont Maid* Butter Lite)	26.0	0
Pancetta, see "Bacon, Italian"		
Pancreas, without added ingredients	0	0
Paneer entree, see "Cheese entree" and "Spinach entree"		
Panera Bread:		
bread, artisan, 2 oz.:		
cheese, three, or cheese demi loaf	21.0	<1.0
country or raisin pecan	25.0	1.0
focaccia, cheese	19.0	1.0

Food and Measure	carb. (gms)	fiber (gms)
French	23.0	<1.0
kalamata olive	26.0	1.0
multigrain or sesame semolina	24.0	1.0
rye, stone-milled	22.0	2.0
three seed	23.0	1.0
bread/rolls, 2 oz., except as noted:		
asiago, demi loaf	21.0	<1.0
bread stick, lower carb, 1.2 oz.	13.0	7.0
ciabatta, 6 oz.	70.0	3.0
cinnamon raisin	31.0	1.0
croissant, 3 oz.	26.0	1.0
focaccio, asiago, basil pesto, or rosemary onion	19.0	1.0
French, baguette, loaf	24.0	1.0
French, roll, 2.25 oz.	28.0	1.0
golden original, lower carb, 1.1-oz. slice	10.0	4.0
honey wheat	25.0	1.0
Italian herb, lower carb, 1.1-oz. slice	10.0	4.0
nine grain	26.0	2.0
rosemary walnut, lower carb, 1.1-oz. slice	9.0	5.0
rye	25.0	1.0
sourdough:		
baguette, loaf, round	25.0	1.0
roll, 2.5 oz.	32.0	1.0
soup bowl, 8 oz.	102.0	4.0
sunflower	24.0	1.0
tomato basil	27.0	1.0
bagel, 1 piece:		
plain	57.0	2.0
plain, lower carb	25.0	12.0
apple, Dutch, raisin	70.0	3.0
asiago	58.0	2.0
asiago, lower carb	20.0	9.0
blueberry	67.0	3.0
chocolate hazelnut	72.0	3.0
chocolate raspberry	67.0	2.0
cinnamon crunch	78.0	3.0
everything	58.0	2.0
French toast	65.0	2.0

Food and Measure	carb. (gms)	fiber (gms)
nine grain	58.0	3.0
pumpkin spice	76.0	3.0
sesame	60.0	3.0
spinach Parmesan	83.0	3.0
cream cheese, plain, 2 oz.	2.0	0
cream cheese, reduced calorie, 2 oz.:		
plain	2.0	<1.0
hazelnut	6.0	<1.0
honey walnut	9.0	<1.0
mocha	10.0	<1.0
raspberry	3.0	0
sun-dried tomato	4.0	<1.0
veggie	4.0	1.0
soup, 8 oz.:		
asparagus chicken Florentine	12.0	3.0
black bean, chicken chorizo	33.0	15.0
black bean, low fat	31.0	11.0
broccoli cheddar	13.0	1.0
chicken, cream of, and wild rice	19.0	<1.0
chicken noodle, low fat	15.0	1.0
clam chowder, Boston	19.0	<1.0
mushroom bisque	17.0	1.0
onion, French	23.0	2.0
potato, baked	23.0	1.0
tomato basil, low fat	17.0	3.0
vegetable, garden, low fat	17.0	2.0
sandwiches:		
asiago roast beef	54.0	2.0
Bacon Turkey Bravo	84.0	5.0
chicken, Tuscan	77.0	6.0
chicken salad, nine grain	56.0	4.0
chicken salad, sesame semolina	80.0	6.0
ham and Swiss, artisan rye	106.0	6.0
ham and Swiss, rye	47.0	4.0
Italian combo	180.0	5.0
peanut butter and jelly, artisan French	90.0	5.0
peanut butter and jelly, French	63.0	3.0
Pepperblue Steak	78.0	4.0

Food and Measure	carb. (gms)	fiber (gms)
pesto Roma club	27.0	11.0
tuna salad, artisan multigrain	78.0	5.0
tuna salad, honey wheat	50.0	4.0
turkey, Sierra	71.0	4.0
turkey breast, smoked, artisan country	73.0	5.0
turkey breast, smoked, sourdough	44.0	3.0
veggie, garden	74.0	5.0
sandwiches, panini:		
carnitas, Coronado	77.0	3.0
Frontago Chicken Panini	71.0	5.0
portobello mozzarella	69.0	7.0
Smokehouse Turkey Panini, artisan three cheese	68.0	4.0
Smokehouse Turkey Panini, asiago focaccia	73.0	5.0
turkey artichoke	76.0	6.0
salad, with dressing:		
Bistro Steak Salad	10.0	4.0
Caesar	22.0	3.0
Caesar, grilled chicken	19.0	3.0
classic café	14.0	4.0
chicken, Asian sesame	34.0	5.0
Fandango Salad	21.0	6.0
Greek	17.0	5.0
tomato mozzarella	50.0	6.0
pastries/sweets:		
apple croissant	34.0	1.0
apple Danish	50.0	2.0
apple raisin strudel	40.0	1.0
banana nut muffin, 3 oz.	34.0	3.0
banana nut muffin, 5.75 oz.	67.0	5.0
bear claw	37.0	1.0
blueberry muffin	73.0	4.0
brownie:		
caramel pecan	60.0	2.0
chocolate raspberry	47.0	2.0
very chocolate	62.0	2.0
butter Danish, gooey	88.0	2.0
carrot walnut mini bundt cake	51.0	2.0
cheese croissant	34.0	1.0

Food and Measure	carb. (gms)	fiber (gms)
cheese Danish	55.0	1.0
cherry Danish	60.0	1.0
cherry strudel	38.0	1.0
chocolate chip muffin, 2.5 oz.	36.0	2.0
chocolate chip muffin, 5.75 oz.	83.0	5.0
chocolate cookie:		
chipper	51.0	2.0
duet, with walnuts	30.0	3.0
nutty chipper	46.0	3.0
chocolate croissant	56.0	4.0
chocolate Danish, German	83.0	4.0
chocolate hazelnut macaroon	30.0	3.0
cinnamon chip scone	70.0	2.0
cinnamon roll	64.0	3.0
cobblestone	100.0	4.0
coffeecake, cherry-cheese	21.0	1.0
lemon poppy mini bundt cake	62.0	1.0
nutty oatmeal raisin cookie	51.0	3.0
orange scone	67.0	3.0
peach Danish, Georgia	67.0	2.0
pecan roll	60.0	2.0
pineapple upside-down mini bundt cake	64.0	2.0
pumpkin muffin, 3 oz.	43.0	1.0
pumpkin muffin, 5.75 oz.	80.0	1.0
raspberry cheese croissant	37.0	1.0
shortbread cookie	36.0	1.0
tripleberry muffin, low fat	63.0	3.0
beverages:		
caffée latte	12.0	0
caffée mocha	47.0	2.0
cappuccino	12.0	0
caramel latte	54.0	0
chai tea latte	37.0	0
hot chocolate	45.0	2.0
house latte	43.0	0
I.C., 16 oz.:		
cappuccino chip	64.0	0
caramel	77.0	0

Food and Measure	carb. (gms)	fiber (gms)
mocha	70.0	2.0
spice	66.0	0
iced chai tea latte	29.0	0
Panko, flakes (*Shirakiku*), ⅓ cup	15.0	0
Papa John's:		
original crust, 12'', ⅛ pizza:		
cheese	27.0	1.0
chicken, barbecued, and bacon	32.0	1.0
chicken, barbecued, Hawaiian	33.0	1.0
chicken Alfredo	26.0	1.0
chicken club	28.0	1.0
garden fresh	28.0	2.0
Italian, spicy	27.0	3.0
meatball, spicy	28.0	1.0
the meats or sausage	27.0	2.0
pepperoni	27.0	1.0
spinach Alfredo	26.0	1.0
spinach Alfredo chicken tomato, or the works	28.0	2.0
original crust, 14'', ⅛ pizza:		
cheese	39.0	2.0
chicken, barbecued, and bacon	44.0	2.0
chicken, barbecued, Hawaiian	46.0	2.0
chicken Alfredo	36.0	2.0
chicken club or garden fresh	40.0	2.0
Italian, spicy	39.0	4.0
meatball, spicy	40.0	2.0
the meats or pepperoni	38.0	2.0
the meats, with beef, or sausage	38.0	3.0
spinach Alfredo	36.0	2.0
spinach Alfredo chicken tomato	37.0	2.0
the works	40.0	3.0
thin crust, 14'', ⅛ pizza:		
cheese	24.0	1.0
chicken, barbecued, and bacon	29.0	<1.0
chicken, barbecued, Hawaiian	31.0	1.0
chicken Alfredo	21.0	1.0
chicken club	25.0	1.0
garden fresh	25.0	2.0

Food and Measure	carb. (gms)	fiber (gms)
Italian, spicy	24.0	3.0
meatball, spicy	25.0	1.0
the meats or sausage	23.0	2.0
pepperoni	23.0	1.0
spinach Alfredo	21.0	1.0
spinach Alfredo chicken tomato	24.0	1.0
the works	25.0	2.0
sides:		
bread sticks, 1 piece	26.0	1.0
cheese sticks, 2 pieces	42.0	2.0
chicken strips, 2 pieces	10.0	0
dipping sauce, 1 oz.:		
barbecue	11.0	0
Buffalo	2.0	0
cheese, blue cheese, or ranch	1.0	0
garlic	0	0
honey mustard	5.0	0
pizza	3.0	0
Papa's wings, Buffalo, spicy, 2 pieces	1.0	<1.0
Papa's wings, chipotle, mild, 2 pieces	5.0	0
Papa's Cinnaple, 2 pieces	29.0	<1.0
Papaya, fresh:		
(*Del Monte*), ½ medium, 4.9 oz.	19.0	2.0
(*Dole*), ½ medium, 4.9 oz.	19.0	2.0
(*Frieda's* Golden Sunrise/Mexican), 1 cup, 5 oz.	14.0	3.0
1 lb., 3½'' × 5⅛''	29.8	5.5
cubed, 1 cup	13.7	2.5
mashed, 1 cup	22.6	4.1
Papaya, dried (*SunRidge Farms* Organic), 1.4-oz. piece	26.0	5.0
Papaya, frozen, (*Goya*), ⅓ pkg.	11.0	2.0
Papaya, in jars, in extra light syrup (*Del Monte Sunfresh*), ½ cup	17.0	1.0
Papaya drink (*Lincoln*), 8 fl. oz.	32.0	0
Papaya juice, 8 fl. oz.:		
(*Ceres*)	30.0	0
(*R.W. Knudsen* Nectar)	35.0	0
creamed (*R.W. Knudsen*)	10.0	0

Food and Measure	carb. (gms)	fiber (gms)
Papaya juice blend, 8 fl. oz.:		
(*L&A* Delight)	32.0	0
pineapple (*L&A* Delight)	31.0	0
Papaya nectar:		
(*Goya*), 12 fl. oz.	56.0	1.0
canned, 8 fl. oz.	36.3	1.5
Paprika, 1 tsp.	1.2	.6
Parsley, fresh:		
10 sprigs	.6	.3
chopped, ½ cup	1.9	1.0
Parsley, dried:		
1 tsp.	.2	.2
freeze-dried, 1 tbsp.	.2	.2
Parsley root (*Frieda's*), ⅔ cup, 3 oz.	2.0	1.0
Parsnip:		
raw, sliced (*Frieda's*), 1 cup	24.0	7.0
raw, sliced, ½ cup	12.1	3.3
boiled, drained, 1 medium, 9''	31.3	6.4
boiled, drained, sliced, ½ cup	15.2	3.1
Passion fruit, fresh:		
(*Frieda's*), 5 oz.	33.0	15.0
purple, 1 medium	4.2	1.9
purple, trimmed, ½ cup	27.5	12.2
Passion fruit, frozen (*Goya*), ⅓ pkg.	15.0	2.0
Passion fruit juice:		
(*Ceres*), 8 fl. oz.	31.0	0
fresh, purple, 8 fl. oz.	33.6	.5
fresh, yellow, 8 fl. oz.	35.7	.5
Passion fruit juice blend, apple and carrot (*Bolthouse Farms*),		
8 fl. oz.	29.0	2.0
Passion fruit nectar (*Goya*), 12 fl. oz.	57.0	0
Passion fruit syrup (*Trader Vic's*), 2 tbsp.	21.0	0
Pasta (see also "Macaroni" and "Noodles"), dry, 2 oz., except as noted:		
plain	42.6	1.4
all styles:		
(*Delverde*)	41.0	1.0
(*Venecia*)	41.0	2.0

Food and Measure	carb. (gms)	fiber (gms)
unflavored (*DeBoles*)	41.0	1.0
unflavored (*DeBoles* Organic)	43.0	1.0
veggie (*Hodgson Mills*)	41.0	1.0
alphabets, vegetable (*Eden* Organic)	40.0	2.0
angel hair:		
garlic and parsley or tomato and basil (*DeBoles*)	41.0	2.0
garlic and parsley (*DeBoles* Organic)	42.0	2.0
tomato and basil (*DeBoles* Organic)	43.0	2.0
tomato and pesto (*DeBoles* Organic)	42.0	1.0
artichoke ribbons (*Eden* Organic)	40.0	2.0
elbows, whole wheat (*Hodgson Mill*)	40.0	6.0
extra fine (*Eden* Organic)	40.0	3.0
corn, angel hair (*Westbrae Natural*)	46.0	0
corn, elbow or spaghetti (*DeBoles*)	43.0	5.0
gemelli twists, pesto (*Eden* Organic)	41.0	4.0
quinoa/kamut (*Eden* Organic)	42.0	5.0
lasagna, spinach (*Westbrae Natural* Organic), 2 pieces	35.0	8.0
lasagna, whole wheat (*Westbrae Natural* Organic), 2 pieces	34.0	7.0
mung bean (*Eden* Harusame)	47.0	0
penne (*Annie's* Organic)	41.0	2.0
penne, whole wheat (*Annie's* Organic)	41.0	5.0
ribbons:		
parsley garlic, pesto, saffron, or vegetable (*Eden* Organic)	40.0	3.0
spelt (*Eden* Organic)	41.0	5.0
spinach (*Eden* Organic)	41.0	4.0
yolkless, whole wheat (*Hodgson Mill*)	34.0	5.0
rice:		
(*Eden* Bifun)	44.0	0
all styles, except lasagna (*DeBoles*)	46.0	<1.0
lasagna (*DeBoles*), ¼ pkg., 2.5 oz.	56.0	1.0
rotini, spaghetti, or penne (*Lundberg* Organic)	44.0	3.0
rigatoni (*Eden* Organic Endless Tubes)	41.0	4.0
rotini (*Annie's* Organic)	41.0	2.0
shells, vegetable (*Eden* Organic)	40.0	3.0
shells, vegetable, small (*Eden* Organic)	40.0	4.0

Food and Measure	carb. (gms)	fiber (gms)
spaghetti:		
(*Annie's* Organic)	41.0	2.0
garlic parsley (*Eden* Organic)	41.0	4.0
kamut (*Eden* Organic)	38.0	6.0
semolina (*Eden* Organic)	40.0	2.0
spinach (*Westbrae Natural* Organic)	38.0	8.0
spinach, whole wheat (*Hodgson Mill*)	35.0	5.0
whole grain, 60% (*Eden* Organic)	41.0	4.0
whole grain, 100% (*Eden* Organic)	40.0	6.0
whole wheat (*Annie's* Organic)	41.0	5.0
whole wheat (*Westbrae Natural* Organic)	39.0	9.0
spelt, white (*Vita Spelt*)	42.0	2.0
spelt, whole grain (*Vita Spelt*)	40.0	5.0
spinach, fettuccine or spaghetti (*DeBoles* Organic)	43.0	0
spirals:		
flax rice (*Eden* Organic)	40.0	4.0
kamut (*Eden* Organic)	33.0	6.0
kamut vegetable (*Eden* Organic)	40.0	6.0
mixed grain (*Eden* Organic)	41.0	7.0
rye (*Eden* Organic)	44.0	8.0
spinach (*Eden* Organic)	41.0	4.0
vegetable (*Eden* Organic)	40.0	3.0
whole wheat, all styles:		
(*DeBoles* Organic)	42.0	5.0
except elbows, spinach spaghetti and yolkless ribbons (*Hodgson Mill*)	34.0	6.0
with flax seed (*Hodgson Mill* Organic)	40.0	6.0
ziti rigati, garlic parsley or spelt (*Eden* Organic)	41.0	5.0
Pasta, cooked (see also "Macaroni"):		
corn, 1 cup	39.1	3.4
spaghetti, 1 cup:		
plain	39.7	2.4
protein fortified	44.3	2.4
spinach	36.6	n.a.
whole wheat	37.2	6.3
Pasta, refrigerated (see also specific listings):		
uncooked:		
with egg, 2 oz.	31.0	2.0

Food and Measure	carb. (gms)	fiber (gms)
spinach (*Azumaya*), 1 cup	42.0	2.0
spinach, with egg, 2 oz.	31.6	n.a.
cooked, with egg, 4 oz.	28.3	n.a.
cooked, spinach, with egg, 4 oz.	28.4	n.a.
Pasta dish, frozen, see "Pasta entree, frozen" and specific pasta listings		
Pasta dish, mix (see also "Pasta salad mix" and specific pasta listings), 1 cup*:		
butter and herb (*Annie's* Organic)	43.0	2.0
with cheese (*Annie's* Bunny)	49.0	1.0
with cheese, Parmesan (*Annie's* Peace Pasta)	48.0	1.0
garlic, roasted, and herb (*Annie's* Organic)	39.0	2.0
Parmesan (*Annie's* Organic)	45.0	2.0
Pasta entree, can or pkg. (see also specific listings):		
Alfredo (*Bowl Appétit!*), 1 cont.	52.0	1.0
chicken flavored (*Bowl Appétit!* Homestyle), 1 cont.	42.0	2.0
garden salsa (*Hormel* Pasta Cup), 1 cont.	23.0	2.0
Italian style (*Hormel* Pasta Cup), 1 cont.	26.0	1.0
lemon pepper (*Hormel* Bowl), 10 oz.	33.0	2.0
lemon pepper (*Hormel* Pasta Cup), 1 cont.	25.0	2.0
Mediterranean (*Hormel* Pasta Cup), 1 cont.	24.0	2.0
pesto primavera, vegetarian (*Fantastic Carb'Tastic*), 1 cont.	22.0	14.0
tomato cheese sauce, 1 cup:		
(*Annie's* Organic All Stars/BernieO's)	31.0	<1.0
(*Annie's Arthur* Organic Loops)	32.0	1.0
with soy "meatballs" (*Annie's* Organic P'Sghetti Loops)	29.0	2.0
Pasta entree, freeze-dried, 1 serving:		
primavera:		
(*Mountain House* Can/Four), 1 cup	32.0	2.0
(*Mountain House* Double), ½ pouch	42.0	3.0
(*Mountain House* Single)	52.0	3.0
Roma (*AlpineAire*)	54.0	3.0
Pasta entree, frozen (see also specific listings), 1 pkg., except as noted:		
Alfredo:		
broccoli (*Green Giant*), 9 oz.	38.0	3.0
broccoli (*Green Giant Pasta Accents*), 1 cup cooked . . .	34.0	3.0

Food and Measure	carb. (gms)	fiber (gms)
chicken and broccoli (*Lean Cuisine Everyday Favorites*), 10 oz.	38.0	3.0
broccoli, Parmesan (*Moosewood*), 10 oz.	48.0	3.0
cheese, three (*Green Giant*), 9 oz.	40.0	3.0
with chicken, wine/mushroom sauce (*Michelina's Lean Gourmet*), 8.5 oz.	46.0	3.0
and beans (*Moosewood* Pasta e Fagioli), 10 oz.	47.0	6.0
peanut, spicy, with vegetarian chicken (*Linda McCartney*), 10 oz.	44.0	4.0
portobello mushroom (*Uncle Ben's* Pasta Bowl Savory), 12 oz.	43.0	3.0
primavera:		
(*Amy's*), 9 oz.	37.0	3.0
(*Green Giant*), 9 oz.	39.0	3.0
(*Michelina's* Zap'ems), 8 oz.	36.0	2.0
with vegetables:		
cheese sauce (*Amy's* Bowls Country Cheddar), 9.5 oz.	41.0	4.0
cheese sauce, creamy (*Birds Eye*), 1 cup	27.0	1.0
garlic, roasted (*Green Giant*), 9 oz.	41.0	3.0
wheels and cheese (*Michelina's* Zap'ems), 8 oz.	48.0	3.0
Pasta flour, see "Semolina flour"		
Pasta salad, refrigerated, Italian (*Reser's*), ½ cup	18.0	3.0
Pasta salad mix:		
(*Suddenly Salad* Classic), approx. 1 cup*	37.0	2.0
Caesar (*Suddenly Salad*), approx. 1 cup*	34.0	1.0
Parmesan, creamy (*Suddenly Salad*), approx. 1 cup*	30.0	1.0
Parmesan, roasted garlic (*Suddenly Salad*), ¾ cup*	34.0	1.0
ranch and bacon (*Suddenly Salad*), ¾ cup*	31.0	1.0
Pasta salad sauce mix, dry:		
Mediterranean (*McCormick*), 1 tbsp.	4.0	0
vinaigrette (*McCormick*), 1 tsp.	2.0	0
Pasta sauce (see also "Tomato sauce" and specific sauce listings), tomato, ½ cup, except as noted:		
(*Amy's* Pomodoro Zucca)	6.0	1.0
(*Del Monte* Traditional)	15.0	3.0
(*Eden* Organic/*Eden* Organic No Salt)	12.0	3.0
(*Healthy Choice* Traditional)	13.0	3.0
(*Hunt's* Light/No Sugar)	9.0	3.0

Food and Measure	carb. (gms)	fiber (gms)
(*Hunt's* Traditional)	10.0	3.0
(*Prego* Chunky Garden)	17.0	3.0
(*Prego* Traditional)	19.0	3.0
(*Prego* Traditional Plastic)	20.0	3.0
(*Ragú* Old World Traditional)	8.0	2.0
(*Red Pack* Spaghetti)	11.0	2.0
(*Tree of Life* Classic Tomato Fat Free/Pasta Sauce)	9.0	<1.0
arrabiata (*Mama Capri*)	6.0	2.0
arrabiata (*Pasta Cosi*)	6.0	1.0
basil, tomato:		
(*Amy's*)	11.0	3.0
(*Classico* di Napoli)	11.0	2.0
(*Del Monte*)	16.0	3.0
(*Muir Glen*)	12.0	0
(*Newman's Own* Bombolina)	13.0	<1.0
(*Walnut Acres*)	9.0	1.0
(*Walnut Acres* Low Sodium)	9.0	<1.0
basil and garlic (*Mama Capri* Basilico)	5.0	2.0
basil and garlic (*Prego*)	17.0	3.0
beef, with onion, garlic (*Classico* Bolognese)	14.0	3.0
with cheese:		
five (*Newman's Own*)	10.0	<1.0
four (*Classico* di Parma)	10.0	1.0
four (*Del Monte*)	15.0	3.0
four (*Hunt's*)	10.0	3.0
three (*Prego*)	17.0	3.0
with cheese and garlic (*Hunt's*)	9.0	2.0
chicken, roasted, with Parmesan and garlic		
(*Classico* di Romagna)	13.0	2.0
garlic (*Prego* Supreme)	17.0	3.0
garlic (*Walnut Acres* Garlic-Garlic)	10.0	1.0
garlic, roasted:		
(*Amy's*)	13.0	3.0
(*Classico* di Sorrento)	11.0	2.0
(*Muir Glen*)	10.0	0
(*Pasta Cosi*)	9.0	2.0
(*Walnut Acres*)	11.0	1.0
and herb (*Prego*)	17.0	2.0

Food and Measure	carb. (gms)	fiber (gms)
and onion (*Hunt's*)	10.0	3.0
Parmesan (*Prego*)	20.0	3.0
and peppers (*Newman's Own*)	11.0	4.0
tomato and (*Newman's Own*)	11.0	<1.0
garlic and:		
basil (*Prego* Pasta Bake), ⅛ jar	11.0	2.0
herb (*Del Monte* Chunky)	11.0	<1.0
herb (*Healthy Choice*)	13.0	3.0
herb (*Hunt's*)	8.0	3.0
mushroom (*Amy's*)	10.0	3.0
onion (*Del Monte*)	16.0	2.0
onion (*Muir Glen*)	12.0	0
onion (*Ragú* Chunky)	21.0	2.0
green pepper and mushroom (*Del Monte*)	16.0	3.0
herb:		
(*Muir Glen/Muir Glen* Italian)	12.0	0
Italian (*Del Monte* Chunky)	12.0	<1.0
seven (*Ragú Robusto*)	12.0	2.0
hot and spicy (*Newman's Own* Fra Diavolo)	10.0	0
marinara:		
(*Amy's* Family)	8.0	3.0
(*Amy's* Low Sodium)	7.0	1.0
(*Mama Capri*)	5.0	2.0
(*Newman's Own*)	12.0	<1.0
(*Pasta Cosi*)	6.0	1.0
(*Prego*)	11.0	4.0
(*Red Pack*)	8.0	6.0
basil, sweet (*Classico* di Campania)	13.0	1.0
Cabernet (*Muir Glen*)	11.0	0
Cabernet, with herbs (*Classico* di Piedmont)	10.0	2.0
with cheese (*Prego*)	11.0	4.0
cheese, three (*Prego* Pasta Bake), ⅛ jar	11.0	2.0
with herbs or zinfadel (*Walnut Acres*)	9.0	1.0
mushroom (*Newman's Own*)	12.0	<1.0
with mushroom (*Prego*)	11.0	4.0
meat:		
(*Del Monte*)	14.0	3.0
(*Hunt's*)	11.0	3.0

Food and Measure	carb. (gms)	fiber (gms)
(*Prego*)	19.0	3.0
(*Prego* Pasta Bakes Hearty), ⅛ jar	12.0	2.0
(*Ragú* Old World)	7.0	2.0
(*Ragú* Rich & Meaty)	10.0	2.0
with fresh mushrooms (*Prego Hearty Meat* Classic)	14.0	2.0
three (*Prego Hearty Meat* Supreme)	12.0	3.0
with meatballs, mini (*Prego*)	20.0	3.0
with meatballs, Parmesan (*Prego Hearty Meat*)	16.0	2.0
mushroom:		
(*Del Monte*)	14.0	2.0
(*Hunt's*)	10.0	3.0
(*Prego* Chunky Garden Supreme)	20.0	4.0
(*Prego* Zesty)	18.0	3.0
(*Ragú* Old World)	8.0	2.0
fresh (*Prego*)	18.0	3.0
fresh (*Prego* Plastic)	21.0	3.0
marinara (*Muir Glen*)	10.0	0
portobello (*Muir Glen*)	11.0	0
tomato and (*Walnut Acres*)	9.0	1.0
triple (*Classico* di Toscana)	12.0	3.0
wild (*Amy's*)	7.0	2.0
mushroom and:		
garlic (*Healthy Choice* Super Chunky)	10.0	3.0
garlic (*Prego*)	20.0	2.0
green pepper (*Prego* Chunky Garden)	17.0	4.0
olive, ripe (*Classico* di Sicillia)	11.0	2.0
Parmesan (*Prego*)	22.0	3.0
onion:		
diced, and garlic (*Prego*)	18.0	3.0
and garlic (*Prego* Chunky Garden)	18.0	4.0
and garlic (*Tree of Life* Fat Free)	8.0	<1.0
roasted, balsamic (*Muir Glen*)	12.0	0
pepper, red:		
roasted, and garlic (*Prego*)	19.0	3.0
spicy (*Classico* di Roma Arrabbiata)	7.0	2.0
tomatoes and spices (*Newman's Own*)	12.0	<1.0
pepper, sweet (*Tree of Life* Fat Free)	8.0	<1.0

Food and Measure	carb. (gms)	fiber (gms)
pepper, sweet, and onion (*Walnut Acres*)	9.0	1.0
puttanesca (*Amy's*)	5.0	1.0
puttanesca (*Pasta Cosi*)	6.0	1.0
ricotta Parmesan (*Prego*)	20.0	3.0
sausage, Italian:		
(*Hunt's*)	10.0	3.0
(*Prego* Pasta Bakes), ⅛ jar	12.0	3.0
(*Prego Hearty Meat*)	16.0	2.0
and garlic (*Prego*)	16.0	3.0
with pepper, onion (*Classico* d'Abruzzi)	13.0	2.0
spinach and cheese (*Classico* di Firenze)	6.0	2.0
steak, hearty, with Burgundy (*Classico*)	13.0	3.0
tomato:		
fire-roasted, and garlic (*Classico* di Siena)	10.0	2.0
spicy, and pesto (*Classico* di Genoa)	11.0	2.0
sun-dried (*Classico* di Capri)	11.0	2.0
sun-dried (*Muir Glen*)	10.0	0
vegetable:		
chunky (*Hunt's*)	11.0	3.0
garden (*Muir Glen*)	10.0	0
garden, primavera (*Classico* di Lazio)	11.0	2.0
primavera (*Healthy Choice* Super Chunky)	13.0	3.0
vodka:		
(*Bove's*)	7.0	1.0
(*Mama Capri*)	5.0	2.0
(*Newman's Own*)	11.0	0
(*Pasta Cosi*)	8.0	2.0
Pasta-sauce, refrigerated (see also specific sauce listings), tomato, ½ cup:		
marinara:		
(*DiGiorno*)	15.0	2.0
garlic, roasted (*Buitoni*)	9.0	1.0
regular or portobello mushroom (*Buitoni*)	11.0	2.0
tomato herb Parmesan (*Buitoni*)	9.0	2.0
Pasta sauce mix, dry, 1 tbsp., except as noted:		
(*Lawry's* Spaghetti Extra Rich & Thick)	7.0	<1.0
(*Lawry's* Spaghetti Original), 1½ tbsp.	6.0	0
(*McCormick* Pasta Rosa)	4.0	0

Food and Measure	carb. (gms)	fiber (gms)
herb and garlic (*McCormick*)	2.0	0
primavera (*McCormick*)	4.0	0
spaghetti sauce (*McCormick* Thick & Zesty)	6.0	0
spaghetti sauce, Italian style or mild (*McCormick*)	5.0	0
tomato basil (*McCormick*)	5.0	0
Pastrami, beef, 2 oz., except as noted:		
(*Black Bear* Brisket)	2.0	0
(*Boar's Head* Brisket)	2.0	0
(*Boar's Head* Red/Round/Top Round Cap-off)	1.0	0
(*Dietz & Watson* Brisket)	0	0
(*Healthy Choice*)	2.0	0
(*Healthy Choice Deli Thin*), 4 slices, 1.8 oz.	2.0	0
(*Healthy Deli*)	3.0	0
(*Hebrew National*)	1.0	0
(*Hormel*)	0	0
(*Sara Lee*)	1.0	0
(*Sara Lee* Pre-sliced), 2 slices, 1.6 oz.	0	0
(*Tyson* Bag), 2 slices, 2.25 oz.	0	0
Pastry, puff (see also "Fillo dough" and "Pie crust"):		
frozen (*Kineret* Ready To Bake), 2-oz. sq.	20.0	<1.0
patty shell (*Pepperidge Farm*), 1 piece	16.0	<1.0
sheet (*Pepperidge Farm*), 1/6 sheet	14.0	<1.0
Pastry filling (see also "Pie filling"), canned, 2 tbsp.:		
almond (*Solo*)	23.0	2.0
apple, Dutch, or cherry (*Solo*)	20.0	1.0
apricot or blueberry (*Solo*)	17.0	1.0
date (*Solo*)	22.0	3.0
nut, fancy (*Solo*)	25.0	5.0
pecan (*Solo*)	24.0	1.0
pineapple or raspberry (*Solo*)	19.0	1.0
poppy seed (*Solo*)	30.0	3.0
prune plum or strawberry (*Solo*)	18.0	1.0
Pâté, can or jar:		
2 oz.	.6	0
1 tbsp.	.2	0
chicken liver, 2 oz.	3.7	0
chicken liver, 1 tbsp.	.9	0
goose liver, smoked, 2 oz.	2.6	0

Food and Measure	carb. (gms)	fiber (gms)
goose liver, smoked, 1 tbsp.	.6	0
truffle flavor, 2 oz.	3.5	0
Pâté, refrigerated (see also "Salmon pâté"), 2 oz.:		
duck mousse, with truffles (*Chef Georges*)	5.0	0
duck mousse, with truffles and port wine (*Marcel & Henri*)	<1.0	0
with goose fat and liver (*Schaller & Weber*)	1.0	0
pork, with champagne (*Marcel & Henri* Pâté de Campagne)	1.0	<1.0
Pea pods, see "Peas, edible-podded"		
Peach, fresh:		
(*Del Monte*), 1 medium, 3.5 oz.	10.0	2.0
(*Dole*), 1 medium, 3.5 oz.	10.0	2.0
(*Frieda's Donut/Frieda's* Late Season), 5 oz.	16.0	3.0
2½'' peach, 4 per lb.	9.7	1.7
sliced, 1 cup	18.9	3.4
Peach, can or jar, halves or slices, ½ cup, except as noted:		
(*Del Monte Carb Clever*)	7.0	1.0
diced (*Dole Fruit Bowls*), 4 oz.	16.0	1.0
in juice:		
(*Del Monte/Del Monte Fruit Naturals*)	15.0	1.0
(*S&W* Natural Style)	19.0	1.0
chunks (*Del Monte Fruit Naturals*)	17.0	<1.0
diced (*Del Monte Fruit Naturals Fruit Cup*), 4.5 oz.	13.0	<1.0
with liquid	14.5	1.6
in extra light syrup:		
(*Del Monte* Lite Cling)	15.0	1.0
(*Del Monte* Lite Freestone)	14.0	1.0
diced (*Del Monte Fruit Cup* Lite), 4.5 oz.	13.0	<1.0
in gelatin:		
peach gel (*Del Monte*), 4.5-oz. cup	22.0	0
raspberry gel (*Del Monte*), 4.5-oz. cup	23.0	0
strawberry-banana (*Del Monte* Lite), 4.5-oz. cup	14.0	0
in light syrup:		
(*Del Monte Orchard Select*)	20.0	<1.0
(*S&W*)	17.0	1.0
with liquid	18.3	1.6
raspberry flavor (*Del Monte*)	20.0	<1.0
spiced (*Del Monte* Harvest Spice)	21.0	<1.0
strawberry-banana flavor (*Del Monte*)	17.0	<1.0

Food and Measure	carb. (gms)	fiber (gms)
in light syrup, chunks:		
(*S&W* Sun)	20.0	1.0
(*S&W* Tropical)	19.0	<1.0
cinnamon (*Del Monte*)	20.0	1.0
cinnamon, brown sugar (*S&W* Sweet Memory)	19.0	<1.0
hybrid (*S&W* Snow)	20.0	1.0
raspberry flavor (*Del Monte*)	20.0	<1.0
in heavy syrup:		
(*Del Monte*)	24.0	1.0
(*S&W*)	24.0	1.0
with liquid	26.1	1.7
diced (*Del Monte*)	20.0	<1.0
diced (*Del Monte Fruit Cup*), 4.5 oz.	20.0	<1.0
spiced, whole (*Del Monte*)	24.0	<1.0
Peach, dried:		
(*Sun•Maid*), ¼ cup	25.0	3.0
(*Sunsweet*), 3 pieces, 1.4 oz.	25.0	3.0
sulfured, halves, ½ cup	49.1	6.6
sulfured, 10 halves, 4.6 oz.	79.7	10.7
Peach, freeze-dried, diced (*AlpineAire*), .4 oz.	9.0	0
Peach, frozen, sliced:		
(*Cascadian Farm*), 1 cup	14.0	1.0
(*C&W*), ⅔ cup	13.0	2.0
sweetened, ½ cup	30.0	1.8
Peach drink:		
(*Snapple* Summer Peach), 8 fl. oz.	30.0	0
(*Snapple-a-Day*), 11.5 fl. oz.	43.0	5.0
(*Walnut Acres*), 8 fl. oz.	32.0	0
nectar:		
(*Goya*), 6 fl. oz.	27.0	1.0
(*Goya*), 12 fl. oz.	54.0	2.0
(*R.W. Knudsen*), 8 fl. oz.	30.0	0
(*Santa Cruz Organic*), 8 fl. oz.	29.0	0
canned, 8 fl. oz.	34.7	1.5
Peach dumpling, frozen (*Pepperidge Farm*), 3-oz. piece	50.0	4.0
Peach glaze (*Litehouse*), 3 tbsp.	18.0	0
Peach juice:		

Food and Measure	carb. (gms)	fiber (gms)
(*After the Fall* Georgia), 8 fl. oz.	31.0	0
(*Ceres*), 8 fl. oz.	30.0	0
Peach nectar, see "Peach drink"		
Peach-mango drink (*V8 Splash* Smoothies), 8 fl. oz.	27.0	0
Peach-orange juice, (*Nantucket Nectars*), 8 fl. oz.	31.0	0
Peanuts, shelled, 1 oz., except as noted:		
(*Beer Nuts* Kettle Cooked)	6.0	2.0
(*Beer Nuts* Original)	7.0	2.0
(*Frito Lay* Salted)	6.0	2.0
(*Planters* Cocktail/Unsalted)	6.0	2.0
(*Planters* Cocktail Lightly Salted)	5.0	2.0
(*Shiloh Farms* Raw Redskin), ¼ cup	7.0	3.0
barbecue (*Beer Nuts* Crunch Nuts)	18.0	2.0
boiled, salted	6.0	2.5
Cajun (*Beer Nuts* Crunch Nuts)	15.0	1.0
dry-roasted:		
(*Fisher*)	6.0	2.0
(*Planters*), 1.75-oz. pkg.	9.0	4.0
(*Planters* Lightly Salted)	5.0	2.0
(*Planters/Planters* Unsalted)	6.0	2.0
½ cup	15.7	5.8
honey (*Planters*)	8.0	2.0
glazed (*Beer Nuts* Old Fashioned)	6.0	2.0
honey mustard (*Beer Nuts* Crunch Nuts)	19.0	1.0
honey roasted:		
(*Fisher*)	7.0	2.0
(*Kettle*)	8.0	2.0
(*Planters*)	8.0	2.0
hot and spicy (*D.L. Jardine's* Texacali), ¼ cup	5.0	2.0
hot and spicy (*Frito Lay*), 1.1 oz.	6.0	2.0
oil-roasted (*Fisher*)	6.0	2.0
oil-roasted, ½ cup	13.6	6.6
sesame (*Beer Nuts* Crunch Nuts)	15.0	2.0
Spanish:		
(*Kettle* Jumbo Salted)	5.0	2.0
(*Planters* Redskin)	5.0	2.0
raw (*Kettle*)	4.0	3.0
raw (*Planters*)	6.0	3.0

Food and Measure	carb. (gms)	fiber (gms)
sweet and crunchy (*Planters*)	16.0	2.0
sweet and crunchy, honey-roasted (*Planters*)	6.0	2.0
Peanut butter (see also "Peanut Spread"), 2 tbsp.:		
(*Simply Jif*)	6.0	2.0
chunky or creamy:		
(*Arrowhead Mills*)	6.0	2.0
(*Smucker's*)	6.0	2.0
(*Tree of Life/Tree of Life* No Salt)	7.0	1.0
blended (*Tree of Life*)	7.0	2.0
chunky/crunchy:		
(*Jif* Reduced Fat)	15.0	2.0
(*Reese's*)	7.0	2.0
(*Skippy Super Chunk*)	7.0	2.0
(*Skippy Super Chunk* Reduced Fat)	14.0	2.0
extra (*Jif*)	7.0	2.0
creamy:		
(*Jif*)	7.0	2.0
(*Jif* Reduced Fat)	15.0	2.0
(*Reese's*)	8.0	2.0
(*Skippy*)	7.0	2.0
(*Skippy* Natural)	6.0	2.0
(*Skippy* Reduced Fat)	15.0	2.0
(*Skippy Carb Options*)	5.0	2.0
(*Smucker's* No Salt)	6.0	2.0
(*Smucker's* Reduced Fat)	12.0	2.0
honey:		
(*Smucker's*)	9.0	2.0
creamy (*Jif*)	11.0	2.0
roasted, chunky or creamy (*Skippy*)	7.0	2.0
Peanut butter baking chips, 1 tbsp., .5 oz.:		
(*Hershey's Bake Shoppe Reese's*)	8.0	<1.0
and milk (*Hershey's Bake Shoppe Reese's*)	8.0	0
Peanut butter sprinkles (*Reese's*) 2 tbsp.	12.0	<1.0
Peanut butter topping (*Reese's* Shell), 2 tbsp.	17.0	1.0
Peanut butter–jelly, grape or strawberry (*Smucker's*		
Goober), 3 tbsp.	24.0	2.0
Peanut butter–jelly sandwich, frozen, grape or strawberry		
(*Smucker's Uncrustables*), 2-oz. piece	25.0	2.0

Food and Measure	carb. (gms)	fiber (gms)
Peanut coating mix (*Thai Kitchen* Peanut Bake), dry,		
.75 oz.	13.9	0
Peanut flour, 1 cup:		
defatted	20.8	9.5
low fat	18.8	9.5
Peanut sauce, 2 tbsp., except as noted:		
(*Annie Chun's*)	10.0	1.0
(*Heaven and Earth*), 1 tbsp.	5.0	0
(*San-J* Thai)	7.0	1.0
satay:		
(*A Taste of Thai*)	9.0	1.0
(*Thai Kitchen*)	7.0	<1.0
spicy (*Thai Kitchen*)	8.0	0
Peanut sauce mix:		
(*Thai Kitchen*), ¼ cup*	7.0	0
plain or spicy Thai bake (*A Taste of Thai*), ¼ pkg.	7.0	1.0
Peanut spread (see also "Peanut butter") (*Peanut Wonder/*		
Peanut Wonder Low Sodium), 2 tbsp.	13.0	0
Pear, fresh, with peel:		
(*Del Monte*), 1 medium, 5.9 oz.	25.0	4.0
(*Dole*), 1 medium, 5.9 oz.	25.0	4.0
1 large, 2 per lb.	31.6	5.0
Bartlett, 1 medium, 2½ per lb.	25.1	4.0
sliced, ½ cup	12.5	2.0
Pear, Asian:		
(*Frieda's*), 5 oz.	15.0	5.0
1 medium, 2¼'' × 2½'' diam.	13.0	4.4
Pear, can or jar, halves or slices, ½ cup, except		
as noted:		
(*Del Monte Carb Clever*)	10.0	1.0
in juice:		
(*Del Monte/Del Monte Fruit Naturals*)	15.0	1.0
(*S&W* Natural Style)	21.0	2.0
with liquid	16.0	2.0
in extra-light syrup:		
(*Del Monte* Lite)	15.0	1.0
diced (*Del Monte* Lite), 4-oz. can	13.0	<1.0
diced (*Del Monte Fruit Cup* Lite), 4.5 oz.	13.0	<1.0

Food and Measure	carb. (gms)	fiber (gms)
in light syrup:		
(*Del Monte Orchard Select*)	20.0	2.0
(*S&W*)	19.0	2.0
with liquid	19.0	2.0
chunks (*S&W* Sun)	20.0	<1.0
cinnamon (*Del Monte*)	21.0	1.0
ginger (*Del Monte*)	22.0	1.0
in heavy syrup:		
(*Del Monte*)	24.0	1.0
(*S&W*)	24.0	1.0
with liquid	25.5	2.1
diced (*Del Monte*), 4-oz. can	20.0	<1.0
diced (*Del Monte Fruit Cup*), 4.5 oz.	20.0	<1.0
Pear, dried:		
2 oz.	39.5	4.3
sulfured, halves, ½ cup	62.7	6.8
sulfured, stewed, ½ cup	43.1	8.2
Pear juice, 8 fl. oz.:		
(*Ceres*)	30.0	0
(*R.W. Knudsen* Organic)	30.0	0
sparkling (*R.W. Knudsen*)	29.0	0
Pear nectar:		
(*Goya*), 12 fl. oz.	59.0	2.0
(*Santa Cruz Organic*), 8 fl. oz.	30.0	0
canned, 8 fl. oz.	39.4	1.5
Peas, see specific listings		
Peas, black-eyed, see "Black-eyed peas"		
Peas, cream, canned (*East Texas Fair*), ½ cup	17.0	5.0
Peas, crowder, canned, ½ cup:		
(*Allens/East Texas Fair*)	19.0	8.0
(*Bush's*)	18.0	5.0
Peas, edible-podded, fresh:		
raw (*Frieda's* Snow), 1 cup, 3 oz.	6.0	2.0
raw, in pods (*Frieda's* Sugar Snap), ⅔ cup, 3 oz.	6.0	2.0
raw, with sauce (*Frieda's* Snow/Sugar Snap), ½ cup	8.0	2.0
boiled, drained, ½ cup	5.6	2.2
Peas, edible-podded, frozen:		
snow peas (*C&W* Baby Pea Pods), ⅔ cup	7.0	3.0

Food and Measure	carb. (gms)	fiber (gms)
sugar snap:		
(*Birds Eye*), ²/₃ cup	7.0	2.0
(*Cascadian Farm* Bag/Box), ¾ cup	6.0	2.0
(*C&W Sugar Snap*), ²/₃ cup	6.0	2.0
(*Green Giant*), ½ cup	10.0	3.0
(*Green Giant Select*), ¾ cup	7.0	3.0
boiled, drained, ½ cup	7.2	2.5
Peas, edible-podded, combinations, frozen, sugar snap, 1 cup:		
baby carrots, cauliflower, broccoli (*C&W*)	5.0	2.0
stir-fry, with carrots, onion, mushrooms (*Birds Eye*)	7.0	2.0
Peas, field, canned, (see also "Peas, crowder" and "Peas, purple hull"), ½ cup:		
with bacon (*Trappey's*)	15.0	5.0
with jalapeños (*East Texas Fair* Pepper Peas)	22.0	6.0
with pork (*East Texas Fair* Peas & Pork)	19.0	5.0
seasoned (*Glory*)	14.0	4.0
with snaps:		
(*Allens East Texas Fair/Sunshine*)	21.0	6.0
(*Bush's*)	17.0	5.0
and bacon (*Trappey's*)	19.0	4.0
seasoned (*Glory*)	12.0	5.0
Peas, field, frozen (*McKenzie's*), ½ cup	21.0	4.0
Peas, green, fresh:		
raw, in pod, 1 lb.	24.9	8.8
raw, shelled, ½ cup	10.4	3.7
boiled, drained, ½ cup	12.5	4.4
Peas, green, can or jar, ½ cup:		
(*Del Monte*)	13.0	4.0
(*Del Monte* No Salt)	11.0	4.0
(*Del Monte* Very Young Small)	10.0	4.0
(*Freshlike* Selects Petite)	16.0	5.0
(*Freshlike* Tender Garden/No Salt)	19.0	6.0
(*Green Giant/Green Giant* 50% Less Sodium)	11.0	3.0
(*LeSueur*)	12.0	3.0
(*S&W* Petit Pois)	10.0	4.0
(*S&W* Young)	13.0	4.0
(*Veg-All* Tender)	10.0	3.0

Food and Measure	carb. (gms)	fiber (gms)
(*Westbrae Natural* Organic)	10.0	3.0
drained	10.7	3.5
in onion sauce (*Glory* Creamed Peas)	13.0	3.0
seasoned, with liquid	10.5	2.8
Peas, green, combinations, can or jar:		
and carrots, ½ cup:		
(*Del Monte*)	11.0	2.0
(*Freshlike*)	11.0	3.0
(*S&W*)	11.0	2.0
(*Veg-All*)	12.0	4.0
with liquid	10.8	2.6
and onions, ½ cup:		
(*Freshlike* Selects)	11.0	3.0
(*Green Giant*)	11.0	3.0
(*S&W*)	11.0	3.0
with liquid	5.1	1.4
Peas, green, combinations, frozen:		
and carrots:		
(*Cascadian Farm*), ⅔ cup	10.0	3.0
(*C&W Early Harvest* Petite/Baby), ⅔ cup	12.0	3.0
boiled, drained, ½ cup	8.1	2.5
and pearl onions:		
(*Cascadian Farm*), ¾ cup	11.0	3.0
(*C&W* Petite), ⅔ cup	11.0	4.0
(*Green Giant*), ½ cup	10.0	3.0
baby (*Birds Eye*), ⅔ cup	12.0	3.0
baby, and vegetables (*Birds Eye*), ¾ cup	7.0	2.0
in sauce (*Birds Eye*), ⅔ cup	17.0	4.0
boiled, drained, ½ cup	7.8	2.0
Peas, green, dried:		
rehydrated (*Frieda's*), ⅓ cup, 3 oz.	22.0	9.0
wasabi (*Anne's House of Nuts*), ⅓ cup	17.0	2.0
Peas, green, freeze-dried:		
(*AlpineAire*), ¾ oz.	14.0	5.0
(*Mountain House* Can), ½ cup	14.0	5.0
Peas, green, frozen, ⅔ cup, except as noted:		
(*Birds Eye* Baby/Garden)	12.0	4.0
(*Cascadian Farm* Garden/Sweet)	12.0	4.0

Food and Measure	carb. (gms)	fiber (gms)
(*Cascadian Farm* Petite)	11.0	4.0
(*C&W Early Harvest*/Organic/Petite)	12.0	4.0
(*Green Giant* Baby Sweet/Sweet)	12.0	4.0
(*Green Giant Select* Early June)	11.0	4.0
(*Tree of Life*)	12.0	4.0
boiled, drained, ½ cup	11.4	4.4
Peas, pigeon, see "Pigeon peas"		
Peas, purple hull, canned, ½ cup:		
(*Allens/East Texas Fair*)	21.0	6.0
(*Bush's*)	18.0	5.0
Peas, purple hull, frozen (*McKenzie's*), ½ cup	21.0	4.0
Peas, split, see "Split peas"		
Peas, sprouted:		
raw, ½ cup	17.0	n.a.
boiled, drained, 4 oz.	24.8	3.7
Peas, sugar snap or snow, see "Peas, edible-podded"		
Peas, sweet, see "Peas, green"		
Peas, wasabi, see "Peas, green, dried"		
Peas, white acre, canned (*East Texas Fair*), ½ cup	17.0	5.0
Peas and carrots or onions, see "Peas, green, combinations"		
Pecan, shelled:		
(*Fisher*), 1 oz.	4.0	2.0
1 oz.	5.2	2.2
halves (*Shiloh Farms*), ⅓ cup, 1.2 oz.	6.0	3.0
halves, 1 cup	19.7	8.2
halves or pieces (*Planters*), 1 oz.	4.0	3.0
halves or pieces (*Planters*), 2-oz. pkg.	9.0	7.0
chips (*Planters*), 2-oz. pkg.	9.0	7.0
chopped, 1 cup	21.7	9.0
dry-roasted, unsalted, 1 oz.	3.8	2.7
dry-roasted, unsalted, 1 cup	14.9	10.5
oil-roasted, unsalted, 1 oz.	3.7	2.7
oil-roasted, unsalted, 1 cup	14.3	10.5
Pecan flour, 1 oz.	14.4	n.a.
Pecan topping, in syrup (*Smucker's* Spoonable), 1 tbsp.	20.0	0
Pectin, see "Fruit pectin"		
Penne, dry, see "Pasta"		
Penne entree, frozen, 1 pkg.:		

Food and Measure	carb. (gms)	fiber (gms)
(*Jeff Nathan Creations* Siciliano), 12 oz.	41.0	5.0
with chicken, see "Chicken entree, frozen"		
puttanesca, spicy (*Moosewood*), 10 oz.	45.0	2.0
with sauce and meatballs (*Organic Classics*), 10 oz.	45.0	4.0
with tomato (*Lean Cuisine Everyday Favorites*), 10 oz.	51.0	5.0
vegetarian (*Yves* Veggie), 10.5 oz.	36.0	4.0
Penne entree, pkg.:		
Alfredo (*Annie's*), 1 cup*	49.0	1.0
Alfredo (*Fantastic Carb'Tastic*), 8-oz. pkg.	25.0	21.0
"meat" sauce, vegetarian (*Fantastic Carb'Tastic*), 8-oz. pkg.	22.0	14.0
tomato Parmesan (*Bowl Appétit!*), 1 cont.	59.0	2.0
Pepeao, raw, sliced, 1 cup	6.7	n.a.
Pepeao, dried, 1 cup	19.5	n.a.
Peppadew (*Frieda's*), ⅓ cup, 1.1 oz.	10.0	3.0
Pepper, seasoning:		
black, ground, 1 tsp.	1.7	.7
black, whole, 1 tsp.	1.9	.8
chili, 1 tsp.	1.2	.7
red or cayenne, 1 tsp.	1.0	.7
seasoned (*Lawry's*), ¼ tsp.	1.0	0
Szechuan blend (*McCormick*), ¼ tsp.	0	0
white, 1 tsp.	1.7	.2
Pepper, ancho, dried, .6-oz. pepper	8.7	3.7
Pepper, banana, fresh, 1.2-oz. piece	1.8	1.1
Pepper, banana, in jars, wax (*Fanci Food*), 2 pieces, 1 oz.	2.0	0
Pepper, bell, see "Pepper, sweet"		
Pepper, cherry, in jars:		
(*Fanci Food*), 2–3 pieces	0	0
(*Vlasic*), 2 pieces, 1 oz.	2.0	0
Pepper, cherry, stuffed, with proscuitto and provolone, marinated (*Boar's Head*), 2 oz.	1.0	0
Pepper, chili, fresh, green and red:		
1 medium, 1.6 oz.	4.3	.7
chopped, ½ cup	7.1	1.1
Pepper, chili, can or jar (see also specific listings):		
whole, green, 1 piece:		
(*Chi-Chi's*), 1.2 oz.	2.0	0
(*La Victoria*), 1.2 oz.	1.0	<1.0

Food and Measure	carb. (gms)	fiber (gms)
(*Las Palmas*), 1.2 oz.	2.0	1.0
(*Old El Paso*), 1.2 oz.	2.0	1.0
mild (*Zapata*)	1.0	0
large, 2.6 oz.	3.7	1.0
whole, green, ½ cup	3.2	1.2
chopped (*Old El Paso*), 2 tbsp.	1.0	1.0
chopped, with liquid, ½ cup	4.2	1.3
diced, green, 2 tbsp.:		
(*Chi-Chi's*)	2.0	0
(*La Victoria*)	<1.0	0
(*Las Palmas*)	1.0	1.0
mild (*Zapata*)	1.0	0
strips, green (*Las Palmas*), 1.3-oz. piece	2.0	1.0
Pepper, chili, dried:		
(*Frieda's* Ancho/Guajillo Chiles), .5 oz.	8.0	2.0
(*Frieda's* California Chiles), 2 tbsp.	2.0	0
(*Frieda's* Japones Chiles), .5 oz.	7.0	2.0
sun-dried, hot, 2 pieces	.8	.3
Pepper, Greek, golden (*Fanci Food*), 3 pieces	2.0	0
Pepper, green or red, sweet, see "Pepper, sweet"		
Pepper, güerito, in jars (*Embasa*), 7 pieces, 1.1 oz.	1.0	2.0
Pepper, Hungarian, fresh, .94-oz. piece	1.8	n.a.
Pepper, jalapeño, fresh, .5-oz. piece	.8	.4
Pepper, jalapeño, can or jar:		
whole:		
(*Chi-Chi's*), 2 pieces, 1.1 oz.	2.0	0
(*Herdez*), 3 pieces, 1.25 oz.	1.0	1.0
(*Las Palmas*), 2 pieces, 1.3 oz.	2.0	0
(*Old El Paso*), 2 pieces, .9 oz.	1.0	0
(*Zapata* Very Hot), 1½ pieces	1.0	0
chopped, with liquid, ¼ cup	1.2	.8
diced (*La Victoria*), 2 tbsp.	<1.0	0
diced (*Zapata*), 4 tbsp.	1.0	0
marinated (*La Victoria*), 1½ tbsp.	2.0	1.0
sliced:		
(*Herdez*), ¼ cup	1.0	0
(*La Victoria* Nacho), 14 pieces, 1.1 oz.	<1.0	0

Food and Measure	carb. (gms)	fiber (gms)
(*Las Palmas*), 3 tbsp.	2.0	0
(*Zapata* Nacho), 4 tbsp.	<1.0	0
with liquid, ¼ cup	1.6	.9
wheels (*Chi-Chi's*), ¼ cup	2.0	0
Pepper, pablanos, in jars (*Herdez*), ½ piece, 1.2 oz.	1.0	0
Pepper, pasilla, dried, 2 pieces, .5 oz.	7.2	3.8
Pepper, poblano, see "Pepper, chili, can or jar"		
Pepper, roasted, see "Pepper, sweet, can or jar"		
Pepper, Serrano, fresh:		
whole, .2-oz. piece	.4	.2
chopped, ½ cup	3.5	1.9
Pepper, Serrano, in jars (*Herdez*), 4 pieces, 1.25 oz.	1.0	0
Pepper, stuffed, entree, frozen, with beef, tomato sauce:		
(*Stouffer's*), 10-oz. pkg.	25.0	2.0
(*Stouffer's*), ½ of 15.5-oz. pkg.	21.0	2.0
(*Stouffer's* Family Style Recipes), ¼ of 32-oz. pkg.	20.0	2.0
Pepper, sweet, fresh:		
green and red:		
raw (*Dole*), 5.2-oz. piece	7.0	2.0
raw, 1 medium, 3¾" × 3" or ½ cup chopped	4.8	1.3
raw, sliced, 1 cup	5.9	1.7
boiled, drained, 1 medium	4.9	.9
boiled, drained, chopped, 1 tbsp.	.8	.1
boiled, drained, strips, ½ cup	4.6	.8
yellow, raw, 1 large, 5" × 3"	11.8	1.7
yellow, raw, 10 strips, 1.8 oz.	3.3	.5
Pepper, sweet, can or jar (see also "Pimento"), red:		
drained, ½ cup	2.7	.8
fire-roasted (*Pompeian*), ½ cup	5.0	1.0
fire-roasted with garlic, oil (*Paesana*), 2 tbsp.	2.0	0
roasted (*Frieda's*), 1-oz. piece	5.0	0
Pepper, sweet, freeze-dried, red or green, ¼ cup	1.1	.3
Pepper, sweet, frozen:		
sliced, stir-fry, with onion (*Birds Eye*), 1 cup	5.0	1.0
strips (*C&W*), ¾ cup	4.0	2.0
chopped, 1 oz.	1.2	.5
Pepper, tempero, see "Pepperoncini"		

Food and Measure	carb. (gms)	fiber (gms)
Pepper relish, 1 tbsp.:		
hot or sweet (*Cains*)	5.0	0
jalapeño (*Old El Paso*)	1.0	0
Pepper rings, marinated (*Vlasic*), 3 pieces, 1 oz.	1.0	0
Pepper sauce, see "Hot sauce," and specific listings		
Pepper spread, red, with eggplant and garlic (*Marco Polo*),		
2 tbsp.	2.0	<1.0
Pepper steak, see "Beef entree, frozen"		
Peppercorns, green (*Fanci Food*), 2 tbsp.	3.0	1.0
Pepperoncini:		
(*Krinos*), ¼ cup	2.0	0
(*Trappey's* Tempero), 1 oz.	1.0	0
(*Zorba*), 5 pieces, 1.1 oz.	2.0	0
Pepperoni, 1 oz., except as noted:		
(*Hansel 'n Gretel*), 2 oz.	2.0	0
(*Hormel* Chunk/Sliced/Twin/*Pillow Pack*)	0	0
(*Rosa Grande*)	0	0
sandwich style:		
(*Boar's Head*)	1.0	0
(*Fiorucci*)	1.0	0
(*Sara Lee* Sliced)	0	0
(*Tyson* Sliced)	0	0
turkey, see "Turkey pepperoni"		
"Pepperoni," vegetarian, pizza slices (*Yves*), 1.7 oz.	4.0	.0
Pepperoni pocket, see "Pizza, stuffed/pocket"		
Perch, without added ingredients	0	0
Persimmon, fresh:		
(*Frieda's* Fuyu/Hachiya/Sharon), 5 oz.	26.0	5.0
Japanese, 1 medium	31.2	6.0
native, 1 medium, 1.1 oz.	8.4	n.a.
Persimmon, dried:		
(*Frieda's* Fuyu), ⅓ cup, 1.4 oz.	35.0	3.0
Japanese, 1 oz.	20.8	4.1
Pesto paste (*Amore*), 2 tbsp.	3.0	0
Pesto sauce, in jars, ¼ cup, except as noted:		
basil:		
(*Bellino*)	3.0	1.0
(*Classico* di Genova)	6.0	1.0

Food and Measure	carb. (gms)	fiber (gms)
(*Sacla*)	2.0	3.0
tomato, sun-dried (*Classico* di Capri)	8.0	1.0
tomato, sun-dried, and garlic (*Scala*)	5.0	1.0
Pesto sauce, refrigerated, ¼ cup:		
basil:		
(*Buitoni* Family Size)	11.0	6.0
(*Buitoni/Buitoni* Reduced Fat)	9.0	2.0
(*DiGiorno*)	2.0	1.0
tomato, sun-dried (*Buitoni*)	9.0	2.0
Pesto sauce mix (*McCormick*), 2 tsp.	1.0	0
Pheasant, without added ingredients	0	0
Phyllo, see "Fillo dough"		
Picante sauce (see also "Salsa"), 2 tbsp.:		
(*Pace*)	2.0	<1.0
(*Taco Bell* Smooth & Zesty Mild)	3.0	1.0
mild or medium (*Chi-Chi's*)	2.0	0
mild or medium (*Old El Paso*)	2.0	0
Piccalilli, see "Tomato relish"		
Pickle, cucumber, 1 oz., except as noted:		
bread and butter:		
(*Cascadian Farm*)	6.0	0
(*Claussen Chips*)	4.0	0
(*D.L. Jardine's* Texas)	14.0	0
(*Mrs. Fannings*), 3 pieces, 1 oz.	6.0	0
(*Vlasic* Chips)	6.0	0
cornichon:		
(*Italica*), 7 pieces, 1.1 oz.	0	0
(*Maille*)	.3	.5
(*Trois Petits Cochons*), 1 oz., about 6 pieces	0	0
dill:		
baby or kosher (*Cascadian Farm*)	1.0	1.0
chips, hamburger (*Del Monte*)	0	0
chips, hamburger (*Vlasic*)	3.0	0
whole or halves (*Del Monte*)	1.0	<1.0
dill, kosher:		
(*Cascadian Farm* Reduced Sodium)	0	0
baby (*Vlasic/Vlasic Snack'mms*)	1.0	0
burger slices or mini (*Claussen*), .8 oz.	1.0	0

Food and Measure	carb. (gms)	fiber (gms)
halves or spears (*Claussen*)	1.0	0
sandwich slices (*Claussen*), 1.2 oz.	1.0	0
tiny (*Del Monte*)	1.0	<1.0
whole (*Hebrew National*), 1 large	4.0	0
whole or spears (*Vlasic*)	1.0	0
garlic, slices (*Claussen* Hearty Deli Style), 1.2 oz.	1.0	0
sour, half (*Claussen* New York Deli Style Wholes)	1.0	0
sweet:		
all styles (*Del Monte*)	10.0	<1.0
gherkins (*Claussen*), .9 oz.	7.0	0
gherkins (*Vlasic*), 3 pieces, 1 oz.	9.0	<0
Pickle relish, cucumber, 1 tbsp.:		
(*Crosse & Blackwell* Branston)	6.0	0
dill (*Vlasic*)	1.0	0
hamburger (*Del Monte*)	6.0	<1.0
hot dog (*Del Monte*)	4.0	<1.0
hot dog (*Heinz*)	4.0	0
India (*Heinz*)	5.0	0
sweet:		
(*Cascadian Farm*)	5.0	0
(*Claussen*)	3.0	0
(*Del Monte*)	5.0	0
(*Heinz*)	5.0	0
(*Vlasic*)	4.0	0
Pickle relish cubes, sweet (*Vlasic*), 1 oz.	5.0	0
Pickling spice (*Tone's*), 1 tsp.	1.2	.3
Pie, fresh, apple (*Entenmann's*), ⅙ pie	57.0	2.0
Pie, frozen (see also "Cobbler"), ⅛ pie, except as noted:		
apple:		
(*Amy's*), ½ of 8-oz. pie	37.0	2.0
(*Mrs. Smith's*)	46.0	2.0
(*Sara Lee Oven Fresh*)	46.0	1.0
cinnamon French, deep dish (*Sara Lee Signature Selection*), ⅒ pie	48.0	2.0
crumb (*Mrs. Smith's*)	52.0	2.0
deep dish (*Mrs. Smith's*), ⅟₁₂ pie	45.0	2.0
deep dish (*Sara Lee Signature Selection Orchard*), ⅒ pie	43.0	3.0

Food and Measure	carb. (gms)	fiber (gms)
Dutch (*Sara Lee Oven Fresh*)	53.0	2.0
berry (*Marie Callender's* Razzleberry), ¹⁄₁₀ pie	43.0	5.0
blueberry (*Sara Lee Oven Fresh*)	53.0	2.0
caramel applenut, deep dish (*Sara Lee Signature Selection*), ¹⁄₉ pie	45.0	2.0
cherry:		
(*Mrs. Smith's*)	45.0	2.0
(*Sara Lee Oven Fresh*)	44.0	0
deep dish (*Sara Lee Signature Selection* Gourmet), ¹⁄₁₀ pie	46.0	2.0
chocolate cream (*Sara Lee* French Silk), ¹⁄₅ pie	34.0	2.0
coconut cream (*Sara Lee*), ¹⁄₅ pie	37.0	2.0
dulce de leche caramel swirl (*Sara Lee Signature Selection*)	37.0	2.0
fruit, mixed, deep dish (*Sara Lee Signature Selection* Fruits of the Forest), ¹⁄₉ pie	41.0	0
lemon meringue (*Mrs. Smith's*)	47.0	<1.0
lemon meringue (*Sara Lee*), ¹⁄₆ pie	41.0	1.0
lime, key (*Smart Ones*), 2.8-oz. piece	34.0	0
lime, key (*Sara Lee Signature Selection*)	41.0	2.0
mince (*Sara Lee Oven Fresh*)	55.0	2.0
Mississippi mud (*Smart Ones*), 2.4-oz. piece	26.0	1.0
peach:		
(*Mrs. Smith's*)	40.0	2.0
(*Sara Lee Oven Fresh*)	50.0	2.0
deep dish (*Sara Lee Signature Selection Golden*), ¹⁄₁₀ pie	46.0	2.0
peanut butter (*Smart Ones*), 2.6-oz. piece	27.0	1.0
pecan (*Mrs. Smith's*), ¹⁄₅ pie	75.0	<2.0
pecan (*Sara Lee Signature Selection* Southern)	70.0	3.0
pumpkin:		
(*Sara Lee Oven Fresh*)	37.0	2.0
(*Sara Lee Signature Selection* Traditional), ¹⁄₁₀ pie	34.0	2.0
custard (*Mrs. Smith's*)	35.0	2.0
raspberry (*Sara Lee Oven Fresh*)	50.0	3.0
strawberry and cream (*Sara Lee Signature Selection*)	33.0	2.0
sweet potato (*Mrs. Smith's*)	44.0	2.0
sweet potato (*Sara Lee Oven Fresh* Southern)	45.0	2.0
Pie, mix, ¹⁄₆ pkg., except as noted:		

Food and Measure	carb. (gms)	fiber (gms)
chocolate silk (*Jell-O* No Bake)	34.0	2.0
cookie (*Jell-O Chips Ahoy!* No Bake)	46.0	1.0
cookie (*Jell-O Oreo* No Bake)	48.0	2.0
peanut butter cup (*Jell-O* No Bake), ⅛ pkg.	38.0	2.0
pumpkin pie style (*Jell-O* No Bake), ⅛ pkg.	29.0	1.0
Pie, snack (see also "Cake, snack"), fruit:		
apple (*Little Debbie*), 4-oz. pie	62.0	1.0
apple or cherry (*Drake's*), 2 pies, 4 oz.	60.0	3.0
cherry (*Little Debbie*), 4-oz. pie	64.0	1.0
lemon (*Drakes*), 4.5-oz. pie	66.0	0
Pie crust (see also "Pastry shell"):		
(*Nilla*), ⅙ crust	18.0	1.0
(*Oreo*), ⅙ crust	18.0	1.0
(*Pet•Ritz*), ⅛ crust	9.0	0
(*Pet•Ritz* Extra Large), ⅛ crust	13.0	0
(*Pillsbury*), ⅛ crust	13.0	0
chocolate (*Ready Crust*), ⅛ crust	14.0	<1.0
deep dish (*Pet•Ritz*), ⅛ crust	11.0	0
graham:		
(*Honey Maid*), ⅙ crust	18.0	1.0
(*Ready Crust* 9''), ⅛ crust	14.0	<1.0
(*Ready Crust* 10''), ⅒ crust	18.0	<1.0
(*Ready Crust* Reduced Fat), ⅛ crust	15.0	0
tart (*Ready Crust*), .8-oz. piece	15.0	<1.0
shortbread (*Ready Crust*), ⅛ crust	14.0	0
Pie crust mix:		
(*Betty Crocker*), ⅛ of 9'' crust*	9.0	0
("*Jiffy*"), ¼ cup mix	19.0	<1.0
Pie filling (see also "Pastry filling"), ⅓ cup, except as noted:		
apple (*Lucky Leaf/Lucky Leaf* Premium)	22.0	2.0
apple (*Lucky Leaf* Lite)	7.0	0
apricot (*Lucky Leaf*)	22.0	0
blueberry (*Lucky Leaf*)	22.0	1.0
blueberry (*Lucky Leaf* Premium)	24.0	1.0
cherry:		
(*Lucky Leaf*)	24.0	0
(*Lucky Leaf* Lite)	8.0	0
(*Lucky Leaf* Premium)	24.0	1.0

Food and Measure	carb. (gms)	fiber (gms)
coconut crème (*Lucky Leaf*)	25.0	3.0
lemon (*Lucky Leaf*)	29.0	0
lemon crème (*Lucky Leaf*)	31.0	0
mince/mincemeat:		
(*Crosse & Blackwell*), ¼ cup	43.0	0
(*None Such* Original)	45.0	0
with brandy and rum (*Crosse & Blackwell*), ¼ cup	43.0	0
with brandy and rum (*None Such*)	47.0	0
condensed (*None Such*), 4 tsp.	36.0	1.0
peach (*Lucky Leaf*)	21.0	0
pineapple (*Lucky Leaf*)	23.0	1.0
pumpkin (*Libby's* Mix)	20.0	3.0
raisin (*Lucky Leaf*)	22.0	1.0
raspberry (*Lucky Leaf* Premium)	19.0	2.0
strawberry (*Lucky Leaf*)	20.0	1.0
Pie filling mix, see "Pudding and pie filling mix"		
Pierogi, frozen, 3 pieces, 4.25 oz., except as noted:		
potato and cheddar:		
bacon, mini (*Mrs. T.'s*), 7 pieces, 3 oz.	25.0	1.0
broccoli (*Mrs. T.'s*)	33.0	2.0
jalapeño (*Mrs. T.'s*)	34.0	1.0
mini (*Mrs. T.'s*), 7 pieces, 3 oz.	25.0	1.0
potato and cheese:		
(*Empire* Kosher), ½ pkg., 5.3 oz.	44.0	.7
American (*Mrs. T.'s*)	32.0	1.0
four (*Mrs. T.'s*)	36.0	1.0
four, mini (*Mrs. T.'s*), 7 pieces, 3 oz.	27.0	1.0
potato and onion (*Empire* Kosher), ½ pkg., 5.3 oz.	47.0	.7
potato and onion (*Mrs. T.'s*)	33.0	1.0
potato, sour cream, and chive (*Mrs. T.'s*)	34.0	1.0
sauerkraut (*Mrs. T.'s*)	30.0	3.0
Pig's feet, pickled, cured, 1 oz.	<.1	0
Pigeon peas, fresh:		
raw, ½ cup	18.4	3.2
boiled, drained, ½ cup	15.0	2.5
Pigeon peas, canned, green (*Goya*), 8 oz.	26.0	8.0
Pigeon peas, dried, boiled, ½ cup	19.5	3.9
Pignolia nuts, see "Pine nuts"		

Food and Measure	carb. (gms)	fiber (gms)
Pike, without added ingredients	0	0
Pili nuts, shelled:		
dried, 1 oz.	1.1	<1.0
dried, 1 cup	4.8	3.4
Pimiento, in jars (*Goya* Fancy), ¼ piece, .5 oz.	1.0	0
Piña colada drink, see "Pineapple drink blend"		
Piña colada drink mixer:		
(*Bacardi*), 3.2 fl. oz.	39.0	0
(*Daily's*), 3 fl. oz.	44.0	0
(*Holland House*), 4 fl. oz.	44.0	0
frozen (*Bacardi*), 2 fl. oz.	35.0	0
Pine nuts, dried:		
(*Frieda's*), ¼ cup, 1.1 oz.	4.0	1.0
(*Planters*), 2-oz. pkg.	8.0	3.0
pignolia:		
(*Shiloh Farms*), ¼ cup, 1.3 oz.	9.0	4.0
1 oz.	4.0	1.3
1 tbsp.	1.2	.4
pinyon, 1 oz.	5.5	3.0
pinyon, 10 kernels	.2	.1
Pineapple, fresh:		
(*Del Monte*), 2 slices, 4 oz.	17.0	1.0
(*Dole* Whole/Cut), 2 slices, 3'' diam × ¾''	16.0	1.0
(*Frieda's* South African Baby), 1 cup, 5 oz.	17.0	2.0
whole, 1 lb.	58.5	5.7
diced, ½ cup	9.6	.9
Pineapple, can or jar, ½ cup, except as noted:		
(*Dole Fruit Bowls*), 4 oz.	16.0	1.0
in juice:		
all styles, except sliced (*Del Monte*)	17.0	1.0
chunks (*Del Monte Fruit Naturals*)	18.0	<1.0
chunks or tidbits (*Dole*)	15.0	1.0
crushed (*Dole*)	17.0	1.0
sliced (*Del Monte*), 2 pieces	16.0	1.0
sliced (*Dole*), 2 pieces	15.0	1.0
sliced (*S&W*), 2 pieces	16.0	1.0
tidbits (*Del Monte* Plastic), 4 oz.	18.0	<1.0
tidbits (*Del Monte* Pull-Top), 4 oz.	15.0	<1.0

Food and Measure	carb. (gms)	fiber (gms)
tidbits (*Del Monte Fruit Cup*), 4.5 oz.	15.0	<1.0
wedges (*Dole*)	15.0	1.0
in light syrup (*Del Monte Sunfresh*)	18.0	<1.0
in light syrup, crushed or chunks	17.0	1.0
in heavy syrup:		
chunks or crushed (*Del Monte*)	24.0	1.0
chunks or tidbits (*Dole*)	24.0	1.0
chunks, tidbits or crushed	25.8	.9
sliced (*Del Monte*), 2 pieces	23.0	1.0
sliced (*Dole*), 2 pieces	24.0	1.0
Pineapple, dried:		
(*Shiloh Farms*), 6–7 rings, 1.4 oz.	32.0	1.0
(*SunRidge Farms*), 1.5 rings, 1.4 oz.	30.0	2.0
(*Sunsweet*), ⅓ cup, 1.4 oz.	34.0	1.0
Pineapple, freeze-dried, chunks (*AlpineAire*), .4 oz.	10.0	1.0
Pineapple, frozen, chunks, sweetened, ½ cup	27.1	1.3
Pineapple drink blend, 8 fl. oz.:		
coconut (*AriZona* Piña Colada)	34.0	0
coconut (*R.W. Knudsen*)	31.0	0
orange (*Hood Carb Countdown*)	5.0	0
orange guava (*Langers*)	30.0	0
orange guava (*Nantucket Nectars*)	31.0	0
Pineapple guava, see "Feijoas"		
Pineapple juice, 8 fl. oz.:		
(*Ceres*)	29.0	2.0
(*Del Monte*)	29.0	2.0
(*Del Monte* From Concentrate)	32.0	1.0
(*Dole*)	29.0	0
(*R.W. Knudsen* Nectar)	34.0	0
(*S&W*)	29.0	2.0
(*Walnut Acres*)	32.0	0
canned	34.5	.5
frozen*	31.9	.5
Pineapple juice blend, 8 fl. oz.:		
coconut (*L&A*)	28.0	0
coconut (*Langers*)	28.0	0
orange banana (*Nantucket Nectars*)	35.0	0
Pineapple topping (*Smucker's*), 2 tbsp.	26.0	0

Food and Measure	carb. (gms)	fiber (gms)
Pink beans, dried, boiled, ½ cup	23.5	4.5
Pinquito beans, canned (*S&W* California), ½ cup	20.0	6.0
Pinto beans:		
dry (*Arrowhead Mills*), ¼ cup	27.0	10.0
dry (*Shiloh Farms*), ¼ cup	31.0	12.0
boiled, ½ cup	21.8	7.3
Pinto beans, canned (see also "Chili Beans" and "Refried beans"), ½ cup:		
(*Allens*)	20.0	7.0
(*Bush's*)	19.0	6.0
(*Eden* Organic)	18.0	6.0
(*Progresso*)	16.0	7.0
(*S&W*)	22.0	7.0
(*Westbrae Natural* Organic)	19.0	7.0
with bacon:		
(*Trappey's*)	20.0	7.0
and jalapeño (*Trappey's Jalapinto*)	22.0	8.0
seasoned (*Bush's*)	17.0	6.0
in chili sauce, red (*Old El Paso* Mexe Beans)	19.0	7.0
with pork (*Bush's*)	17.0	6.0
seasoned (*Glory*)	15.0	5.0
spicy (*Eden* Organic)	24.0	7.0
with tomato, corn, and chili (*Del Monte Savory Sides* Rio Grande)	14.0	2.0
Pinto beans, frozen, boiled, drained, ⅓ of 10-oz. pkg. . .	29.0	8.1
Pipian sauce (*Doña María*), 2 tbsp.	5.0	3.0
Pistachio nut, shelled, except as noted:		
(*Shiloh Farms*), ¼ cup	9.0	1.0
(*Sunkist*), ½ cup in shell, ¼ cup shelled	9.0	3.0
dried, 1 oz.	7.1	3.1
dry-roasted:		
(*Planters*), 1 oz.	7.0	3.0
unsalted, 1 oz.	7.8	2.9
unsalted, ¼ cup	8.9	3.3
Pita, see "Bread"		
Pitanga:		
1 medium, .3 oz.	.5	<1.0
½ cup	6.5	<1.0

Food and Measure	carb. (gms)	fiber (gms)
Pizza, frozen, 1 pie or pkg., except as noted:		
artichoke and roasted garlic (*Linda McCartney*), ½ pie	33.0	4.0
bacon burger (*Totino's Crisp Crust Party Pizza*), ½ pie	35.0	2.0
Canadian bacon (*Jenos Crisp 'n Tasty*)	51.0	2.0
Canadian bacon (*Totino's Crisp Crust Party Pizza*), ½ pie	35.0	1.0
cheese:		
(*Amy's*), ⅓ pie	38.0	2.0
(*Elio's*), ⅓ pie	47.0	2.0
(*Elio's* Rectangle 24 oz.), ⅑ pie	25.0	2.0
(*Ian's* Natural), ⅙ pie	14.0	1.0
(*Linda McCartney*), ½ pie	35.0	4.0
(*Michelina's* Zap'ems)	44.0	2.0
(*Totino's* Family Size), ⅓ pie	39.0	2.0
(*Totino's Crisp Crust Party Pizza*), ½ pie	34.0	2.0
extra (*Tombstone* Original)	74.0	4.0
rice crust (*Amy's*), ⅓ pie	31.0	2.0
cheese, five, tomato:		
(*California Pizza Kitchen* 12.58 oz.), ⅓ pie	29.0	1.0
(*California Pizza Kitchen* 27.2 oz.), ⅙ pie	35.0	2.0
cheese, four:		
(*DiGiorno* Thin Crispy Crust), ⅕ pie	34.0	3.0
(*DiGiorno Rising Crust*), ⅙ pie	40.0	3.0
(*DiGiorno Rising Crust* Microwave), ½ pie	44.0	3.0
(*Health is Wealth*)	54.0	6.0
(*Ian's* Natural Low Carb), ⅓ pie	8.0	3.0
(*Lean Cuisine* Cafe Classics)	60.0	3.0
(*Smart Ones*)	49.0	3.0
(*South Beach Diet*)	33.0	14.0
cheese, three (*Heaven's Bistro*), ⅓ pie	42.0	4.0
cheese, three, cornmeal crust (*Amy's*), ⅓ pie	41.0	2.0
"cheese," vegetarian (*Amy's* Soy Cheeze), ⅓ pie	37.0	2.0
"cheese," vegetarian (*Tofutti* Pizza Pizzaz), ⅓ pkg.	24.0	0
cheese and pesto, whole wheat crust (*Amy's*), ⅓ pie	37.0	2.0
chicken:		
barbecue (*California Pizza Kitchen* 12.96 oz.), ⅓ pie	33.0	1.0
barbecue (*California Pizza Kitchen* 28 oz.), ⅙ pie	38.0	2.0
barbecue (*Heaven's Bistro*), ⅓ pie	48.0	4.0
grilled, and vegetable (*South Beach Diet*)	34.0	14.0

Food and Measure	carb. (gms)	fiber (gms)
Jamaican jerk (*California Pizza Kitchen*), ⅓ pie	33.0	2.0
sausage (*Heaven's Bistro*), ⅓ pie	42.0	4.0
Thai (*California Pizza Kitchen* 12.98 oz.), ⅓ pie	33.0	3.0
Thai (*California Pizza Kitchen* 27.9 oz.), ⅙ pie	38.0	2.0
tomato and spinach, grilled (*DiGiorno* Thin Crispy Crust), ⅕ pie	33.0	2.0
deluxe:		
(*Lean Cuisine* Cafe Classics)	55.0	3.0
(*Smart Ones*)	47.0	4.0
(*South Beach Diet*)	34.0	14.0
ham and shrimp, Hawaiian (*Contessa*), ⅓ pie	45.0	2.0
hamburger (*Jenos Crisp 'n Tasty*)	51.0	2.0
hamburger (*Totino's Crisp Crust Party Pizza*), ½ pie	35.0	2.0
Margherita (*Lean Cuisine* Cafe Classics)	48.0	4.0
meat, four (*DiGiorno* Thin Crispy Crust), ⅕ pie	37.0	2.0
meat, three:		
(*DiGiorno Rising Crust* Microwave), ½ pie	44.0	3.0
(*Lean Cuisine* Cafe Classics)	48.0	4.0
(*Jenos Crisp 'n Tasty*)	49.0	2.0
(*Totino's Crisp Crust Party Pizza*), ½ pie	35.0	2.0
cheese stuffed (*DiGiorno*), ⅙ pie	37.0	3.0
Mexican style (*Health is Wealth*)	50.0	3.0
mushroom and olive (*Amy's*), ⅓ pie	33.0	2.0
mushroom and spinach (*Linda McCartney*), ½ pie	34.0	4.0
pepperoni:		
(*DiGiorno* Deep Dish), ⅙ pie	33.0	2.0
(*DiGiorno* Thin Crispy Crust), ⅕ pie	34.0	2.0
(*DiGiorno Rising Crust*), ⅙ pie	40.0	2.0
(*DiGiorno Rising Crust* Microwave), ½ pie	43.0	3.0
(*Elio's* Rectangle 24 oz.), ⅑ pie	24.0	1.0
(*Heaven's Bistro*), ⅓ pie	42.0	4.0
(*Jenos Crisp 'n Tasty*)	50.0	2.0
(*Lean Cuisine* Cafe Classics)	55.0	3.0
(*Michelina's* Zap'ems)	44.0	2.0
(*Smart Ones*)	49.0	3.0
(*South Beach Diet*)	33.0	14.0
(*Tombstone* Brick-oven), ¼ pie	29.0	2.0
(*Totino's* Family Size), ⅓ pie	38.0	2.0

Food and Measure	carb. (gms)	fiber (gms)
(*Totino's Crisp Crust Party Pizza*), ½ pie	34.0	2.0
and cheese (*DiGiorno Rising Crust* Half & Half), ⅙ pie	40.0	3.0
cheese (*Tombstone* Deep Dish), ½ pie	51.0	3.0
sliced (*Totino's Crisp Crust Party Pizza*), ½ pie	35.0	1.0
"pepperoni," meatless (*Boca*), ⅓ pie	36.0	2.0
"pepperoni," meatless, and "sausage" (*Boca*), ⅓ pie	36.0	2.0
pesto (*Amy's*), ⅓ pie	39.0	2.0
sausage:		
(*Jenos Crisp 'n Tasty*)	51.0	2.0
(*Totino's* Family Size), ¼ pie	29.0	1.0
(*Totino's Crisp Crust Party Pizza*), ½ pie	36.0	2.0
spicy (*Smart Ones*)	48.0	4.0
sausage and mushroom (*Totino's Crisp Crust Party Pizza*), ½ pie	34.0	2.0
sausage and pepperoni:		
(*Jenos Crisp 'n Tasty*)	50.0	2.0
(*Tombstone* Brick-oven), ¼ pie	30.0	3.0
(*Totino's* Family Size), ¼ pie	29.0	1.0
(*Totino's Crisp Crust Party Pizza*), ½ pie	19.0	2.0
zesty Italiano (*Totino's Crisp Crust Party Pizza*), ½ pie	36.0	2.0
shrimp, basil pesto (*Contessa*), ⅓ pie	37.0	2.0
shrimp, roasted red pesto or vegetables (*Contessa*), ⅓ pie	38.0	2.0
spinach:		
(*Amy's*), ⅓ pie	38.0	2.0
and 4 cheese (*Ian's* Natural Low Carb), ⅓ pie	8.0	4.0
and mushroom (*Lean Cuisine* Cafe Classics)	46.0	4.0
supreme:		
(*DiGiorno* Deep Dish), ⅛ pie	25.0	2.0
(*DiGiorno Rising Crust* 14.3 oz.), ⅓ pie	35.0	3.0
(*DiGiorno Rising Crust* 32.7 oz.), ⅙ pie	41.0	3.0
(*DiGiorno Rising Crust* Microwave), ½ pie	44.0	3.0
(*Jenos Crisp 'n Tasty*)	50.0	2.0
(*Tombstone* Brick-oven), ¼ pie	30.0	3.0
(*Totino's Crisp Crust Party Pizza*), ½ pie	35.0	2.0
vegetable/veggie:		
(*Heaven's Bistro*), ⅓ pie	42.0	4.0
(*Smart Ones* Ultimate)	50.0	4.0
combo (*Amy's*), ⅓ pie	36.0	1.0

Food and Measure	carb. (gms)	fiber (gms)
roasted (*Amy's*), ⅓ pie	42.0	2.0
roasted (*Lean Cuisine* Cafe Classics)	57.0	3.0
Thai, spicy (*Linda McCartney*), ½ pie	36.0	4.0
Pizza, bagel, frozen:		
(*Health is Wealth*), 4 pieces, 3.1 oz.	28.0	3.0
(*Dr. Praeger's*), 2-oz. piece	20.0	2.0
cheese, three (*Bagel Bites*), 4 pieces, 3 oz.	28.0	2.0
Pizza, French bread, frozen, 1 piece:		
cheese:		
(*Healthy Choice*)	57.0	5.0
(*Lean Cuisine*)	47.0	3.0
(*Stouffer's*)	43.0	3.0
extra (*Stouffer's*)	44.0	3.0
five (*Stouffer's*)	47.0	3.0
deluxe (*Lean Cuisine*)	44.0	3.0
deluxe (*Stouffer's*)	45.0	3.0
meat, three (*Stouffer's*)	47.0	4.0
pepperoni:		
(*Healthy Choice*)	56.0	6.0
(*Lean Cuisine*)	44.0	2.0
(*Stouffer's*)	44.0	3.0
pepperoni and mushroom (*Stouffer's*)	47.0	4.0
sausage (*Stouffer's*)	45.0	3.0
sausage and pepperoni (*Stouffer's*)	47.0	4.0
supreme (*Healthy Choice*)	51.0	6.0
vegetable (*Healthy Choice*)	50.0	4.0
vegetable, grilled (*Stouffer's*)	49.0	3.0
white (*Stouffer's*)	44.0	4.0
Pizza, stuffed/pocket, frozen, 1 piece, 4.5 oz.,		
except as noted:		
cheese:		
(*Amy's*)	42.0	4.0
(*Amy's* Toaster Pops), 1.9 oz.	23.0	<1.0
(*Jack's Pizza Bursts Super*), 3 oz.	25.0	1.0
five (*Croissant Pockets*)	37.0	3.0
"cheese," soy (*Amy's* Cheeze)	39.0	6.0
pepperoni:		
(*Croissant Pockets*)	39.0	3.0

Food and Measure	carb. (gms)	fiber (gms)
(*Hot Pockets*)	41.0	3.0
(*Jack's Pizza Bursts*), 3 oz.	25.0	1.0
(*Lean Pockets*)	42.0	4.0
(*Smart Ones Smartwich*)	39.0	2.0
sausage and pepperoni (*Jack's Pizza Bursts*), 3 oz.	25.0	1.0
sausage and pepperoni (*Lean Pockets*)	41.0	3.0
supreme (*Jack's Pizza Bursts*), 3 oz.	25.0	1.0
supreme (*Lean Pockets* Ultra)	19.0	7.0
vegetarian (*Amy's*)	39.0	4.0
Pizza crust, frozen, dough (*Rhodes*), ⅙ pkg.	32.0	1.0
Pizza crust mix:		
(*Betty Crocker*), ¼ crust*	33.0	1.0
("*Jiffy*"), ⅓ cup mix	31.0	2.0
Pizza entree, frozen, with dessert (*Ian's* Natural Kids Meal),		
9 oz.	60.0	4.0
Pizza Hut:		
Dippin' Strips, 2 pieces:		
cheese only	29.0	2.0
ham, quartered, or pepperoni	28.0	2.0
Meat Lover's/Pepperoni Lover's	29.0	2.0
Pepperoni Trio	30.0	1.0
supreme, super supreme, or chicken supreme	30.0	2.0
Veggie Lover's	30.0	2.0
dipping sauce:		
garlic, 1½ oz.	3.0	0
marinara, 3 oz.	9.0	2.0
ranch, 1½ oz.	4.0	0
Fit 'N Delicious, 12", 1 slice:		
chicken, onion, and pepper	23.0	2.0
chicken, ham, or tomato and mushroom	22.0	2.0
ham and pineapple or pepper and onion	24.0	2.0
Fit 'N Delicious, 14", 1 slice:		
chicken, onion and pepper	22.0	2.0
chicken and mushroom	20.0	2.0
ham and mushroom or tomato and		
mushroom	21.0	2.0
ham and pineapple	22.0	1.0
pepper and onion	22.0	2.0

Food and Measure	carb. (gms)	fiber (gms)
extra large, 16", 1 slice:		
cheese only	51.0	3.0
chicken supreme	52.0	3.0
ham, quartered, or pepperoni	50.0	3.0
Meat Lover's/Pepperoni Lover's/Sausage Lover's	51.0	3.0
supreme	52.0	4.0
super supreme or *Veggie Lover's*	53.0	4.0
hand-tossed, 12", 1 slice:		
cheese only	30.0	2.0
ham, quartered, or pepperoni	29.0	2.0
Meat Lover's	29.0	2.0
Pepperoni Lover's/Pepperoni Trio/Sausage Lover's	30.0	2.0
supreme or chicken supreme	30.0	2.0
super supreme or *Veggie Lover's*	31.0	2.0
hand-tossed, 14", 1 slice:		
cheese only or quartered ham	27.0	1.0
Meat Lover's/Pepperoni Lover's/Sausage Lover's	27.0	2.0
pepperoni	27.0	2.0
Pepperoni Trio/Veggie Lover's	28.0	2.0
supreme, super supreme, or chicken supreme	28.0	2.0
pan pizza, 12", 1 slice:		
cheese only or quartered ham	29.0	1.0
Meat Lover's/Pepperoni Lover's/Sausage Lover's	29.0	2.0
pepperoni	29.0	2.0
Pepperoni Trio	29.0	1.0
supreme, super supreme, or chicken supreme	30.0	2.0
Veggie Lover's	30.0	4.0
pan pizza, 14", 1 slice:		
cheese only	27.0	1.0
ham, quartered, or pepperoni	26.0	1.0
Meat Lover's/Pepperoni Lover's/Sausage Lover's	27.0	2.0
Pepperoni Trio	27.0	1.0
supreme or chicken supreme	27.0	2.0
super supreme	28.0	2.0
Veggie Lover's	28.0	4.0
***Personal Pan Pizza,* ¼ of 6" pie:**		
cheese only or quartered ham	18.0	<1.0
chicken supreme	19.0	<1.0

Food and Measure	carb. (gms)	fiber (gms)
Meat Lover's/Pepperoni Lover's/Sausage Lover's	18.0	1.0
pepperoni	18.0	<1.0
supreme, super supreme, or Veggie Lover's	19.0	1.0
stuffed crust, 14", 1 slice:		
cheese only	43.0	2.0
ham, quartered	42.0	2.0
Meat Lover's/Pepperoni Lover's/Sausage Lover's	43.0	3.0
pepperoni	42.0	3.0
Pepperoni Trio	45.0	3.0
supreme or chicken supreme	44.0	3.0
super supreme or Veggie Lover's	45.0	3.0
stuffed crust, 3Cheese, 1 slice		
cheese only	43.0	3.0
chicken supreme	44.0	3.0
ham, quartered, or pepperoni	42.0	3.0
Meat Lover's/Pepperoni Lover's	43.0	3.0
supreme	43.0	4.0
super supreme	45.0	4.0
Veggie Lover's	45.0	3.0
The Full House XL Pizza, 1 slice:		
cheese, ham, quartered, or pepperoni	30.0	3.0
Meat Lover's/Pepperoni Lover's/Pepperoni Trio	30.0	3.0
supreme or chicken supreme	31.0	3.0
super supreme or Veggie Lover's	32.0	3.0
Thin 'N Crispy, 12", 1 slice:		
cheese	21.0	1.0
chicken supreme	22.0	1.0
ham, quartered, or pepperoni	21.0	1.0
Meat Lover's/Pepperoni Lover's/Sausage Lover's	21.0	2.0
Pepperoni Trio	21.0	1.0
supreme	22.0	2.0
super supreme or Veggie Lover's	23.0	2.0
Thin 'N Crispy, 14", 1 slice:		
cheese	20.0	1.0
chicken supreme	21.0	1.0
ham, quartered, or pepperoni	19.0	1.0
Meat Lover's	20.0	2.0
Pepperoni Trio	19.0	1.0

Food and Measure	carb. (gms)	fiber (gms)
Pepperoni Lover's/Sausage Lover's	20.0	1.0
supreme, super supreme, or *Veggie Lover's*	21.0	2.0
appetizers:		
bread stick, regular, 1 piece	20.0	<1.0
bread stick, cheese, 1 piece	21.0	<1.0
bread stick dipping sauce	11.0	2.0
wings, hot, 2 pieces	1.0	0
wings, mild, 2 pieces	<1.0	0
wings dipping sauce, blue cheese	2.0	0
wings dipping sauce, ranch	4.0	0
desserts:		
apple pizza, 1 slice	53.0	1.0
cherry pizza, 1 slice	47.0	1.0
cinnamon sticks, 2 pieces	27.0	<1.0
icing dipping	46.0	0
Pizza kit, taco, cheesy (*Old El Paso* Dinner Kit), ⅛ pizza*	17.0	1.0
Pizza pocket, see "Pizza, stuffed/pocket"		
Pizza rolls, see "Pizza snack"		
Pizza sauce, ¼ cup, except as noted:		
(*Contadina* Original/Squeeze)	6.0	1.0
(*Eden* Organic Pizza/Pasta), ½ cup	12.0	3.0
(*Hunt's* Family Favorites)	5.0	1.0
(*Muir Glen*)	6.0	2.0
with basil (*Red Pack*)	6.0	1.0
with cheese, four (*Contadina*)	6.0	<1.0
pepperoni flavor (*Contadina*)	5.0	<1.0
Pizza snack, frozen:		
(*Cedarlane* Mini Bistro), 3 pieces, 4 oz.	27.0	2.0
(*Health is Wealth*), 2 pieces, 3 oz.	32.0	3.0
(*Health is Wealth* Supreme), 10 pieces, 5 oz.	46.0	7.0
(*Ian's Pizzetta*), 7 pieces, 4.75 oz.	38.0	4.0
(*Michelina's* Zap'ems), 5-oz. pkg.	41.0	2.0
cheese (*Amy's*), 5–6 pieces	22.0	2.0
cheese, double (*Pizza Mini's*), 5 pieces, 3 oz.	30.0	2.0
pepperoni (*Pizza Mini's*), 5 pieces, 3 oz.	29.0	2.0
"pepperoni," meatless (*Health is Wealth*), 10 pieces, 5 oz.	46.0	6.0
rolls, 6 pieces, 3 oz.:		
cheese (*Totino's* Pizza Rolls)	26.0	1.0

Food and Measure	carb. (gms)	fiber (gms)
cheesy taco or sausage and pepperoni (*Totino's* Pizza Rolls)	23.0	1.0
hamburger and three meat, pepperoni, spicy pepperoni sausage, or pepperoni supreme and sausage (*Totino's* Pizza Rolls)	24.0	1.0
supreme (*Totino's* Pizza Rolls)	25.0	1.0
sausage and pepperoni (*Pizza Mini's*), 5 pieces, 3 oz.	29.0	2.0
spinach (*Amy's*), 5–6 pieces	26.0	<1.0
Plantain, fresh:		
raw:		
(*Del Monte*), ½ medium, 3.9 oz.	22.0	5.0
(*Frieda's*), 3 oz.	27.0	2.0
1 medium, 6.3 oz.	57.1	4.1
sliced, ½ cup	23.6	1.7
cooked, sliced, ½ cup	24.0	1.8
Plantain, frozen:		
baked, ripe (*Goya* Plátanos Maduros Horneados), 3 pieces, 3 oz.	56.0	3.0
fried (*Goya* Tostones), 3 pieces, 3 oz.	37.0	9.0
fried, ripe (*Goya* Plátanos Maduros), 2 pieces, 2 oz.	22.0	2.0
Plum, fresh:		
(*Del Monte*), 2 medium, 4.7 oz.	19.0	2.0
Japanese or hybrid, 2⅛'' fruit	8.6	<1.0
sliced, ½ cup	10.7	1.2
Plum, can or jar, purple:		
in juice, ½ cup	19.1	1.3
in juice, 3 plums and 2 tbsp. liquid	14.4	1.0
in light syrup, ½ cup	20.5	1.3
in light syrup, 3 plums and 2¾ tbsp. liquid	21.7	1.3
in heavy syrup, ½ cup	30.0	1.3
in extra heavy syrup, whole (*S&W*), ½ cup	33.0	2.0
Plum, dried (prune):		
(*Dole*), ¼ cup, 1.4 oz.	26.0	2.0
with pits (*Sunsweet*), 3 extra large, 5 large, or 6 medium, 1.4 oz.	26.0	3.0
pitted:		
(*Shiloh Farms*), 5 pieces, 1.4 oz.	29.0	3.0
(*Sunsweet*), ⅓ cup, 1.4 oz.	24.0	3.0

Food and Measure	carb. (gms)	fiber (gms)
10 pieces	52.7	6.0
bite size (*Sunsweet*), 7 pieces, 1.4 oz.	26.0	3.0
cherry, lemon, or orange essence (*Sunsweet*), 5 pieces, 1.4 oz.	26.0	3.0
stewed, with pits, unsweetened, ½ cup	29.8	7.0
Plum, dried, canned, in heavy syrup:		
pitted, 4 oz.	31.5	4.3
½ cup	32.5	4.4
5 pieces and 2 tbsp. liquid	23.9	3.3
Plum, pickled, see "Umeboshi plum"		
Plum butter (*Lost Acres*), 1 tbsp.	11.0	0
Plum drink, red (*Nantucket Nectars*), 8 fl. oz.	31.0	0
Plum pudding (*Crosse & Blackwell*), ⅓ pkg.	87.0	5.0
Plum sauce, 2 tbsp., except as noted:		
(*Ka•Me*)	16.0	0
(*Kikkoman*)	18.0	0
(*Ty Ling* Duck)	20.0	0
dipping (*Trader Vic's*)	16.0	0
light, sweet (*Thai Kitchen*), 1 tbsp.	<1.0	0
Poi, ½ cup	32.7	.5
Pocket sandwich, see specific listings		
Pokeberry shoots:		
raw, ½ cup	3.0	1.4
boiled, drained, ½ cup	2.5	1.2
Pole beans, see "Green beans"		
Polenta (see also "Cornmeal"), ¼ cup:		
(*Shiloh Farms*)	22.0	1.0
instant (*Bellino*)	32.0	4.0
Polenta, refrigerated, prepared, 3.5 oz.:		
(*Frieda's* Organic Traditional), 2 slices, ½"	15.0	1.0
basil and garlic or traditional (*San Gennaro*), 2½" slice	15.0	1.0
sun-dried tomato and garlic (*San Gennaro*), 2½" slice	16.0	1.0
Polish sausage, see "Sausage"		
Pollock, without added ingredients	0	0
Pomegranate:		
(*Frieda's*), 5 oz.	24.0	1.0
with peel, 9.7-oz. fruit	26.4	.9

Food and Measure	carb. (gms)	fiber (gms)
Pomegranate drink blend, 8 fl. oz.:		
cranberry (*SoBe Elixir 3C*)	26.0	0
pear (*Nantucket Nectars*)	28.0	0
Pomegranate juice, 8 fl. oz.:		
(*Pom*)	35.0	0
(*R.W. Knudsen*)	37.0	0
(*R.W. Knudsen* Just Pomegranate)	38.0	0
Pomegranate juice blend, 8 fl. oz.:		
blueberry or mango (*Pom*)	34.0	0
cherry (*Pom*)	33.0	0
tangerine (*Pom*)	37.0	0
Pomegranate juice concentrate (*Tree of Life*), 8 tsp.	41.0	0
Pomegranate syrup, see "Grenadine syrup"		
Pompano, Florida, without added ingredients	0	0
Ponzu sauce (*Eden*), 1 tbsp.	1.0	0
Popcorn, unpopped, 2 tbsp., except as noted:		
(*America's Best*)	23.0	9.0
(*Arrowhead Mills*), ¼ cup	33.0	7.0
(*B.K. Heuermann's* Kettle Korn)	17.0	3.0
(*B.K. Heuermann's Exclusive*)	16.0	4.0
(*Healthy Choice* Natural Flavor), 3 tbsp.	26.0	5.0
(*Jolly Time* Mallow Magic)	15.0	3.0
(*Jolly Time* Crispy 'n White)	16.0	6.0
(*Jolly Time* Crispy 'n White Light)	20.0	7.0
(*Jolly Time* Healthy Pop Kettle Corn Regular/Minis)	23.0	8.0
(*Jolly Time* KettleMania)	15.0	3.0
(*Newman's Own* Natural), 1.1 oz., 3½ cups*	16.0	3.0
(*Orville Redenbacher's*), 3 tbsp.	29.0	6.0
(*Orville Redenbacher's* Corn on the Cob)	15.0	4.0
(*Orville Redenbacher's* Natural)	17.0	4.0
(*Orville Redenbacher's* Natural Light)	19.0	4.0
(*Orville Redenbacher's* Smart Pop! Kettle Korn), 3 tbsp.	27.0	6.0
(*Pop•Secret* Homestyle), 3 tbsp.	17.0	3.0
(*Pop•Secret* Kettle Corn), 3 tbsp.	15.0	3.0
(*Simple Snacks* Organic Lightly Salted 94% Fat Free), 1 oz., 4 cups*	21.0	5.0
butter flavor:		
(*B.K. Heuermann's Exclusive*/Low Fat)	16.0	4.0

Food and Measure	carb. (gms)	fiber (gms)
(*B.K. Heuermann's Exclusive* Intense Butter Taste)	16.0	4.0
(*Healthy Choice*), 3 tbsp.	25.0	5.0
(*Jolly Time Blast O Butter Light*)	21.0	6.0
(*Jolly Time Blast O Butter Minis*), 3 tbsp.	21.0	10.0
(*Jolly Time Blast O Butter Ultimate Theater Style Butter*)	19.0	9.0
(*Jolly Time Butter•Licious*)	16.0	5.0
(*Jolly Time Butter•Licious Light*)	22.0	4.0
(*Jolly Time Healthy Pop* Regular or Minis)	23.0	9.0
(*Jolly Time White & Buttery*)	16.0	4.0
(*Newman's Own*), 1.1 oz., 3½ cups*	16.0	3.0
(*Newman's Own* Butter Boom), 1.1 oz., 3½ cups*	15.0	3.0
(*Newman's Own* Light), 1.1 oz., 3½ cups*	20.0	3.0
(*Newman's Own* 99% Fat Free), 1.1 oz., 3½ cups*	22.0	2.0
(*Orville Redenbacher's*)	17.0	4.0
(*Orville Redenbacher's* Kettle Korn)	16.0	3.0
(*Orville Redenbacher's* Light)	19.0	4.0
(*Orville Redenbacher's* Movie Theater Light)	19.0	5.0
(*Orville Redenbacher's* Movie Theater Pour Over)	14.0	3.0
(*Orville Redenbacher's* Old Fashioned)	17.0	4.0
(*Orville Redenbacher's* Pour Over)	14.0	3.0
(*Orville Redenbacher's* Smart Pop!), 3 tbsp.	26.0	6.0
(*Orville Redenbacher's* Smart Pop! Movie Theater), 3 tbsp.	28.0	7.0
(*Orville Redenbacher's* Sweet'n Buttery)	16.0	3.0
(*Orville Redenbacher's* Ultimate!)	16.0	4.0
(*Pop•Secret*), 3 tbsp.	17.0	3.0
(*Pop•Secret* Jumbo Pop), 3 tbsp.	18.0	3.0
(*Pop•Secret* Jumbo Pop Movie Theater), 3 tbsp.	18.0	3.0
(*Pop•Secret* Light), 3 tbsp.	23.0	4.0
(*Pop•Secret* Movie Theater), 3 tbsp.	17.0	3.0
(*Pop•Secret* 94% Fat Free), 3 tbsp.	26.0	4.0
(*Simple Snacks* Organic), 1 oz., 4 cups*	19.0	3.0
extra (*Orville Redenbacher's* Movie Theater)	16.0	4.0
extra (*Pop•Secret*), 3 tbsp.	17.0	3.0
caramel (*Orville Redenbacher's*)	23.0	2.0
caramel apple (*Jolly Time Healthy Pop*)	23.0	6.0
cheddar (*Orville Redenbacher's* Pour Over)	12.0	3.0
cheddar, white (*Newman's Own*), 1.1 oz., 3½ cups*	18.0	3.0

Food and Measure	carb. (gms)	fiber (gms)
cheese (*Jolly Time The Big Cheez*)	17.0	6.0
cinnamon butter (*Orville Redenbacher's Cinnabon*)	15.0	2.0
honey butter (*Orville Redenbacher's*)	16.0	3.0
honey or toffee butter (*Pop•Secret*), 3 tbsp.	15.0	3.0
yellow (*Shiloh Farms*), ¼ cup	27.0	6.0
yellow or white (*Jolly Time*)	24.0	6.0
white (*Orville Redenbacher's*), 3 tbsp.	29.0	6.0
Popcorn, popped:		
(*Chester's*), 3 cups	12.0	3.0
(*Hain PureSnax* Kettle Corn), 1½ cups	24.0	3.0
(*Shiloh Farms* Organic No Salt/Lite), 3½ cups	19.0	3.0
butter flavor:		
(*Orville Redenbacher's*), 2¾ cups	10.0	3.0
(*Snyder's*), ⅝ oz.	6.0	n.a.
(*Wise*), .5 oz.	7.0	1.0
caramel (*Jays* Fat Free), ¾ cup	26.0	1.0
caramel nut (*Cracker Jack*), ½ cup	23.0	1.0
caramel nut (*Orville Redenbacher's* Clusters), ½ cup	22.0	1.0
cheddar, white:		
(*Cape Cod*), 3 cups	13.0	2.0
(*Orville Redenbacher's*), 2¾ cups	16.0	2.0
(*Shiloh Farms*), 3 cups	18.0	3.0
(*Smartfood*), 3 cups	19.0	3.0
(*Wise*), .5 oz.	6.0	1.0
cheddar, zesty (*Orville Redenbacher's*), 2¾ cups	15.0	2.0
cheese:		
(*Chester's*), 3 cups	17.0	2.0
(*O-Ke-Doke*), 1 oz.	13.0	2.0
hot (*Wise*), .5 oz.	7.0	1.0
chocolate, milk (*Orville Redenbacher's* Drizzlers), ⅔ cup .	23.0	2.0
fudge, white (*Orville Redenbacher's* Drizzlers), ⅔ cups ...	24.0	<1.0
toffee, butter (*Cracker Jack*), ¾ cup	22.0	1.0
toffee, butter (*Orville Redenbacher's* Clusters), ½ cup	20.0	1.0
white (*Orville Redenbacher's* Tender), 2 tbsp.	14.0	2.0
Popcorn cake:		
butter (*Orville Redenbacher's*), 2 pieces, .6 oz.	14.0	2.0
butter, mini (*Orville Redenbacher's*), 6 pieces, .5 oz.	12.0	1.0
caramel (*Orville Redenbacher's*), .4-oz. piece	10.0	<1.0

Food and Measure	carb. (gms)	fiber (gms)
caramel, mini (*Orville Redenbacher's*), 6 pieces, .5 oz. ...	13.0	1.0
cheddar, white (*Orville Redenbacher's*), 2 pieces, .6 oz. ..	13.0	2.0
chocolate (*Orville Redenbacher's*), .4-oz. piece	10.0	<1.0
chocolate peanut crunch, mini (*Orville Redenbacher's*),		
6 pieces, .5 oz.	12.0	2.0
peanut caramel crunch, mini (*Orville Redenbacher's*),		
6 pieces, .5 oz.	12.0	1.0
and rice (*Lundberg* Organic), .7-oz. piece	16.0	0
sour cream and onion, mini (*Orville Redenbacher's*),		
6 pieces, .5 oz.	12.0	2.0
Popcorn seasoning:		
butter flavor (*Fanci Food*), ½ tsp.	0	0
butter flavor (*Fanci Food Pop'n Topper*), ½ tsp.	2.0	0
buttery (*Jolly Time*), ¼ tsp.	0	0
cheddar flavor (*Fanci Food*), ½ tsp.	<1.0	0
Poppy seeds:		
(*Shiloh Farms*), 1 tsp.	1.0	1.0
1 tsp.	.7	.8
Porgy, see "Scup"		
Pork, fresh, meat only, without added ingredients	0	0
Pork, cured (see also "Ham"):		
arm (picnic), roasted, 4 oz.	0	0
blade roll, lean with fat, roasted, 4 oz.	.4	0
Pork, freeze-dried, cooked, diced (*Mountain House*),		
¾ cup	1.0	0
Pork, frozen or refrigerated, raw, 4 oz., except as noted:		
all cuts, without added ingredients	0	0
chop, boneless, center cut, marinated, all varieties		
(*Hatfield Simply Tender*), 4.25-oz. chop	0	0
chop, breaded (*Tyson*), 6.25-oz. chop	10.0	0
chop, breaded, lemon pepper (*Tyson*), 6.25-oz. chop	5.0	2.0
loin fillet, marinated, honey mustard (*Always Tender*)	4.0	0
loin fillet, marinated, mojo (*Always Tender*)	3.0	0
shoulder roast, onion garlic (*Always Tender*)	2.0	0
tenderloin, marinated:		
garlic (*Always Tender*)	1.0	0
mesquite or peppercorn (*Always Tender*)	2.0	0
teriyaki (*Always Tender*)	5.0	0

Food and Measure	carb. (gms)	fiber (gms)
Pork, frozen or refrigerated, cooked:		
with barbecue sauce:		
pulled (*Hormel*), 2 oz.	10.0	0
pulled, with sauce (*Smithfield*), 2 oz.	7.0	0
shredded, honey sauce with (*Lloyd's*), ¼ cup	13.0	0
shredded, original sauce with (*Lloyd's*), ¼ cup	11.0	0
sliced (*Hormel*), 5 oz.	23.0	0
carnitas, Southwestern (*Hormel*), 2 oz.	2.0	0
patties, breaded (*Tyson*), 3.2-oz. patty	17.0	2.0
ribs, barbecue sauce:		
baby back (*Lloyd's*), 2 ribs with honey hickory sauce, 4.1 oz.	16.0	0
baby back (*Lloyd's*), 2 ribs with original sauce, 5 oz.	18.0	0
spareribs (*Boar's Head*), 3 ribs with sauce, 5 oz.	9.0	0
spareribs (*Lloyd's*), 2 ribs with original sauce, 4.25 oz.	13.0	0
roast (*Hormel*), 5 oz.	0	0
roast, in gravy (*Tyson*), 5 oz.	3.0	0
chops, with gravy (*Hormel*), 5 oz.	3.0	0
strips, teriyaki (*Tyson*), 3 oz.	0	0
sweet and sour (*Simply Simmered*), 5 oz.	21.0	5.0
Pork, pickled (see also "Pig's feet"), (*Hormel*), 2 oz.	0	0
Pork backfat or belly, 2 oz.	0	0
Pork coating mix, seasoned:		
(*Oven Fry* Extra Crispy), ⅛ pkg.	11.0	0
(*Shake 'n Bake*), 1⁄16 of 6-oz. pkg.	8.0	0
chops (*McCormick Bag 'n Season*), 2 tsp.	4.0	0
herb roasted tenderloin (*McCormick Bag 'n Season*), ⅛ pkg.	0	0
Pork entree, freeze-dried, sweet and sour, with rice:		
(*Mountain House* Can), 1 cup	43.0	2.0
(*Mountain House*), ½ pouch	56.0	3.0
Pork entree, frozen, 1 pkg.:		
apple glazed medallions (*Healthy Choice*), 10.8 oz.	46.0	4.0
boneless, with potato and corn (*Swanson*), 10.5 oz.	67.0	4.0
with cherry sauce (*Lean Cuisine Spa Cuisine*), 8.25 oz.	38.0	4.0
cutlet, boneless, breaded (*Stouffer's* Homestyle), 10 oz.	33.0	4.0
roast (*Stouffer's* Homestyle), 9.5 oz.	43.0	4.0
roast, honey (*Lean Cuisine* Cafe Classics), 9.5 oz.	18.0	5.0

Food and Measure	carb. (gms)	fiber (gms)
sweet and sour (*Contessa* Minute Meal Bowl), 10.5 oz. . .	58.0	2.0
Pork entree mix:		
chops, breaded, mashed potato (*Pork Helper Oven Favorites*), ⅙ pkg.*	28.0	1.0
chops, with herb stuffing (*Campbell's Supper Bakes*), ⅙ pkg. mix	31.0	2.0
chops and stuffing (*Pork Helper*), 1 cup*	23.0	1.0
fried rice (*Pork Helper*), 1 cup*	24.0	<1.0
Pork gravy, in jars, golden (*Campbell's*), ¼ cup	3.0	0
Pork gravy mix (*McCormick*), ¼ cup*	4.0	0
Pork lunch meat (see also "Ham lunch meat"), roast, 2 oz.:		
all varieties (*Hatfield Deli Choice*)	1.0	0
barbecue flavor (*Dietz & Watson*)	3.0	0
Italian style (*Dietz & Watson*)	1.0	0
oven roasted (*Sara Lee*)	1.0	0
sirloin (*Dietz & Watson*)	0	0
Pork rind snack, .5 oz., except as noted:		
(*Baken-ets* Cracklins)	<1.0	<1.0
(*Baken-ets* Fried Skins)	0	0
all varieties (*Wise* Original), .6 oz.	1.0	0
barbecue (*Baken-ets* Sweet & Tangy)	1.0	1.0
hot (*Baken-ets* Hot 'n Spicy Cracklins/Skins)	<1.0	<1.0
Pork seasoning mix, see "Pork coating mix"		
Pork tidbits, pickled (*Hormel*), 2 oz.	0	0
Portugese sausage, see "Linguica sausage"		
Pot pie, see specific entree listings		
Pot roast, see "Beef dinner, frozen" and "Beef entree, frozen"		
Pot stickers, see "Dumplings" and "Chicken entree, frozen"		
Potato:		
raw:		
(*Del Monte*), 1 medium, 5.2 oz.	26.0	3.0
(*Frieda's* Baby/Fingerling/Red/Purple/Yukon Gold/Yellow Finnish), ½ cup, 3 oz.	15.0	1.0
(*Frieda's* Fingerling Bag), 4 pieces, 5.2 oz.	25.0	3.0
unpeeled, 1 large, 6.5 oz.	33.1	2.9
unpeeled, 1 long, 7.1 oz.	36.3	3.2
peeled, 2½" potato	20.1	1.8
peeled, diced, ½ cup	13.5	1.2

Food and Measure	carb. (gms)	fiber (gms)
baked:		
in skin, 4¾'' × 2⅓''	51.0	4.8
without skin, 2⅓''	33.6	2.3
without skin, ½ cup	13.2	.9
skin only, 1 oz.	13.1	2.2
boiled in skin, peeled, 2½'' potato, 4.8 oz.	27.4	2.4
boiled in skin, peeled, ½ cup	15.7	1.4
boiled without skin, 2½'' potato	27.0	2.4
boiled without skin, ½ cup	15.6	1.4
microwaved in skin:		
with skin, 4¾'' × 2⅓'' potato	48.7	4.7
peeled, ½ cup	18.2	1.2
skin only, 2 oz.	16.8	3.2
mashed, with whole milk:		
½ cup	18.4	2.1
with butter, ½ cup	17.5	2.1
with margarine, ½ cup	17.5	2.1
Potato, can or jar:		
with liquid, 1 cup	29.7	4.2
drained, 1 cup	24.5	4.1
whole:		
(*Butterfield* New), 3½ pieces	20.0	2.0
(*Del Monte* New), 2 pieces	13.0	2.0
(*Sunshine*), 3 pieces	20.0	2.0
(*S&W* Small), 2 pieces	13.0	2.0
1.2-oz. potato	4.8	.8
diced (*Butterfield* New), ⅔ cup	22.0	3.0
diced (*Del Monte* New), ½ cup	11.0	<1.0
sliced (*Butterfield* New), ½ cup	22.0	4.0
sliced (*Del Monte* New), ⅔ cup	13.0	2.0
Potato, dried, see "Potato dish, freeze-dried" and "Potato dish, mix"		
Potato, frozen (see also "Potato dish, frozen"), 3 oz., except as noted:		
whole, baby (*Birds Eye*), 7 pieces, 4 oz.	17.0	1.0
fried/fries:		
(*Cascadian Farm* Oven French Fries)	14.0	0
(*Ian's* Natural Harvest Fries), 2.5 oz.	13.0	1.0

Food and Measure	carb. (gms)	fiber (gms)
(*Ian's* Natural Quick Fries)	23.0	2.0
(*Ian's Alphatots* Natural), 3.5 oz.	23.0	.5
(*McCain Smiles*)	24.0	2.0
(*Ore-Ida Golden Fries*)	17.0	2.0
(*Tree of Life*)	19.0	1.0
cheddar cheese (*Ian's* Natural)	29.0	2.0
crinkle cut (*Kineret*)	20.0	2.0
crinkle cut (*McCain*)	21.0	2.0
crinkle cut (*McCain Premium Golden Crisp*)	23.0	2.0
crinkle cut (*Ore-Ida* Golden Crinkles)	17.0	2.0
crinkle cut, seasoned (*McCain Premium Golden Crisp*)	20.0	2.0
cross cut, with skin (*McCain Premium Golden Crisp*)	21.0	2.0
shoestring (*Cascadian Farm*)	21.0	2.0
shoestring (*McCain*)	21.0	2.0
shoestring (*McCain* 5 Minute Fries!)	32.0	3.0
shoestring (*McCain Premium Golden Crisp*)	20.0	2.0
shoestring (*Ore-Ida*)	19.0	2.0
spirals, seasoned (*McCain Premium Golden Crisp*)	18.0	2.0
steak (*McCain*)	21.0	2.0
steak (*McCain Premium Golden Crisp*)	23.0	1.0
steak (*Ore-Ida*)	17.0	2.0
straight cut (*McCain*)	20.0	2.0
straight cut (*McCain Premium Golden Crisp*)	23.0	2.0
waffle (*Ore-Ida*)	22.0	2.0
wedges, with skin (*McCain Premium Golden Crisp*)	17.0	2.0
hash browns (*Cascadian Farm*)	17.0	2.0
hash browns (*Ore-Ida Golden Patties*), 2.4-oz. patty	15.0	2.0
with onions and peppers (*Cascadian Farm* Country Style)	9.0	2.0
mashed:		
(*Ore-Ida*), ⅔ cup	18.0	2.0
creamy (*Reser's* Deluxe), ½ cup	18.0	2.0
garlic (*Reser's*), ½ cup	19.0	2.0
garlic or plain (*Diner's Choice*), ⅔ cup	19.0	1.0
onion, caramelized (*Reser's*), ½ cup	21.0	2.0
puffs:		
(*Cascadian Farm Spud Puppies*)	14.0	0
(*McCain Tasti Tater*)	20.0	3.0
(*Ore-Ida Tater Tots*)	20.0	2.0

Food and Measure	carb. (gms)	fiber (gms)
roasting, seasoned (*McCain Roasters* All-American)	21.0	2.0
roasting, seasoned (*McCain Roasters* South of the Border).	25.0	2.0
and vegetable blend (*Birds Eye*), ¾ cup	8.0	1.0
Potato, mix, see "Potato dish, mix"		
Potato, sweet, see "Sweet potato"		
Potato chips/crisps (see also "Potato soy crisps" and "Sweet potato chips"), 1 oz., except as noted:		
(*Barbara's* Unsalted/*Barbara's/Barbara's* Ripple)	15.0	1.0
(*Cape Cod* Classic/Whole Earth Classic)	17.0	1.0
(*Cape Cod* 40% Reduced Fat)	18.0	1.0
(*Cape Cod* No Salt)	14.0	1.0
(*Cape Cod* Robust Russet)	16.0	1.0
(*Garden of Eatin'*)	16.0	1.0
(*Herr's/Herr's* Ripples)	16.0	1.0
(*Jays*)	14.0	1.0
(*Kettle Chips* Lightly Salted/Unsalted)	15.0	1.0
(*Kettle Chips* Lightly Salted Low Fat)	22.0	2.0
(*Krunchers!* Original)	16.0	1.0
(*Lay's* Classic/Chicago Steakhouse/Original Wavy)	15.0	1.0
(*Lay's* Deli Style)	16.0	1.0
(*Lay's* Original Baked!)	23.0	2.0
(*Lay's* Original Light)	18.0	1.0
(*Lay's Stax* Original)	16.0	1.0
(*Miss Vickie's* Original), 1 pkg.	22.0	1.0
(*Munchos*)	16.0	1.0
(*Pringles* Original)	15.0	1.0
(*Pringles* Reduced Fat)	19.0	1.0
(*Ruffles* Original)	14.0	1.0
(*Ruffles* Original Baked!)	21.0	2.0
(*Ruffles* Original Light)	17.0	1.0
(*Snyder's/Snyder's* Unsalted)	19.0	n.a.
(*Snyder's* Coney Island)	20.0	n.a.
(*Snyder's* Ripple)	18.0	n.a.
(*Terra* Potpourri)	17.0	4.0
(*Terra* Yukon Gold)	19.0	0
(*Terra Blues*)	17.0	1.0
(*Terra Red Bliss*)	18.0	2.0

Food and Measure	carb. (gms)	fiber (gms)
(*Wise* Original)	14.0	1.0
(*Wise Choice* Crisps)	19.0	1.0
(*Wise New York Deli*)	13.0	1.0
aioli (*Terra Frites*)	18.0	3.0
au gratin (*Lay's* Wavy)	14.0	1.0
barbecue:		
(*Cape Cod* Beachside)	17.0	1.0
(*Kettle Chips* Classic)	16.0	1.0
(*Kettle Chips Chipotle Chili Barbecue* Organic)	16.0	2.0
(*Lay's* Country Natural/*Lay's KC Masterpiece*)	15.0	1.0
(*Lay's KC Masterpiece* Baked!)	22.0	2.0
(*Lay's KC Masterpiece* Light)	17.0	1.0
(*Ruffles KC Masterpiece*)	16.0	1.0
(*Snyder's*)	21.0	n.a.
(*Snyder's* Rib)	17.0	n.a.
(*Terra* Yukon Gold)	19.0	2.0
(*Wise*)	15.0	1.0
hickory (*Kettle Chips* Low Fat)	22.0	2.0
hickory (*Lay's* Wavy)	16.0	1.0
mesquite (*Lay's* Kettle Cooked)	16.0	<1.0
mesquite, with soy (*Wise Choice* Crisps)	14.0	3.0
mesquite, sweet (*Pringles*)	15.0	1.0
Cajun (*Pringles*)	14.0	1.0
cheddar, white (*Pringles*)	15.0	0
cheddar with herbs (*Kettle Chips* New York)	15.0	1.0
cheddar and bacon (*T.G.I. Friday's*)	17.0	1.0
cheddar and sour cream:		
(*Ruffles*)	14.0	1.0
(*Ruffles* Baked!)	22.0	2.0
(*Ruffles* Light)	16.0	1.0
(*Wise* Ridgies)	15.0	1.0
cheese flavor (*Pringles* Cheezums)	15.0	0
cheese flavor (*Wise Cheez Doodles*)	14.0	1.0
chili cheese (*Pringles*)	15.0	1.0
chipotle (*Wise*)	14.0	1.0
cottage cut (*Wise*)	12.0	1.0
dill:		
(*Snyder's* Kosher)	20.0	n.a.

Food and Measure	carb. (gms)	fiber (gms)
pickle (*Lay's*)	13.0	1.0
and sour cream (*Kettle Chips* Krinkle Cut)	15.0	1.0
garlic, roasted, and chive (*Wise Choice* Crisps)	20.0	1.0
garlic, roasted, Parmesan (*Yukon Red Bliss*)	16.0	2.0
guacamole (*Lay's Cool Guacamole*)	15.0	1.0
herb:		
fine (*Terra Red Bliss*)	18.0	3.0
garden (*Cape Cod*)	19.0	1.0
Italian, with soy (*Wise Choice* Crisps)	13.0	3.0
honey Dijon (*Kettle Chips*)	16.0	1.0
hot:		
(*Lay's Flamin' Hot*)	15.0	1.0
(*Pringles* Fiery)	15.0	1.0
(*Snyder's* Louisiana), 1.5 oz.	30.0	n.a.
(*Wise* Mighty Hot)	15.0	1.0
Buffalo wing (*Snyder's*)	20.0	n.a.
jalapeño:		
(*Lay's* Kettle Cooked)	16.0	1.0
(*Miss Vickie's*), 1 pkg.	22.0	1.0
(*Snyder's*)	20.0	n.a.
cheddar (*Cape Cod*)	16.0	2.0
cheddar (*Kettle Chips* Krinkle Cut)	16.0	1.0
with tequila and lime (*Kettle Chips*)	16.0	2.0
ketchup (*Herr's Heinz*)	15.0	1.0
lime (*Lay's Limón*)	15.0	1.0
malt vinegar (*Terra Frites*)	18.0	3.0
mustard and honey or French onion (*Kettle Chips* Low Fat)	22.0	2.0
onion and garlic:		
(*Garden of Eatin'*)	16.0	1.0
(*Terra* Yukon Gold)	19.0	1.0
(*Wise*)	14.0	1.0
Parmesan garlic (*Garden of Eatin'*)	16.0	1.0
pepper, cracked (*Snyder's*)	20.0	n.a.
pizza (*Pringles* Pizza-licious)	14.0	1.0
ranch (*Lay's Hidden Valley Ranch* Wavy)	16.0	1.0
ranch (*Pringles* RanchRageous)	15.0	1.0
red pepper, roasted, with goat cheese (*Kettle Chips*)	16.0	1.0
salsa with mesquite (*Kettle Chips*)	15.0	1.0

Food and Measure	carb. (gms)	fiber (gms)
salt and pepper:		
(*Terra* Yukon Gold)	19.0	1.0
fresh ground (*Kettle Chips*)	16.0	2.0
fresh ground (*Kettle Chips* Krinkle Cut)	15.0	1.0
sea salt (*Kettle Chips* Organic)	16.0	2.0
sea salt (*Terra* Kettles)	18.0	<1.0
sea salt, cracked pepper (*Cape Cod* Nantucket Spice)	16.0	1.0
salt and vinegar:		
(*Garden of Eatin'*)	16.0	1.0
(*Lay's*)	15.0	1.0
(*Pringles*)	15.0	1.0
(*Snyder's*)	19.0	1.0
(*Terra* Yukon Gold)	20.0	2.0
(*Wise*)	14.0	1.0
sea salt (*Cape Cod*)	17.0	1.0
sea salt (*Kettle Chips*)	15.0	1.0
sea salt (*Lay's* Kettle Cooked)	17.0	1.0
sea salt (*Miss Vickie's*), 1 pkg.	24.0	1.0
sea salt:		
(*Lay's* Natural)	15.0	1.0
(*Ruffles* Natural Reduced Fat)	17.0	1.0
with blue potato or sweet potato (*Terra* Kettles)	18.0	<1.0
seasoned salt (*Terra* Frites)	18.0	3.0
shoestring (*Jays*)	16.0	1.0
sour cream and onion:		
(*Kettle Chips*)	16.0	2.0
(*Lay's*)	12.0	1.0
(*Lay's* Baked!)	21.0	2.0
(*Pringles*)	15.0	1.0
(*Pringles* Reduced Fat)	18.0	1.0
(*Ruffles*)	14.0	1.0
(*Snyder's*)	19.0	1.0
(*Wise* Ridgies)	14.0	1.0
sun-dried tomato and balsamic vinegar (*Terra* Red Bliss)	18.0	3.0
taco (*Snyder's* Fiesta)	20.0	1.0
tomato and onion (*Terra* Frites Américaine)	18.0	2.0
yogurt and green onion:		
(*Barbara's*)	15.0	1.0

Food and Measure	carb. (gms)	fiber (gms)
(*Kettle Chips*)	15.0	1.0
(*Terra* Yukon Gold)	19.0	1.0
Potato dish, can or pkg.:		
au gratin (*Del Monte Savory Sides*), ½ cup	13.0	1.0
au gratin, with ham (*Hormel Cure 81* Bowl), 10 oz.	32.0	1.0
with chickpeas (*Tasty Bite* Bombay), ½ pkg.	13.0	3.0
scalloped (*Glory*), ½ cup	14.0	1.0
scalloped and ham (*Dinty Moore* Cup), 1 cont.	20.0	2.0
smothered, beef or chicken gravy or herbs and garlic (*Glory*), ½ cup	11.0	1.0
Potato dish, freeze-dried, 1 serving:		
and beef or cheese (*Mountain House*), ½ pouch	38.0	3.0
and cheese, cheddar, with chives (*AlpineAire*)	39.0	3.0
hash browns (*AlpineAire* Red & Green)	24.0	0
mashed (*AlpineAire* Instant)	22.0	0
mashed, garlic (*AlpineAire*)	5.0	0
Potato dish, frozen, 1 pkg., except as noted:		
au gratin (*Stouffer's*), ½ cup	18.0	2.0
baked, twice, butter flavor (*Ore-Ida*), 5 oz.	26.0	2.0
cheddar (*Lean Cuisine Everyday Favorites*), 10⅜ oz.	36.0	5.0
cheddar, bake (*Stouffer's*), 10 oz.	19.0	1.0
cheddar broccoli (*Healthy Choice*), 10.5 oz.	41.0	6.0
pancakes, see "Potato pancakes"		
roasted, with broccoli, cheese sauce:		
(*Birds Eye*), ⅔ cup	15.0	1.0
(*Green Giant*), ¾ cup	19.0	2.0
(*Lean Cuisine Everyday Favorites*), 10.25 oz.	35.0	5.0
(*Smart Ones*), 10 oz.	33.0	4.0
roasted, with garlic and herbs (*Green Giant*), 1¼ cups	33.0	4.0
whipped, and gravy (*Stouffer's*), ½ of 10-oz. pkg.	17.0	2.0
Potato dish, mix:		
au gratin (*Betty Crocker*), ⅔ cup*	22.0	1.0
au gratin, cheesy (*Velveeta*), 2.1 oz. mix	26.0	2.0
bacon and cheddar, twice baked (*Betty Crocker*), ¾ cup*	21.0	1.0
broccoli au gratin (*Betty Crocker*), ⅔ cup*	20.0	2.0
cheddar, au gratin, cheesy (*Betty Crocker* Deluxe), ½ cup*	22.0	1.0
cheddar bacon or three cheese (*Betty Crocker*), ⅔ cup*	21.0	1.0
garlic, roasted (*Betty Crocker*), ½ cup*	19.0	1.0

Food and Measure	carb. (gms)	fiber (gms)
hash browns (*Betty Crocker*), ½ cup*	26.0	2.0
julienne (*Betty Crocker*), ⅔ cup*	19.0	1.0
mashed:		
(*Barbara's*), ⅓ cup mix	17.0	1.0
with beef gravy, hearty (*Betty Crocker* Homestyle), ¾ cup*	24.0	2.0
butter, creamy (*Betty Crocker* Homestyle), ½ cup*	21.0	1.0
butter and herb, cheddar and bacon, or four cheese (*Betty Crocker*), ½ cup*	20.0	1.0
with chicken gravy, roasted (*Betty Crocker* Homestyle), ¾ cup*	25.0	1.0
chicken and herb (*Betty Crocker*), ½ cup*	21.0	1.0
garlic, roasted (*Betty Crocker*), ½ cup*	20.0	1.0
garlic, roasted, and cheddar (*Betty Crocker*), ½ cup*	20.0	1.0
sour cream and chive (*Betty Crocker*), ½ cup*	21.0	1.0
ranch (*Betty Crocker*), ⅔ cup*	23.0	1.0
scalloped:		
(*Betty Crocker*), ½ cup*	22.0	1.0
bacon, cheesy (*Velveeta*), 2.1 oz. mix	26.0	2.0
cheesy (*Betty Crocker*), ½ cup*	21.0	2.0
creamy roasted garlic (*Betty Crocker* Deluxe), ⅔ cup*	25.0	1.0
sour cream and chive (*Betty Crocker*), ⅔ cup*	21.0	1.0
Potato entree, see "Potato dish"		
Potato flour:		
(*Shiloh Farms*), ¼ cup	23.0	2.0
1 cup	132.9	9.4
Potato nuggets, frozen, with cheese and dill, breaded (*Kineret*), 3½ pieces, 2.8 oz.	19.0	5.0
Potato pancake, frozen:		
(*Dr. Praeger's*), 1.5-oz. piece	10.0	1.0
(*Dr. Praeger's* Bombay), 1.45-oz. piece	10.0	1.0
(*Kineret* Latkas), 1.5-oz. piece	9.0	1.0
mini (*Kineret* Latkas), 11 pieces, 3 oz.	21.0	2.0
nuggets (*Dr. Praeger's*), 4 pieces 1.4 oz.	7.0	<1.0
Potato pancake mix (*Carmel*), 3 tbsp.	18.0	2.0
Potato salad, refrigerated:		
(*Blue Ridge Farm*), 4 oz.	22.0	1.0
(*Hellmann's* Classic), 4.9 oz.	27.0	3.0

Food and Measure	carb. (gms)	fiber (gms)
(*Reser's* Regular/Homestyle), ½ cup	28.0	3.0
bacon cheese (*Hellmann's*), 4.9 oz.	24.0	2.0
with egg (*Reser's*), ½ cup	29.0	3.0
Potato salad mix (*Suddenly Salad*), ¾ cup*	24.0	2.0
Potato salad seasoning (*Watkins*), ¼ tsp.	0	0
Potato seasoning mix, dry:		
French fries (*Shake 'n Bake*), ¹⁄₁₂ pkg.	3.0	0
roasted Italian herb (*Produce Partners*), 2 tsp.	2.0	0
topping (*Produce Partners* Potato Toppers), 1 tbsp.	4.0	0
Potato soy crisps, 1 oz.:		
barbecue (*GeniSoy*)	17.0	2.0
Parmesan garlic, ranch, or sea salt and pepper (*GeniSoy*)	16.0	2.0
Potato starch (*Manischewitz*), 1 tbsp.	8.0	0
Potato sticks (see also "Potato chips/crisps"), canned:		
(*Butterfield*), ⅔ cup	16.0	2.0
(*Butterfield* Single Serve), 1 cup	26.0	3.0
Poultry seasoning (see also "Chicken seasoning"):		
1 tsp.	1.0	.2
and game pepper rub (*Ducks Unlimited*), ¼ tsp.	0	0
Pout, ocean, without added ingredients	0	0
Praline sauce (*Trader Vic's*), 2 tbsp.	21.0	0
Pretzel, 1 oz., except as noted:		
(*Cape Cod*)	27.0	<1.0
(*Goldfish*)	22.0	<1.0
(*Mr. Salty*), 1.1 oz.	25.0	0
(*Rold Gold* Thins)	23.0	1.0
(*Snyder's* Homestyle/Snaps)	25.0	<1.0
(*Snyder's* Olde Tyme)	24.0	<1.0
(*Snyder's* Snack Mix)	16.0	<1.0
(*Snyder's* Thins)	23.0	<1.0
butter (*Rold Gold* Checkers)	22.0	1.0
butter (*Snyder's* Snaps/Tiny Sticks)	25.0	<1.0
cheddar (*Rold Gold* Tiny Twists)	22.0	1.0
hard (*Snyder's* Unsalted)	22.0	<1.0
honey mustard (*Rold Gold* Tiny Twists)	23.0	1.0
honey wheat, sticks (*Snyder's* Organic)	24.0	<1.0
honey wheat, twists (*Rold Gold* Tiny)	22.0	1.0
mini (*Quinlan* Low Fat), 1.5 oz.	34.0	1.0

Food and Measure	carb. (gms)	fiber (gms)
mini (*Snyder's*/Organic Classic/Unsalted)	25.0	<1.0
multigrain, five, sticks (*Snyder's*)	23.0	1.0
mustard, deli style (*Gardetto's* Mix), ½ cup, 1.1 oz.	24.0	1.0
oat bran (*Shiloh Farms/Shiloh Farms* No Salt)	21.0	2.0
oat bran, sticks (*Snyder's* Organic)	25.0	1.0
pumpernickel onion, sticks (*Snyder's*)	23.0	1.0
pumpernickel onion, sticks (*Snyder's* Organic)	24.0	1.0
rods (*Rold Gold*)	22.0	1.0
rods (*Snyder's*)	24.0	<1.0
sourdough:		
(*Rold Gold* Specials)	23.0	1.0
(*Snyder's* Nibblers Fat Free/Unsalted)	25.0	<1.0
hard (*Rold Gold*)	21.0	1.0
hard (*Snyder's*)	22.0	1.0
sourdough, seasoned:		
(*Snyder's* Pieces New York Deli)	16.0	<1.0
buttermilk ranch (*Snyder's* Pieces)	19.0	1.0
cheddar (*Snyder's* Pieces)	18.0	<1.0
garlic bread (*Snyder's* Nibblers)	24.0	<1.0
honey barbecue (*Snyder's* Pieces)	17.0	<1.0
honey mustard onion (*Snyder's* Nibblers)	23.0	<1.0
honey mustard onion (*Snyder's* Pieces)	18.0	<1.0
jalapeño (*Snyder's* Pieces)	20.0	<1.0
spelt:		
(*Shiloh Farms* Big), .8-oz. piece	18.0	2.0
(*Shiloh Farms* Big No Salt), .8-oz. piece	17.0	2.0
(*Shiloh Farms* Mini/No Salt)	23.0	3.0
sticks:		
(*Rold Gold*)	23.0	1.0
(*Snyder's*)	25.0	<1.0
(*Snyder's* Dipping/Old Fashioned)	23.0	<1.0
sesame (*Snyder's* Old Fashioned)	23.0	<1.0
twists (*Rold Gold* Braided)	22.0	1.0
twists (*Rold Gold* Tiny/Fat Free)	23.0	1.0
whole wheat (*Shiloh Farms*)	20.0	3.0
whole wheat (*Shiloh Farms* No Salt)	18.0	3.0
Pretzel, soft, frozen:		
(*SuperPretzel*), 2.25-oz. piece	36.0	2.0

Food and Measure	carb. (gms)	fiber (gms)
(*SuperPretzel*), 2.5-oz. piece	40.0	2.0
(*SuperPretzel Soft Pretzel Bites*), 5 pieces, 1.9 oz.	29.0	<1.0
filled, 2 pieces, 1.8 oz.:		
cheddar (*SuperPretzel Softstix*)	23.0	<1.0
onion veggie cream cheese or pepperjack (*SuperPretzel*		
Pretzelfils)	22.0	1.0
pizza (*SuperPretzel Pretzelfils*)	23.0	1.0
Pretzel dip, honey mustard:		
(*Nance's*), 2 tbsp.	18.0	0
(*Snyder's*), 1 oz.	15.0	0
Pretzel sandwich, cheddar or peanut butter (*Snyder's*),		
1 oz.	16.0	<1.0
Prickly pear:		
(*Andy Boy* Cactus Pear), 1 large, trimmed, 3.6 oz.	8.0	2.0
(*Frieda's* Cactus Pear), 5 oz.	13.0	5.0
4.8-oz. fruit, 3.6 oz. trimmed	9.9	3.7
1 cup	14.3	5.4
Prosciutto:		
(*Boar's Head* Riserva Stradolce), 1 oz.	0	0
(*Fiorucci*), 1 oz.	0	0
Prune, see "Plum, dried"		
Prune juice, 8 fl. oz.:		
(*L&A*)	41.0	0
(*Langers* Plus)	41.0	1.0
(*R.W. Knudsen* Organic)	46.0	3.0
(*Sunsweet*)	42.0	3.0
(*S&W*)	41.0	1.0
(*Tree of Life Pure Fruit*)	43.0	2.0
canned	44.7	2.6
Psyllium husk (*Shiloh Farms*), 2 tbsp.	8.0	8.0
Pudding (see also specific listings), ready-to-eat,		
1 cont.:		
banana, creamy (*Kozy Shack*), 4 oz.	22.0	0
banana crème pie (*Hunt's Dessert Favorites*), 3.5 oz.	20.0	0
butterscotch (*Hunt's Snack Packs*), 3.5 oz.	20.0	0
chocolate:		
(*Handi-Snacks* Mega Cup), 5.25 oz.	31.0	1.0
(*Hunt's Snack Packs*), 3.5 oz.	22.0	0

Food and Measure	carb. (gms)	fiber (gms)
(*Jell-O*), 4 oz.	27.0	1.0
(*Jell-O*), ⅕ of 22-oz. cont.	33.0	1.0
(*Jell-O* Fat Free), 4 oz.	23.0	1.0
(*Jell-O* Sugar Free), 3.75 oz.	14.0	1.0
(*Kozy Shack* Real), 4 oz.	24.0	<1.0
chocolate brownie (*Hunt's Dessert Favorites*), 3.5 oz.	28.0	0
chocolate chip cookie (*Handi-Snacks* Doubles), 3.5 oz.	22.0	1.0
chocolate fudge (*Hunt's Snack Packs*), 3.5 oz.	23.0	0
chocolate fudge sundae (*Jell-O*), 4 oz.	25.0	0
chocolate marshmallow (*Hunt's Snack Packs*), 3.5 oz.	21.0	0
chocolate mud pie (*Hunt's Dessert Favorites*), 3.5 oz.	25.0	0
chocolate peanut butter pie (*Hunt's Dessert Favorites*), 3.5 oz.	27.0	0
chocolate/vanilla (*Handi-Snacks*), 3.5 oz.	21.0	1.0
chocolate/vanilla (*Handi-Snacks* Doubles), 3.5 oz.	22.0	0
chocolate/vanilla swirl:		
(*Jell-O*), 4 oz.	26.0	1.0
(*Jell-O* Fat Free), 4 oz.	23.0	1.0
(*Jell-O* Sugar Free), 3.75 oz.	13.0	1.0
cookie (*Jell-O Oreo*), 4 oz.	27.0	1.0
crème caramel flan (*Kozy Shack*), 4 oz.	23.0	<1.0
devil's food (*Jell-O* Fat Free), 4 oz.	22.0	1.0
dulce de leche (*Hunt's Dessert Favorites*), 3.5 oz.	23.0	0
dulce de leche (*Kozy Shack*), 4 oz.	25.0	0
lemon (*Hunt's Snack Packs*), 3.5 oz.	23.0	0
orange or strawberry cream swirl (*Jell-O Creme Savers*), 4 oz.	25.0	0
tapioca:		
(*Hunt's Snack Packs*), 3.5 oz.	20.0	0
(*Jell-O*), 4 oz.	25.0	0
(*Jell-O* Fat Free), 4 oz.	23.0	0
(*Kozy Shack* Old Fashioned), 4 oz.	23.0	0
vanilla:		
(*Hunt's Snack Packs*), 3.5 oz.	21.0	0
(*Jell-O*), 4 oz.	24.0	0
(*Kozy Shack* Natural), 4 oz.	22.0	0
vanilla caramel sundae (*Jell-O* Fat Free), 4 oz.	23.0	0
vanilla/chocolate (*Jell-O* Fat Free), 4 oz.	24.0	0

Food and Measure	carb. (gms)	fiber (gms)
Pudding bar, frozen, all varieties (*Jell-O* Pops),		
1.75-fl.-oz. bar	16.0	<1.0
Pudding and pie filling mix, dry mix, ¼ pkg. or 1 serving:		
banana cream:		
(*Jell-O* Cook & Serve)	20.0	0
(*Jell-O* Instant)	23.0	0
(*Jell-O* Sugar/Fat Free)	6.0	0
butter cream (*Jell-O* Instant)	23.0	0
butterscotch (*Jell-O* Cook & Serve)	24.0	1.0
butterscotch (*Jell-O* Instant)	23.0	0
cheesecake (*Jell-O* Instant)	24.0	0
chocolate:		
(*Jell-O* Cook & Serve)	22.0	1.0
(*Jell-O* Cook & Serve Sugar Free)	7.0	1.0
(*Jell-O* Instant)	25.0	1.0
(*Jell-O* Instant Sugar/Fat Free)	8.0	1.0
milk (*Jell-O* Cook & Serve)	22.0	1.0
white (*Jell-O* Instant)	23.0	0
white (*Jell-O* Instant Sugar/Fat Free)	6.0	0
chocolate cherry (*Jell-O* Instant)	25.0	1.0
chocolate fudge:		
(*Jell-O* Cook & Serve)	22.0	1.0
(*Jell-O* Instant)	25.0	1.0
(*Jell-O* Instant Sugar/Fat Free)	8.0	1.0
chocolate mint (*Jell-O* Instant)	25.0	1.0
coconut cream (*Jell-O* Cook & Serve)	18.0	1.0
coconut cream (*Jell-O* Instant)	21.0	1.0
cookies and cream (*Jell-O Oreo* Instant)	28.0	0
devil's food (*Jell-O* Instant)	25.0	1.0
lemon (*Jell-O* Cook & Serve)	12.0	0
lemon (*Jell-O* Instant)	24.0	0
pistachio (*Jell-O* Instant)	23.0	0
pistachio (*Jell-O* Instant Sugar/Fat Free)	6.0	0
tapioca (*Jell-O* Americana)	22.0	0
vanilla:		
(*Jell-O* Cook & Serve)	20.0	0
(*Jell-O* Cook & Serve Sugar Free)	5.0	0
(*Jell-O* Instant)	23.0	0

Food and Measure	carb. (gms)	fiber (gms)
(*Jell-O* Instant Sugar/Fat Free)	6.0	0
French (*Jell-O* Instant)	23.0	0
Pudding, plum (*Crosse & Blackwell*), ⅓ pkg.	91.0	4.0
Puff pastry shell, see "Pastry, puff"		
Pummelo (see also "Melogold"):		
(*Frieda's*), 5 oz.	13.0	1.0
1 lb. 3 oz., without rind	58.6	6.1
sections, 1 cup	18.3	1.9
Pumpkin, fresh:		
mini (*Frieda's* Orange/White), ¾ cup, 3 oz.	6.0	1.0
pulp, raw, 1'' cubes, ½ cup	3.8	1.0
pulp, boiled, drained, mashed, ½ cup	6.0	1.0
Pumpkin, canned, ½ cup:		
(*Libby's* Pure)	9.0	5.0
with or without winter squash	9.9	3.4
Pumpkin butter (*Lost Acres*), 1 tbsp.	11.0	0
Pumpkin flower:		
raw, ½ cup	.5	1.0
boiled, drained, ½ cup	2.2	.6
Pumpkin leaf:		
raw, ½ cup	.5	1.0
boiled, drained, ½ cup	1.2	.9
Pumpkin pie spice, 1 tsp.	1.2	.3
Pumpkin seeds:		
in shell, roasted:		
1 oz. or 85 seeds	15.3	n.a.
1 cup	34.4	n.a.
salted, 1 oz.	15.3	n.a.
shelled (*Shiloh Farms*), ¼ cup	4.0	3.0
shelled, 1 oz., 142 kernels	5.1	n.a.
shelled, dry-roasted (*Eden* Organic), ¼ cup	5.0	5.0
shelled, roasted:		
(*Tree of Life* Salted), ¼ cup, 2 oz.	8.0	4.0
1 oz.	3.8	1.8
salted, 1 oz.	3.8	1.8
Purslane, ½ cup:		
raw	.7	<1.0
boiled, drained	2.1	<1.0

Q

Food and Measure	carb. (gms)	fiber (gms)
Quail, meat only, without added ingredients	0	0
Quesadilla, frozen, 3.5-oz. piece, except as noted:		
beefsteak, shredded (*El Monterey* Carb Friendly)	15.0	9.0
cheese, three (*Cedarlane*), 3-oz. piece	25.0	0
chicken (*Tyson* Meal Kit), 3.9-oz. piece*	26.0	3.0
chicken and cheese:		
(*El Monterey* Carb Friendly)	16.0	9.0
char-broiled (*El Monterey* Mexican Grill)	20.0	1.0
three-cheese (*El Monterey*)	20.0	1.0
three-cheese, fried (*El Monterey Cruncheros*), 2 pieces,		
6 oz.	34.0	1.0
Quiche, frozen, 6 oz.:		
broccoli cheddar (*Cedarlane Carb Buster*)	7.0	2.0
cheese, four (*Cedarlane Carb Buster*)	5.0	<1.0
spinach artichoke (*Cedarlane Carb Buster*)	7.0	2.0
Quince:		
(*Frieda's*), 5 oz.	21.0	3.0
1 medium, 5.3 oz.	14.1	1.7
peeled, seeded, 1 oz.	4.3	.5
Quinoa, dry, ¼ cup, except as noted:		
(*Arrowhead Mills*), ⅓ cup	30.0	3.0
(*Eden* Organic)	29.0	11.0
(*Shiloh Farms*)	28.0	4.0
red (*Shiloh Farms*)	29.0	4.0
Quinoa flour (*Shiloh Farms*), ¼ cup	30.0	4.0
Quinoa seeds (*Arrowhead Mills*), ¼ cup	25.0	4.0

R

Food and Measure	carb. (gms)	fiber (gms)
Rabbit, meat only, without added ingredients	0	0
Raccoon, meat only, without added ingredients	0	0
Radiatore pasta entree, frozen, Romano (*Smart Ones*),		
10.4-oz. pkg.	40.0	4.0
Radiatore pasta mix,		
basil and herb (*Near East*), 1 cup*	41.0	3.0
and cheese (*Velveeta*), 4 oz. mix	46.0	2.0
with sun-dried tomato, basil sauce (*Annie's*), 1 cup*	52.0	1.0
Radicchio, fresh:		
(*Frieda's*), 2 cups, 3 oz.	4.0	1.0
1 medium leaf, .3 oz.	.4	0
shredded, 1 cup	1.8	.4
Radish:		
(*Dole*), 3 oz.	3.0	0
10 medium, ¾"–1" diam.	1.6	.7
sliced, ½ cup	2.1	.9
Radish, black (*Frieda's*), ¾ cup, 3 oz.	3.0	1.0
Radish, Oriental:		
(*Frieda's* Chinese Lo Bok), ⅔ cup, 3 oz.	5.0	2.0
(*Frieda's* Daikon), ½ cup, 1.1 oz.	1.0	0
(*Frieda's* Korean Moo), ⅔ cup, 3 oz.	3.0	1.0
7" piece, 11.9 oz.	12.8	5.4
sliced, ½ cup	1.8	.7
boiled, drained, sliced, ½ cup	2.5	1.2
Radish, Oriental, dried:		
shredded (*Eden* Daikon), 2 tbsp.	9.0	3.0
shredded, ½ cup, .5 oz.	36.8	4.8
Radish, pickled, see "Daikon, picked"		

Food and Measure	carb. (gms)	fiber (gms)
Radish, white-icicle:		
1 medium, .6 oz.	.5	.2
sliced, ½ cup	1.3	.7
Radish sprouts (*Jonathan's*), 1 cup	3.0	2.0
Raisin sauce, in jars (*Reese*), ¼ cup	36.0	0
Raisins, ¼ cup, except as noted:		
seeded, not packed	28.5	2.5
seedless:		
(*Dole*)	31.0	2.0
(*Shiloh Farms*), ⅓ cup	31.0	2.0
(*Tree of Life*	31.0	2.0
not packed	28.7	1.5
seedless, golden, not packed	28.9	1.5
vine-dried (*Frieda's* Raisins on the Vine), 4 oz.	77.0	6.0
chocolate/yogurt coated, see "Candy"		
cinnamon (*Dole CinnaRaisins*)	32.0	2.0
Rambuten, canned, in syrup, ½ cup	15.7	1.4
Ranch dip, 2 tbsp:		
(*Cabot*)	1.0	0
(*Litehouse*)	2.0	0
(*Ott's* Dipping Sauce)	1.0	0
(*Ruffles*)	1.0	<1.0
creamy (*Kraft*)	3.0	0
creamy (*Reser's*)	1.0	0
salsa (*Litehouse*)	2.0	0
Ranch dip mix (*McCormick*), ¾ tsp. dry	0	0
Rapini, see "Broccoli rabe"		
Raspberry, fresh:		
(*Dole*), 1 cup	17.0	8.0
½ cup	7.1	4.2
Raspberry, canned, in heavy syrup (*Oregon*), ½ cup	30.0	5.0
Raspberry, dried (*Frieda's*), ⅓ cup, 1.4 oz.	36.0	1.0
Raspberry, frozen:		
(*Cascadian Farm*), 1¼ cup	15.0	7.0
(*C&W*), ¾ cup thawed	7.0	7.0
(*Tree of Life*), ⅔ cup	12.0	2.0
sweetened, ½ cup	32.7	5.5

Food and Measure	carb. (gms)	fiber (gms)
Raspberry drink, 8 fl. oz.:		
(*Nantucket Nectars* Organic Very)	30.0	0
(*Newman's Own* Razz-Ma-Tazz)	28.0	0
(*Walnut Acres*)	32.0	0
Raspberry juice, frozen* (*Cascadian Farm*), 8 fl. oz.	29.0	0
Raspberry mist, blue, drink mixer (*Rose's* Cocktail Infusions),		
1.5 fl. oz.	15.0	0
Raspberry syrup, red (*Smucker's*), ¼ cup	52.0	0
Raspberry topping (*Smucker's PlateScapers*), 2 tbsp. . . .	25.0	0
Raspberry-peach drink (*Snapple*), 8 fl. oz.	29.0	0
Raspberry-peach juice (*R.W. Knudsen*), 8 fl. oz.	31.0	0
Raspberry-tamarind sauce, dipping (*Helen's Tropical Exotics*),		
2 tbsp.	11.0	1.0
Ravioli, frozen or refrigerated, 1 cup, except as noted:		
artichoke lemon parsley (*Cafferata* Oki Doki)	31.0	2.0
cheese:		
five, and soy (*Cafferata* 10 Carb)	14.0	4.0
four (*Buitoni*), 1¼ cups	40.0	3.0
four (*Buitoni* Light), 1¼ cups	37.0	2.0
four, and chive (*Monterey Carb Smart*), 3.5 oz.	18.0	5.0
three, mini (*Buitoni*)	43.0	2.0
cheese and sun-dried tomato (*Cafferata* Sunny)	22.0	0
chicken, Parmesan (*Buitoni*), 1¼ cups	45.0	2.0
chicken, roasted garlic (*Buitoni*), 1¼ cups	47.0	2.0
beef (*Buitoni* Classic), 1¼ cups	48.0	2.0
beef, mini (*Buitoni*)	46.0	2.0
butternut squash (*Cafferata* Squash By Gosh)	33.0	1.0
edamame and roasted corn (*Cafferata* Soy Good 4 U)	31.0	1.0
lobster (*Andrea*), 3 pieces cooked, 4.7 oz.	30.0	2.0
mozzarella herb (*Buitoni* Double Stuffed), 1½ cups	43.0	3.0
mushroom (*Cafferata* Magical)	31.0	0
pesto (*Cafferata* Manifesto)	24.0	0
seafood or spinach ricotta (*Monterey Carb Smart*),		
3.5 oz.	18.0	5.0
spinach and roasted garlic (*Andrea*), 3 pieces cooked,		
4.7 oz.	27.0	1.0
vegetable, garden (*Buitoni*)	39.0	2.0

Food and Measure	carb. (gms)	fiber (gms)
walnut and gorgonzola (*Cafferata* Nutty Gorgonzola)	25.0	2.0
whole wheat pasta:		
chicken, roasted, sun-dried tomato (*Monterey*)	34.0	4.0
tomato, basil, and mozzarella (*Monterey*)	34.0	4.0
vegetable and cheese (*Monterey*)	35.0	4.0
Ravioli entree, can or pkg., 1 cup:		
beef:		
meat sauce (*SpaghettiOs* Raviolios)	39.0	3.0
meat sauce (*SpaghettiOs* Superior)	43.0	5.0
mini (*Kid's Kitchen*)	35.0	1.0
cheese, tomato sauce (*Annie's* Organic Cheesy)	31.0	3.0
Ravioli entree, frozen, 1 pkg.:		
butternut squash (*Linda McCartney*), 10 oz.	49.0	3.0
cheese:		
(*Amy's*), 8 oz.	43.0	3.0
(*Contessa* Minute Meal Bowl), 9 oz.	33.0	6.0
(*Lean Cuisine Everyday Favorites*), 8.5 oz.	38.0	3.0
(*Stouffer's*), 10⅝ oz.	55.0	4.0
with Alfredo broccoli sauce (*Michelina's* Authentico),		
8 oz.	42.0	2.0
and rigatoni, Italian style (*Stouffer's*), 8.25 oz.	52.0	3.0
chicken, roasted, Italian style (*Stouffer's*), 8.25 oz.	42.0	2.0
Florentine (*Smart Ones*), 8.5 oz.	34.0	3.0
meatless (*Hain Vegetarian Classics*), 10 oz.	40.0	8.0
Recaito (*Goya*), 1 tsp.	0	0
Red bean (see also "Kidney beans"), canned, ½ cup:		
(*Allens*)	19.0	9.0
(*Bush's*)	19.0	6.0
(*Eden* Organic Small)	17.0	5.0
(*Glory* New Orleans)	22.0	7.0
(*S&W* Louisiana)	20.0	5.0
(*Westbrae Natural Organic*)	19.0	7.0
with rice (*Glory*)	18.0	3.0
Red bean dish, frozen, seasoned, and rice		
(*Glory* Savory Accents), ½ cup	17.0	3.0
Red kuri squash (*Frieda's*), ¾ cup, 3 oz.	7.0	1.0
Red snapper, see "Snapper"		

Redfish, see "Ocean perch"
Refried beans, canned, ½ cup:

Food and Measure	carb. (gms)	fiber (gms)
(*Allens*)	24.0	11.0
(*Amy's* Traditional)	21.0	6.0
(*Bush's/Bush's* Fat Free)	24.0	7.0
(*Las Palmas*)	23.0	9.0
(*Old El Paso* Fat Free)	18.0	6.0
(*Old El Paso* Traditional)	17.0	6.0
(*Pace* Traditional)	16.0	5.0
(*Taco Bell* Fat Free)	21.0	6.0
(*Taco Bell* Vegetarian Blend)	23.0	7.0
(*Zapata*)	22.0	7.0
black beans:		
(*Allens* No Fat)	23.0	8.0
(*Amy's*)	20.0	6.0
(*Ducal*)	26.0	6.0
(*Eden* Organic)	18.0	7.0
(*Goya*)	25.0	8.0
(*Zapata*)	20.0	5.0
and black soybean (*Eden* Organic)	13.0	6.0
spicy (*Eden* Organic)	18.0	7.0
green chilies (*Amy's*)	20.0	6.0
kidney beans (*Eden* Organic)	15.0	6.0
pinto beans (*Goya* Traditional)	24.0	7.0
pinto beans, regular or spicy (*Eden* Organic)	19.0	7.0
red beans (*Ducal*)	20.0	10.0
spicy:		
(*Old El Paso* Fat Free)	18.0	6.0
(*Pace*)	17.0	5.0
(*Zapata*)	24.0	8.0
Refried beans, mix, instant (*Fantastic*), ¼ cup	23.0	8.0

Relish, see "Pickle relish" and specific listings

Food and Measure	carb. (gms)	fiber (gms)
Relish, mixed, hot, Indian (*Patak's*), 1 tbsp.	<1.0	0
Remoulade dressing, in jars:		
dressing (*Louisiana* New Orleans), 1 tbsp.	2.0	0
sauce (*Zatarain's*), 2 tbsp.	4.0	<1.0
Rennet (*Junket*), 1 tablet	0	0

Food and Measure	carb. (gms)	fiber (gms)
Rhubarb, fresh:		
1 stalk	2.3	.9
diced, ½ cup	2.8	1.1
Rhubarb, canned, in extra heavy syrup (*Oregon*), ½ cup	44.0	3.0
Rhubarb, frozen, sweetened, cooked, ½ cup	37.4	2.4
Rice (see also "Wild rice"), dry, ¼ cup, except as noted:		
Arborio:		
(*Fantastic*)	36.0	<1.0
(*Goya*)	36.0	1.0
(*Lundberg Nutra-Farmed*)	35.0	1.0
(*S&W*)	35.0	<1.0
basmati, brown:		
(*Arrowhead Mills*)	31.0	2.0
(*Lundberg* Organic)	34.0	2.0
(*Lundberg Nutra-Farmed*/Royal)	38.0	2.0
(*Shiloh Farms*)	33.0	2.0
basmati, white:		
(*Arrowhead Mills*)	33.0	<1.0
(*Fantastic*)	36.0	<1.0
(*Lundberg* Organic)	38.0	1.0
(*Lundberg Nutra-Farmed*)	41.0	0
(*Mahatma* Indian)	36.0	0
(*S&W* Indian)	36.0	0
blends:		
(*Lundberg Jubilee*)	39.0	3.0
(*Lundberg Wild Blend/Countrywild*)	35.0	3.0
basmati/wild (*Lundberg*)	34.0	2.0
basmati/wild (*Shiloh Farms*)	32.0	2.0
brown/wild (*Fanci Food*)	34.0	1.0
brown/wlld (*Gourmet House*)	34.0	1.0
field rice (*Lundberg Black Japonica*)	38.0	3.0
white/wild (*Gourmet House*)	35.0	1.0
white/wild (*S&W*)	31.0	<1.0
wild rice garden (*Fanci Food*)	40.0	1.0
wild rice garden (*Gourmet House*)	40.0	1.0
brown:		
(*Carolina*)	32.0	1.0

Food and Measure	carb. (gms)	fiber (gms)
(*Lundberg Christmas*)	37.0	<3.0
(*Lundberg Wehani*)	38.0	3.0
(*Success* Boil-in-Bag), ½ cup	33.0	2.0
(*S&W*)	32.0	1.0
(*Uncle Ben's* Whole Grain Instant)	34.0	2.0
(*Uncle Ben's* Whole Grain Original)	35.0	2.0
precooked (*Uncle Ben's Ready Rice*), 1 cup*	41.0	1.0
brown, long grain:		
(*Arrowhead Mills*)	32.0	1.0
(*Lundberg* Organic)	38.0	3.0
(*Lundberg Nutra-Farmed*)	37.0	3.0
(*Mahatma*)	32.0	1.0
(*River Maid*)	32.0	<1.0
brown, medium grain (*Lundberg* Organic Golden Rose)	34.0	1.0
brown, short grain (*Arrowhead Mills*)	38.0	2.0
brown, short grain (*Lundberg Nutra-Farmed/Organic*)	40.0	3.0
glutinous or sweet	37.8	1.3
jasmine:		
(*Fantastic*)	36.0	<1.0
(*Mahatma* Thai)	36.0	0
(*A Taste of Thai* Soft)	36.0	0
(*Thai Kitchen*), 1 cup*	36.0	<1.0
(*Success* Boil-in-Bag), ½ cup	43.0	0
(*S&W* Thai)	36.0	0
white (*Lundberg Nutra-Farmed/Organic*)	36.0	0
sushi (*Lundberg* Organic)	36.0	1.0
white (*Success* Boil-in-Bag), ½ cup	43.0	0
white (*Success* Boil-in-Bag, 14 oz.), ½ cup	43.0	<1.0
white, long grain:		
(*Shiloh Farms*)	32.0	2.0
(*S&W*)	35.0	0
(*Uncle Ben's* Instant)	36.0	0
(*Uncle Ben's Converted Original*)	38.0	0
extra (*Carolina*)	35.0	0
extra (*Mahatma*)	35.0	0
parboiled (*Carolina Gold*)	32.0	1.0
parboiled (*Mahatma Gold*)	35.0	0

Food and Measure	carb. (gms)	fiber (gms)
precooked (*Uncle Ben's* Boil-in-Bag), ⅓ cup	41.0	0
precooked (*Uncle Ben's Ready Rice*), 1 cup*	44.0	1.0
white, medium grain (*Water Maid*)	37.0	<1.0
white, short grain:		
(*Goya* Valencia)	33.0	0
(*Mahatma* Valencia)	36.0	0
(*Shiloh Farms*)	36.0	2.0
Rice and beans, see "Rice dish, mix"		
Rice beverage (see also "Rice-soy beverage"), 8 fl. oz.:		
(*AmaZake* Gimme Green)	37.0	0
(*AmaZake* Oh So Original)	34.0	0
(*AmaZake* Rice Nog)	39.0	0
(*Lundberg Drink Rice* Original)	22.0	<1.0
(*Rice Dream/Rice Dream* Enriched)	25.0	0
(*Rice Dream* Heartwise)	27.0	3.0
(*Westbrae*)	20.0	0
almond (*AmaZake* Shake)	36.0	0
banana (*AmaZake* Appeal)	35.0	0
chai (*AmaZake* Tiger)	35.0	0
carob (*Rice Dream*)	32.0	0
chocolate:		
(*AmaZake* Chimp)	35.0	0
(*Rice Dream* Enriched)	36.0	0
almond (*AmaZake*)	36.0	0
mango (*AmaZake*)	35.0	0
mocha java (*AmaZake*)	37.0	0
hazelnut (*AmaZake*)	36.0	0
vanilla:		
(*AmaZake* Gorilla)	35.0	0
(*Lundberg Drink Rice*)	22.0	<1.0
(*Rice Dream* Heartwise)	30.0	3.0
(*Rice Dream/Rice Dream* Enriched)	28.0	0
(*Westbrae*)	20.0	0
vanilla pecan pie (*AmaZake*)	36.0	0
Rice bran (*Shiloh Farms*), ¼ cup	30.0	8.0
Rice cake (see also "Popcorn cake"), 1 piece, except as noted:		
apple cinnamon, buttery caramel, or honey nut		
(*Lundberg Nutra-Farmed*), .75 oz.	18.0	<1.0

Food and Measure	carb. (gms)	fiber (gms)
brown rice:		
(*Lundberg Nutra-Farmed*/Organic), .7 oz.	15.0	0
(*Lundberg Nutra-Farmed*/Organic Salt Free), .7 oz.	16.0	0
koku seaweed (*Lundberg* Organic), .75 oz.	17.0	1.0
mochi (*Lundberg Nutra-Farmed* Organic), .7 oz.	15.0	0
multigrain (*Lundberg* Organic), .7 oz.	16.0	<1.0
sesame:		
all varieties (*Westbrae Natural*), 2 pieces, .5 oz.	10.0	0
koku (*Lundberg* Organic), .75 oz.	17.0	2.0
tamari (*Lundberg Nutra-Farmed*/Organic), .7 oz.	16.0	2.0
toasted (*Lundberg Nutra-Farmed*), .7 oz.	14.0	1.0
tamari seaweed (*Lundberg* Organic), .7 oz.	15.0	0
wild rice (*Lundberg Nutra-Farmed*/Organic), .7 oz.	15.0	0
Rice chips/puffs, see "Rice snacks"		
Rice dish, canned, Spanish (*Zapata*), ⅔ cup	21.0	3.0
Rice dish, frozen, see "Rice entree, frozen"		
Rice dish, mix (see also "Grains, mixed, dish"):		
almond, toasted, pilaf (*Near East*), 2 oz. or 1 cup*	40.0	2.0
and beans:		
black (*Carolina*), 2 oz.	39.0	5.0
black (*Mahatma*), 2 oz.	42.0	2.0
red (*Carolina/Mahatma*), 2 oz.	40.0	6.0
red (*Goya*), ¼ cup	35.0	3.0
red (*Success* Boil-in-Bag), 2 oz.	51.0	8.0
beef (*Mahatma*), 2 oz.	41.0	<1.0
beef (*Success* Boil-in-Bag), 2 oz.	43.0	2.0
biryani (*Neera's*), 1 cup*	29.0	1.0
broccoli au gratin (*Uncle Ben's Country Inn*), 1 cup*	43.0	1.0
broccoli and cheese:		
(*Mahatma*), 2 oz.	41.0	2.0
(*Success* Boil-in-Bag), 2 oz.	40.0	1.0
cheddar (*Annie's* Organic), 1 cup*	40.0	2.0
brown rice:		
(*Lundberg* Quick Hearty Harvest), 1 cup*	30.0	3.0
and wild (*Success* Boil-in-Bag), 2 oz.	41.0	3.0
wild and mushroom (*Lundberg* Quick), 1 cup*	53.0	4.0
picante Spanish (*Lundberg* Quick Fiesta), 1 cup*	53.0	5.0
pilaf (*Near East*), 2 oz. or 1 cup*	41.0	3.0

Food and Measure	carb. (gms)	fiber (gms)
roasted garlic pesto (*Lundberg* Quick), 1 cup*	52.0	5.0
vegetarian chicken (*Lundberg* Quick Savory), 1 cup*	53.0	5.0
butter flavor (*Uncle Ben's Ready Rice*), 1 cup*	47.0	1.0
butter flavor, herb pilaf (*Marrakesh Express*), 1 cup*	43.0	0
Cantonese (*Health Valley Cup*), ½ cup	27.0	2.0
cheddar broccoli pilaf (*Marrakesh Express*), 1 cup*	40.0	0
cheese:		
(*Success* Boil-in-Bag), 2 oz.	39.0	1.0
four (*Uncle Ben's Flavorful Rice*), 1 cup*	43.0	1.0
nacho (*Mahatma*), 2.5 oz.	49.0	<1.0
three (*Uncle Ben's Country Inn*), 1 cup*	40.0	1.0
chicken/chicken flavor:		
(*Carolina*), 2 oz.	42.0	<1.0
(*Health Valley* Cup), ½ cup	26.0	3.0
(*Mahatma*), 2 oz.	41.0	1.0
(*Success* Boil-in-Bag), 1.5 oz.	32.0	1.0
(*Uncle Ben's Country Inn*), 1 cup*	41.0	1.0
herb or roasted (*Uncle Ben's Flavorful Rice*), 1 cup*	44.0	<1.0
pilaf (*Near East*), 2 oz.	43.0	2.0
pilaf (*Near East*), 1 cup*	43.0	2.0
roasted (*Uncle Ben's Ready Rice*), 1 cup*	44.0	1.0
roasted, and broccoli (*Success* Boil-in-Bag), 2 oz.	42.0	1.0
roasted, and garlic pilaf (*Near East*), 2 oz. or 1 cup*	44.0	2.0
chicken and broccoli (*Uncle Ben's Country Inn*), 1 cup*	42.0	1.0
chicken and vegetable (*Uncle Ben's Country Inn*), 1 cup*	41.0	1.0
chicken and wild rice (*Uncle Ben's Country Inn*), 1 cup*	42.0	1.0
chili, Thai, 1 cup*:		
green, and garlic (*Thai Kitchen* Jasmine)	39.0	<1.0
spicy (*Thai Kitchen* Jasmine)	43.0	0
sweet, and onion (*Thai Kitchen* Jasmine)	42.0	0
coconut ginger (*A Taste of Thai*), ¾ cup*	42.0	2.0
coconut ginger, Thai (*Lundberg* Sensations), ½ cup	22.0	2.0
curry:		
with carrots, onion (*Goya*), ¼ cup	34.0	3.0
with lentils (*Lundberg* One-Step), 1 cup*	38.0	5.0
pilaf (*Near East*), 2 oz. or 1 cup*	44.0	2.0
yellow, Thai (*Thai Kitchen* Jasmine), 1 cup*	41.0	0
dirty rice (*Lipton Cajun Sides*), 1 cup*	50.0	2.0

Food and Measure	carb. (gms)	fiber (gms)
dirty rice (*Neera's* Jamaican), 1 cup*	28.0	2.0
fried, Oriental (*Uncle Ben's Country Inn*), 1 cup*	42.0	1.0
garlic, roasted, and chili (*Thai Kitchen* Jasmine), 1 cup*	42.0	<1.0
garlic, roasted, herb (*Annie's* Organic), 1 cup*	43.0	1.0
garlic basil (*A Taste of Thai*), ¾ cup*	35.0	0
garlic basil, with lentils (*Lundberg* One-Step), 1 cup*	37.0	5.0
garlic butter (*Lipton Cajun Sides*), 1 cup*	48.0	1.0
garlic butter (*Uncle Ben's Flavorful Rice*), 1 cup*	44.0	<1.0
garlic and herb pilaf (*Near East*), 2 oz. or 1 cup*	44.0	1.0
ginger miso (*Lundberg* Sensations), ½ cup	24.0	1.0
jambalaya (*Mahatma*), 1.5 oz.	32.0	<1.0
lemon herb (*Uncle Ben's Flavorful Rice*), 1 cup*	45.0	<1.0
lemon grass and ginger (*Thai Kitchen* Jasmine), 1 cup*	42.0	0
long grain and wild rice:		
(*Carolina/Mahatma*), 2 oz.	41.0	2.0
(*Success* Boil-in-Bag), 2 oz.	42.0	1.0
(*Uncle Ben's* Fast Cook Recipe), 1 cup*	43.0	1.0
(*Uncle Ben's* Original Recipe), 1 cup*	42.0	1.0
(*Uncle Ben's Ready Rice*), 1 cup*	44.0	1.0
all varieties (*Near East*), 2 oz. or 1 cup*	43.0	2.0
butter and herb (*Uncle Ben's*), 1 cup*	40.0	1.0
garlic, roasted (*Uncle Ben's*), 1 cup*	42.0	1.0
mushroom (*Uncle Ben's*), 1 cup*	41.0	3.0
vegetable and herb (*Uncle Ben's*), 1 cup*	42.0	1.0
Mexican:		
(*Goya*), ¼ cup	37.0	0
(*Uncle Ben's Country Inn* Fiesta), 1 cup*	42.0	1.0
cheesy (*Old El Paso*), ⅓ pkg.*	55.0	2.0
mushroom, portobello, risotto (*Buitoni*), 1 serving	48.0	0
mushroom, shiitake (*Health Valley* Cup), ½ cup	26.0	2.0
mushroom, wild:		
herb pilaf (*Near East*), 2 oz. or 1 cup*	44.0	2.0
risotto (*Marrakesh Express*), 1 cup*	42.0	1.0
Parmesan and butter (*Uncle Ben's Flavorful Rice*), 1 cup*	44.0	<1.0
Parmesan pilaf (*Marrakesh Express*), 1 cup*	42.0	1.0
pilaf (see also specific listings):		
(*Carolina/Mahatma* Classic), 2 oz.	43.0	1.0
(*Near East*), 2 oz. or 1 cup*	44.0	1.0

Food and Measure	carb. (gms)	fiber (gms)
(*Success* Boil-in-Bag), 2 oz.	44.0	2.0
(*Uncle Ben's Country Inn*), 1 cup*	43.0	1.0
(*Uncle Ben's Ready Rice*), 1 cup*	44.0	1.0
Moroccan (*Lundberg* Sensations), ½ cup	22.0	1.0
pilau (*Neera's* Shahi), 1 cup*	48.0	2.0
primavera (*Goya*), ¼ cup	35.0	1.0
primavera (*Health Valley* Cup), ½ cup	26.0	2.0
risotto, (see also specific listings):		
Alfredo or Florentine (*Lundberg* Risotto), ¼ pkg.	31.0	1.0
garlic primavera (*Lundberg* Risotto), ¼ pkg.	29.0	1.0
Italian herb (*Lundberg* Risotto), ¼ pkg.	28.0	1.0
Milano (*Lundberg* Risotto), ¼ pkg.	34.0	1.0
Parmesan, creamy (*Lundberg Risotto*), ¼ pkg.	27.0	1.0
Parmesan or red pepper (*Marrakesh Express*), 1 cup*	42.0	1.0
rosemary and potato (*Buitoni*), 1 serving	47.0	2.0
Tuscan (*Lundberg* RIsotto), ¼ pkg.	31.0	1.0
vegetable, garden (*Buitoni*), 1 serving	47.0	0
saffron, see "yellow," below		
Southwestern, zesty (*Lundberg* Sensations), ½ cup	22.0	1.0
Spanish:		
(*Carolina/Mahatma* Authentic), 2 oz.	42.0	2.0
(*Old El Paso*), ⅓ pkg.*	55.0	2.0
(*Success* Boil-in-Bag), 2 oz.	43.0	1.0
(*Uncle Ben's Flavorful Rice*), 1 cup*	45.0	<1.0
(*Uncle Ben's Ready Rice*), 1 cup*	44.0	1.0
pilaf (*Near East*), 2 oz. or 1 cup*	54.0	2.0
teriyaki:		
(*Lipton Asian Sides*), ½ cup	51.0	1.0
(*Uncle Ben's Ready Rice*), 1 cup*	51.0	1.0
stir-fry (*Kraft*), ¼ pkg.	46.0	2.0
Thai (*Health Valley* Cup), ½ cup	27.0	2.0
Thai, seasoned (*A Taste of Thai* Golden), ¾ cup*	38.0	0
tomato, herb (*Uncle Ben's Flavorful Rice*), 1 cup*	45.0	<1.0
tomato, sun-dried, herb risotto (*Marrakesh Express*), 1 cup*	42.0	1.0
tomato basil:		
pilaf (*Marrakesh Express*), 1 cup*	41.0	0

Food and Measure	carb. (gms)	fiber (gms)
risotto (*Buitoni*), 1 serving	46.0	0
risotto (*Lundberg* Risotto), ¼ pkg.	30.0	1.0
yellow:		
(*Carolina/Mahatma* Saffron), 2 oz.	43.0	<1.0
(*Carolina/Mahatma* Spicy), 2 oz.	41.0	<1.0
(*Goya*), 2 oz.	40.0	0
(*Success* Boil-in-Bag), 1.5 oz.	33.0	<1.0
Spanish style (*Goya*), ¼ cup	37.0	1.0
Spanish style (*Vigo* Saffron), ⅓ cup	43.0	.5
Rice entree, freeze-dried, 1 serving:		
black beans and (*AlpineAire* Santa Fe)	69.0	10.0
Mexican, with cheese (*AlpineAire*)	39.0	3.0
mushroom pilaf, with vegetables (*AlpineAire*)	66.0	4.0
wild rice pilaf:		
with almonds (*AlpineAire*)	58.0	7.0
mushroom (*Mountain House* Can), 1 cup	44.0	2.0
mushroom (*Mountain House* Double), ½ pouch	55.0	3.0
Rice entree, frozen, 1 pkg., except as noted:		
and beans, Santa Fe:		
(*Lean Cuisine Everyday Favorites*), 10⅜ oz.	50.0	5.0
(*Michelina's Lean Gourmet*), 9 oz.	56.0	3.0
(*Smart Ones*), 10 oz.	49.0	6.0
and beans, Southwest (*Linda McCartney*), 10 oz.	43.0	4.0
broccoli, cheese sauce (*Birds Eye*), 10 oz.	49.0	1.0
broccoli, cheese sauce (*Green Giant* Cheesy), 10 oz.	56.0	2.0
brown, with vegetables:		
(*Amy's* Bowls), 10 oz.	36.0	5.0
black-eyed peas (*Amy's* Bowls), 9 oz.	38.0	8.0
teriyaki (*Amy's* Bowls), 9.5 oz.	52.0	4.0
chicken and, see "Chicken entree, frozen"		
fried rice:		
chicken (*Contessa*), 1¾ cups*	49.0	4.0
chicken (*Lean Cuisine* Cafe Classics Bowl), 10 oz.	45.0	3.0
chicken (*Tyson* Meal Kit), ½ of 28-oz. pkg.	69.0	5.0
chicken (*Uncle Ben's* Rice Bowl), 12 oz.	65.0	3.0
shrimp (*Ethnic Gourmet*), 11 oz.	63.0	4.0
shrimp (*Gorton's* Shrimp Bowl), 10.5 oz.	68.0	1.0
shrimp (*Michelina's Yu Sing* Bowls), 11 oz.	76.0	3.0

Food and Measure	carb. (gms)	fiber (gms)
paella, with chicken and seafood (*Contessa*), 1½ cups* ..	28.0	2.0
pilaf, with vegetables (*Green Giant*), 10 oz.	44.0	3.0
pilaf, with vegetables, herb butter sauce (*Birds Eye*),		
1 cup.	34.0	1.0
Thai stir-fry (*Amy's*), 9.5 oz.	45.0	5.0
and vegetables (*Green Giant* Medley), 10 oz.	52.0	4.0
and vegetables, Creole (*Glory* Savory Accents), ½ cup ...	25.0	2.0
white/wild, green beans (*Green Giant*), 10 oz.	51.0	3.0
Rice entree, pkg., 1 pkg. or cont.:		
black beans and (*Hormel* Bowl Southwest), 10 oz.	34.0	4.0
cheddar broccoli (*Bowl Appétit!*)	51.0	2.0
with chicken, see "Chicken entree"		
herb roasted (*Hormel* Cup), 7.5 oz.	28.0	2.0
Masala beans, basmati (*Tasty Bite*), 12 oz.	75.0	13.0
mushroom risotto, Tuscan (*Fantastic Fast Naturals*),		
8 oz.	50.0	2.0
paella, Spanish (*Fantastic Fast Naturals*), 8 oz.	55.0	4.0
Southwestern (*Bowl Appétit!*)	52.0	3.0
Southwestern (*Hormel* Cup), 7.5 oz.	25.0	2.0
sweet and sour (*Hormel* Bowl), 10 oz.	49.0	3.0
sweet and sour (*Hormel* Cup), 7.5 oz.	37.0	2.0
teriyaki:		
(*Bowl Appétit!*)	54.0	2.0
(*Hormel* Bowl), 10 oz.	47.0	3.0
(*Hormel* Cup), 7.5 oz.	35.0	2.0
Rice flour, ¼ cup, except as noted:		
brown:		
(*Arrowhead Mills*), ⅓ cup	27.0	2.0
(*Hodgson Mill*), <¼ cup	23.0	1.0
(*Lundberg* Organic)	22.0	2.0
(*Lundberg Nutra-Farmed*)	26.0	1.0
(*Shiloh Farms*)	27.0	2.0
1 cup	120.8	7.3
white (*Arrowhead Mills*), ⅓ cup	28.0	<1.0
white, 1 cup	126.6	3.9
Rice pasta, see "Pasta"		
Rice pudding, ready-to-eat, ½ cup, 4 oz., except as noted:		
(*Kozy Shack* European Style/Original)	22.0	0

Food and Measure	carb. (gms)	fiber (gms)
chocolate and vanilla (*Handi-Snacks*), 3.5 oz.	19.0	0
cinnamon raisin (*Kozy Shack*)	24.0	0
Rice pudding mix, dry:		
(*Uncle Ben's*), ¼ pkg.	23.0	0
(*Watkins*), 1½ tsp.	12.0	0
cinnamon raisin (*Lundberg* Elegant), ½ cup	16.0	1.0
cinnamon raisin (*Uncle Ben's*), ⅓ pkg.	37.0	0
coconut (*Lundberg* Elegant), ½ cup	13.0	1.0
honey almond (*Lundberg* Elegant), ½ cup	15.0	1.0
vanilla, French (*Uncle Ben's*), ⅓ pkg.	28.0	1.0
Rice seasoning, Mexican (*Lawry's*), 1⅓ tbsp.	6.0	0
Rice snacks (see also "Crackers" and "Rice cake"):		
(*Grainaissance Mochi* Bake & Serve), 1.5 oz., ⅛ pkg.:		
all varieties, except raisin-cinnamon, sesame-garlic and		
super seed	24.0	0
raisin-cinnamon	25.0	0
sesame-garlic or super seed	23.0	0
chips, brown rice (*Eden*), 1.1 oz.	19.0	0
puffs, five-flavor arare (*Eden*), 1.1 oz.	24.0	2.0
Rice syrup, brown (*Lundberg Sweet Dreams Nutra-*		
*Farmed/*Organic), ¼ cup	42.0	0
Rice-soy beverage:		
(*EdenBlend* Organic), 8 fl. oz.	18.0	0
(*EdenBlend* Organic), 8.45-oz. cont.	19.0	0
Rigatoni pasta dinner, frozen, jumbo, and meatballs		
(*Lean Cuisine Dinnertime Selections*), 15⅜-oz. pkg. . . .	50.0	6.0
Rigatoni pasta entree, frozen, 1 pkg.:		
with broccoli and chicken (*Healthy Choice*), 9 oz.	34.0	3.0
with broccoli and chicken, creamy (*Smart Ones*), 9 oz. . .	39.0	4.0
with chicken, white meat (*Stouffer's*), 8⅜ oz.	46.0	3.0
and ravioli, see "Ravioli entree, frozen"		
stuffed:		
cheese (*Michelina's* Authentico), 8.5 oz.	42.0	3.0
cheese (*Michelina's* Homestyle Bowls), 11 oz.	53.0	5.0
cheese (*Michelina's Lean Gourmet*), 8.5 oz.	37.0	3.0
cheese, three (*Lean Cuisine* Cafe Classics Bowl), 10 oz.	38.0	4.0
sausage, Italian style (*Stouffer's*), 9⅛ oz.	46.0	3.0

Food and Measure	carb. (gms)	fiber (gms)
Risotto, see "Rice dish, mix"		
Rockfish, without added ingredients	0	0
Roe (see also "Caviar"), mixed species:		
raw, 1 oz., 2 tbsp.	.4	0
baked, broiled, or microwaved, 1 oz.	.5	0
Roll (see also "Biscuit"), 1 roll, except as noted:		
brown and serve or plain, 2 oz.	28.6	1.7
club (*Pepperidge Farm* Hot & Crusty)	24.0	1.0
dinner (*Pepperidge Farm* Parker House)	14.0	<1.0
dinner, soft (*Pepperidge Farm* Country Style)	17.0	1.0
egg, 2 oz.	29.5	2.1
French:		
(*Pepperidge Farm* Hot & Crusty)	20.0	1.0
2 oz.	28.5	1.8
7-grain (*Pepperidge Farm* Hot & Crusty)	19.0	2.0
hamburger:		
(*Pepperidge Farm*)	21.0	1.0
(*Pepperidge Farm Carb Style*)	17.0	3.0
wheat (*Sara Lee* Classic)	38.0	3.0
wheat (*Sara Lee* Classic Heart Healthy)	37.0	3.0
2 oz.	28.5	1.5
hoagie, soft, with sesame seeds (*Pepperidge Farm*)	33.0	2.0
hot dog:		
(*Pepperidge Farm*)	24.0	<1.0
(*Pepperidge Farm Carb Style*)	20.0	3.0
(*Sara Lee* Gourmet)	23.0	<1.0
2 oz.	28.5	1.5
mixed grain, 2 oz.	25.3	2.2
kaiser or hard, 2 oz.	29.9	1.3
oat bran, 2 oz.	22.8	2.3
party, round (*Pepperidge Farm*), 3 pieces	26.0	1.0
rye, 2 oz.	30.0	2.8
sandwich bun:		
onion (*Anzio & Sons*)	34.0	1.0
onion, with poppy seeds (*Pepperidge Farm*)	25.0	1.0
potato, golden (*Pepperidge Farm Farmhouse*)	36.0	<1.0
sesame seed (*Pepperidge Farm*)	22.0	1.0

Food and Measure	carb. (gms)	fiber (gms)
sesame white (*Pepperidge Farm Farmhouse*)	36.0	5.0
wheat (*Pepperidge Farm Farmhouse* Country)	36.0	1.0
white (*Pepperidge Farm Farmhouse* Hearty)	35.0	<1.0
sourdough (*Pepperidge Farm* Hot & Crusty)	19.0	1.0
wheat, 2 oz.	26.1	2.2
wheat, whole, 2 oz.	29.0	4.3
Roll, frozen or refrigerated (see also "Biscuit, frozen or refrigerated"), ready-to-bake, 1 piece:		
butter swirl (*Rhodes Anytime!*)	16.0	0
butter swirl, with frosting* (*Rhodes Anytime!*)	21.0	0
crescent:		
(*Grands!*)	29.0	<1.0
(*Pillsbury* Big & Flaky)	18.0	<1.0
(*Pillsbury* Original/Butter Flake)	11.0	0
(*Pillsbury* Reduced Fat)	12.0	0
dinner:		
(*Pillsbury* Oven Baked Butter Flake)	20.0	0
(*Pillsbury Carb Monitor* Oven Baked)	11.0	4.0
French, crusty (*Pillsbury Home Baked Classics*)	19.0	0
sourdough, crusty (*Pillsbury Home Baked Classics*)	18.0	<1.0
white (*Pillsbury*)	18.0	<1.0
white, soft (*Pillsbury* Microwave)	25.0	<1.0
white, soft (*Pillsbury* Oven Baked)	17.0	<1.0
whole wheat (*Pillsbury* Oven Baked)	17.0	2.0
egg twists (*Kineret* Chall-Ettes)	27.0	<1.0
wheat, cracked (*Rhodes*)	24.0	3.0
white:		
(*Rhodes* Fat Free)	17.0	1.0
dinner (*Rhodes*)	17.0	0
Texas (*Rhodes*)	27.0	1.0
Roll, sweet, see "Bun, sweet"		
Romaine, see "Lettuce" and "Salad blend"		
Roman beans, canned (*Goya*), ½ cup	19.0	6.0
Roseapple, 1 oz.	1.6	<1.0
Roselle, 1 oz., ½ cup	3.2	<1.0
Rosemary, fresh, 1 oz.	5.9	4.0
Rosemary, dried, 1 tsp.	.8	.2

Food and Measure	carb. (gms)	fiber (gms)
Rotelle pasta dish, frozen, and vegetables, herb butter sauce (*Birds Eye*), 1 cup	26.0	1.0
Rotini pasta entree, three cheese (*Bowl Appétit!*), 1 pkg.	56.0	2.0
Rotini pasta mix:		
and cheese (*Velveeta*), ½ of 9.4-oz. pkg.	49.0	2.0
four cheese sauce (*Annie's*), 1 cup*	49.0	1.0
white cheddar sauce (*Annie's* Creamy Deluxe), 1 cup*	44.0	2.0
Roughy, orange, without added ingredients	0	0
Rowal, ½ cup, 4 oz.	27.2	7.1
Rum runner, drink mixer, frozen (*Bacardi*), 2 fl. oz.	32.0	0
Rutabaga, fresh:		
1 large, 1.7 lbs.	62.8	19.3
cubed, ½ cup, raw	5.7	1.8
cubed, ½ cup, boiled, drained	7.4	1.5
boiled, drained, mashed, ½ cup	10.5	2.2
Rutabaga, canned, diced (*Sunshine*), ½ cup	7.0	1.0
Rye, whole grain:		
(*Shiloh Farms*), ¼ cup	34.0	6.0
1 cup	117.9	24.7
Rye flour:		
(*Arrowhead Mills*), ¼ cup	23.0	4.0
(*Hodgson Mill/Hodgson Mill* Organic), <¼ cup	22.0	5.0
dark, 1 cup	88.0	28.9
light, 1 cup	81.8	14.9
medium, 1 cup	79.0	14.9
Rye malt, see "Malt syrup"		

S

Food and Measure	carb. (gms)	fiber (gms)
Sablefish, fresh or smoked, without added ingredients ..	0	0
Safflower kernels, dried, 1 oz.	9.7	1.0
Safflower meal, partially defatted, 1 oz.	13.8	<3.0
Saffron, 1 tsp.	.5	0
Sage, ground, 1 tsp.	.4	0
Sake, see "Wine"		
Salad blend (see also "Lettuce" and "Salad kit"), fresh, 3 oz., except as noted:		
(*Dole* American/European/Italian)	3.0	1.0
(*Dole* French)	4.0	2.0
(*Dole* Mediterranean)	3.0	2.0
(*Dole Very Veggie*)	4.0	1.0
(*Fresh Express* American)	3.0	1.0
(*Fresh Express* Italian/*Fresh Express Riviera*)	2.0	1.0
(*Fresh Express* Royal Blend)	5.0	2.0
(*Fresh Express Greener European*)	3.0	1.0
(*Fresh Express Veggie Lover's*)	4.0	1.0
(*Ready Pac* All American), 3 cups, 3.2 oz.	3.0	1.0
(*Ready Pac* Bordeaux), 5-oz. pkg.	5.0	2.0
(*Ready Pac* Continental)	4.0	2.0
(*Ready Pac* Costa Brava/Milano/Monterey Organic)	3.0	2.0
(*Ready Pac* Parisian)	4.0	1.0
(*Ready Pac* Portofino), 5-oz. pkg.	4.0	2.0
(*Ready Pac* Santa Barbara)	3.0	<1.0
(*Ready Pac Lafayette*)	3.0	1.0
butter, leaf (*Dole* Butter Mix)	3.0	1.0
with carrots, double (*Fresh Express* Green & Crisp)	4.0	1.0
coleslaw:		
(*Dole* Angel Hair/Classic)	5.0	2.0

Food and Measure	carb. (gms)	fiber (gms)
(*Fresh Express* Angel Hair), ⅓ of 10-oz. pkg.	5.0	2.0
(*Fresh Express* Old Fashioned), 3.2 oz.	5.0	2.0
3-color (*Fresh Express*), 3.2. oz.	5.0	2.0
field greens (*Dole*)	4.0	2.0
field greens (*Fresh Express Fancy Field Greens*)	3.0	2.0
iceberg blend (*Ready Pac* Classic Crisp/Hearty Green)	2.0	<1.0
iceberg, carrots, red cabbage:		
(*Dole* Classic Iceberg)	4.0	1.0
(*Fresh Express Iceberg Garden Salad* Zip Bag)	3.0	4.0
romaine (*Dole Greener Selection*)	3.0	1.0
iceberg and romaine (*Fresh Express* Green & Crisp),		
3.4 oz.	3.0	1.0
leafy greens (*Ready Pac*)	2.0	2.0
mesclun blend (*Ready Pac* Organic), 4.5-oz. pkg.	7.0	3.0
romaine blend:		
carrots, red cabbage (*Dole* Classic)	4.0	1.0
iceberg (*Dole Just Lettuce*)	3.0	1.0
leaf (*Dole* Leafy)	3.0	1.0
spring mix (*Ready Pac*), 5-oz. pkg.	7.0	3.0
Salad bowl, fresh, with dressing (*Ready Pac Bistro To Go*), 1 bowl:		
chef salad, 10 oz.	9.0	2.0
Cobb salad, 8.75 oz.	7.0	2.0
chicken Caesar, 7.8 oz.	8.0	2.0
Greek salad, 10.2 oz.	5.0	3.0
spinach bacon, 5.9 oz.	22.0	1.0
veggie, spring mix, 6.5 oz.	18.0	3.0
Salad kit, fresh, with dressing, 3.5 oz., except as noted:		
Caesar:		
(*Dole*)	8.0	2.0
(*Dole* Light)	8.0	1.0
(*Fresh Express*)	9.0	1.0
(*Fresh Express* Light)	14.0	1.0
(*Fresh Express* Supreme)	8.0	1.0
creamy garlic (*Dole*)	8.0	1.0
coleslaw (*Fresh Express*), ⅓ of 11-oz. pkg.	12.0	2.0
Oriental (*Fresh Express*)	13.0	2.0
ranch (*Fresh Express*)	8.0	1.0

Food and Measure	carb. (gms)	fiber (gms)
ranch, sunflower (*Dole*)	5.0	2.0
Romano (*Dole*)	9.0	2.0
taco (*Fresh Express Taco Fiesta*)	7.0	1.0
Salad dressing, 2 tbsp., except as noted:		
(*Albert's* Steakhouse)	4.0	0
(*Annie's Naturals* Goddess)	2.0	0
(*Ott's* Famous/Reduced Calorie)	8.0	0
(*Ott's* Famous Fat Free)	9.0	0
(*Wish-Bone Western* Fat Free)	12.0	0
(*Wish-Bone* Western Original Sweet & Smooth)	10.0	0
(*Wish-Bone Western Just 2 Good!*)	13.0	0
bacon (*Wish-Bone Western*)	10.0	0
basil, garlic vinaigrette (*Annie's Naturals*)	<1.0	0
basil, Parmesan (*Bernstein's*)	2.0	0
balsamic vinaigrette:		
(*Annie's Naturals*)	3.0	0
(*Cains*)	6.0	0
(*Kraft* Special Collection)	4.0	0
(*Litehouse* Natural)	4.0	0
(*Litehouse* Organic)	3.0	0
(*Newman's Own*)	3.0	0
(*Newman's Own Lighten Up!*)	2.0	0
(*Wish-Bone*)	3.0	0
basil (*Ken's*)	12.0	0
Italian (*Wish-Bone*)	5.0	0
berry vinaigrette (*Wish-Bone*)	2.0	0
blue/bleu cheese:		
(*Cains*)	2.0	0
(*Kraft Roka*)	2.0	0
(*Kraft Roka Carb Well*)	0	0
(*Kraft Roka Light Done Right*)	3.0	0
(*Litehouse* Big Bleu/Chunky/Original)	1.0	0
(*Litehouse* Lite/Organic)	2.0	0
(*Litehouse One Carb Plus*)	1.0	0
(*Ott's*)	3.0	0
(*Wish-Bone Just 2 Good*)	6.0	0
(*Wish-Bone Western*)	9.0	0
chunky (*Bernstein's*)	2.0	0

Food and Measure	carb. (gms)	fiber (gms)
chunky (*Ken's*)	1.0	0
chunky (*Marie's*)	0	0
chunky (*Wish-Bone*)	2.0	0
chunky (*Wish-Bone* Fat Free)	7.0	<1.0
vinaigrette (*La Martinique*)	0	0
vinaigrette (*Litehouse* Natural)	3.0	0
buttermilk (*Annie's Naturals* Organic)	1.0	0
Caesar:		
(*Annie's Naturals*)	1.0	0
(*Cains* Fat Free)	7.0	0
(*Cains* Light)	5.0	0
(*Kraft Carb Well*)	0	0
(*Litehouse*)	1.0	0
(*Litehouse* Fat Free)	2.0	0
(*Litehouse* Organic/*Litehouse One Carb Plus*)	1.0	0
(*Marie's*)	1.0	0
(*Newman's Own*)	1.0	0
(*Ott's*)	2.0	0
(*Wish-Bone Just 2 Good* Classic)	5.0	0
asiago, creamy (*Brianna's*)	1.0	0
cilantro pepita (*El Torito*)	2.0	0
creamy (*Bernstein's*)	1.0	0
creamy (*Cains*)	1.0	0
creamy (*Ken's*)	0	0
creamy (*Newman's Own*)	1.0	0
creamy (*Wish-Bone*)	1.0	0
creamy (*Wish-Bone Just 2 Good*)	7.0	0
creamy garlic (*Litehouse* Natural)	1.0	0
Italian, with oregano (*Kraft* Special Collection)	2.0	0
vinaigrette with Parmesan (*Kraft* Special Collection)	1.0	0
cheese (*Bernstein's* Fantastico)	2.0	0
cilantro lime vinaigrette (*Annie's Naturals*)	2.0	0
citrus vinaigrette (*Wish-Bone Citrus Splash*)	7.0	0
coleslaw:		
(*Hidden Valley*)	5.0	0
(*Kraft* Coleslaw Maker)	7.0	0
(*Litehouse*)	7.0	0
(*Marie's*)	8.0	0

Food and Measure	carb. (gms)	fiber (gms)
cranberry vinaigrette (*Litehouse* Natural/Fat Free)	6.0	0
Dijon, honey (*Cains* Fat Free)	9.0	0
Dijon, lime (*Newman's Own* Parisienne)	0	0
dill cucumber, creamy (*Cains* Fat Free)	8.0	0
feta, chunky (*Marie's*)	1.0	0
French:		
(*Annie's Naturals*)	3.0	0
(*Cains*)	7.0	0
(*Cains* Light)	5.0	0
(*Ken's* Country)	10.0	0
(*Kraft Catalina*)	8.0	0
(*Kraft Catalina* Fat Free)	8.0	1.0
(*Wish-Bone* Deluxe/*Just 2 Good* Deluxe)	8.0	<1.0
creamy (*Kraft*)	5.0	0
creamy (*Kraft Carb Well*)	0	0
creamy (*Kraft Light Done Right*)	9.0	0
creamy (*Wish-Bone Western*)	9.0	0
herb garden (*Bernstein's*)	8.0	0
sweet honey (*Kraft Catalina* Special Collection)	8.0	0
sweet red (*Litehouse*)	11.0	0
sweet and spicy (*Wish-Bone*)	6.0	0
sweet and spicy (*Wish-Bone Just 2 Good*)	9.0	0
vinaigrette (*La Martinique* True)	0	0
garlic, green (*Annie's Naturals* Organic)	2.0	0
garlic, roasted:		
creamy (*Bernstein's*)	3.0	0
vinaigrette (*Kraft* Special Collection)	3.0	0
vinaigrette (*Wish-Bone*)	3.0	0
garlic and herb vinaigrette (*Wish-Bone*)	5.0	0
ginger (*Makoto*)	2.0	0
ginger vinaigrette (*Annie's Naturals* Low Fat)	4.0	0
green goddess (*Annie's Naturals* Organic)	2.0	0
green goddess (*Seven Seas*)	1.0	0
Greek (*Cains*)	2.0	0
Greek vinaigrette (*Kraft* Special Collection)	2.0	0
honey bacon (*Litehouse* Fat Free)	11.0	0
honey Dijon:		
(*Kraft*)	6.0	0

Food and Measure	carb. (gms)	fiber (gms)
(*Kraft* Fat Free)	10.0	1.0
(*Litehouse* Fat Free)	9.0	0
(*Wish-Bone Just 2 Good*)	8.0	<1.0
vinaigrette (*Wish-Bone*)	6.0	0
honey mustard:		
(*Annie's Naturals* Low Fat)	6.0	0
(*Litehouse*)	3.0	0
(*Ott's*)	8.0	0
huckleberry vinaigrette (*Litehouse* Natural/Fat Free)	4.0	0
Italian:		
(*Annie's Naturals* Tuscany)	5.0	0
(*Bernstein's* Dressing & Marinade/Restaurant Recipe)	1.0	0
(*Cains*)	3.0	0
(*Cains* Bellissimo)	2.0	0
(*Cains* Fat Free/Robust)	4.0	0
(*Ken's*)	1.0	0
(*Kraft* Fat Free)	4.0	0
(*Kraft* House/*Kraft Light Done Right* House)	3.0	0
(*Kraft Carb Well/Kraft Carb Well* Light)	0	0
(*Litehouse One Carb Plus*)	1.0	0
(*Newman's Own* Family Recipe)	1.0	0
(*Newman's Own Lighten Up!*)	0	0
(*Ott's* Fat Free)	5.0	0
(*Ott's* St. Louis Style)	6.0	0
(*Seven Seas Viva*/Fat Free/Reduced Fat/Robust)	2.0	0
(*Wish-Bone*)	3.0	0
(*Wish-Bone* Fat Free)	4.0	0
(*Wish-Bone* House/Robusto)	3.0	0
(*Wish-Bone Just 2 Good*)	4.0	0
(*Wish-Bone Just 2 Good* Country)	3.0	0
balsamic (*Bernstein's*)	2.0	0
cheese, five (*Wish-Bone*)	6.0	0
cheese, three (*Kraft*)	1.0	0
creamy (*Cains*)	4.0	0
creamy (*Kraft*)	2.0	0
creamy (*Litehouse*)	3.0	0
creamy (*Ott's*)	1.0	0
creamy (*Seven Seas*)	2.0	0

Food and Measure	carb. (gms)	fiber (gms)
creamy (*Wish-Bone*)	4.0	0
herb, sweet (*Bernstein's*)	8.0	0
herb and garlic (*Bernstein's*)	3.0	0
Parmesan basil (*Wish-Bone Just 2 Good*)	7.0	0
pesto (*Kraft* Special Collection)	5.0	0
red wine and garlic (*Bernstein's*)	2.0	0
roasted red pepper, with Parmesan (*Kraft*)	4.0	0
with Romano (*Ken's*)	1.0	0
vinaigrette (*Kraft* Special Collection Classic)	4.0	0
vinegar and oil (*Ott's*)	1.0	0
zesty (*Kraft/Kraft Light Done Right*)	2.0	0
lemon chive (*Annie's Naturals*)	1.0	0
olive oil vinaigrette (*Wish-Bone*)	4.0	0
olive oil and vinegar (*Newman's Own*)	1.0	0
onion, Vidalia:		
(*Albert's/Ott's*)	7.0	0
honey mustard (*Albert's*)	13.0	0
sweet (*Ken's*)	9.0	0
papaya poppy seed (*Annie's Naturals* Organic)	4.0	0
Parmesan:		
(*Newman's Own* Parmesano Italiano)	2.0	0
with cracked peppercorns (*Ken's*)	2.0	0
garlic (*Litehouse*)	1.0	0
Italian, with basil (*Kraft* Special Collection)	2.0	0
and roasted garlic (*Newman's Own*)	2.0	0
Parmesan Romano (*Cains*)	3.0	0
Parmesan Romano (*Kraft* Special Collection)	1.0	0
peanut, Thai (*Litehouse*)	4.0	0
peppercorn Parmesan (*Cains*)	2.0	0
poppy seed:		
(*Albert's/Ott's/Albert's* Light)	7.0	0
(*La Martinique*)	8.0	0
(*Litehouse*)	6.0	0
(*Marie's*)	8.0	0
(*Ott's* Fat Free)	12.0	0
creamy (*Kraft* Special Collection)	8.0	0
ranch:		
(*Annie's Naturals* Cowgirl)	3.0	0

Food and Measure	carb. (gms)	fiber (gms)
(*Cains*)	1.0	0
(*Cains* Light)	6.0	0
(*Ken's*)	2.0	0
(*Kraft*)	2.0	0
(*Kraft* Fat Free)	11.0	0
(*Kraft Carb Well*)	0	0
(*Kraft Light Done Right*)	3.0	0
(*Litehouse* Country/*Litehouse One Carb Plus*)	1.0	0
(*Litehouse/Litehouse* Fat Free/Lite/Organic)	2.0	0
(*Hidden Valley* Original)	1.0	0
(*Newman's Own*)	2.0	0
(*Ott's*)	2.0	0
(*Ott's* Dipping Sauce)	1.0	0
(*Wish-Bone*)	1.0	0
(*Wish-Bone* Fat Free)	7.0	<1.0
(*Wish-Bone Just 2 Good*)	5.0	<1.0
(*Wish-Bone Ranch Up!* Classic/Zesty)	2.0	0
buttermilk (*Ken's*)	1.0	0
buttermilk (*Kraft*)	2.0	0
buttermilk (*Kraft Carb Well Light*)	0	0
cheesy (*Wish-Bone Ranch Up!*)	2.0	0
chipotle (*Litehouse* Natural)	1.0	0
garlic (*Kraft*)	1.0	0
garlic or spring onion (*Wish-Bone*)	2.0	0
jalapeño (*Litehouse*)	1.0	0
jalapeño (*Marie's*)	1.0	0
Parmesan garlic (*Bernstein's*)	2.0	0
Parmesan peppercorn (*Wish-Bone Just 2 Good*)	7.0	<1.0
peppercorn (*Cains* Fat Free)	10.0	0
peppercorn (*Litehouse*)	2.0	0
salsa (*Litehouse* Lite)	2.0	0
Serrano (*El Torito*)	2.0	0
Southwest (*Litehouse One Carb Plus*)	1.0	0
raspberry vinaigrette:		
(*Albert's*)	8.0	0
(*Annie's Naturals* Low Fat)	5.0	0
(*Cains* Fat Free/Light)	8.0	0
(*Kraft Light Done Right*)	5.0	0

Food and Measure	carb. (gms)	fiber (gms)
(*Litehouse* Fat Free)	6.0	0
red (*Ott's*)	2.0	0
raspberry and walnut (*Newman's Own Lighten Up!*)	7.0	0
red pepper, roasted:		
(*Litehouse* Natural)	2.0	0
with Parmesan (*Kraft*)	4.0	0
vinaigrette (*Annie's Naturals*)	3.0	0
red wine vinaigrette:		
(*Seven Seas*)	2.0	0
(*Seven Seas* Fat Free/Reduced Fat)	3.0	0
(*Wish-Bone*)	9.0	0
(*Wish-Bone* Fat Free)	7.0	0
Chianti (*Cains*)	5.0	0
olive oil (*Annie's Naturals*)	1.0	0
red wine vinegar and oil (*Newman's Own*)	3.0	0
Russian (*Wish-Bone*)	14.0	0
Russian, creamy (*Seven Seas*)	3.0	0
sea veggie and sesame vinaigrette (*Annie's Naturals*)	1.0	0
sesame, Asian:		
(*Annie's Naturals*)	4.0	0
cilantro (*Annie Chun's* Noodle/Salad), 1 tbsp.	4.0	0
ginger (*Litehouse* Asian/Fat Free)	8.0	0
ginger vinaigrette (*Annie's Naturals*)	4.0	0
soy (*Trader Vic's*)	3.0	0
shiitake sesame vinaigrette (*Annie's Naturals*)	1.0	0
sweet and sour (*Old Dutch*)	13.0	0
tamari:		
mustard or sesame (*San-J*)	5.0	0
peanut (*San-J*)	9.0	0
vinaigrette (*San-J*)	4.0	0
Thousand Island:		
(*Annie's Naturals* Organic)	5.0	0
(*Ken's*)	4.0	0
(*Kraft*)	5.0	0
(*Kraft* Fat Free)	10.0	0
(*Litehouse*)	3.0	0
(*Newman's Own* Two)	4.0	0
(*Ott's*)	6.0	0

Food and Measure	carb. (gms)	fiber (gms)
(*Wish-Bone*)	6.0	0
(*Wish-Bone Just 2 Good*)	9.0	0
tomato, sun-dried (*Kraft* Special Collection)	4.0	0
tomato bacon, tangy (*Kraft* Special Collection)	8.0	0
tuna salad (*Kraft* Tuna Salad Maker), 1 tbsp.	2.0	0
vinaigrette (see also specific listings):		
(*Litehouse* Fat Free)	1.0	0
blush wine (*Cains* Fat Free)	9.0	0
blush wine (*Cains* Light)	8.0	0
Mediterranean (*Litehouse One Carb Plus*)	1.0	0
olive oil (*Bernstein's*)	3.0	0
vinegar free (*Annie's Naturals* Garden-style)	2.0	0
yogurt with dill (*Annie's Naturals* Organic Nonfat)	3.0	0
Salad dressing mix, ⅛ pkt. dry mix, except as noted:		
Caesar, gourmet (*Good Seasons*)	2.0	0
cheese garlic or garlic herb (*Good Seasons*)	1.0	0
Italian:		
(*Good Seasons* Cruet Kit)	1.0	0
(*Good Seasons* Fat Free)	3.0	0
mild or Parmesan (*Good Seasons*)	2.0	0
zesty (*Good Seasons*)	1.0	0
peanut (*A Taste of Thai*), 2 tbsp.*	7.0	1.0
sesame, Oriental (*Good Seasons*)	3.0	0
Salad dressing/topping kit, approx. ⅕ pkg.:		
balsamic Italian (*Linsey Et Tu Caesar*)	9.0	1.0
Caesar (*Linsey Et Tu Caesar*)	8.0	<1.0
Caesar (*Linsey Et Tu Caesar* Light)	9.0	0
Greek (*Linsey Et Tu Caesar* Authentic)	6.0	0
Oriental (*Linsey Et Tu Caesar*)	14.0	<1.0
spinach (*Linsey Et Tu Caesar*)	8.0	0
Salad toppers (see also "Bacon bits" and "Croutons"):		
(*McCormick Salad Toppins*), 1⅓ tbsp.	2.0	0
(*Produce Partners* Crunchies), 1 tbsp.	2.0	0
garden vegetable (*McCormick Salad Toppins*), 1⅓ tbsp.	3.0	0
Salami:		
(*Hatfield Deli Choice*), 2 oz.	2.0	0
beef, 2 oz.:		
(*Boar's Head*)	0	0

Food and Measure	carb. (gms)	fiber (gms)
(*Hansel 'n Gretel*)	4.0	0
(*Hebrew National*/Chub)	0	0
lean (*Hebrew National*)	1.0	0
cooked, 2 oz.:		
(*Boar's Head*)	0	0
(*Deli Delight*)	4.0	0
regular or hot (*Hansel 'n Gretel*)	4.0	0
cotto, 1 oz.:		
(*Oscar Mayer*)	1.0	0
(*Oscar Mayer* 50% Less Fat)	0	0
beef (*Oscar Mayer*)	1.0	0
dry, Italian (*Boar's Head Bianco D'Oro*), 1 oz.	1.0	0
Genoa:		
(*Boar's Head*), 2 oz.	1.0	0
(*Hansel 'n' Gretel*), 2 oz.	3.0	0
(*Hormel Pillow Pack*), 2 oz.	0	0
(*Sara Lee* Sliced), 4 slices, 1 oz.	1.0	0
(*Tyson* Sliced), 4 slices, 1 oz.	1.0	0
hard:		
(*Boar's Head*), 1 oz.	<1.0	0
(*Hansel 'n' Gretel*), 2 oz.	2.0	0
(*Oscar Mayer*), 1 oz.	1.0	0
(*Sara Lee* Sliced), 4 slices, 1 oz.	0	0
(*Tyson* Sliced), 4 slices, 1 oz.	1.0	0
"Salami," vegetarian:		
(*Worthington*), 3 slices, 2 oz.	3.0	2.0
slices (*Yves*), 2.2 oz.	5.0	1.0
Salisbury steak, see "Beef dinner" and "Beef entree"		
Salmon, fresh or canned, without added ingredients	0	0
Salmon, baked (*Acme*), 2 oz.	1.0	0
Salmon, marinated (*Spence & Co.* Gravlax), 2 oz.	<1.0	<1.0
Salmon, smoked, 2 oz.		
(*Acme*)	0	0
(*Echo Falls*)	2.0	0
all varieties (*Ducktrap River*)	0	0
Chinook	0	0
keta (*SeaBear* Beer Garden)	4.7	1.9
king, wild, Nova style (*SeaBear*)	0	0

Food and Measure	carb. (gms)	fiber (gms)
lox or Nova (*Vita*)	<1.0	0
pastrami style (*Spence & Co.*)	<1.0	<1.0
sockeye, wild (*SeaBear*)	0	0
sockeye, wild, Nova style (*SeaBear*)	1.0	0
Salmon, smoked, canned, in oil (*Bumble Bee*), 1 can drained, 3 oz.	0	0
Salmon, smoked, spread:		
(*Sau•Sea*), 2 tbsp.	1.0	0
(*SeaBear*), 8 oz.	6.5	.5
Salmon burger, frozen (*Dr. Praeger's*), 2.75-oz. piece	11.0	3.0
Salmon cake, frozen (*Dr. Praeger's*), 2.9-oz. piece	14.0	<1.0
Salmon entree, frozen:		
with basil (*Lean Cuisine Spa Cuisine*), 9.5-oz. pkg.	31.0	5.0
grilled:		
(*Gorton's* Classic), 3.8-oz. piece	1.0	0
lemon butter (*Gorton's*), 3.8-oz. piece	1.0	0
lemon butter (*Mrs. Paul's* Meals), 11-oz. pkg.	35.0	3.0
stuffed, with spinach and cheese (*Oven Poppers*), 5-oz. piece	10.0	0
Salmon entree, pkg., poached sockeye (*SeaBear*), 2 oz. ..	0	0
Salmon frankfurter, see "Frankfurter"		
Salmon gefilte fish, see "Gefilte fish, frozen"		
Salmon oil, 2 tbsp.	0	0
Salmon pastrami (*A&B Famous*), 2 oz.	1.0	0
Salmon pâté:		
(*Trois Petits Cochons*), 2 oz.	2.0	0
smoked (*Ducktrap River*), ¼ cup	1.0	0
Salmon salami (*A&B Famous*), 2 oz.	2.0	0
Salmon seasoning mix (*Old Bay* Classic), ⅕ pkg.	3.0	0
Salsa (see also "Picante sauce"), 2 tbsp., except as noted:		
(*Cedar's Boston*), 2 tsp.	<1.0	0
(*D.L. Jardine's* Bobos)	3.0	<1.0
(*D.L. Jardine's* Texacante)	2.0	<1.0
(*El Torito* Original Restaurant)	2.0	0
(*Guiltless Gourmet* Southwestern Grill)	2.0	0
(*Herdez* Casera/Ranchera/Verde)	1.0	0
(*Herdez* Taquera)	2.0	0
(*La Victoria* Ranchera/Salsa Victoria)	2.0	0

Food and Measure	carb. (gms)	fiber (gms)
(*La Victoria* Suprema)	1.0	0
(*La Victoria* Thick 'N Chunky/Verde)	2.0	0
(*Neera's* Caribbean), 1 tbsp.	7.0	0
(*Newman's Own* Bandito)	2.0	1.0
(*Pace* Chunky)	2.0	1.0
(*Pace* Dip)	2.0	<1.0
(*Tostitos* Restaurant Style)	3.0	<1.0
artichoke (*D.L. Jardine's* Cowpoke)	2.0	0
artichoke (*Jose Goldstein*)	2.0	0
black bean and corn:		
(*Amy's*)	3.0	1.0
(*Fiesta*)	2.0	0
(*Frontier Traders*)	3.0	1.0
(*Muir Glen*)	2.0	0
(*Walnut Acres* Midnight Sun)	3.0	1.0
cheese (con queso), see "Cheese dip"		
with cheese (*Kaukauna*)	3.0	0
cherry (*D.L. Jardine's* Cowboy)	6.0	0
chipotle (*D.L. Jardine's* Olé)	2.0	<1.0
chipotle (*Pace* Chunky)	2.0	1.0
cilantro:		
(*Pace* Chunky)	2.0	1.0
(*Walnut Acres* Fiesta)	2.0	0
olive (*D.L. Jardine's*)	2.0	<1.0
corn (*Garden of Eatin'*)	3.0	0
cranberry orange (*D.L. Jardine's*)	4.0	<1.0
fire-roasted tomato:		
(*Pace* Chunky)	2.0	1.0
(*Tostitos*)	2.0	1.0
mild or medium (*El Torito*)	2.0	0
mild, medium, or hot (*Zapata* Roja/Verde)	2.0	0
garlic:		
(*Jose Goldstein* XXX)	2.0	0
(*Garden of Eatin'*)	2.0	0
(*Pace* Chunky Grande)	3.0	1.0
cactus or chipotle (*Jose Goldstein*)	2.0	0
chipotle or cilantro (*Muir Glen*)	2.0	0

Food and Measure	carb. (gms)	fiber (gms)
garlic, roasted (*Newman's Own*)	2.0	1.0
garlic, roasted, and olive (*Jose Goldstein*)	1.0	0
green chili (*Pace* Territorial House)	2.0	<1.0
habañero:		
(*D.L. Jardine's*)	2.0	0
(*Frontier Traders* Wild & Hot)	2.0	0
garlic (*Pain is Good*)	2.0	0
hot:		
(*Chi-Chi's*/Fiesta)	2.0	0
(*Herdez*)	1.0	0
(*Old El Paso Gotta Have Hot* Thick n' Chunky)	3.0	0
jalapeño:		
green or red (*La Victoria*)	2.0	0
smoked (*Fiesta*)	2.0	0
smoked (*Frontier Traders*)	2.0	0
lime cilantro (*D.L. Jardine's*)	3.0	0
lime and garlic (*Pace* Chunky)	3.0	1.0
mango (*D.L. Jardine's* Mariachi)	3.0	0
medium:		
(*Garden of Eatin'*)	4.0	0
(*Herdez*)	1.0	0
(*Litehouse*)	3.0	0
(*Muir Glen*)	2.0	0
(*Taco Bell* Thick 'n Chunky)	2.0	1.0
medium or mild:		
(*Amy's*)	2.0	0
(*Cape Cod*)	3.0	1.0
(*Chi-Chi's*/Chi-Chi's All Natural)	2.0	0
(*Herdez* Casera)	1.0	0
(*Old El Paso* Salsa Verde)	2.0	0
(*Old El Paso* Thick n' Chunky)	3.0	0
(*Red Gold*)	2.0	1.0
(*Tostitos*)	3.0	1.0
mild (*Old El Paso Wild for Mild* Thick 'n Chunky)	2.0	0
mild (*Taco Bell* Thick 'n Chunky)	3.0	1.0
peach:		
(*D.L. Jardine's*)	5.0	0

	carb. (gms)	fiber (gms)
(*Frontier Traders* Wild & Mild)	4.0	0
(*Newman's Own*)	6.0	1.0
Southwest, sweet (*Walnut Acres*)	5.0	0
pepper, garden (*Old El Paso*)	2.0	<1.0
pepper, roasted, and garlic (*Pace* Chunky)	2.0	1.0
pineapple:		
(*D.L. Jardine's*)	4.0	0
(*Newman's Own*)	3.0	1.0
chipotle (*D.L. Jardine's*)	3.0	0
Jamaican (*Pain is Good*)	3.0	0
raspberry:		
(*D.L. Jardine's*)	4.0	<1.0
(*Frontier Traders* Wild & Mild)	4.0	0
Chardonnay (*D.L. Jardine's*)	4.0	0
red pepper, roasted (*Guiltless Gourmet*)	2.0	0
red pepper, roasted, and garlic (*Pace* Chunky)	2.0	<1.0
Southwest Tex-Mex (*Frontier Traders*)	2.0	0
sweet (*Snyder's* Garden Style)	5.0	0
tequila lime (*Chi-Chi's*)	3.0	0
tomatillo, fire-roasted (*Fiesta*)	12.0	0
tomato, roasted (*Chi-Chi's*)	2.0	0
Salsa dip (see also "Cheese dip"), sour cream (*Cabot* Salsa Grande), 2 tbsp.	1.0	0
Salsa seasoning mix, fresh (*Lawry's*), ½ tsp.	1.0	0
Salsify:		
raw (*Frieda's*), ¾ cup, 3 oz.	16.0	3.0
raw, sliced, ½ cup	12.5	2.2
boiled, drained, sliced, ½ cup	10.5	2.1
Salt, regular or seasoned, 1 tbsp.	0	0
Salt, substitute, 1 tbsp.	0	0
Salt pork, raw	0	0
Sandwich, see specific listings		
Sandwich sauce, canned:		
(*Hormel Not-So-Sloppy-Joe*), ¼ cup	13.0	1.0
sloppy Joe, ¼ cup:		
(*Del Monte*)	11.0	0
(*Heinz*)	10.0	1.0
(*Manwich* Original)	6.0	1.0

Food and Measure	carb. (gms)	fiber (gms)
hickory smoke (*Del Monte*)	14.0	0
vegetarian (*Worthington*), ½ cup	23.0	3.0
Sandwich sauce seasoning mix, see "Sloppy Joe seasoning mix"		
Sandwich spread (see also "Meat spread"):		
(*Black Bear*), 1 tbsp.	3.0	0
(*Cains*), 1 tbsp.	2.0	0
(*Hellmann's*), 1 tbsp.	2.0	0
burger (*Kraft*), 2 tbsp.	4.0	0
Sapodilla:		
(*Frieda's*), 3-oz. fruit	17.0	5.0
1 medium, 3'' × 2½'', 6 oz.	33.9	9.0
pulp, ½ cup	24.1	6.4
Sapote:		
(*Frieda's*), 5 oz.	47.0	4.0
11.2-oz. fruit, 7.9 oz. trimmed	76.0	5.9
trimmed, 1 oz.	9.6	.7
Sardine, fresh, see "Herring"		
Sardine, canned (see also "Herring, canned"):		
Atlantic, in oil, 4 oz.	0	0
all varieties (*Bela*), ¼ cup	0	0
in hot sauce (*Beach Cliff/Brunswick* Louisiana), 3.75 oz.	2.0	0
in hot sauce (*Bumble Bee*), 2 oz.	0	0
in mustard sauce:		
(*Beach Cliff/Brunswick*), 3.75-oz. can	2.0	0
(*Bumble Bee*), 2 oz.	1.0	1.0
(*Crown Prince* Brisling), 3.7-oz. can	2.0	2.0
(*Yankee Clipper*), ¼ cup	1.0	0
in olive or soy oil, 4 oz.	0	0
in soy oil, with green chili (*Beach Cliff* 3.75 oz.), 3.4 oz.	1.0	0
spiced (*Goya*), ¼ cup	0	0
in tomato sauce:		
(*Beach Cliff*), 3.75-oz. can	2.0	0
(*Beach Cliff* Oval), 2 oz.	1.0	0
(*Brunswick*), 3.75-oz. can	3.0	0
(*Goya*), ¼ cup	1.0	0
(*Yankee Clipper*), ¼ cup	1.0	0

Food and Measure	carb. (gms)	fiber (gms)
Sardine oil, 2 tbsp.	0	0
Satsuma, see "Tangerine"		
Sauce, see specific sauce listings		
Sauce, all purpose, 2 tbsp.:		
(*Ott's* Famous)	8.0	0
(*Silver Dollar City*)	8.0	0
Sauerbraten seasoning mix (*Knorr Recipe Classics*),		
1 tbsp.	6.0	0
Sauerkraut, 2 tbsp., except as noted:		
(*Boar's Head*)	1.0	<1.0
(*Claussen*)	1.0	1.0
(*Del Monte*)	<1.0	<1.0
(*Eden* Organic), ½ cup	4.0	3.0
(*Hebrew National*)	1.0	1.0
(*S&W*)	1.0	<1.0
Bavarian style (*Bush's*)	3.0	1.0
Bavarian style (*Del Monte*)	4.0	0
chopped or shredded (*Bush's*)	1.0	1.0
Sausage (see also specific listings), cooked, except as noted:		
beef, smoked, regular or hot (*Arnold's*), 1.8-oz. link	1.0	0
beef, spicy (*Johnsonville* Hot Links), 2.7-oz. link	2.0	0
chicken, 1 link, 2-oz., except as noted:		
Andouille, Cajun (*Bilinski*)	1.0	0
apple, smoked (*Aidells*), 3.5 oz.	1.0	0
apple, smoked, minis (*Aidells*), 5 links, 2 oz.	1.0	0
apple Chardonnay (*Bilinski*)	2.5	0
cilantro (*Bilinski*)	1.0	1.0
garlic, roasted (*Bell & Evans*), 2.25 oz.	2.0	0
Italian, mild, with pepper and onion (*Bilinski*)	1.0	0
Italian, sweet (*Bell & Evans*), 2.25 oz.	2.0	0
jalapeño or pesto (*Bilinski*)	0	0
lemon, smoked (*Aidells*), 3.5 oz.	1.0	0
mango (*Aidells*), 3.5 oz.	6.0	0
mango, breakfast (*Aidells*), 2 links, 2 oz.	3.0	0
maple apple (*Bell & Evans*), 2.25 oz.	8.0	0
spinach (*Bilinski*)	1.0	1.0
sun-dried tomato (*Bilinski*)	2.0	0
sun-dried tomato and basil (*Bell & Evans*), 2.25 oz. . . .	2.0	0

Food and Measure	carb. (gms)	fiber (gms)
chicken, raw, Italian (*Organic Valley*), 3 oz.	0	0
chicken/turkey, see "turkey/chicken," below		
duck, smoked (*Aidells*), 3.5-oz. link	1.0	0
garlic (*Johnsonville* Irish O' Garlic), 3-oz. link	1.0	0
garlic (*Trois Petits Cochons* Saucisson a l'Ail), 2 oz.	1.0	0
Italian:		
(*Johnsonville* Heat & Serve), 2.7-oz. link	3.0	0
hot (*Hatfield* Burgers), 3-oz. patty	3.0	0
hot (*Hatfield* Rope), 2 oz.	2.0	0
hot or mild, ground (*Johnsonville*), 2-oz. patty	1.0	0
hot or sweet (*Hatfield* Grillers), 2-oz. link	2.0	0
hot, sweet, or mild, fresh (*Johnsonville*), 3-oz. link	1.0	0
mild, precooked (*Johnsonville*), 2.7-oz. link	2.0	0
sweet (*Hatfield* Burgers), 3-oz. patty	2.0	0
sweet (*Hatfield* Rope), 2 oz.	1.0	0
Italian, raw (*Organic Valley*), 3-oz. link	<1.0	0
Polish, fresh, grilled (*Johnsonville*), 3-oz. link	1.0	0
Polish, precooked (*Johnsonville*), 2.7-oz. link	2.0	0
pork, chub (*Jimmy Dean*), 2 oz.	0	0
pork, fresh:		
ground, grilled (*Johnsonville*), 2 oz.	1.0	0
link, 1 oz. raw or .5 oz. cooked	.3	0
patty, raw, 2 oz.	.6	0
pork, link, 3 links, except as noted:		
(*Johnsonville* Breakfast Original)	1.0	0
(*Little Sizzlers*)	0	0
(*Patrick Cudahy* Pre-cooked), 2 links	<1.0	0
brown sugar honey (*Johnsonville* Breakfast Links)	5.0	0
hickory smoke (*Johnsonville*)	2.0	0
hot and spicy (*Little Sizzlers*)	0	0
maple (*Johnsonville* Vermont Breakfast Links)	1.0	0
maple (*Little Sizzlers*)	2.0	0
mild (*Jones Dairy Farm* Golden Brown Precooked),		
2 links	1.0	0
pepper and onion, pan fried (*Hatfield* Grillers), 1 link . . .	3.0	0
pork, patty, 2 pieces, except as noted:		
(*Johnsonville* Breakfast Patties)	1.0	0
(*Jones Dairy Farm* Golden Brown Precooked), 1 piece .	1.0	0

Food and Measure	carb. (gms)	fiber (gms)
(*Little Sizzlers*)	0	0
(*Patrick Cudahy* Pre-cooked)	<1.0	0
(*Swift Premium Brown 'N Serve* Original)	2.0	0
pork, raw (*Organic Valley* Breakfast), 2 links	0	0
pork, raw ,chub (*Organic Valley*), 4 oz.	<1.0	0
pork and beef, fresh, .5-oz. link	.8	0
pork and turkey (*Healthy Choice* Breakfast), 3 links or 3 patties	3.0	0
smoked, 1 link, except as noted::		
(*Boar's Head* Natural Casing), 4 oz.	2.0	0
(*Healthy Choice*), 2 oz.	6.0	0
(*Johnsonville*), 2.7 oz.	2.0	0
(*Johnsonville* Little Smokies), 6 links, 2 oz.	1.0	0
(*Oscar Mayer* Little Smokies), 6 links, 2 oz.	1.0	0
Andouille (*Aidells* Cajun), 3.5 oz.	1.0	0
Andouille (*Johnsonville* New Orleans), 2.7 oz.	2.0	0
cheese (*Johnsonville* Bedder with Cheddar/Swisswurst), 2.7 oz.	2.0	0
cheese (*Oscar Mayer* Little Smokies), 6 links, 2 oz.	2.0	0
hot (*Boar's Head*), 3.2 oz.	<1.0	0
turkey:		
raw (*Louis Rich* Chub), 2.5 oz.	1.0	0
raw (*Shady Brook Farms* Breakfast), 2.3 oz.	0	0
raw (*Wampler* Breakfast), 4 oz.	1.0	0
smoked (*Louis Rich*), 2-oz. link	2.0	0
turkey, Italian, hot (*Perdue*), 2.9-oz. link	1.0	0
turkey, Italian, sweet (*Perdue*), 2.4-oz. link	1.0	0
turkey, Italian, raw:		
hot (*Perdue*), 3.2 oz.	1.0	0
hot (*Shady Brook Farms* 92% Fat Free), 3 oz.	1.0	0
sweet (*Perdue*), 2.7 oz.	1.0	0
sweet (*Shady Brook Farms* 92% Fat Free), 3 oz.	1.0	0
turkey/chicken, 3.5-oz. link, except as noted:		
Andouille, Cajun, mini (*Aidells*), 5 links, 2 oz.	1.0	0
artichoke and garlic, smoked (*Aidells*)	3.0	0
black bean, Cuban (*Aidells*)	6.0	0
curry, Burmese, smoked (*Aidells*)	3.0	0
habañero green chili, smoked (*Aidells*)	2.0	0

Food and Measure	carb. (gms)	fiber (gms)
New Mexico, smoked or pesto, smoked (*Aidells*)	2.0	0
portobello mushroom (*Aidells*)	3.0	0
roasted red pepper with corn (*Aidells*)	2.0	0
sun-dried tomato, smoked (*Aidells*)	1.0	0
sun-dried tomato, smoked, mini (*Aidells*), 5 links, 2 oz.	1.0	0
Sausage, canned:		
pickled, regular or hot (*Hormel*), 6 links, 2 oz.	1.0	0
Vienna:		
(*Armour*), 3 links	0	0
(*Goya*), 3 links	1.0	0
regular or chicken (*Hormel*), 2 oz.	0	0
Sausage, freeze-dried, pork (*Mountain House*),		
2 patties	2.0	0
"Sausage," vegetarian, canned (see also specific listings):		
(*Loma Linda* Linkettes), 1.2-oz. link	1.0	1.0
(*Loma Linda* Little Links), 2 links, 1.6 oz.	3.0	2.0
(*Loma Linda* Veja-Links), 1.1-oz. link	3.0	0
(*Worthington* Saucettes), 1.3-oz. link	1.0	1.0
(*Worthington* Super-Links), 1.7-oz. link	2.0	1.0
"Sausage," vegetarian, frozen (see also specific listings):		
crumbles (*Morningstar Farms*), ⅔ cup	5.0	1.0
links:		
(*Boca* Breakfast), 2 links, 1.6 oz.	5.0	2.0
(*Morningstar Farms*), 2 links, 1.6 oz.	3.0	2.0
(*Quorn*), 2 links, 1.6 oz.	2.0	1.0
(*Worthington Prosage*), 2 links, 1.6 oz.	3.0	2.0
(*Yves*), 2 oz.	3.0	2.0
.9-oz. link	2.5	.7
Italian or smoked (*Boca*), 2.5-oz. link	6.0	1.0
patties:		
(*Boca* Breakfast), 1.3-oz. piece	5.0	2.0
(*Morningstar Farms*), 1.3-oz. piece	3.0	2.0
(*Worthington Prosage*), 1.4-oz. piece	3.0	2.0
(*Yves*), 1.7-oz. piece	4.0	2.0
1.3-oz. piece	3.7	1.1
Sausage seasoning (*Tone's*), 1 tsp.	2.7	.7
Sausage stick (see also "Beef jerky"), beef or spicy		
(*Johnsonville* Snack Stix), 1 oz.	0	0

Food and Measure	carb. (gms)	fiber (gms)
Sausage sub, frozen, Italian, and peppers (*Michelina's Hot Subs*), 2.1-oz. piece	39.0	2.0
Savory, ground, 1 tsp.	1.0	<1.0
Sbarro, 1 slice or serving:		
pizza:		
cheese or fresh tomato	60.0	3.0
chicken vegetable	69.0	5.0
mushroom	62.0	4.0
pepperoni	61.0	3.0
sausage	60.0	3.0
supreme	63.0	3.0
white	59.0	2.0
pizza, gourmet:		
broccoli spinach	88.0	6.0
cheese or meat delight	84.0	4.0
ham, pineapple, and bacon	88.0	4.0
mushroom	85.0	5.0
mushroom, spinach	87.0	6.0
spinach, yellow pepper	86.0	5.0
tomato basil	87.0	5.0
pizza, low carb, all varieties	18.0	n.a.
pizza, stuffed:		
pepperoni	89.0	4.0
Philly cheesesteak	94.0	5.0
spinach broccoli	89.0	5.0
calzone, cheese	87.0	3.0
stromboli, pepperoni	82.0	3.0
stromboli, spinach, tomato, broccoli	84.0	5.0
salads:		
Caesar	6.0	1.0
cucumber tomato	9.0	2.0
fruit	32.0	3.0
Greek	3.0	<1.0
mixed garden	7.0	3.0
pasta primavera	21.0	2.0
string bean tomato	9.0	2.0
dinner plates:		
baked ziti with sauce	43.0	4.0

Food and Measure	carb. (gms)	fiber (gms)
chicken Francese	8.0	2.0
chicken Parmesan	16.0	2.0
chicken Portofino	7.0	1.0
chicken Vesuvio	8.0	1.0
eggplant rollatini, with cheese	40.0	4.0
garlic rolls	28.0	<1.0
lasagna, meat	36.0	3.0
meatballs	10.0	1.0
pasta Milano	41.0	6.0
pasta rustica	39.0	5.0
penne with sausage, peppers	33.0	4.0
penne alla vodka	67.0	5.0
sausage and peppers	19.0	4.0
spaghetti with:		
chicken Parmesan	75.0	6.0
chicken Vesuvio	64.0	4.0
meatballs	96.0	9.0
sauce	120.0	10.0
vegetables, mixed	14.0	4.0
dessert, cake:		
Black Forest	59.0	1.0
carrot	64.0	1.0
cheesecake	42.0	1.0
milk chocolate	59.0	1.0
Scallion, see "Onion, green"		
Scallop, meat only:		
raw, 4 oz.	2.7	0
raw, 2 large or 5 small, 1.1 oz.	.7	0
steamed, 4 oz.	0	0
Scallop, frozen (*Contessa*), 4 oz.	<1.0	0
"Scallop," imitation:		
(*Louis Kemp Scallop Delights* Bay Style), ½ cup, 3 oz.	12.0	0
from surimi, 4 oz.	12.1	0
Scallop, smoked (*Ducktrap River*), ¼ cup	0	0
"Scallop," vegetarian, canned (*Worthington Skallops*), ½ cup, 3 oz.	4.0	3.0
Scallop dish, frozen:		
breaded, fried (*Mrs. Paul's*), 3.5 oz., 13 pieces	27.0	1.0

Food and Measure	carb. (gms)	fiber (gms)
cakes (*Yankee Trader*), 3-oz. cake	10.0	1.0
ceviche (*Sau•Sea*), ½ cup	5.0	1.0
Scallop squash (see also "Sunburst Squash"), ½ cup:		
raw, sliced	2.5	1.2
boiled, drained, sliced	3.0	1.1
boiled, drained, mashed	4.0	1.4
Scampi sauce, cooking (*Golden Dipt*), 2 tbsp.	4.0	0
Scarlet runner beans, canned (*Westbrae Natural* Organic		
Heirloom Beans), ½ cup	20.0	7.0
Schlotzsky's Deli, 1 serving:		
sandwich, on sourdough bun, except as noted:		
BLT, regular	70.0	3.0
BLT, small	47.0	2.0
chicken, Dijon, on wheat, regular	74.0	6.0
chicken, Dijon, on wheat, small	49.0	4.0
chicken, fiesta, on jalapeño cheese, regular	79.0	4.0
chicken, fiesta, on jalapeño cheese, small	53.0	3.0
chicken, pesto, regular	73.0	4.0
chicken, pesto, small	49.0	2.0
chicken, Santa Fe, on jalapeño cheese, regular	81.0	5.0
chicken, Santa Fe, on jalapeño cheese, small	54.0	3.0
chicken breast, regular	80.0	4.0
chicken breast, small	54.0	3.0
chicken club, regular	75.0	4.0
chicken club, small	50.0	3.0
corned beef, on dark rye, regular	78.0	4.0
corned beef, on dark rye, small	52.0	3.0
pastrami and Swiss, on dark rye, regular	81.0	4.0
pastrami and Swiss, on dark rye, small	54.0	3.0
The Philly, regular	86.0	4.0
The Philly, small	57.0	2.0
Reuben, on dark rye:		
corned beef, regular	82.0	4.0
corned beef, small	55.0	3.0
pastrami, regular	83.0	4.0
pastrami, small	56.0	3.0
turkey, regular	80.0	4.0
turkey, small	54.0	3.0

Food and Measure	carb. (gms)	fiber (gms)
roast beef, regular	78.0	3.0
roast beef, small	52.0	2.0
roast beef and cheese, regular	83.0	4.0
roast beef and cheese, small	56.0	3.0
Texas Schlotsky's, on jalapeño cheese, regular	76.0	3.0
Texas Schlotsky's, on jalapeño cheese, small	51.0	2.0
tuna, on wheat, regular	77.0	5.0
tuna, on wheat, small	52.0	3.0
tuna melt, on wheat, regular	83.0	6.0
tuna melt, on wheat, small	56.0	4.0
turkey, smoked, regular	75.0	3.0
turkey, smoked, small	50.0	2.0
turkey and bacon club, on wheat, regular	79.0	5.0
turkey and bacon club, on wheat, small	53.0	3.0
turkey guacamole, regular	84.0	3.0
turkey guacamole, small	56.0	2.0
vegetable club, regular	76.0	5.0
vegetable club, small	50.0	3.0
The Vegetarian, on wheat, regular	79.0	5.0
The Vegetarian, on wheat, small	53.0	4.0
Western vegetarian, regular	76.0	4.0
Western vegetarian, small	51.0	3.0
sandwich, *The Original:*		
large, family size	152.0	7.0
regular	79.0	4.0
small	53.0	3.0
deluxe, regular	84.0	4.0
deluxe, small	57.0	3.0
ham and cheese, regular	82.0	4.0
ham and cheese, small	55.0	3.0
turkey, original, regular	81.0	4.0
turkey, original, small	54.0	3.0
wraps:		
chicken, Asian almond	72.0	4.0
chicken, Caesar	40.0	3.0
chicken salsa, with cheddar	44.0	3.0
tuna, zesty albacore	45.0	3.0

Food and Measure	carb. (gms)	fiber (gms)
soup, 8-oz. cup:		
black bean, Monterey	42.0	17.0
broccoli cheese	23.0	1.0
cheese, Wisconsin	26.0	1.0
chicken noodle	18.0	1.0
chicken gumbo	13.0	2.0
chicken tortilla	13.0	1.0
chicken with wild rice	36.0	0
chili, Timberline	24.0	7.0
clam chowder, Boston	24.0	1.0
corn chowder	38.0	1.0
minestrone	17.0	3.0
potato with bacon	31.0	2.0
ravioli tomato	21.0	1.0
red beans and rice	32.0	4.0
tomato basil, Tuscan	13.0	3.0
vegetable beef, gourmet	14.0	2.0
vegetarian vegetable	20.0	6.0
salad, deli, small:		
chicken	6.0	2.0
coleslaw	24.0	3.0
fresh fruit	21.0	3.0
macaroni	23.0	2.0
pasta, California	10.0	1.0
pasta, chicken pesto	40.0	3.0
potato	35.0	4.0
potato, mustard	31.0	4.0
tuna, albacore	2.0	0
salad, leaf, without dressing, croutons, noodles:		
Caesar	3.0	2.0
chef, ham and turkey or smoked turkey	13.0	3.0
chicken, Caesar	4.0	2.0
chicken, Chinese	10.0	2.0
garden	7.0	3.0
garden, small	3.0	2.0
Greek	10.0	4.0
salad dressing, 1 pkt.:		
balsamic vinaigrette, Greek	2.0	0

Food and Measure	carb. (gms)	fiber (gms)
Caesar or ranch	1.0	0
Italian, light	3.0	0
ranch, spicy	2.0	0
ranch, spicy, light	9.0	0
sesame ginger vinaigrette	8.0	0
Thousand Island	6.0	0
salad extras, chow mein noodles, 1 pkt.	1.0	1.0
salad extras, garlic cheese croutons, 1 pkt.	5.0	0
pizza, 8'' sourdough:		
bacon, tomato, and mushroom	78.0	4.0
cheese, double	76.0	4.0
cheese, double, and pepperoni	77.0	4.0
chicken, barbecue	93.0	2.0
chicken, kung pao	92.0	5.0
chicken, Thai	89.0	5.0
chicken and pesto	78.0	4.0
combination, the original	79.0	5.0
herb, Tuscan	80.0	5.0
meat, three	74.0	3.0
Mediterranean	72.0	3.0
smoked turkey and jalapeño	80.0	4.0
tomato and pesto	76.0	4.0
vegetarian special	76.0	4.0
buns:		
dark rye, regular	68.0	3.0
dark rye, small	45.0	2.0
jalapeño cheese, regular	66.0	2.0
jalapeño cheese, small	44.0	2.0
sourdough, large	136.0	5.0
sourdough, regular	68.0	2.0
sourdough, small	46.0	2.0
wheat, regular	66.0	4.0
wheat, small	45.0	2.0
desserts, 1 piece:		
cheesecake:		
cookies & crème	36.0	1.0
New York	31.0	0
strawberry swirl	30.0	0

Food and Measure	carb. (gms)	fiber (gms)
cookie:		
chocolate chip	23.0	0
fudge chocolate chip	22.0	1.0
oatmeal raisin	24.0	1.0
peanut butter	21.0	1.0
sugar	23.0	0
white chocolate macadamia	22.0	0
fudge brownie cake	46.0	3.0
Schnitzel, vegetarian, frozen (*Garden Gourmet*), 2.9-oz. piece	5.0	6.0
Scone, all fruit varieties (*Health Valley*), 2.1-oz. piece	43.0	5.0
Scorpion drink mixer (*Trader Vic's*), 4 fl. oz.	21.0	0
Scrapple, 2 oz.:		
(*Dietz & Watson*)	7.0	0
(*Hatfield*)	5.0	0
beef (*Hatfield*)	6.0	0
Scrod, fresh, see "Cod, Atlantic"		
Scup, without added ingredients	0	0
Sea bass, without added ingredients	0	0
Sea trout, without added ingredients	0	0
Sea vegetables, see "Seaweed"		
Seafood, see specific listings		
Seafood coating mix (see also "Batter and breading mix" and "Fish coating mix"):		
Cajun (*Luzianne*), 2 tbsp.	22.0	1.0
fry mix (*Golden Dipt* Fry Easy), 1⅔ tbsp.	9.0	0
shrimp and seafood (*Golden Dipt Oven Easy*), 2 tbsp.	8.0	0
Seafood salad kit, with crab and crackers:		
(*Bumble Bee*), 1 pkg.:		
2.75-oz. can salad	15.0	1.0
6 crackers, .6 oz.	12.0	0
Seafood sauce (see also specific listings), cocktail, ¼ cup, except as noted:		
(*Crosse & Blackwell*)	23.0	0
(*Del Monte*)	24.0	0
(*Heinz*)	15.0	1.0
(*Kraft*)	13.0	1.0
(*Litehouse*), 2 tbsp.	5.0	0

Food and Measure	carb. (gms)	fiber (gms)
(*Old Bay*)	18.0	0
(*Red Gold*)	17.0	1.0
(*S&W*), 1 tbsp.	5.0	0
hot and spicy (*Kraft*)	11.0	1.0
Seafood seasoning (see also "Seafood coating mix"),		
all varieties (*Old Bay*), ¼ tsp.	0	0
Seasoning (see also specific listings):		
(*Ac'cent*), ⅛ tsp.	0	0
(*Sa-són* con Cilantro/*Sa-són Ac'cent*), ¼ tsp.	0	0
(*Sazón Goya* con Achiote/Azafran), ¼ tsp.	0	0
blend, all varieties (*Mrs. Dash*), ¼ tsp.	0	0
Seaweed:		
agar:		
raw, 2 tbsp.	.7	<.1
dried, 1 oz.	2.9	2.2
freeze-dried, bar or flakes (*Eden* Agar Agar), .5 oz.	2.0	2.0
arame (*Eden*), ½ cup, .4 oz.	7.0	7.0
dulse flakes (*Maine Coast Sea Vegetables*), 1 tbsp.	2.0	2.0
hiziki (*Eden*), ½ cup	6.0	6.0
Irish moss, raw, 1 oz.	3.5	.4
kelp, raw, 1 oz.	2.7	.4
kombu (*Eden*), ½ of 7'' piece	2.0	1.0
laver, raw, 1 oz.	1.4	4.1
nori, 1 sheet (*Eden/Eden* Sushi)	1.0	1.0
nori, 1 sheet (*Sushi Chef*)	2.0	1.0
spirulina, raw, 1 oz.	.7	n.a.
spirulina, dried, 1 oz.	6.8	1.0
wakame:		
(*Eden*), ½ cup	4.0	4.0
raw, 1 oz.	2.6	.1
flakes, instant (*Eden*), 1 tsp.	0	0
Seaweed chips (*Eden* Sea Vegetable), 1.1 oz.	23.0	0
Seitan:		
(*White Wave* Traditional), 3 oz.	3.0	1.0
chicken style:		
(*White Wave* Box), 3 oz.	9.0	3.0
(*White Wave* Water Pack), 1 piece with broth, 5 oz.	12.0	10.0
strips, stir-fry (*White Wave*), 3 oz.	2.0	0

Food and Measure	carb. (gms)	fiber (gms)
Semolina, whole grain, 1 cup	121.6	6.5
Semolina flour (*Hodgson Mill* Pasta Flour), <¼ cup	22.0	2.0
Sesame butter (*Kettle Roaster Fresh*), 1 oz.	6.0	0
Sesame flour, 1 oz.:		
high fat	7.6	1.8
partially defatted	10.0	1.7
low fat	10.1	1.4
Sesame meal, partially defatted, 1 oz.	7.4	1.1
Sesame nut mix (*Planters*), 1 oz.	9.0	2.0
Sesame paste (see also "Tahini"), from whole seeds,		
1 tbsp.	4.1	.9
Sesame salt, regular or garlic (*Eden* Organic Seaweed		
Gomasio), ½ tsp.	0	0
Sesame seed condiment (*Eden Shake*), ½ tsp.	1.0	1.0
Sesame seeds:		
black (*Shiloh Farms*), ¼ cup	6.0	3.1
whole:		
(*Arrowhead Mills*), ¼ cup	8.0	4.0
(*Shiloh Farms*), ¼ cup	8.0	5.0
dried, 1 tbsp.	2.1	1.1
roasted, toasted, 1 oz.	7.3	4.0
kernels:		
(*Arrowhead Mills*), ¼ cup	3.0	1.0
(*Shiloh Farms*), ¼ cup	5.0	5.0
dried, 1 tsp.	.3	<1.0
toasted, 1 oz.	7.4	4.8
Sesame spread, see "Sesame butter"		
Sesame stick snack, 1.1 oz.:		
cheddar (*Shiloh Farms*)	15.0	3.0
garlic (*Shiloh Farms*)	13.0	3.0
oat bran (*Shiloh Farms*)	15.0	5.0
poppy onion (*Shiloh Farms*)	12.0	3.0
spelt (*Shiloh Farms*)	13.0	5.0
Sesbania flower:		
raw, 1 cup	1.4	n.a.
steamed, ½ cup...................................	2.7	n.a.
Shad, without added ingredients	0	0

Food and Measure	carb. (gms)	fiber (gms)
Shallot, fresh:		
(*Frieda's*), 1.1 oz.	5.0	0
peeled, 1 oz.	4.8	<1.0
chopped, 1 tbsp.	1.7	<1.0
Shallot, freeze-dried, 1 tbsp.	.7	<1.0
Shark, without added ingredients	0	0
Sheepshead, without added ingredients	0	0
Shellie beans, canned with liquid, ½ cup	7.6	4.1
Shells, pasta, entree, frozen, 1 pkg.:		
and cheese (*Michelina's* Zap'ems), 8 oz.	46.0	2.0
stuffed (*Amy's* Bowls), 10 oz.	30.0	5.0
stuffed (*Healthy Choice*), 11.15 oz.	40.0	5.0
vegetables and, garlic butter sauce (*Birds Eye*), 9 oz.	32.0	3.0
Shells, pasta, mix:		
Alfredo (*Annie's* Natural), 1 cup*	49.0	1.0
Alfredo (*Annie's* Organic), 1 cup*	47.0	1.0
cheddar, 1 cup*:		
Mexican (*Annie's* Organic)	49.0	1.0
white (*Annie's* Natural Family)	49.0	1.0
white (*Annie's* Organic)	48.0	1.0
white (*Annie's* Organic Family)	47.0	2.0
white or Wisconsin (*Annie's* Natural)	49.0	1.0
whole wheat shells (*Annie's* Organic)	47.0	5.0
Wisconsin (*Annie's* Creamy Deluxe)	46.0	2.0
Wisconsin (*Annie's* Organic)	49.0	1.0
cheese, 4 oz. mix:		
(*Velveeta* Light)	53.0	2.0
(*Velveeta* Original 12 oz.)	48.0	2.0
(*Velveeta* Original Family Size)	46.0	2.0
bacon (*Velveeta*)	47.0	2.0
cheese, salsa (*Velveeta*), ½ of 10.85-oz. pkg.	47.0	2.0
"cheese," nondairy (*Road's End Organics Shells & Chreese*),		
¾ cup mix	62.0	7.0
Shepherd's pie, see "Beef entree, frozen"		
Shepherd's pie, meatless, frozen (*Amy's*), 8-oz. pkg.	27.0	5.0
Sherbet (see also "Sorbet"), ½ cup, except as noted:		
berry rainbow (*Dreyer's/Edy's*)	29.0	0

Food and Measure	carb. (gms)	fiber (gms)
cherry amaretto (*Turkey Hill* Orchard)	28.0	0
cherry chip (*Darigold*)	28.0	<1.0
lime (*Dreyer's/Edy's*)	28.0	0
lime, orange, lemon (*Hood Fruit Scoops*)	26.0	0
orange:		
(*Breyer's*)	28.0	0
(*Darigold*)	26.0	0
(*Turkey Hill* Grove)	26.0	0
Swiss (*Dreyer's/Edy's*)	30.0	0
orange, and ice cream:		
(*Breyer's* Take Two)	21.0	0
(*Breyer's Creamsicle*)	20.0	0
(*Darigold* Float)	21.0	0
(*Dreyer's/Edy's*)	23.0	0
(*Peak Pleasures*)	19.0	0
swirl (*Turkey Hill*)	20.0	0
rainbow, fruit:		
(*Breyer's*)	27.0	0
(*Darigold*)	26.0	0
(*Turkey Hill*)	26.0	0
raspberry (*Darigold*)	26.0	0
raspberry (*Dreyer's/Edy's*)	28.0	0
tropical rainbow (*Dreyer's/Edy's*)	29.0	0
Sherbet bar, see "Iced confection bar"		
Shiso leaf powder (*Eden*), 1 tsp.	0	2.0
Shortening, soy and cottonseed, 2 tbsp.	0	0
Shrimp, meat only:		
raw, 4 oz.	1.0	0
raw, 4 large, 1 oz.	.3	0
boiled or steamed, 4 oz.	0	0
boiled or steamed, 4 large, .8 oz.	0	0
Shrimp, canned, drained:		
all varieties (*Bumble Bee/Orleans*), 2 oz., ¼ cup	0	0
small (*Crown Prince*), ½ can	2.0	1.0
1 cup	1.3	0
Shrimp, frozen, cleaned, tail-on:		
raw, all sizes (*Chicken of the Sea*), 4 oz.	1.0	0

Food and Measure	carb. (gms)	fiber (gms)
raw or cooked (*Contessa*), 3 oz.	0	0
cooked (*Chicken of the Sea*), 3 oz.	0	0
"Shrimp," imitation, from surimi, 4 oz.	10.4	0
Shrimp, smoked (*Ducktrap River*), ¼ cup	0	0
Shrimp appetizer, frozen or refrigerated:		
ceviche (*Sau•Sea*), ½ cup	5.0	1.0
cocktail (*Margaritaville* Paradise), ½ pkg.	0	0
with cocktail sauce:		
(*Contessa* Party Platter), 4 oz.	6.0	0
(*Sau•Sea*), 4-oz. jar	20.0	3.0
(*Sau•Sea*), 6-oz. jar	30.0	4.0
coconut (*Margaritaville* Calypso), ½ pkg.:		
shrimp, 4 oz.	25.0	0
sauce, 2 tbsp.	14.0	0
Shrimp coating mix, see "Seafood coating mix"		
Shrimp cocktail, see "Shrimp appetizer"		
Shrimp dinner, frozen, creamy garlic (*Healthy Choice* Dinners), 11.5 oz.	35.0	6.0
Shrimp entree, freeze-dried, 1 serving:		
Alfredo (*AlpineAire*)	44.0	2.0
Newburg (*AlpineAire*)	50.0	2.0
Shrimp entree, frozen, 1 pkg., except as noted:		
Alfredo:		
(*Gorton's* Shrimp Bowl), 10.5 oz.	39.0	4.0
(*Michelina's* Homestyle Bowls), 10 oz.	42.0	2.0
(*Michelina's Signature*), 8 oz.	31.0	2.0
and vegetables (*Michelina's* Homestyle Bowls), 11 oz.	53.0	3.0
and angel-hair pasta (*Lean Cuisine* Cafe Classics), 10 oz.	35.0	2.0
arrabiata (*Contessa* Minute Meal Bowl), 10.5 oz.	36.0	5.0
fajita (*Contessa*), 2 pieces, 8 oz.	29.0	4.0
fried rice, see "Rice entree, frozen"		
garlic (*Birds Eye Voila!*), 1 cup*	27.0	2.0
garlic butter (*Gorton's* Shrimp Bowl), 10.5 oz.	38.0	2.0
jerk (*Margaritaville* Jammin'), ½ of 8-oz. pkg.	4.0	0
kung pao (*Contessa*), 1¾ cups*	30.0	3.0
lime (*Margaritaville* Island), ½ of 8-oz. pkg.	2.0	0

Food and Measure	carb. (gms)	fiber (gms)
marinara, with linguine (*Smart Ones*), 9 oz.	28.0	4.0
Mediterranean (*Contessa*), 8 oz.	27.0	3.0
pad Thai (*Ethnic Gourmet*), 10 oz.	64.0	3.0
Parmesan penne (*Uncle Ben's* Pasta Bowl), 12 oz.	58.0	2.0
with pasta, vegetables (*Michelina's Lean Gourmet*), 8 oz.	37.0	2.0
penne (*Contessa* Minute Meal Bowl), 10 oz.	33.0	4.0
primavera (*Contessa*), 1½ cups*	30.0	2.0
primavera (*Gorton's* Shrimp Bowl), 10.5 oz.	41.0	1.0
Santa Fe (*Contessa*), 1½ cups*	30.0	3.0
scampi:		
(*Contessa*), 4 oz.	5.0	0
(*Margaritaville* Sunset), ½ pkg.	10.0	0
(*SeaPak* Traditional), ⅓ of 12-oz. pkg.	4.0	0
Parmesan sauce (*SeaPak*), ⅓ of 12-oz. pkg.	2.0	0
soy ginger (*Contessa* Minute Meal Bowl), 11 oz.	53.0	4.0
stir-fry (*Contessa*), 1¾ cups*	26.0	4.0
sweet and sour (*Contessa*), 1½ cups*	40.0	3.0
teriyaki (*Gorton's* Shrimp Bowl), 10.5 oz.	57.0	2.0
Shrimp sauce (*Crosse & Blackwell*), ¼ cup	25.0	0
Shrimp spread, with roasted garlic (*Sau•Sea*), 2 tbsp.	1.0	0
Sloppy Joe sauce, see "Sandwich sauce"		
Sloppy Joe seasoning:		
(*Fantastic*), ¼ cup	11.0	3.0
(*Lawry's*), 2 tsp.	5.0	0
(*McCormick*), 1 tsp.	3.0	0
Smelt, rainbow, without added ingredients	0	0
Smoothie, mix, 1⅔ tbsp.:		
banana frost, chocolate banana, or pineapple (*Produce Partners*)	18.0	0
orange (*Produce Partners*)	14.0	0
strawberry (*Produce Partners*)	19.0	0
Smoothie snack, all fruit flavors (*Jell-O* Snacks), 4 oz.	18.0	0
Snack chips (see also "Snack mix" and specific grain and vegetable listings):		
(*Ritz* Original), 1.1 oz.	23.0	1.0
all varieties (*Guiltless Carbs*), 1 oz.	9.0	3.0
cheddar or sour cream and onion (*Ritz*), 1.1 oz.	20.0	1.0

Food and Measure	carb. (gms)	fiber (gms)
Snack mix (see also "Trail mix"):		
(*Cheez-It* Party Mix), ½ cup	19.0	1.0
(*Chex* Bold Party Blend), ½ cup	20.0	<1.0
(*Chex* Traditional), ⅔ cup	22.0	1.0
(*Gardetto's* Original/Reduced Fat), ½ cup	20.0	1.0
(*Munchies* Mini Mix), 1 oz., 1 cup	18.0	<1.0
(*Munchies* Flamin' Hot), 1 oz., ¾ cup	17.0	<1.0
(*Nabisco Mixers*), 1.1 oz.	21.0	1.0
cheese:		
cheddar (*Chex*), ⅔ cup	22.0	<1.0
cheddar (*Nabisco Mixers*), 1 oz.	17.0	1.0
blend, Italian (*Gardetto's*), ½ cup	20.0	<1.0
honey nut (*Chex*), ½ cup	23.0	1.0
hot and spicy (*Chex*), ⅔ cup	22.0	1.0
Italian recipe (*Gardetto's*), ½ cup	20.0	1.0
Oriental (*New England Naturals* Party Mix), ⅓ cup	14.0	2.0
peanut lovers (*Chex*), ½ cup	19.0	1.0
sweet and salt (*Chex* Trail Mix), ½ cup	22.0	1.0
Tex-Mex (*New England Naturals*), ⅓ cup	13.0	3.0
Snail, fresh, raw, 1 oz.	<.1	0
Snail, canned (*Fanci Food* Very Large), 6 pieces	0	0
Snail, sea, see "Whelk"		
Snap beans (see also "Green beans"), fresh, all varieties		
(*Frieda's*), ⅔ cup, 3 oz.	6.0	3.0
Snapper, without added ingredients	0	0
Snow pea, see "Peas, edible-podded"		
Snow pea sprouts (*Jonathan's*), 1 cup	8.0	3.0
Soft drinks, carbonated, 12 fl. oz., except as noted:		
all flavors (*Clearly Canadian*), 8 fl. oz.	10.0	0
all flavors (*Ocean Spray Juice Spritzers*), 11.75 fl. oz.	40.0	0
birch beer (*Pennsylvania Dutch*), 8 fl. oz.	28.0	0
blackberry (*Nantucket Nectars NectarFizz*), 8 fl. oz.	21.0	0
boysenberry (*R.W. Knudsen* Spritzer)	40.0	0
cherries and cream (*Stewart's*)	49.0	0
cherry:		
(*Santa Cruz Organic* Spritzer)	34.0	0
black (*R.W. Knudsen* Spritzer)	42.0	0
sparkling (*R.W. Knudsen* Spritzer)	28.0	0

Food and Measure	carb. (gms)	fiber (gms)
coconut (*Goya*)	45.0	0
cola:		
(*Coca-Cola* Classic)	39.0	0
(*Coca-Cola* Classic), 8 fl. oz.	27.0	0
(*Goya* Champagne)	47.0	0
(*Pepsi/Pepsi* Free)	41.0	0
(*Pepsi/Pepsi* Free), 8 fl. oz.	27.0	0
(*Pepsi Edge*), 8 fl. oz.	13.0	0
(*RC*), 8 fl. oz.	29.0	0
cherry (*Dr Pepper*)	40.0	0
cherry (*R.W. Knudsen* Spritzer)	42.0	0
cherry, lemon, or vanilla (*Pepsi*), 8 fl. oz.	28.0	0
lime (*Coca-Cola*)	39.0	0
citrus, 8 fl. oz.:		
(*Mountain Dew/Code Red/Livewire*)	31.0	0
(*7UP*)	26.0	0
(*7Up Plus*)	2.0	0
Collins mixer (*Canada Dry*), 8 fl. oz.	22.0	0
cranberry:		
(*Nantucket Nectars NectarFizz*), 8 fl. oz.	23.0	0
(*R.W. Knudsen* Spritzer)	45.0	0
sparkling (*R.W. Knudsen* Spritzer)	30.0	0
cream:		
(*A&W*), 8 fl. oz.	31.0	0
(*Mug*), 8 fl. oz.	32.0	0
(*Stewart's*)	45.0	0
vanilla (*R.W. Knudsen* Spritzer)	35.0	0
vanilla (*Santa Cruz Organic* Spritzer)	40.0	0
fruit punch (*Goya*)	49.0	0
ginger ale:		
(*Canada Dry*)	33.0	0
(*Canada Dry*), 8 fl. oz.	25.0	0
(*Health Valley*)	40.0	0
(*R.W. Knudsen* Spritzer)	40.0	0
(*Santa Cruz Organic* Spritzer)	37.0	0
(*Schweppes*)	34.0	0
(*Schweppes*), 8 fl. oz.	23.0	0
(*Seagram's*), 8 fl. oz.	24.0	0

Food and Measure	carb. (gms)	fiber (gms)
(*White Rock*), 8 fl. oz.	21.0	0
grape (*Schweppes*), 8 fl. oz.	26.0	0
ginger beer:		
(*Goya*)	43.0	0
(*Old Tyme*), 10 fl. oz.	34.0	0
(*Reed's* Jamaican Brew Premium/Extra Ginger)	37.4	0
(*Stewart's*)	50.0	0
grape:		
(*Goya*)	59.0	0
(*R.W. Knudsen* Spritzer)	41.0	0
(*Stewart's*)	48.0	0
(*Welch's*)	51.0	0
Concord (*Santa Cruz Organic* Spritzer)	36.0	0
grapefruit, pink (*Nantucket Nectars NectarFizz*), 8 fl. oz.	24.0	0
kiwi lime (*R.W. Knudsen* Spritzer)	32.0	0
lemon ginger (*Tré Limone*), 8 fl. oz.	22.0	0
lemon lime:		
(*Goya*)	42.0	0
(*R.W. Knudsen* Spritzer)	42.0	0
(*Santa Cruz Organic* Spritzer)	33.0	0
(*Sierra Mist*), 8 fl. oz.	26.0	0
(*Sprite/Sprite Remix*)	38.0	0
(*Sprite/Sprite Remix*), 8 fl. oz.	26.0	0
lemonade (see also "Lemonade"):		
(*Nantucket Nectars NectarFizz*), 8 fl. oz.	24.0	0
(*Santa Cruz Organic* Spritzer)	26.0	0
Jamaican (*R.W. Knudsen* Spritzer)	41.0	0
raspberry (*Santa Cruz Organic* Spritzer)	29.0	0
lime, mandarin (*R.W. Knudsen* Spritzer)	42.0	0
mango (*R.W. Knudsen* Spritzer Fandango)	45.0	0
orange:		
(*Fanta*), 8 fl. oz.	30.0	0
(*Slice*)	50.0	0
(*Sunkist*), 8 fl. oz.	35.0	0
mandarin (*Goya*)	44.0	0
orange and cream (*Stewart's*)	48.0	0
orange mango (*Nantucket Nectars NectarFizz*), 8 fl. oz.	24.0	0
orange mango (*Santa Cruz Organic* Spritzer)	33.0	0

Food and Measure	carb. (gms)	fiber (gms)
orange passion fruit (*R.W. Knudsen* Spritzer)	40.0	0
peach (*R.W. Knudsen* Spritzer)	37.0	0
pineapple (*Goya*)	43.0	0
raspberry, red (*R.W. Knudsen* Spritzer)	38.0	0
raspberry lime (*Nantucket Nectars NectarFizz*),		
8 fl. oz.	24.0	0
root beer:		
(*A&W*), 8 fl. oz.	31.0	0
(*Barq's*), 8 fl. oz.	30.0	0
(*Mug*), 8 fl. oz.	29.0	0
(*Santa Cruz Organic* Spritzer)	36.0	0
old-fashioned or sarsaparilla (*Health Valley*)	40.0	0
sangria (*Goya*)	43.0	0
strawberry:		
(*Fanta*), 8 fl. oz.	33.0	0
(*Goya*)	48.0	0
(*R.W. Knudsen* Spritzer)	42.0	0
tangerine (*R.W. Knudsen* Spritzer)	40.0	0
tonic:		
(*Canada Dry*), 8 fl. oz.	24.0	0
(*Schweppes*)	35.0	0
(*Schweppes*), 8 fl. oz.	23.0	0
(*Seagram's*), 8 fl. oz.	22.0	0
vanilla cream, see "cream," above		
Sofrito (*Goya* Jar), 1 tsp.	0	0
Sole, without added ingredients	0	0
Sole entree, frozen, 5-oz. piece, except as noted:		
with garlic, shrimp, and almonds (*Oven Poppers*)	16.0	0
with shrimp and lobster, in Newberg sauce:		
(*Oven Poppers*)	7.0	0
(*Oven Poppers*), 6-oz. piece	4.0	<1.0
with spinach and cheese (*Oven Poppers*)	13.0	0
stuffed:		
with broccoli and cheese (*Oven Poppers*)	4.0	1.0
with crab (*Oven Poppers*)	15.0	0
with crab, miniature (*Oven Poppers*), 2-oz. piece	8.0	0
with lump crabmeat (*Oven Poppers*)	9.0	0

Food and Measure	carb. (gms)	fiber (gms)
Sonic, 1 serving:		
breakfast:		
burrito	29.0	2.0
pancake on a stick, with sausage	22.0	n.a.
Toaster, egg and cheese, with bacon	28.0	3.0
Toaster, egg and cheese, with ham	33.0	3.0
Toaster, egg and cheese, with sausage	24.0	3.0
burgers:		
cheeseburger, bacon or *Sonic* No. 1/No. 2	44.0	2.0
Jr. burger	27.0	1.0
Sonic No. 1 or No. 2	43.0	2.0
SuperSonic No. 1	45.0	2.0
SuperSonic No. 2	46.0	3.0
Toaster sandwich:		
bacon cheddar burger	60.0	4.0
BLT	42.0	3.0
chicken club	75.0	3.0
grilled cheese	39.0	2.0
sandwiches:		
chicken, breaded	66.0	2.0
chicken, grilled	31.0	2.0
steak, country fried	56.0	2.0
chicken:		
Jumbo Popcorn Chicken, family	142.0	7.0
Jumbo Popcorn Chicken, large	36.0	2.0
Jumbo Popcorn Chicken, snack	24.0	1.0
Jumbo Popcorn Chicken Wacky Pack	18.0	1.0
strip, dinner	86.0	5.0
strip, snack	22.0	0
coney:		
plain	22.0	1.0
plain, extra long	44.0	1.0
cheese	24.0	1.0
cheese, extra long	47.0	2.0
corn dog	23.0	1.0
wraps:		
chicken, grilled	40.0	2.0

Food and Measure	carb. (gms)	fiber (gms)
chicken, grilled, without dressing	38.0	2.0
chicken strip	55.0	2.0
chicken strip, without dressing	53.0	2.0
Fritos chili cheese	68.0	5.0
salad, without dressing:		
chicken, grilled	20.0	3.0
chicken, Santa Fe	33.0	6.0
Jumbo Popcorn Chicken	38.0	4.0
salad dressing, 2 oz.:		
honey mustard or light ranch	14.0	0
ranch	0	0
Faves & Craves:		
Ched 'R' Peppers	29.0	4.0
fries:		
large	30.0	5.0
regular	22.0	4.0
SuperSonic	44.0	7.0
fries, cheese:		
large	31.0	5.0
regular	23.0	4.0
chili, large	32.0	5.0
chili, regular	24.0	4.0
Fritos chili pie	36.0	3.0
mozzarella sticks	35.0	0
onion rings:		
large	102.0	10.0
regular	66.0	7.0
SuperSonic	141.0	11.0
tater tots:		
large	40.0	4.0
regular	27.0	3.0
SuperSonic	53.0	5.0
tater tots, cheese:		
large	41.0	4.0
regular	28.0	3.0
chili, large	43.0	5.0
chili, regular	28.0	3.0

Food and Measure	carb. (gms)	fiber (gms)
add-ons:		
add bacon	0	0
add cheese	1.0	0
dressing, 1 oz.:		
honey mustard	9.0	0
ranch dressing	2.0	0
1000 Island	3.0	0
jalapeños-nacho	1.0	1.0
marinara sauce	3.0	0
pickle relish	11.0	0
slaw, .9 oz.	4.0	1.0
Sonic chili	1.0	0
Sonic green chilies	3.0	0
Sonic hickory barbecue sauce	10.0	0
Sopressata, hot or sweet (*Boar's Head*), 1 oz.	<1.0	0
Sorbet (see also "Sherbet"), ½ cup:		
apple cinnamon (*Whole Fruit*)	34.0	1.0
berry, mixed (*Sharon's*)	23.0	1.0
blueberry (*Whole Fruit*)	32.0	1.0
boysenberry (*Whole Fruit*)	37.0	1.0
chocolate:		
(*Häagen-Dazs*)	28.0	2.0
(*Sharon's*)	22.0	1.0
Belgian dark (*Godiva*)	32.0	2.0
raspberry swirl (*Godiva*)	36.0	2.0
coconut (*Sharon's*)	22.0	1.0
coconut (*Whole Fruit*)	28.0	0
grapefruit, pink (*Whole Fruit*)	32.0	0
lemon:		
(*Häagen-Dazs* Zesty)	25.0	<1.0
(*Sharon's*)	19.0	0
(*Whole Fruit*)	35.0	0
(*Whole Fruit* No Sugar)	23.0	7.0
mango:		
(*Häagen-Dazs*)	37.0	0
(*Sharon's*)	20.0	1.0
(*Whole Fruit*)	33.0	0

Food and Measure	carb. (gms)	fiber (gms)
orange (*Whole Fruit* Mandarin)	31.0	0
passion fruit (*Sharon's*)	20.0	0
peach:		
(*Häagen-Dazs*)	33.0	<1.0
(*Whole Fruit*)	32.0	1.0
(*Whole Fruit* No Sugar)	23.0	7.0
raspberry:		
(*Häagen-Dazs*)	30.0	2.0
(*Sharon's*)	20.0	2.0
(*Whole Fruit*)	33.0	1.0
(*Whole Fruit* No Sugar)	23.0	7.0
strawberry:		
(*Häagen-Dazs*)	30.0	<1.0
(*Whole Fruit*)	31.0	0
(*Whole Fruit* No Sugar)	22.0	6.0
strawberry banana (*Whole Fruit*)	31.0	<1.0
tropical (*Häagen-Dazs*)	38.0	0
tropical (*Whole Fruit*)	38.0	0
Sorbet bar (see also "Fruit bar"), 1 bar:		
marshmallow swirl (*Cool Cotton Candy*)	20.0	0
mocha fudge (*Healthy Choice*)	17.0	1.0
orange, with vanilla ice cream:		
(*Tropicana* Light)	12.0	0
(*Tropicana* Real Fruit)	14.0	0
chocolate dipped (*Tropicana*)	19.0	0
orange or raspberry, with vanilla ice cream:		
(*Tropicana* Swirls)	12.0	0
(*Tropicana* Swirls No Sugar)	11.0	0
(*Tropicana* Swirls Single)	20.0	0
raspberry, with vanilla yogurt (*Häagen-Dazs*)	21.0	<1.0
raspberry orange swirl (*Healthy Choice*)	18.0	1.0
strawberry:		
with banana yogurt (*Häagen-Dazs*)	20.0	0
with strawberry sorbet (*Healthy Choice*)	13.0	0
with vanilla ice cream (*Tropicana* Light)	12.0	0
Sorghum, whole grain, 1 cup.	143.3	n.a.
Sorghum syrup:		
½ cup	123.7	0

Food and Measure	carb. (gms)	fiber (gms)
1 tbsp.	15.7	0
Sorrel, see "Dock"		
Soup, ready-to-serve, 1 cup, except as noted:		
alphabet (*Amy's*)	16.0	2.0
bean:		
(*Westbrae Natural* Great Plains Savory)	23.0	7.0
(*Westbrae Natural* Louisiana Stew)	25.0	7.0
five, vegetable (*Health Valley*)	32.0	10.0
with bacon (*Campbell's Kitchen Classics*)	28.0	8.0
and ham (*Campbell's Chunky* Hearty)	30.0	8.0
and ham (*Campbell's Select*)	30.0	7.0
and ham (*Healthy Choice*)	29.0	6.0
bean, black:		
(*Health Valley/Health Valley* No Salt)	25.0	5.0
(*Progresso* Hearty)	30.0	10.0
(*Walnut Acres* Cuban)	30.0	8.0
(*Westbrae Natural* Alabama Gumbo)	26.0	6.0
vegetable (*Amy's*)	25.0	5.0
vegetable (*Health Valley*)	24.0	9.0
beef:		
barley (*Progresso* 97% Fat Free)	20.0	4.0
barley (*Progresso* Steak Soup)	16.0	3.0
barley, roasted (*Campbell's Select*)	24.0	4.0
mushroom (*Progresso* Steak Soup)	14.0	1.0
mushroom medley (*Campbell's Carb Request Savory*)	7.0	1.0
with portobello, rice (*Campbell's Select*)	15.0	2.0
with portobello, rice (*Campbell's Select* Micro Cup)	13.0	2.0
and potato, baked (*Progresso* Steak Soup)	15.0	1.0
and potato, chunky (*Healthy Choice*)	19.0	2.0
with rice, white/wild (*Campbell's Chunky*)	24.0	2.0
slow roasted, with mushrooms (*Campbell's Chunky*)	18.0	3.0
vegetable (*Progresso* Steak Soup)	16.0	2.0
with vegetables, country (*Campbell's Chunky*)	22.0	4.0
with vegetables, country (*Campbell's Chunky* Micro Bowl)	18.0	3.0
beef broth:		
(*College Inn/College Inn* Fat Free Lower Sodium)	0	0
(*Kitchen Basics* Stock)	0	0

Food and Measure	carb. (gms)	fiber (gms)
(*Swanson* Clear)	0	0
(*Swanson* Lower Sodium)	1.0	0
(*Tyson*)	1.0	0
with onion (*Swanson*)	2.0	0
beef flavor broth (*Health Valley/Health Valley* No Salt)	0	0
beef flavor broth (*Health Valley* Organic)	2.0	0
broccoli:		
carotene (*Health Valley* Super)	16.0	7.0
cream of (*Campbell's Soup at Hand*), 1 cont.	16.0	3.0
creamy (*Imagine*)	10.0	2.0
butternut squash (*Amy's*/Light Sodium)	20.0	2.0
butternut squash, creamy (*Imagine*)	23.0	2.0
cheddar chicken chowder (*Progresso*)	25.0	2.0
chicken:		
(*Healthy Choice* Hearty)	20.0	3.0
(*Progresso* Homestyle White Meat)	11.0	<1.0
Alfredo (*Campbell's Select*)	15.0	2.0
barley (*Progresso* White Meat)	15.0	3.0
creamy (*Campbell's Soup at Hand*), 1 cont.	15.0	2.0
and dumplings (*Campbell's Chunky*)	17.0	2.0
and dumplings (*Campbell's Chunky* Micro Bowl)	18.0	3.0
and dumplings (*Healthy Choice*)	19.0	4.0
with meatballs (*Progresso* Chickarina)	12.0	<1.0
rosemary, with roasted potato (*Campbell's Select*)	17.0	2.0
rotini, hearty (*Progresso* White Meat)	12.0	<1.0
pasta, with roasted garlic (*Campbell's Select*)	18.0	2.0
and stars (*Campbell's Soup at Hand*), 1 cont.	11.0	2.0
tortilla, Mexican style (*Campbell's Select*)	22.0	4.0
chicken, grilled:		
(*Progresso* Italiano White Meat)	14.0	1.0
sausage gumbo (*Campbell's Chunky*)	21.0	3.0
with sun-dried tomatoes and mushrooms (*Campbell's Select*)	18.0	2.0
with vegetables, pasta (*Campbell's Chunky*)	15.0	2.0
with vegetables, pasta (*Campbell's Chunky* Micro Bowl)	13.0	2.0
chicken, roasted:		
(*Healthy Choice* Italian)	19.0	4.0
(*Progresso* Italiano White Meat)	10.0	<1.0

Food and Measure	carb. (gms)	fiber (gms)
with garlic (*Healthy Choice*)	21.0	2.0
herb, garden (*Progresso* White Meat)	9.0	1.0
herb, with potatoes and garlic (*Campbell's Chunky*)	17.0	3.0
honey, with potato (*Campbell's Select*)	19.0	3.0
with penne, garden vegetables (*Campbell's Carb Request*)	7.0	2.0
and rotini (*Progresso* White Meat)	11.0	<1.0
with rotini and penne (*Campbell's Select*)	16.0	2.0
with white/wild rice (*Campbell's Select*)	18.0	2.0
with wild rice (*Progresso* 97% Fat Free)	12.0	<1.0
chicken broccoli cheese (*Campbell's Carb Request*)	8.0	5.0
chicken broccoli cheese and potato (*Campbell's Chunky*)	14.0	1.0
chicken broth:		
(*Allens*)	0	0
(*Campbell's* Low Sodium), 1 can	1.0	0
(*College Inn*)	0	0
(*Health Valley* Fat Free/Low Fat/No Salt)	0	0
(*Health Valley* Organic)	2.0	0
(*Imagine* Free Range)	2.0	<1.0
(*Kitchen Basics* Stock)	1.0	0
(*Pacific* Free Range)	1.0	0
(*Swanson/Swanson Natural Goodness*)	1.0	0
(*Tyson/Tyson* Reduced Sodium)	2.0	0
with ginger (*Annie Chun's*)	3.0	0
with Italian herbs (*Swanson*)	3.0	0
roasted (*Tyson*)	2.0	0
with roasted garlic (*College Inn*)	3.0	0
with roasted garlic (*Swanson*)	2.0	0
chicken flavor broth (*Imagine* No-Chicken)	4.0	<1.0
chicken gumbo (*Healthy Choice* Zesty)	16.0	3.0
chicken noodle:		
(*Campbell's* Low Sodium), 1 can	17.0	2.0
(*Campbell's Chunky* Classic)	16.0	2.0
(*Campbell's Chunky* Classic Micro Bowl)	15.0	1.0
(*Campbell's Kitchen Classics*)	13.0	1.0
(*Health Valley* 99% Fat Free	20.0	2.0
(*Health Valley* Rich & Hearty)	13.0	2.0

Food and Measure	carb. (gms)	fiber (gms)
(*Healthy Choice* Old Fashioned)	16.0	3.0
(*Progresso* 97% Fat Free)	13.0	<1.0
(*Progresso* White Meat)	9.0	<1.0
egg noodles (*Campbell's Select*)	14.0	1.0
egg noodles (*Campbell's Select* Micro Cup)	12.0	2.0
mini noodles (*Campbell's Soup at Hand*), 1 cont.	12.0	2.0
chicken rice:		
(*Campbell's Select*)	18.0	2.0
(*Healthy Choice*)	12.0	2.0
(*Healthy Choice* Fiesta)	17.0	3.0
white/wild (*Campbell's Kitchen Classics*)	18.0	2.0
white/wild, savory (*Campbell's Chunky*)	19.0	2.0
wild (*Progresso* White Meat)	15.0	1.0
with vegetables (*Progresso* White Meat)	13.0	1.0
chicken vegetable:		
(*Campbell's Select*)	19.0	3.0
(*Progresso* White Meat)	13.0	2.0
hearty (*Campbell's Chunky*)	14.0	2.0
herbed, roasted vegetables (*Campbell's Select*)	15.0	2.0
clam chowder, Manhattan (*Campbell's Chunky*)	19.0	2.0
clam chowder, Manhattan (*Progresso*)	17.0	2.0
clam chowder, New England:		
(*Campbell's Chunky*)	21.0	2.0
(*Campbell's Kitchen Classics*)	20.0	3.0
(*Campbell's Select*)	16.0	2.0
(*Campbell's Select* 98% Fat Free)	18.0	2.0
(*Campbell's Select* 98% Fat Free Micro Bowl)	16.0	3.0
(*Campbell's Soup at Hand*), 1 cont.	12.0	4.0
(*Healthy Choice*)	21.0	3.0
(*Progresso*)	23.0	1.0
(*Progresso* 97% Fat Free)	18.0	2.0
coconut ginger (*Thai Kitchen*), 7 oz.	11.0	1.0
consommé, madrilène, clear (*Dominique's*)	<1.0	0
consommé, madrilène, red (*Dominique's*)	2.0	<1.0
corn, creamy (*Imagine*)	15.0	1.0
corn, vegetable (*Health Valley*)	17.0	7.0
corn chowder:		
(*Walnut Acres*)	28.0	2.0

Food and Measure	carb. (gms)	fiber (gms)
chicken (*Campbell's Chunky*)	19.0	2.0
Southwestern (*Progresso*)	29.0	3.0
escarole in chicken broth (*Progresso*)	3.0	1.0
ginger carrot (*Walnut Acres*)	22.0	3.0
ham, honey roasted, with potato (*Campbell's Chunky*)	20.0	3.0
hot and sour (*Thai Kitchen*), 7 oz.	7.0	1.5
Italian style wedding (*Campbell's Select*)	16.0	2.0
Italian style wedding (*Campbell's Select* Micro Cup)	15.0	2.0
lentil:		
(*Amy's*)	19.0	9.0
(*Campbell's Kitchen Classics*)	23.0	5.0
(*Campbell's Select* Savory)	27.0	6.0
(*Campbell's Select* Savory Micro Cup)	24.0	5.0
(*Health Valley* Organic/No Salt)	21.0	8.0
(*Progresso*)	22.0	7.0
(*Progresso* Vegetable Classics 99% Fat Free)	20.0	6.0
(*Walnut Acres* Mediterranean)	26.0	8.0
(*Westbrae Natural* Mediterranean)	24.0	10.0
carrot (*Health Valley*)	25.0	7.0
vegetable (*Amy's*)	23.0	9.0
vegetable (*Amy's* Light Sodium)	23.0	6.0
macaroni and bean (*Progresso*)	23.0	6.0
meatball, Mediterranean (*Campbell's Carb Request*)	5.0	2.0
Mexican style (*Campbell's Soup at Hand* Fiesta), 1 cont.	22.0	3.0
minestrone:		
(*Amy's*)	17.0	3.0
(*Campbell's Kitchen Classics*)	22.0	3.0
(*Campbell's Select*)	20.0	4.0
(*Campbell's Select* Micro Cup)	19.0	4.0
(*Health Valley* Italian)	21.0	8.0
(*Health Valley* Organic/No Salt)	17.0	3.0
(*Progresso*)	21.0	5.0
(*Progresso* 97% Fat Free)	19.0	4.0
(*Walnut Acres*)	22.0	3.0
(*Westbrae Natural* Hearty Milano)	24.0	6.0
herb and shells (*Progresso*)	22.0	4.0
miso broth (*Annie Chun's*)	5.0	1.0
mushroom barley (*Health Valley*/No Salt)	17.0	3.0

Food and Measure	carb. (gms)	fiber (gms)
mushroom, portobello, creamy (*Imagine*)	10.0	2.0
mushroom, cream of:		
(*Amy's*)	13.0	2.0
(*Campbell's* Low Sodium), 1 can	19.0	3.0
creamy (*Campbell's Soup at Hand*), 1 cont.	8.0	2.0
creamy (*Progresso*)	12.0	<1.0
mushroom broth (*Health Valley*)	2.0	0
mushroom broth, shiitake (*Annie Chun's*)	3.0	0
penne, in chicken broth (*Progresso*)	14.0	<1.0
noodle (*Amy's* No Chicken)	12.0	2.0
noodle (*Westbrae Natural* New York Un-Chicken)	10.0	<1.0
onion, French (*Progresso*)	9.0	1.0
pasta, cacciatore or Romano (*Health Valley*)	20.0	4.0
pasta and bean (*Health Valley* Fagioli)	25.0	4.0
pasta and bean, 3-bean (*Amy's*)	19.0	4.0
pea, split:		
(*Amy's*)	19.0	4.0
(*Campbell's* Low Sodium), 1 can	38.0	6.0
(*Health Valley*/No Salt)	23.0	8.0
(*Westbrae Natural* Old World)	28.0	6.0
carrot (*Health Valley*)	17.0	4.0
green (*Progresso*)	25.0	5.0
with ham (*Campbell's Chunky*)	27.0	4.0
with ham (*Campbell's Select*)	29.0	5.0
with ham (*Healthy Choice*)	30.0	4.0
with ham (*Progresso*)	20.0	5.0
pepper steak (*Campbell's Chunky*)	18.0	3.0
pizza (*Campbell's Soup at Hand*), 1 cont.	27.0	2.0
potato:		
(*Campbell's Soup at Hand* Velvety), 1 cont.	21.0	4.0
cheddar, white (*Progresso* 97% Fat Free)	20.0	2.0
cream of (*Campbell's Kitchen Classics*)	20.0	2.0
creamy, with roasted garlic (*Campbell's Select*)	20.0	2.0
potato, baked:		
with bacon bits and chives (*Campbell's Chunky*)	21.0	1.0
with cheddar and bacon bits (*Campbell's Chunky*)	23.0	2.0

Food and Measure	carb. (gms)	fiber (gms)
with steak and cheese (*Campbell's Chunky*)	21.0	3.0
potato chowder:		
with broccoli and cheese (*Progresso*)	21.0	1.0
with ham (*Campbell's Chunky* Old Fashioned)	17.0	2.0
with ham and cheese (*Progresso*)	21.0	1.0
roasted garlic (*Progresso*)	23.0	2.0
potato leek (*Health Valley/Health Valley* No Salt)	15.0	3.0
potato leek, creamy (*Imagine*)	14.0	2.0
pumpkin potato (*Walnut Acres* Autumn Harvest)	19.0	2.0
ravioli, with vegetables:		
three cheese (*Campbell's Select*)	20.0	4.0
tomato cheese (*Campbell's Chunky*)	27.0	4.0
rib roast, seasoned, with potatoes and herbs (*Campbell's Chunky*)	17.0	3.0
Salisbury steak, mushrooms, onions (*Campbell's Chunky*)	18.0	2.0
sausage with chicken, spicy (*Campbell's Carb Request*) ..	7.0	2.0
seafood stock (*Kitchen Basics*)	0	0
sirloin burger, with country vegetables:		
(*Campbell's Chunky*)	17.0	3.0
(*Campbell's Chunky* Micro Bowl)	18.0	3.0
sirloin steak, grilled, with hearty vegetables:		
(*Campbell's Chunky*)	19.0	4.0
(*Campbell's Chunky* Micro Bowl)	18.0	3.0
steak, grilled (*Progresso* Steak Soup)	13.0	1.0
steak and potato (*Campbell's Chunky*)	18.0	2.0
tomato:		
(*Campbell's* 32 oz.)	21.0	2.0
(*Campbell's Kitchen Classics*)	24.0	1.0
(*Campbell's Soup at Hand* Classic), 1 cont.	27.0	2.0
(*Health Valley/Health Valley* No Salt)	18.0	1.0
(*Progresso* Hearty)	23.0	2.0
basil (*Progresso*)	29.0	2.0
chunky (*Health Valley/Health Valley* No Salt)	18.0	2.0
garden (*Campbell's Select*)	21.0	3.0
with roasted garlic, herbs (*Campbell's* 32 oz.)	28.0	2.0
rotini (*Progresso*)	30.0	2.0
savory (*Walnut Acres*)	23.0	2.0

Food and Measure	carb. (gms)	fiber (gms)
with tomato pieces (*Campbell's* Low Sodium), 1 can ..	25.0	4.0
vegetable (*Health Valley*)	17.0	5.0
tomato, cream of:		
(*Amy's*)	17.0	4.0
(*Amy's* Sodium Light)	17.0	3.0
creamy (*Campbell's* 32 oz.)	26.0	2.0
creamy (*Campbell's Kitchen Classics*)	24.0	2.0
creamy (*Campbell's Soup at Hand*), 1 cont.	34.0	4.0
creamy (*Healthy Choice*)	22.0	2.0
creamy (*Imagine*)	17.0	2.0
creamy (*Progresso*)	30.0	1.0
tomato bisque (*Amy's*)	21.0	2.0
tortellini, cheese, with chicken, vegetables (*Campbell's Chunky*)	18.0	2.0
tortellini, herb (*Progresso*)	23.0	2.0
turkey:		
chili, with beans (*Campbell's Chunky*)	27.0	6.0
noodle (*Progresso* White Meat)	11.0	<1.0
pot pie (*Campbell's Chunky*)	18.0	3.0
rice, with vegetables (*Progresso* White Meat)	18.0	1.0
vegetable:		
(*Campbell's Chunky*)	22.0	4.0
(*Campbell's Kitchen Classics*)	22.0	3.0
(*Campbell's Select*)	21.0	3.0
(*Campbell's Select* Fiesta)	24.0	2.0
(*Health Valley*/No Salt)	18.0	4.0
(*Healthy Choice* Country)	22.0	4.0
(*Progresso*)	17.0	2.0
(*Progresso* Italiano)	15.0	4.0
(*Westbrae Natural* Santa Fe)	31.0	8.0
(*Westbrae Natural* Spicy Southwest)	35.0	6.0
barley (*Amy's*)	13.0	3.0
barley (*Health Valley*)	19.0	4.0
blended medley (*Campbell's Soup at Hand*), 1 cont.	21.0	3.0
14, garden (*Health Valley*)	17.0	4.0
garden (*Healthy Choice*)	25.0	4.0
herb and rotini (*Progresso*)	19.0	5.0

Food and Measure	carb. (gms)	fiber (gms)
with pasta (*Campbell's Chunky*)	23.0	3.0
vegetarian (*Progresso*)	20.0	4.0
vegetable beef:		
(*Campbell's Chunky* Old Fashioned)	18.0	6.0
(*Campbell's Select*)	16.0	3.0
(*Campbell's Soup at Hand*), 1 cont.	10.0	2.0
(*Healthy Choice*)	24.0	4.0
chunky (*Campbell's* Low Sodium), 1 can	17.0	6.0
vegetable broth:		
(*College Inn* Garden)	6.0	0
(*Health Valley*)	5.0	0
(*Health Valley* Organic)	4.0	0
(*Imagine*)	5.0	1.0
(*Kitchen Basics* Stock)	0	0
(*Pacific* Stock)	3.0	0
(*Swanson*)	3.0	0
Soup, condensed, undiluted, ½ cup:		
asparagus, cream of (*Campbell's*)	10.0	1.0
bean, with bacon (*Campbell's*)	25.0	8.0
bean, black (*Campbell's*)	19.0	5.0
beef, with vegetables and barley (*Campbell's*)	15.0	3.0
beef broth or beef consommé (*Campbell's*)	1.0	0
beef noodle (*Campbell's*)	9.0	<1.0
broccoli, cream of (*Campbell's*)	12.0	1.0
broccoli, cream of (*Campbell's* 98% Fat Free)	12.0	2.0
broccoli cheese (*Campbell's*)	12.0	0
broccoli cheese (*Campbell's* 98% Fat Free)	12.0	1.0
celery, cream of:		
(*Campbell's*)	10.0	1.0
(*Campbell's* 98% Fat Free)	8.0	1.0
(*Campbell's Healthy Request*)	11.0	0
cheddar cheese (*Campbell's*)	12.0	1.0
cheese, nacho (*Campbell's* Fiesta)	10.0	1.0
chicken:		
alphabet (*Campbell's*)	11.0	1.0
dumplings or gumbo (*Campbell's*)	10.0	1.0
and stars (*Campbell's*)	12.0	1.0
vegetable (*Campbell's*)	15.0	2.0

Food and Measure	carb. (gms)	fiber (gms)
vegetable, creamy (*Campbell's* Southwest Style)	21.0	4.0
won ton (*Campbell's*)	6.0	0
chicken, cream of:		
(*Campbell's*)	11.0	1.0
(*Campbell's* 98% Fat Free)	10.0	<1.0
(*Campbell's Healthy Request*)	12.0	1.0
with herbs (*Campbell's*)	10.0	1.0
and mushrooms (*Campbell's*)	9.0	1.0
chicken broth (*Campbell's*)	1.0	0
chicken noodle:		
(*Campbell's/Campbell's* 26 oz.)	8.0	<1.0
(*Campbell's Healthy Request*/Homestyle)	8.0	1.0
(*Campbell's Noodle O's*)	12.0	1.0
creamy (*Campbell's*)	13.0	0
chicken, with rice:		
(*Campbell's*)	14.0	1.0
(*Campbell's Healthy Request*)	13.0	1.0
white/wild (*Campbell's*)	12.0	1.0
white/wild, hearty (*Campbell's Healthy Request*)	17.0	2.0
chili beef (*Campbell's* Fiesta)	25.0	8.0
clam bisque (*Chincoteague*)	13.0	1.0
clam chowder, Manhattan (*Campbell's*)	12.0	2.0
clam chowder, Manhattan (*Chincoteague*)	13.0	1.0
clam chowder, New England:		
(*Campbell's/Campbell's* 98% Fat Free)	13.0	1.0
(*Chincoteague*)	10.0	<1.0
(*Chincoteague* 99% Fat Free)	12.0	<1.0
corn chowder (*Chincoteague*)	16.0	1.0
crab:		
(*Chincoteague* She Crab)	7.0	0
and cheddar (*Chincoteague*)	10.0	0
cream of (*Chincoteague*)	23.0	0
red, vegetable (*Chincoteague*)	12.0	2.0
lobster bisque, regular or cheddar (*Chincoteague*)	10.0	0
minestrone (*Campbell's*)	17.0	3.0
minestrone (*Campbell's Healthy Request*)	15.0	3.0
mushroom, beefy (*Campbell's*)	6.0	0
mushroom, golden (*Campbell's*)	10.0	1.0

Food and Measure	carb. (gms)	fiber (gms)
mushroom, cream of:		
(*Campbell's*)	9.0	1.0
(*Campbell's* 98% Fat Free)	9.0	2.0
(*Campbell's Healthy Request*)	10.0	1.0
with roasted garlic (*Campbell's*)	11.0	1.0
noodle:		
(*Campbell's* Fun Shapes)	12.0	2.0
curly (*Campbell's*)	11.0	1.0
double, in chicken broth (*Campbell's*)	17.0	2.0
mega, in chicken broth (*Campbell's*)	14.0	2.0
onion, cream of (*Campbell's*)	12.0	1.0
onion, French (*Campbell's*)	6.0	1.0
oyster stew (*Campbell's*)	5.0	0
oyster stew (*Chincoteague*)	11.0	0
pasta (*Campbell's* Goldfish)	28.0	1.0
pasta, with chicken and broth (*Campbell's* Goldfish)	11.0	1.0
pea, green (*Campbell's*)	28.0	4.0
pea, split, with ham and bacon (*Campbell's*)	27.0	5.0
pepper pot (*Campbell's*)	9.0	1.0
potato, cream of (*Campbell's*)	15.0	1.0
Scotch broth (*Campbell's*)	9.0	2.0
shrimp, cream of (*Campbell's*)	8.0	1.0
shrimp bisque (*Chincoteague*)	10.0	0
tomato:		
(*Campbell's*)	20.0	1.0
(*Campbell's Healthy Request*)	18.0	1.0
bisque (*Campbell's*)	23.0	1.0
noodle (*Campbell's*)	25.0	2.0
rice (*Campbell's* Old Fashioned)	23.0	1.0
turkey noodle (*Campbell's*)	9.0	1.0
vegetable:		
(*Campbell's*)	20.0	3.0
(*Campbell's* California Style)	13.0	2.0
(*Campbell's* Old Fashioned)	14.0	2.0
(*Campbell's Healthy Request*)	20.0	3.0
beef (*Campbell's/Campbell's Healthy Request*)	15.0	3.0
with pasta, hearty (*Campbell's*)	19.0	2.0
vegetarian (*Campbell's*)	18.0	2.0

Food and Measure	carb. (gms)	fiber (gms)
Soup, semicondensed, undiluted:		
broth, vegetarian (*Westbrae Natural* California Un-Chicken), ¾ cup	2.0	0
clam chowder, Manhattan (*Bookbinder's*), ½ cup	10.0	<1.0
lobster bisque (*Bookbinder's*), ½ cup	10.0	0
mushroom, creamy (*Westbrae Natural* Monte Carlo), ¾ cup	10.0	0
pepperpot, seafood (*Bookbinder's*), ½ cup	23.0	1.0
seafood bisque (*Bookbinder's*), ½ cup	9.0	0
shrimp bisque (*Bookbinder's*), ½ cup	10.0	0
snapper (*Bookbinder's*), ½ cup	12.0	<1.0
tomato (*Westbrae Natural* Tuscany), ¾ cup	16.0	0
Soup, freeze-dried (see also "Soup, mix"), 1 serving:		
bean, multi (*AlpineAire*)	28.0	8.0
broccoli, cream of (*AlpineAire*)	21.0	2.0
corn chowder (*AlpineAire* Kernel's)	36.0	9.0
minestrone (*AlpineAire* Alpine)	34.0	6.0
potato cheddar, creamy (*AlpineAire*)	36.0	3.0
seafood chowder (*Mountain House*)	19.0	1.0
split pea (*AlpineAire* Soup-er)	34.0	9.0
Soup, frozen, 1 cup:		
asparagus, creamy (*Impromptu Gourmet*)	14.0	1.0
bean, white, and vegetable (*Moosewood* Tuscan)	24.0	5.0
broccoli and cheese, creamy (*Moosewood*)	7.0	3.0
chicken noodle (*Organic Classics*)	15.0	2.0
clam chowder, New England (*Boston Chowda*)	20.0	1.0
crab, Charleston (*Boston Chowda* She-Crab)	16.0	<1.0
lobster bisque (*Boston Chowda* Rockport)	12.0	1.0
lobster bisque (*Impromptu Gourmet*)	10.0	0
mushroom barley (*Moosewood* Hearty)	14.0	3.0
potato and corn chowder (*Moosewood*)	26.0	3.0
salmon, smoked, chowder (*Impromptu Gourmet*)	21.0	1.0
seafood chowder (*Organic Classics*)	17.0	1.0
shrimp and sausage gumbo (*Boston Chowda*)	38.0	2.0
tomato and rice (*Moosewood* Mediterranean)	16.0	2.0
Soup, mix (see also "Soup, freeze-dried"), dry, 1 cont. or pkg., except as noted:		

Food and Measure	carb. (gms)	fiber (gms)
bean:		
3-bean (*Bean Cuisine* Bouillabaisse), 1 cup*	17.0	5.0
5-bean (*Fantastic Big Soup*), ½ cont.	33.0	9.0
and ham (*Hormel* Micro Cup)	29.0	2.0
bean, black:		
(*Bean Cuisine* Island), 1 cup*	17.0	7.0
(*Fantastic Big Soup* Jumpin'), ½ cont.	41.0	19.0
with couscous, spicy (*Health Valley* Cup), ⅓ cup	29.0	5.0
with rice (*Health Valley* Cup Zesty), ⅓ cup	22.0	4.0
and rice (*Uncle Ben's* Hearty), ⅓ pkg.	28.0	7.0
bean, white (*Bean Cuisine* Provençal), 1 cup*	32.0	11.0
beef, vegetarian:		
barley (*Fantastic Carb'Tastic*)	14.0	6.0
noodle (*Fantastic Big Soup* Noodle Bowl), ½ cont.	21.0	2.0
beef stew, hearty (*Wyler's Soup Starter*), 1 cup* with water	19.0	2.0
beef vegetable (*Hormel* Micro Cup)	15.0	1.0
beef vegetable, beefy (*Instant Gourmet*)	6.0	1.0
broccoli:		
cheddar (*Fantastic Carb'Tastic*)	13.0	7.0
cheddar (*Instant Gourmet*)	6.0	2.0
cheddar (*Produce Partners*), 2 tbsp.	5.0	0
cheddar (*Wyler's Soup Starter*), 1 cup*	19.0	2.0
cheddar, creamy (*Fantastic Big Soup*), ½ cont.	21.0	2.0
cheese (*Cup-a-Soup*)	17.0	0
cheese and rice (*Uncle Ben's* Hearty), ⅓ pkg.	19.0	1.0
cream of (*Produce Partners*), 1⅓ tbsp.	4.0	0
ginger, Asian (*Fantastic Carb'Tastic*)	11.0	9.0
Mandarin (*Fantastic Big Soup* Noodle Bowl), ½ cont.	20.0	2.0
cheese (*Watkins* Soup and Sauce Base), 2½ tbsp.	14.0	0
chicken:		
with asparagus (*Instant Gourmet*)	5.0	1.0
cream of (*Cup-a-Soup*)	14.0	0
spicy Thai (*Cup-a-Soup*)	12.0	0
"chicken," vegetarian, gumbo (*Fantastic Carb'Tastic*)	9.0	4.0
"chicken," vegetarian, Mandarin (*Fantastic Carb'Tastic*)	13.0	10.0
chicken noodle:		
(*Fantastic Big Soup* Noodle Bowl), ½ cont.	19.0	1.0

Food and Measure	carb. (gms)	fiber (gms)
(*Fantastic* Simmer), ⅓ cup	22.0	2.0
(*Hormel* Micro Cup)	12.0	0
(*Wyler's Soup Starter*), 1 cup* with water	13.0	1.0
chicken rice (*Hormel* Micro Cup)	18.0	1.0
chili (*Fantastic Big Soup* Cha Cha), ½ cont.	37.0	11.0
clam chowder, New England (*Hormel* Micro Cup)	18.0	1.0
corn chowder:		
bean (*Bean Cuisine* Santa Fe), 1 cup*	18.0	6.0
and potato (*Fantastic Big Soup*), ½ cont.	26.0	2.0
with tomato (*Health Valley* Cup), ½ cup	21.0	3.0
couscous, with lentils (*Fantastic Big Soup*), ½ cont.	35.0	5.0
cream (*Watkins* Soup Base), 2½ tbsp.	4.0	0
garlic herb (*Fantastic* Soup/Dip), 2¼ tsp.	5.0	0
hot and sour (*Fantastic Big Soup* Noodle Bowl), ½ cont.	22.0	1.0
hot and sour (*Fantastic Carb'Tastic*)	7.0	1.0
lentil:		
(*Bean Cuisine* Lots of Lentils), 1 cup*	17.0	5.0
(*Fantastic Big Soup* Country), ½ cont.	32.0	9.0
with couscous (*Health Valley* Cup), ⅓ cup	28.0	5.0
minestrone (*Fantastic Big Soup*), ½ cont.	27.0	4.0
miso:		
dark (*San-J*)	3.0	1.0
mild (*San-J*)	5.0	1.0
red or white (*Westbrae Natural* Instant)	3.0	0
with tofu (*Fantastic Big Soup* Noodle Bowl), ½ cont.	19.0	<1.0
sesame (*Fantastic Big Soup* Noodle Bowl), ½ cont.	17.0	<1.0
white (*San-J*)	3.0	0
mushroom:		
(*Watkins Soup* and Sauce Base), 2 tbsp.	9.0	0
shiitake (*Fantastic Carb'Tastic*)	9.0	7.0
and chicken, with garlic (*Instant Gourmet*)	8.0	2.0
noodle:		
beef flavor (*Cup-a-Soup* Asian)	14.0	0
chicken flavor (*Cup-a-Soup*)	17.0	0
chicken flavor, with vegetables (*Health Valley* Cup), ½ cup	24.0	3.0
thin cut (*Azumaya* Asian), 1 cup	24.0	<1.0
wide cut (*Azumaya* Asian), 1 cup	24.0	<1.0

Food and Measure	carb. (gms)	fiber (gms)
noodle, ramen, ½ pkg. or cont.:		
buckwheat or brown rice (*Westbrae Natural*)	30.0	2.0
chicken free, vegetarian (*Fantastic Big Soup*)	19.0	2.0
curry or 5 spice (*Westbrae Natural*)	30.0	3.0
miso (*Westbrae Natural*)	29.0	4.0
mushroom or seaweed (*Westbrae Natural*)	30.0	3.0
spinach (*Westbrae Natural*)	29.0	3.0
vegetable curry (*Fantastic Big Soup*)	20.0	2.0
vegetable miso (*Fantastic Big Soup*)	19.0	1.0
onion (*Fantastic* Soup/Dip), 2½ tsp.	6.0	1.0
onion, mushroom (*Fantastic* Soup & Dip), 1½ tbsp.	6.0	<1.0
pasta (*Health Valley* Cup Italiano), ½ cup	31.0	3.0
pasta, marinara, Mediterranean, or Parmesan (*Health Valley* Cup), ½ cup	20.0	1.0
pea, split:		
(*Fantastic* Simmer), ¼ cup	2.0	6.0
(*Fantastic Big Soup*), ½ cont.	7.0	7.0
garden, with carrots (*Health Valley* Cup), ⅓ cup	22.0	2.0
potato, cream of (*Produce Partners*), 1 tbsp.	3.0	0
potato, creamy (*Fantastic* Simmer), ¼ cup	22.0	1.0
potato broccoli, creamy (*Health Valley* Cup), ⅓ cup	17.0	3.0
rice noodles, 1 cup*:		
curry (*Thai Kitchen*)	28.0	0
curry (*Thai Kitchen* Bangkok Instant)	16.0	0
garlic, roasted (*Thai Kitchen* Soup Bowls)	25.0	0
garlic and vegetables (*Thai Kitchen* Instant)	17.0	0
ginger (*Thai Kitchen* Instant)	16.0	0
ginger (*Thai Kitchen* Soup Bowls)	24.0	0
hot and sour (*Thai Kitchen*)	30.0	0
hot and sour (*Thai Kitchen* Soup Bowls)	24.0	0
lemon grass and chili (*Thai Kitchen*)	60.0	0
lemon grass and chili (*Thai Kitchen* Instant)	17.0	0
mushroom (*Thai Kitchen* Soup Bowls)	25.0	0
onion, spring (*Thai Kitchen* Instant)	16.0	0
onion, spring (*Thai Kitchen* Soup Bowls)	25.0	0
shrimp bisque (*Instant Gourmet* Bay Shrimp)	7.0	1.0
Thai:		
with mushrooms (*Tasty Bite* Tom Yum), ½ pkg.	5.0	<1.0

Food and Measure	carb. (gms)	fiber (gms)
spicy (*Fantastic Big Soup* Noodle Bowl), ½ cont.	22.0	1.0
with vegetables (*Tasty Bite* Gang Pha), ½ pkg.	4.0	1.0
tomato:		
with croutons (*Cup-a-Soup*)	16.0	<1.0
noodle, Italian (*Fantastic Big Soup* Noodle Bowl),		
½ cont.	26.0	2.0
sun-dried, basil (*Fantastic Carb'Tastic*)	10.0	7.0
tortilla (*Chi-Chi's* Fiesta), ⅕ pkg.	13.0	1.9
vegetable:		
(*Fantastic* Soup & Dip), 1½ tsp.	5.0	<1.0
barley (*Fantastic* Simmer), ¼ cup	26.0	3.0
barley (*Fantastic Big Soup*), ½ cont.	27.0	5.0
spring (*Cup-a-Soup*)	11.0	<1.0
spring (*Fantastic Big Soup* Noodle Bowl), ½ cont.	19.0	<1.0
wakame (*San-J*)	12.0	0
Sour cream, see "Cream, sour"		
Soursop, ½ cup	18.9	3.7
Soy, cultured, see "Yogurt, soy"		
Soy bean, see "Soybean"		
Soy beverage, 8 fl. oz., except as noted:		
(*Edensoy* Extra Organic Original)	13.0	3.0
(*Edensoy* Light Organic Original)	14.0	0
(*Edensoy* Organic Original)	14.0	2.0
(*Edensoy* Organic Unsweetened)	5.0	2.0
(*8ᵗʰ Continent*)	11.0	0
(*Organic Valley* Original)	11.0	3.0
(*Pearl* Organic Original)	12.0	1.0
(*Power Dream*), 11 fl. oz.	48.0	2.0
(*Silk*)	8.0	1.0
(*Silk*), 11 fl. oz.	11.0	1.0
(*Silk* Enhanced/Light)	8.0	1.0
(*Silk* Unsweetened/Unsweetened Aseptic)	5.0	1.0
(*Soy Dream* Original).............................	17.0	n.a.
(*WestSoy* Lite)	15.0	2.0
(*WestSoy* Low Fat)	14.0	2.0
(*WestSoy* Non Fat)	10.0	<1.0
(*WestSoy* Organic Original)	18.0	3.0

Food and Measure	carb. (gms)	fiber (gms)
(*WestSoy* Organic Unsweetened)	5.0	4.0
(*WestSoy Plus*)	17.0	3.0
(*WestSoy Smart Plus*)	22.0	5.0
banana berry (*WestSoy* Smoothie)	28.0	2.0
cappucino (*WestSoy* Soy Slender)	4.0	3.0
carob (*Edensoy* Organic)	27.0	0
carob (*Soy Dream*)	36.0	1.0
chai:		
(*Power Dream* Sky High), 11 fl. oz.	42.0	<1.0
(*Silk*)	19.0	0
(*WestSoy* Original)	25.0	<1.0
chocolate:		
(*Edensoy* Organic)	28.0	1.0
(*8th Continent*)	23.0	1.0
(*8th Continent* Light)	11.0	<1.0
(*Organic Valley*)	19.0	3.0
(*Silk*)	23.0	2.0
(*Silk*), 6.5 fl. oz.	19.0	2.0
(*Silk*), 11 fl. oz.	32.0	2.0
(*Soy Dream* Enriched)	37.0	1.0
(*WestSoy* Lite)	25.0	2.0
(*WestSoy* Low Fat)	24.0	3.0
(*WestSoy* Organic Unsweetened)	6.0	5.0
(*WestSoy* Shake)	30.0	4.0
(*WestSoy* Soy Slender)	5.0	4.0
(*WestSoy VigorAid*), 1 cont.	42.0	6.0
coffee:		
(*Power Dream* Java Jolt), 11 fl. oz.	42.0	2.0
(*Silk* Soylatte)	25.0	1.0
(*Silk* Soylatte), 11 fl. oz.	34.0	1.0
green tea (*Pearl* Organic)	13.0	1.0
kefir blend, all flavors (*Lifeway Soy Treat*)	23.0	0
mango (*Power Dream* Passion), 11 fl. oz.	65.0	1.0
mango (*Silk Live!*), 10 fl. oz.	41.0	4.0
mocha (*Silk*)	22.0	0
peach (*Soy Live!*), 10 fl. oz.	38.0	4.0
raspberry (*Silk Live!*), 10 fl. oz.	40.0	4.0

Food and Measure	carb. (gms)	fiber (gms)
spice (*Silk* Soylatte), 11 fl. oz.	27.0	1.0
strawberry (*Silk*), 6.5 fl. oz.	21.0	1.0
strawberry (*Silk Live!*), 10 fl. oz.	40.0	4.0
tropical (*Pearl* Organic Delight)	14.0	0
tropical (*WestSoy* Smoothie Whip)	28.0	2.0
vanilla:		
(*Edensoy* Organic)	24.0	1.0
(*Edensoy* Extra Organic)	23.0	1.0
(*Edensoy* Light Organic)	20.0	0
(*8th Continent*)	11.0	0
(*8th Continent* Light)	4.0	0
(*Organic Valley*)	14.0	3.0
(*Pearl* Organic Creamy)	11.0	0
(*Power Dream* Blast), 11 fl. oz.	39.0	2.0
(*Silk*)	10.0	1.0
(*Silk* Light)	10.0	1.0
(*Silk* Very)	19.0	1.0
(*Soy Dream*/Enriched)	22.0	0
(*WestSoy* Lite)	19.0	2.0
(*WestSoy* Low Fat)	21.0	2.0
(*WestSoy* Non Fat)	12.0	<1.0
(*WestSoy* Organic Unsweetened)	5.0	4.0
(*WestSoy* Shake)	28.0	3.0
(*WestSoy* Soy Slender)	4.0	3.0
(*WestSoy* Plus)	19.0	3.0
(*WestSoy* Smart Plus)	25.0	5.0
(*WestSoy* VigorAid), 1 cont.	37.0	5.0
chai tea (*Bolthouse Farms* Perfectly Protein)	25.0	0
Soy butter, see "Soy spread"		
Soy chips/crisps (see also "Potato soy crisps"), 1 oz., except as noted:		
apple cinnamon (*GeniSoy* Crisps)	17.0	2.0
barbecue (*GeniSoy* Crisps Zesty)	17.0	2.0
caramel (*Hain PureSnax* Munchies), 7 pieces, .5 oz.	8.0	<1.0
cheddar, white (*Hain PureSnax* Munchies), 9 pieces, .5 oz.	6.0	1.0
cheese, nacho (*GeniSoy* Crisps)	15.0	2.0
cheese, rich (*GeniSoy* Crisps)	14.0	2.0

Food and Measure	carb. (gms)	fiber (gms)
garlic, roasted, onion (*GeniSoy* Crisps)	14.0	2.0
Parmesan, garlic, olive oil (*Synder's* Crisps)	11.0	1.0
ranch (*GeniSoy* Crisps)	15.0	2.0
ranch (*Hain PureSnax* Munchies), 9 pieces, .5 oz.	8.0	1.0
salt and vinegar or sea salted (*GeniSoy* Crisps)	14.0	2.0
tomato, Romano, olive oil (*Snyder's* Crisps)	12.0	n.a.
Soy flour, see "Soybean flour"		
Soy meal, defatted, raw, 1 cup	49.0	14.0
Soy milk, see "Soy beverage"		
Soy nuts, roasted:		
(*Frieda's*), ⅓ cup, 1.1 oz.	9.0	1.0
(*GeniSoy* Unsalted), 1 oz.	9.0	5.0
(*Tree of Life*), 1.1 oz.	9.0	3.0
barbecue (*GeniSoy* Zesty), 1 oz.	9.0	5.0
barbecue, honey, or wasabi (*Frieda's*), ¼ cup	11.0	5.0
hickory smoked (*GeniSoy*), 1 oz.	9.0	5.0
sea salted (*GeniSoy*), 1 oz.	9.0	2.0
toasted, 1 oz. or 95 kernels	8.7	1.0
toasted, whole, 1 cup	33.0	3.9
Soy protein, concentrate, w/alcohol or acid/water wash, 1 oz.	8.8	<2.0
Soy sauce, 1 tbsp.:		
(*House of Tsang* Low Sodium/Mandarin Marinade)	0	0
(*Kikkoman*)	0	0
(*Kikkoman* Lite)	1.0	0
(*World Harbors Angostura*)	1.0	0
(*World Harbors Angostura* All Natural)	2.0	0
ginger flavor (*House of Tsang*)	4.0	0
ginger flavor (*House of Tsang* Low Sodium)	2.0	0
shoyu or tamari:		
(*Eden* Imported/Organic/Imported Reduced Sodium) ..	2.0	0
(*San-J* Organic/Reduced Sodium/Wheat Free Organic) .	1.0	0
(*Tree of Life* Wheat Free Organic)	0	0
Soy spread, creamy or crunchy (*Soy Wonder*), 2 tbsp. ...	10.0	1.0
Soybean, fresh (see also "Edamame"):		
raw, shelled, ½ cup	14.1	5.4
boiled, drained, ½ cup	10.0	3.8

Food and Measure	carb. (gms)	fiber (gms)
Soybean, canned, ½ cup:		
(*Westbrae Natural Organic*)	11.0	3.0
black (*Eden Organic*)	8.0	7.0
Soybean, dried:		
dry, ¼ cup:		
(*Arrowhead Mills*)	11.0	4.0
black or yellow (*Shiloh Farms*)	14.0	10.0
dry-roasted	14.1	3.5
roasted	14.5	3.5
boiled, ½ cup	8.5	5.2
Soybean, frozen:		
in pod, see "Edamame"		
shelled (*C&W* Sweet), ½ cup	16.0	10.0
Soybean curd or cake, see "Tofu"		
Soybean flakes (*Shiloh Farms*), ½ cup	18.0	0
Soybean flour, ¼ cup:		
(*Arrowhead Mills*)	9.0	4.0
(*Hodgson Mill*), <¼ cup	9.0	6.0
(*Hodgson Mill Organic*), <¼ cup	9.0	4.0
(*Shiloh Farms*)	7.0	3.5
stirred:		
full fat, raw	7.5	2.1
defatted	9.6	4.4
lowfat	8.4	2.3
Soybean grits, roasted (*Shiloh Farms*), ¼ cup	7.0	3.5
Soybean kernels, roasted, see "Soy nuts"		
Soybean sprouts,		
(*Jonathan's*), 1 cup	8.0	2.0
steamed, ½ cup	3.1	.4
Spaghetti, see "Pasta"		
Spaghetti entree, can or pkg., 1 cup, except as noted:		
(*SpaghettiOs*)	37.0	3.0
(*SpaghettiOs* A to Z's)	36.0	3.0
(*SpaghettiOs* Fun Shapes Smilers)	33.0	3.0
(*SpaghettiOs* Plus Calcium)	35.0	3.0
(*SpaghettiOs* Spaghetti)	40.0	3.0
with franks:		
(*SpaghettiOs*)	27.0	5.0

Food and Measure	carb. (gms)	fiber (gms)
(*SpaghettiOs* A to Z's)	33.0	2.0
rings (*Kid's Kitchen*)	32.0	1.0
with meat sauce:		
(*Hormel* Bowl), 10 oz.	41.0	4.0
(*Hormel* Meal), 1 cont.	31.0	2.0
(*SpaghettiOs*)	31.0	3.0
with meatballs:		
(*Kid's Kitchen*)	28.0	2.0
(*SpaghettiOs* Fun Shapes Smilers)	32.0	3.0
(*SpaghettiOs* A to Z's)	33.0	3.0
rings (*Kid's Kitchen*)	31.0	1.0
tomato cheese sauce (*SpaghettiOs*)	40.0	2.0
Spaghetti entree, dried, 1 serving:		
marinara, with mushrooms (*AlpineAire*)	53.0	6.0
meat and sauce:		
(*Mountain House* Can/Four), 1 cup	32.0	2.0
(*Mountain House* Double), ½ pouch	37.0	2.0
(*Mountain House* Single)	46.0	3.0
Spaghetti entree, frozen, 1 pkg.:		
Bolognese (*Smart Ones*), 11.5 oz.	43.0	5.0
cheese bake (*Stouffer's*), 12 oz.	45.0	4.0
marinara (*Michelina's* Zap'ems), 8 oz.	46.0	4.0
marinara (*Smart Ones*), 9 oz.	46.0	4.0
with meat sauce:		
(*Healthy Choice*), 10 oz.	36.0	5.0
(*Lean Cuisine Everyday Favorites*), 9.5 oz.	48.0	3.0
(*Michelina's* Authentico), 8.5 oz.	45.0	4.0
(*Michelina's Lean Gourmet*), 9 oz.	45.0	4.0
(*Stouffer's*), 12 oz.	51.0	4.0
with meatballs:		
(*Lean Cuisine Everyday Favorites*), 9.5 oz.	38.0	3.0
(*Michelina's* Authentico), 9 oz.	44.0	4.0
(*Michelina's* Zap'ems), 8 oz.	38.0	4.0
(*Stouffer's*), 12⅝ oz.	58.0	4.0
tomato basil sauce (*Michelina's* Zap'ems), 8 oz.	47.0	4.0
Spaghetti sauce, see "Pasta sauce"		
Spaghetti squash:		
raw (*Frieda's*), ¾ cup, 3 oz.	6.0	1.0

Food and Measure	carb. (gms)	fiber (gms)
baked or boiled, drained, ½ cup	5.0	1.1
Spanakopita, see "Spinach entree, frozen" and "Spinach snack rolls/nuggets"		
Spareribs, see "Pork" and "Pork, frozen or refrigerated"		
Spelt, grain, ¼ cup:		
(*Purity Foods* Berries)	32.0	8.0
(*Shiloh Farms*)	32.0	8.0
Spelt chips (*VitaSpelt* Flatchips), 1 oz.	15.0	.5
Spelt flakes, see "Cereal, ready-to-eat"		
Spelt flour:		
(*Arrowhead Mills*), ⅓ cup	25.0	4.0
(*Hodgson Mill* Organic), <¼ cup	21.0	5.0
(*Shiloh Farms*), ¼ cup	23.0	2.0
white (*Shiloh Farms*), ¼ cup	21.0	1.0
Spinach, fresh:		
raw:		
(*Dole/Dole* Baby), 3 oz.	3.0	2.0
baby (*Dole* Organic), 3 oz.	9.0	4.0
baby (*Fresh Express*), 1½ cups, 3 oz.	3.0	2.0
baby (*Ready Pac*), 4 cups, 3 oz.	10.0	5.0
flat leaf (*Fresh Express*), 1½ cups, 3 oz.	10.0	5.0
boiled, drained, (*Ready Pac*), ½ cup	3.0	<1.0
boiled, drained, ½ cup	3.4	2.2
Spinach, canned, ½ cup:		
leaf:		
(*Popeye* No Salt)	5.0	2.0
(*S&W*)	4.0	2.0
cut (*Freshlike*)	5.0	3.0
leaf or chopped (*Del Monte*/No Salt)	4.0	2.0
leaf or chopped (*Popeye*)	4.0	2.0
seasoned (*Glory*)	3.0	2.0
drained	3.6	2.6
Spinach, frozen (see also "Spinach dish"):		
leaf (*Birds Eye*), ⅓ cup	3.0	1.0
leaf (*C&W*), ⅓ cup	2.0	2.0
cut leaf:		
(*Birds Eye*), 1 cup	3.0	1.0

Food and Measure	carb. (gms)	fiber (gms)
(*Cascadian Farm* Bag), ⅓ cup	3.0	3.0
(*Cascadian Farm* Box), ⅓ cup	3.0	1.0
(*Green Giant*), ⅓ cup cooked	2.0	2.0
(*Tree of Life*), 1 cup	2.0	2.0
cut leaf, in butter sauce (*Green Giant*), ½ cup	4.0	2.0
cut leaf or chopped (*Seabrook Farms*), ⅓ cup	2.0	2.0
chopped:		
(*Birds Eye*), ⅓ cup	3.0	1.0
(*C&W*), ⅓ cup	2.0	2.0
(*Green Giant*), ½ cup	3.0	2.0
chopped or leaf, drained, ½ cup	5.1	2.6
Spinach, malabar, cooked, 1 cup	1.2	.9
Spinach, New Zealand, chopped:		
raw, 1 oz. or ½ cup	.7	n.a.
boiled, drained, ½ cup	2.0	n.a.
Spinach dip, frozen, with cheese and artichoke (*T.G.I. Friday's*), 2 tbsp.	2.0	0
Spinach dip mix, dry (*McCormick*), 1 tsp.	1.0	0
Spinach dish, frozen, ½ cup, except as noted:		
creamed:		
(*Birds Eye*)	7.0	1.0
(*Boston Market*)	7.0	3.0
(*C&W*)	5.0	2.0
(*Green Giant*)	9.0	1.0
(*Seabrook Farms*)	10.0	3.0
(*Stouffer's*), ½ of 9-oz. pkg.	10.0	2.0
pancake:		
(*Dr. Praeger's*), 1.3-oz. piece	5.0	<1.0
(*Dr. Praeger's* Bombay), 1.3-oz. piece	8.5	1.0
nuggets (*Dr. Praeger's*), 4 pieces, 1.4 oz.	5.0	1.0
soufflé (*Stouffer's*), ⅓ of 12-oz. pkg.	9.0	1.0
Spinach entree, frozen, 1 pkg., except as noted:		
with cheese, palak paneer:		
(*Amy's*), 10 oz.	38.0	5.0
(*Deep*), ½ of 10-oz. pkg.	7.0	4.0
(*Ethnic Gourmet*), 12 oz.	42.0	7.0
feta pie (*Cedarlane* Spanakopita), ½ of 10-oz. pkg.	38.0	2.0

Food and Measure	carb. (gms)	fiber (gms)
Spinach entree, pkg.:		
with cheese and rice:		
(*Tamarind Tree* Palak Paneer), 9.25-oz. pkg.	46.0	6.0
(*Tasty Bite* Kashmir), ½ of 10-oz. pkg.	8.0	3.0
dal, with rice (*Tasty Bite*), 12-oz. pkg.	62.0	8.0
with garbanzos and rice (*Tamarind Tree* Saag Chole),		
9.25-oz. pkg.	55.0	13.0
Spinach snack rolls/nuggets, frozen:		
(*Health is Wealth Munchees*), 2 pieces, 1 oz.	9.0	1.0
with cheese, breaded (*Kineret*), 3½ pieces, 2.8 oz.	19.0	6.0
with feta cheese:		
(*Amy's*), 5–6 pieces	24.0	2.0
(*Athens/Apollo* Spanakopita), 2 pieces, 2 oz.	17.0	<1.0
(*Health is Wealth Munchees*), 2 pieces, 1 oz.	9.0	1.0
Spinach-feta pocket, frozen (*Amy's*), 4.5-oz. piece	34.0	3.0
Spiny lobster, meat only:		
raw, 4 oz.	2.8	0
boiled or steamed, 2 lbs. in shell	5.1	0
boiled or steamed, 4 oz.	3.5	0
Spleen, braised, without added ingredients	0	0
Split peas:		
dry, ¼ cup:		
green (*Arrowhead Mills*)	24.0	4.0
green (*Goya*)	27.0	11.0
green or yellow (*Shiloh Farms*)	27.0	11.0
yellow (*Goya*)	28.0	12.0
boiled, ½ cup	20.7	8.1
Sports bar, see "Granola/cereal bar"		
Sports drink, all flavors, 8 fl. oz.:		
(*Gatorade*)	14.0	0
(*Recharge*)	18.0	0
Spot, without added ingredients	0	0
Spring roll (see also "Egg roll"), frozen, 2 pieces, 1.6 oz.:		
(*Health is Wealth*)	10.0	5.0
hot and spicy (*Health is Wealth*)	16.0	1.0
Thai (*Health is Wealth*)	15.0	1.0
SpriteMelon (*Frieda's*), 10.6-oz. melon	29.0	2.0
Sprouts, see "Bean sprouts" and specific listings		

Food and Measure	carb. (gms)	fiber (gms)
Sprouts, mixed, 1 cup:		
(*Jonathan's*)	21.0	4.0
(*Jonathan's* Gourmet)	3.0	2.0
hot and spicy (*Jonathan's*)	4.0	2.0
salad (*Jonathan's*)	10.0	4.0
Squab, meat only, without added ingredients	0	0
Squid, fresh, meat only, raw, 4 oz.	3.5	0
Squirrel, meat only, without added ingredients	0	0
Star fruit, see "Carambola"		
Star spangled squash (*Frieda's*), ⅔ cup, 3 oz.	3.0	1.0
Starbucks, 1 serving		
Chantico, 6 fl. oz.	51.0	6.0
Classics, without cream/topping, 12 fl. oz.:		
caramel apple cider	55.0	0
chocolate milk or hot chocolate, whole milk	33.0	1.0
chocolate milk or hot chocolate, nonfat milk	35.0	1.0
pumpkin spice crème, whole milk	38.0	0
toffee nut crème, whole milk	31.0	0
vanilla crème, whole milk	29.0	0
white hot chocolate, whole milk	49.0	0
coffee, brewed, coffee of week, 12 fl. oz.	1.0	0
coffee, brewed, iced, shaken, 12 fl. oz.	15.0	0
espresso, hot, whole milk, without cream/topping, 12 fl. oz.:		
caffé Americano	2.0	0
caffé latte	16.0	0
caffé misto/café au lait	8.0	0
caffé mocha	31.0	.0
cappuccino	10.0	0
caramel macchiato	28.0	0
caramel mocha	46.0	1.0
cinnamon spice mocha	30.0	0
pumpkin spice latte	38.0	0
syrup latte	29.0	0
toffee nut latte	30.0	0
vanilla latte	29.0	0
white chocolate mocha	43.0	0
espresso, iced, whole milk, without cream/topping, 12 fl. oz.:		
caffé Americano	2.0	0

Food and Measure	carb. (gms)	fiber (gms)
caffé latte	6.0	0
caffé mocha	26.0	1.0
caramel macchiato	24.0	0
caramel mocha	42.0	0
syrup or vanilla latte	23.0	0
white chocolate mocha	42.0	0
Frappuccino coffee blend, without cream/topping, 12 fl. oz.:		
caffé vanilla	51.0	0
caramel or toffee nut	43.0	0
caramel mocha	52.0	0
coffee	38.0	0
espresso	33.0	0
java chip	51.0	1.0
mocha	44.0	0
pumpkin spice	47.0	0
white chocolate mocha	48.0	0
Frappuccino crème blend, without cream/topping, 12 fl. oz.:		
caramel chocolate	62.0	<1.0
double chocolate chip	57.0	2.0
strawberries/crème	65.0	0
Tazo chai crème	52.0	0
toffee nut	48.0	0
vanilla bean	51.0	0
Tazo tea, whole milk, chai latte/iced, 12 fl. oz.	36.0	0
Tazo tea, iced	16.0	0
Tazo tea lemonade	23.0	0
drink extras:		
syrup, flavored, 1 pump	5.0	0
syrup, mocha, 1 pump	6.0	0
toppings:		
chocolate	1.0	0
caramel	2.0	0
sprinkles	<1.0	0
whipped cream, cold drinks	2.0	0
whipped cream, hot drinks	1.0	0
bagels, 5 oz.:		
plain	92.0	3.0

Food and Measure	carb. (gms)	fiber (gms)
cinnamon raisin	96.0	3.0
sesame	92.0	6.0
bars:		
caramel apple	38.0	2.0
caramel brownie	60.0	2.0
carrot cake	46.0	<1.0
chocolate marshmallow	61.0	2.0
chocolate peanut butter stack	67.0	4.0
cranberry bliss	38.0	<1.0
espresso brownie	43.0	2.0
espresso brownie, enrobed or fudge	48.0	3.0
lemon	44.0	0
milk chocolate peanut butter brownie	45.0	2.0
oatmeal cranberry mountain	49.0	3.0
Oreo dream bar	33.0	2.0
pecan almond	38.0	2.0
peppermint brownie	48.0	2.0
raspberry sammy	41.0	1.0
seven layer	63.0	4.0
toffee cream cheese chew	38.0	2.0
toffee crunch	56.0	1.0
biscotti, chocolate hazelnut or vanilla almond	15.0	1.0
cakes:		
apple harvest torte	53.0	4.0
bundt, chocolate big baby	45.0	4.0
bundt, lemon yogurt	56.0	<1.0
coffee cake:		
apple walnut	41.0	1.0
blueberry walnut	43.0	1.0
cinnamon walnut	46.0	1.0
classic	75.0	2.0
crumble berry	69.0	2.0
hazelnut	74.0	2.0
sour cream	43.0	1.0
crumb cake	89.0	1.0
gingerbread, holiday	81.0	1.0
key lime crumb	71.0	1.0

Food and Measure	carb. (gms)	fiber (gms)
pound cake:		
banana	47.0	1.0
cranberry walnut	45.0	1.0
carrot, iced	101.0	3.0
lemon, iced	69.0	<1.0
marble	49.0	<1.0
orange poppy cheese	55.0	2.0
pumpkin	47.0	2.0
zucchini	47.0	2.0
pullman:		
banana	57.0	2.0
chocolate	54.0	2.0
cranberry walnut	53.0	2.0
lemon glazed	55.0	<1.0
marble chocolate chip	61.0	1.0
orange poppy cheese	55.0	1.0
pumpkin	51.0	2.0
cookies:		
black and white	68.0	2.0
cinnamon twist	9.0	0
double chocolate chunk	58.0	3.0
graham, dark or milk chocolate	17.0	<1.0
Madeline	11.0	0
oatmeal raisin	65.0	3.0
shortbread	12.0	0
white chocolate macadamia	54.0	2.0
croissants:		
almond filled	39.0	2.0
butter, apricot glaze	37.0	1.0
chocolate filled	43.0	2.0
raspberry cream cheese filled	34.0	1.0
muffins:		
blueberry	49.0	1.0
chocolate cream cheese	53.0	1.0
cranberry orange	53.0	2.0
morning sunrise	54.0	2.0
scones:		
apricot currant	67.0	3.0

Food and Measure	carb. (gms)	fiber (gms)
blueberry	68.0	3.0
butterscotch pecan	64.0	2.0
cinnamon chip, iced	71.0	2.0
maple oat, iced	69.0	2.0
raspberry	65.0	2.0
sweet rolls:		
caramel pecan sticky	75.0	7.0
cinnamon	80.0	3.0
cinnamon twist	37.0	1.0
danish, mocha swirl:		
apple	44.0	2.0
cheese	44.0	1.0
raspberry	45.0	1.0
Steak sauce, 1 tbsp.:		
(*A.1.*)	3.0	0
(*A.1.* Bold and Spicy with *Tabasco*)	5.0	0
(*A.1.* Carb Well)	1.0	0
(*Crosse & Blackwell*)	7.0	0
(*Heinz 57*)	4.0	0
(*HP*)	3.0	0
(*Kikkoman*)	5.0	0
(*Lawry's*)	3.0	0
(*Newman's Own*)	4.0	0
(*Peter Luger*)	7.0	0
(*Pickapeppa*)	4.0	0
(*San-J* Japanese)	2.0	0
(*Watkins*)	4.0	0
and burger (*TryMe* Bullfighter)	4.0	0
garlic, roasted or teriyaki (*A.1.*)	5.0	0
Steak sauce, cooking, see "Grilling sauce"		
Steak seasoning:		
(*D.L. Jardine's*), 1 tbsp.	4.0	<1.0
broiled (*McCormick*), ¼ tsp.	0	0
Stir-fry sauce (see also "Marinade," and specific listings), 1 tbsp., except as noted:		
(*House of Tsang Classic/Bangkok Padang*)	4.0	0
(*House of Tsang Saigon Sizzle*)	7.0	0
(*Kikkoman*)	4.0	0

Food and Measure	carb. (gms)	fiber (gms)
(*Litehouse*), 2 tbsp.	10.0	0
citrus (*House of Tsang* Imperial)	5.0	0
garlic, and rib sauce (*Mikee*)	10.0	0
oyster flavored (*House of Tsang*)	7.0	0
teriyaki (*House of Tsang Korean*)	5.0	0
sweet and sour (*House of Tsang*)	38.0	0
Szechuan, spicy (*House of Tsang*)	4.0	0
Stir-fry seasoning mix (*Produce Partners*), 2 tsp.	2.0	0
Stomach, pork, without added ingredients	0	0
Strawberry, fresh:		
(*Del Monte*), 8 medium, 5.2 oz.	12.0	4.0
(*Dole*), 8 medium	12.0	4.0
halves, ½ cup	5.3	1.8
pureed, ½ cup	8.1	2.7
Strawberry, canned, in heavy syrup, ½ cup	29.9	2.2
Strawberry, dried (*Frieda's*), ½ cup, 1.4 oz.	34.0	3.0
Strawberry, frozen:		
whole:		
(*Cascadian Farm*), 1 cup	13.0	3.0
(*C&W*), ⅔ cup	12.0	2.0
(*Tree of Life*), ¾ cup	13.0	2.0
unsweetened, ½ cup	10.1	2.3
Strawberry drink, 8 fl. oz., except as noted:		
(*Capri Sun*), 6.75 fl. oz.	25.0	0
(*Hi-C Blast*)	32.0	0
(*Yoo-hoo*)	29.0	0
sparkling (*R.W. Knudsen*)	28.0	0
Strawberry drink blend, 8 fl. oz., except as noted:		
all varieties (*Langers*)	30.0	0
banana:		
(*Snapple-a-Day*), 11.5 fl. oz.	43.0	5.0
(*V8 Splash*)	27.0	0
(*V8 Splash* Smoothies)	30.0	1.0
daiquiri (*SoBe Lizard Lava*)	32.0	0
kiwi:		
(*Capri Sun*), 6.75 fl. oz.	26.0	0
(*Hi-C Blast*)	31.0	0
(*V8 Splash*)	27.0	0

Food and Measure	carb. (gms)	fiber (gms)
passion fruit (*Minute Maid*)	31.0	0
passion fruit (*Minute Maid*), 12-fl.-oz. can	46.0	0
raspberry (*Minute Maid*)	33.0	0
Strawberry glaze:		
(*Great Expectations*), ⅓ cup	38.0	0
(*Litehouse*), 3 tbsp.	26.0	0
(*Litehouse* Sugar Free), 3 tbsp.	8.0	0
Strawberry juice (*Ceres*), 8 fl. oz.	28.0	1.0
Strawberry milk, see "Milk, flavored"		
Strawberry milk mix (*Nesquik*), 2 tbsp.	21.0	0
Strawberry syrup:		
(*Hershey's*), 2 tbsp.	26.0	0
(*Nesquik*), 2 tbsp.	27.0	0
(*Smucker's*), ¼ cup	52.0	0
(*Smucker's Sundae Syrup*), 2 tbsp.	26.0	0
Strawberry topping (*Smucker's*), 2 tbsp.	24.0	0
Strawberry-banana juice, 8 fl. oz.:		
(*Bolthouse Farms*)	29.0	<1.0
(*Juicy Juice*)	30.0	0
String beans, see "Green beans"		
Stuffing, ¾ cup:		
corn bread (*Pepperidge Farm*)	33.0	2.0
cube (*Pepperidge Farm* Country Style)	27.0	2.0
herb (*Pepperidge Farm*)	33.0	3.0
sage and onion (*Pepperidge Farm*)	26.0	3.0
Stuffing, frozen, corn bread (*Glory* Savory Accents Dressing), ½ cup	33.0	1.0
Stuffing mix, dry:		
chicken:		
(*Pepperidge Farm* One-Step), ½ cup	12.0	<1.0
(*Stove Top*), ⅙ 6-oz. pkg.	20.0	1.0
(*Stove Top*), ⅛ of 8-oz. cont.	19.0	1.0
(*Stove Top* Lower Sodium), ⅙ of 6-oz. pkg.	21.0	1.0
cornbread:		
(*Mrs. Cubbison's*), ¾ cup	24.0	2.0
(*Pepperidge Farm* One-Step), ½ cup	26.0	2.0
(*Stove Top*), ⅙ of 6-oz. pkg.	21.0	1.0
(*Stove Top*), ⅛ of 8-oz. cont.	19.0	1.0

Food and Measure	carb. (gms)	fiber (gms)
herb (*Stove Top* Homestyle), ⅛ of 8-oz. cont.	19.0	1.0
herb, garden (*Pepperidge Farm* One-Step), ½ cup	14.0	<1.0
herb seasoned cube (*Mrs. Cubbison's*), ¾ cup	24.0	1.0
pork (*Stove Top*), ⅙ of 6-oz. pkg.	20.0	1.0
seasoned (*Mrs. Cubbison's* Dressing), ¾ cup	24.0	1.0
turkey (*Pepperidge Farm* One-Step), ½ cup	14.0	<1.0
turkey (*Stove Top*), ⅙ of 6-oz. pkg.	20.0	1.0
Sturgeon, fresh or smoked, without added		
ingredients	0	0
Subway, 1 serving:		
breakfast, French toast, with syrup	57.0	2.0
breakfast, omelet:		
bacon, cheese, or ham	2.0	0
steak	3.0	1.0
vegetable or Western	4.0	1.0
breakfast sandwich:		
on deli round:		
bacon and egg or cheese and egg	34.0	3.0
ham and egg or steak and egg	35.0	3.0
vegetable and egg or Western and egg	36.0	3.0
on 6″ white/wheat:		
bacon and egg or cheese and egg	42.0	3.0
ham and egg or steak and egg	43.0	3.0
vegetable and egg or Western and egg	44.0	4.0
6″ sub, cold:		
cold cut combo	47.0	4.0
Subway seafood	51.0	5.0
tuna, classic	45.0	4.0
6″ sub, toasted:		
cheese steak	47.0	5.0
cheese steak, chipotle Southwest	48.0	6.0
chicken and bacon ranch	47.0	5.0
Italian BMT	47.0	4.0
meatball marinara	63.0	7.0
turkey, ham, and bacon melt	48.0	4.0
6″ sub, 6 grams fat or less:		
chicken breast, roasted	47.0	4.0
chicken teriyaki	59.0	4.0

Food and Measure	carb. (gms)	fiber (gms)
ham, honey mustard	53.0	4.0
roast beef	45.0	4.0
Subway Club	47.0	4.0
turkey breast	46.0	4.0
turkey breast and ham	47.0	4.0
Veggie Delite	44.0	4.0
6'' double meat (DM):		
cheese steak	50.0	6.0
cheese steak, chipotle Southwest	51.0	7.0
chicken, roasted	50.0	4.0
chicken teriyaki	68.0	4.0
cold cut combo	49.0	4.0
ham	57.0	4.0
Italian BMT	49.0	4.0
meatball marinara	82.0	10.0
roast beef	46.0	4.0
Subway Club	50.0	4.0
Subway seafood	58.0	5.0
tuna, classic	45.0	4.0
turkey breast	48.0	4.0
turkey breast and ham	50.0	4.0
turkey breast, ham, and bacon melt	51.0	4.0
deli-style sandwich, ham or turkey breast	36.0	3.0
deli-style sandwich, roast beef or classic tuna	35.0	3.0
wraps:		
chicken and bacon ranch, with cheese	18.0	9.0
tuna, with cheese	16.0	9.0
turkey breast	18.0	9.0
turkey and bacon melt, with cheese	20.0	9.0
condiments/extras:		
bacon, 2 slices	0	0
chipotle sauce	1.0	0
honey mustard sauce	7.0	0
mayo, 1 tbsp.	0	0
mayo, light, 1 tbsp.	1.0	0
mustard, 2 tsp.	1.0	0
olive oil blend, 1 tsp.	0	0
onion sauce, sweet	9.0	0

Food and Measure	carb. (gms)	fiber (gms)
ranch dressing	0	0
red wine vinaigrette	6.0	0
salad, without dressing:		
chicken, grilled, baby spinach	11.0	4.0
Subway Club	15.0	4.0
tuna, with cheese, or *Veggie Delite*	12.0	4.0
salad dressing, 2 oz.:		
Greek vinaigrette	3.0	0
honey mustard	1.0	0
Italian, fat free	7.0	0
ranch	1.0	.5
soup, 1 cup:		
broccoli, cream of	15.0	2.0
broccoli cheese	16.0	2.0
brown and wild rice, with chicken	17.0	2.0
cheese, with ham and bacon	17.0	1.0
chicken dumpling	16.0	1.0
chicken noodle or minestrone	7.0	1.0
chicken rice, Spanish	13.0	1.0
chili con carne	23.0	8.0
clam chowder	16.0	1.0
potato, with bacon	21.0	2.0
tomato vegetable rotini	20.0	2.0
vegetable beef	15.0	3.0
Fruzie Express, small:		
berry lishus	28.0	1.0
berry lishus, banana	35.0	2.0
pineapple delight	33.0	1.0
peach pizzazz	26.0	0
pineapple delight, banana	40.0	2.0
sunrise refresher	29.0	1.0
cookies/dessert:		
apple pie	37.0	1.0
chocolate chip or chocolate chunk	30.0	1.0
double chocolate chip	30.0	1.0
fruit roll, 1 piece	12.0	0
M&M's	30.0	1.0

Food and Measure	carb. (gms)	fiber (gms)
oatmeal raisin	26.0	2.0
peanut butter	26.0	1.0
sugar	28.0	0
white chip macadamia	37.0	1.0
Succotash, canned:		
(*Glory*), ½ cup	17.0	3.0
cream style, ½ cup	23.4	4.0
Succotash, frozen, boiled, drained, ½ cup	17.0	4.6
Sucker, white, without added ingredients	0	0
Sugar, beet or cane:		
brown:		
(*Hain* Organic), 1 tsp.	4.0	0
1 oz.	27.6	0
1 cup, not packed	141.0	0
1 cup, packed	214.0	0
granulated:		
(*Hain* Organic), 1 tsp.	3.0	0
1 oz.	28.3	0
1 cup	99.8	0
1 tbsp.	12.0	0
1 tsp.	4.0	0
powdered/confectioner's:		
(*Hain* Organic), ¼ cup	37.0	0
1 cup, sifted	99.5	0
1 tbsp., unsifted	8.0	0
Sugar, date (*Shiloh Farms*), 1½ tsp.	3.0	0
Sugar, maple, 1 oz.	25.5	0
Sugar, substitute (see also "Fructose"):		
(*Equal*), 1 pkt.	<1.0	0
(*NutraSweet*), 1 tsp.	<1.0	0
(*Splenda*), 1 pkt.	<1.0	0
(*Sugar Twin*), 1 pkt.	<1.0	0
(*Sweet'n Low*), 1 pkt.	1.0	0
white or brown (*Sugar Twin*), 1 tsp.	0	0
Sugar, turbinado:		
(*Hain*), 1 tsp.	4.0	0
(*Tree of Life*), 1 tsp.	4.0	0

Food and Measure	carb. (gms)	fiber (gms)
Sugar apple:		
1 medium, 9.9 oz.	36.6	6.8
½ cup	29.6	5.5
Sugar snap peas, see "Peas, edible-podded"		
Sugarcane juice drink (*Foco*), 11.8-fl.-oz. can	37.0	0
Summer sausage, 2 oz.:		
(*Johnsonville* Old World/Original/Beef)	1.0	0
(*Old Smokehouse*)	2.0	0
beef (*Hickory Farms Beef Stick* Original/Smoked)	1.0	0
garlic (*Johnsonville*)	1.0	0
Summer squash (see also specific listings), all varieties, 1 cup:		
raw, sliced	4.9	2.2
boiled, drained, sliced	7.8	2.5
Sun choke, see "Jerusalem artichoke"		
Sunburst squash, baby (*Frieda's*), ⅔ cup, 3 oz.	3.0	1.0
Sunfish, pumpkin seed, without added ingredients	0	0
Sunflower butter:		
(*Kettle Roaster Fresh* Unsalted), 1 oz.	5.0	0
1 tbsp.	4.4	.8
Sunflower seed, shelled:		
(*Arrowhead Mills*), ¼ cup	6.0	3.0
(*Frito Lay*), 3 tbsp., 1 oz.	5.0	2.0
(*Shiloh Farms*), ¼ cup	6.0	2.0
unsalted, 1 oz.:		
dry-roasted	6.8	3.2
oil-roasted	4.2	4.2
toasted	5.8	3.3
roasted, salted (*Planters*), 1 oz.	5.0	2.0
roasted, salted (*Planters*), ½ of 3-oz. pkg.	8.0	4.0
tamari (*New England Naturals*), ¼ cup, 1.2 oz.	7.0	5.0
Sunflower seed flour, partially defatted, 1 cup	28.7	4.2
Sunflower sprouts, (*Jonathan's*), 1 cup	2.0	1.0
Surimi, pollock, 4 oz.	7.8	0
Sushi, supermarket (*Southern Tsunami Sushi Bar*), rolls, except as noted:		
California, 9 pieces	54.0	3.0

Food and Measure	carb. (gms)	fiber (gms)
carrot and cucumber, 12 pieces	51.5	2.3
combo rolls:		
fullmoon, 6 pieces	50.1	2.2
marina, 6 pieces	73.4	.6
meteor special, 11 pieces	66.7	2.1
shoreline, 10 pieces	84.0	2.4
crab, ocean, 9 pieces	53.6	3.9
"crab" and cucumber, 12 pieces	51.6	1.6
cream cheese, 9 pieces	53.1	2.4
cucumber, 12 pieces	50.0	1.8
dragon, 9 pieces	62.9	7.3
eel, 9 pieces	55.5	2.2
eel and carrot, 12 pieces	51.6	2.1
inari, 4 pieces	46.0	1.0
orange, 9 pieces	65.0	3.9
rainbow, 9 pieces	92.0	4.0
salads:		
calamari, 4 oz.	20.2	0
edamame, plain, 4 oz.	12.5	4.8
edamame mixed, 4 oz.	4.5	.6
harusame, 2 oz.	13.2	0
seaweed, seabreeze, 2 oz.	11.3	0
salmon, grilled, 9 pieces	54.4	3.3
salmon, spicy, 9 pieces	52.4	2.4
shrimp, crunchy, 9 pieces	83.0	4.0
shrimp, spicy, 9 pieces	52.4	2.4
shrimp and avocado, 12 pieces	50.4	2.5
tempura, 9 pieces	92.6	4.4
tofu, 9 pieces	48.0	3.0
tsunami, 9 pieces	63.2	2.7
tuna, spicy, 9 pieces	45.0	3.0
tuna and cucumber, 12 pieces	49.4	1.7
vegetable combo, 9 pieces	45.0	1.0
Swamp cabbage:		
raw, 6-oz. shoot	.4	.3
boiled, drained, chopped, ½ cup	1.8	.9
Sweet dumpling squash (*Frieda's*), ¾ cup, 3 oz.	7.0	1.0

Food and Measure	carb. (gms)	fiber (gms)
Sweet peas, see "Peas, green"		
Sweet potato:		
raw, 5" × 2" potato	31.6	3.9
raw, cut (*Glory*), 4.9 oz.	36.0	4.0
baked in skin, 5" × 2" potato	27.7	3.4
baked in skin, mashed, ½ cup	24.3	3.0
boiled, without skin, 4 oz.	20.1	2.8
boiled, without skin, mashed, ½ cup	31.7	4.5
Sweet potato, canned, ½ cup, except as noted:		
candied:		
(*Glory*)	52.0	1.0
(*Royal Prince*)	50.0	2.0
(*S&W*)	46.0	4.0
cut (*Princella/Sugary Sam*), ⅔ cup	39.0	3.0
mashed (*Glory* Casserole)	43.0	2.0
mashed (*Princella/Sugary Sam*), ⅔ cup	28.0	3.0
in syrup:		
(*Sylvia's* Yams)	30.0	2.0
light syrup (*Glory*)	30.0	2.0
whole (*Royal Prince/Trappey's*), 3 pieces	48.0	4.0
with liquid	23.9	2.8
drained	24.9	2.9
orange pineapple (*Royal Prince*)	50.0	3.0
Sweet potato, frozen:		
baked, cubed, ½ cup	20.6	2.6
candied (*Green Giant*), ¾ cup	41.0	3.0
casserole (*Glory* Savory Accents), ½ cup	37.0	0
fries (*Ian's* Natural), 2.5 oz.	13.0	1.0
fries, straight cut (*McCain Premium Golden Crisp*), 3 oz.	22.0	2.0
Sweet potato chips, 1 oz.:		
regular or jalapeño (*Terra*)	18.0	1.0
Southern recipe (*Terra Frites*)	15.0	2.0
spiced (*Terra*)	16.0	3.0
Sweet potato leaf:		
raw, chopped, ½ cup	1.1	<1.0
steamed, ½ cup	2.3	.6
Sweet and sour drink mixer (*Angostura*), 2 fl. oz.	17.0	0

Food and Measure	carb. (gms)	fiber (gms)
Sweet and sour sauce, 2 tbsp., except as noted:		
(*Contadina*), 1 tbsp.	8.0	0
(*Kikkoman*)	9.0	0
(*Kraft*)	13.0	0
(*Port Arthur*)	13.0	0
(*Sagawa's* Sweet & Sour/Sassy)	11.0	0
(*San-J* Sweet & Tangy)	13.0	0
(*World Harbors* Sweet & Sour/Sweet & Tangy)	14.0	0
barbecue, see "Barbecue sauce"		
duck sauce:		
(*Ka•Me*)	15.0	0
(*La Choy*)	15.0	0
(*Mee Tu*)	19.0	1.0
(*Mikee*), 1 tbsp.	6.0	0
with ginger (*Ka•Me*)	13.0	0
Sweetbreads, see "Pancreas" and "Thymus"		
Swiss chard, fresh:		
raw (*Frieda's*), 1 cup, 3 oz.	3.0	1.0
raw, chopped, ½ cup	.7	.3
boiled, drained, chopped, ½ cup	3.6	1.8
Swiss chard, frozen (*C&W*), ½ cup	3.0	2.0
Swordfish, without added ingredients	0	0
Syrup, see specific syrup listings		
Szechuan sauce (see also "Stir-fry sauce"):		
(*Ka•Me*), 1 tbsp.	2.0	0
(*San-J*), 1 tsp.	1.0	0

T

Food and Measure	carb. (gms)	fiber (gms)
Tabouli salad:		
(*Cedar's*), 2 tbsp.	3.0	1.0
(*Joseph's*), 2 tbsp.	5.0	1.0
Tabouli salad mix:		
(*Fantastic*), 2 tbsp.	15.0	4.0
(*Near East*), 1 oz.	21.0	5.0
(*Near East*), ⅔ cup*	23.0	5.0
Taco, frozen, 5.5-oz. piece, except as noted:		
beef, mini (*El Monterey* Fiesta Minis), 4 pieces, 4 oz.	27.0	3.0
beef and cheese (*El Monterey* Soft Taco)	42.0	3.0
beef and cheese, spicy (*El Monterey* Soft Taco)	40.0	2.0
chicken and cheese, spicy (*El Monterey* Soft Taco)	44.0	4.0
Taco, breakfast, sausage, egg, and cheese (*El Monterey* Soft), 4.5-oz. piece	29.0	1.0
Taco entree kit, pkg.:		
(*Old El Paso* Dinner Kit), with chicken breast or lean beef, ⅙ pkg.*	19.0	1.0
(*Old El Paso* Hard & Soft Dinner Kit):		
hard, with lean beef, 2 pieces*	19.0	2.0
soft, with lean beef, 2 pieces*	32.0	1.0
(*Old El Paso* Soft Dinner Kit), with chicken breast or lean ground beef, ⅕ pkg.*	32.0	2.0
(*Taco Bell* Dinner), ⅙ pkg.	19.0	2.0
cheesy (*Taco Bell* Dinner Double Decker), ⅙ pkg.	29.0	2.0
cheesy, with shells, sauce (*Taco Bell* Dinner), ⅙ pkg.	20.0	1.0
Taco filling, vegetarian (*SoyTaco*), 1 oz.	3.0	2.0
Taco filling mix (*Fantastic*), ¼ cup	10.0	4.0

Taco Bell, 1 serving:
Big Bell Value Menu:

	carb. (gms)	fiber (gms)
burrito, bean especial	82.0	12.0
burrito, beef combo	52.0	5.0
burrito, beef and potato	65.0	4.0
burrito, chicken, spicy	50.0	4.0
caramel apple empanada	37.0	1.0
cheesy potatoes	27.0	2.0
taco, chicken, spicy	21.0	2.0
taco, *Double Decker*	39.0	5.0
taco, *Double Decker Supreme*	41.0	5.0
taco, soft, grande	44.0	2.0
burritos:		
bean	55.0	8.0
beef, fiesta	50.0	3.0
beef, grilled *Stuft*	79.0	7.0
beef, *Supreme*	52.0	5.0
chicken, fiesta	48.0	3.0
chicken, grilled *Stuft*	76.0	7.0
chicken *Supreme*	50.0	5.0
chili cheese	40.0	3.0
steak, fiesta	48.0	4.0
steak, grilled *Stuft*	76.0	8.0
steak, *Supreme*	50.0	6.0
7-layer	66.0	10.0
chalupas:		
beef, *Baja*	32.0	2.0
beef, nacho	33.0	1.0
beef, *Supreme*	31.0	1.0
chicken, *Baja*	30.0	2.0
chicken, nacho	31.0	1.0
chicken, *Supreme*	30.0	1.0
steak, *Baja*	30.0	2.0
steak, nacho	31.0	2.0
steak, *Supreme*	29.0	2.0
gorditas:		
beef, *Baja*	31.0	2.0
beef, nacho	32.0	2.0

Food and Measure	carb. (gms)	fiber (gms)
beef, *Supreme*	30.0	2.0
chicken, nacho	30.0	2.0
chicken or steak, *Baja*	29.0	2.0
chicken or steak, *Supreme*	28.0	2.0
steak, nacho	30.0	2.0
taco, regular	13.0	<1.0
taco, *Supreme*	14.0	1.0
taco, soft:		
beef	21.0	<1.0
beef, *Supreme*	23.0	1.0
chicken, Ranchero	21.0	2.0
steak, grilled	21.0	1.0
specialties:		
Border Bowl, chicken	65.0	12.0
Border Bowl, chicken, no dressing	60.0	12.0
Enchirito, beef	35.0	5.0
Enchirito, chicken or steak	33.0	5.0
express taco salad	58.0	10.0
express taco salad, no chips	32.0	8.0
Fiesta Taco Salad	80.0	12.0
Fiesta Taco Salad, without shell	42.0	10.0
Fiesta Taco Salad, without shell and strips	34.0	9.0
Mexican pizza	47.0	5.0
MexiMelt	23.0	2.0
quesadilla, cheese	39.0	3.0
quesadilla, chicken or steak	40.0	3.0
Southwest steak bowl	73.0	13.0
tostada	29.0	7.0
nachos and sides:		
cinnamon twists	28.0	0
Mexican rice	23.0	3.0
nachos	33.0	2.0
nachos *BellGrande*	80.0	11.0
nachos supreme	42.0	5.0
pintos 'n cheese	20.0	6.0
Taco John's, 1 serving:		
burritos:		
bean	53.0	10.0

Food and Measure	carb. (gms)	fiber (gms)
beef, grilled	49.0	9.0
beefy	41.0	8.0
chicken, grilled	47.0	8.0
chicken and potato	54.0	8.0
chicken and potato, crunchy	62.0	8.0
combination	47.0	9.0
meat and potato	55.0	9.0
super	49.0	10.0
quesadilla, cheese	39.0	6.0
quesadilla, chicken	41.0	7.0
tacos:		
chicken, softshell	19.0	4.0
crispy	13.0	3.0
softshell	21.0	4.0
Taco Bravo	39.0	8.0
taco burger	28.0	3.0
local favorites:		
Beefy Cheesy Taco Bravo	35.0	6.0
burrito:		
chicken fajita	39.0	7.0
chicken festiva	58.0	8.0
el grande	67.0	10.0
el grande, chicken	64.0	9.0
platter, smothered	102.0	16.0
ranch, beef	41.0	8.0
ranch, chicken	40.0	7.0
smothered	56.0	11.0
enchilada:		
chili	71.0	8.0
double	54.0	11.0
platter, beef	80.0	11.0
platter, chicken	73.0	9.0
cheese crisp	11.0	1.0
chilito	38.0	7.0
chili *Potato Olés*	59.0	7.0
chimi platter, beef and bean	88.0	9.0
Mexi Rolls	33.0	3.0
Mexi Rolls, without nacho cheese	29.0	3.0

Food and Measure	carb. (gms)	fiber (gms)
taco, el grande	32.0	4.0
tostada	14.0	3.0
tostada, bean	19.0	3.0
salad, without dressing:		
chicken festiva	60.0	11.0
chicken festiva, without tortilla	25.0	5.0
chicken festiva, crunchy	71.0	10.0
chicken festiva, crunchy, without tortilla	36.0	4.0
chicken taco	45.0	3.0
side salad	6.0	1.0
taco	46.0	4.0
nachos and sides:		
chicken, crunchy	24.0	0
chili, Texas style	26.0	4.0
Mexican rice	36.0	1.0
nachos	38.0	<1.0
nachos, super	73.0	5.0
nachos, super, chicken	62.0	3.0
Potato Olés:		
large	86.0	8.0
medium	67.0	6.0
small	48.0	5.0
super	82.0	10.0
with nacho cheese	52.0	5.0
refried beans	50.0	11.0
condiments, 2 oz., except as noted:		
barbecue sauce	15.0	0
chipotle cream sauce	4.0	0
dressing:		
Italian, creamy, or ranch	4.0	0
house	3.0	0
ranch, bacon	14.0	0
guacamole	6.0	0
jalapeños	3.0	1.0
pico de gallo	4.0	<1.0
sauce, hot or mild, 1 oz.	1.0	0
sauce, super hot, 1 oz.	2.0	<1.0
sour cream	2.0	0

Food and Measure	carb. (gms)	fiber (gms)
desserts:		
apple grande	36.0	0
choco taco	38.0	1.0
churro	31.0	1.0
Taco sauce, 1 tbsp., except as noted:		
(*Chi-Chi's* Fiesta Squeezable)	1.0	0
(*La Victoria* Salsa Brava)	0	0
(*Pace* Taco Topper)	2.0	0
(*Pace Mexican Creations*), 2 tbsp.	3.0	0
green (*Pace* Taco Topper)	1.0	0
green (*La Victoria*)	<1.0	0
hot, medium, or mild (*Old El Paso*)	1.0	0
medium (*Taco Bell*), 2 tbsp.	2.0	1.0
mild (*Taco Bell*), 2 tbsp.	3.0	1.0
hot (*La Victoria*)	1.0	0
Taco seasoning mix, 2 tsp., except as noted:		
(*Chi-Chi's* Fiesta), ⅕ pkg.	4.0	1.0
(*Ducks Unlimited*)	3.0	0
(*Lawry's*/Family Pack/Hot)	3.0	<1.0
(*McCormick* 30% Less Sodium)	3.0	0
(*Old El Paso/Old El Paso* 40% Less Sodium)	4.0	0
(*Taco Bell*)	3.0	1.0
(*Wick Fowler's*)	3.0	0
chicken (*Lawry's*)	5.0	<1.0
chicken (*McCormick*)	4.0	0
hot (*McCormick*)	3.0	0
mild (*McCormick*)	4.0	0
mild (*Old El Paso*)	4.0	0
Taco shell (see also "Tortilla" and "Tostada shell"):		
(*Old El Paso*), 3 pieces	20.0	1.0
(*Old El Paso* Super Stuffer), 2 pieces	23.0	2.0
(*Taco Bell*), 1.1-oz. piece	21.0	2.0
(*Zapata*), 2 pieces	14.0	1.0
corn, blue or yellow (*Garden of Eatin'*), 2 pieces	17.0	1.0
corn, white (*Old El Paso*), 3 pieces	20.0	1.0
mini (*Old El Paso* Fun Shells), 7 pieces	19.0	1.0
salad shell (*Old El Paso*), .8-oz. piece	14.0	<1.0

Food and Measure	carb. (gms)	fiber (gms)
Taco snack, frozen (*Michelina's* Zap'ems Rockin'),		
5.5-oz. pkg.	34.0	2.0
TacoTime, 1 serving:		
burritos:		
bean, crisp	53.0	9.0
bean, soft	58.0	13.0
beef, Big Juan	71.0	15.0
beef, bean and cheese	66.0	18.0
Casita Burrito	54.0	16.0
chicken, Big Juan	69.0	12.0
chicken, crisp	32.0	2.0
chicken and black bean	45.0	5.0
chicken BLT	38.0	5.0
meat, crisp	39.0	7.0
meat, soft	48.0	12.0
veggie	70.0	10.0
tacos:		
crisp	16.0	5.0
soft	23.0	5.0
soft, ½ lb.	46.0	12.0
soft, chicken, ½ lb.	41.0	7.0
soft, super	50.0	11.0
salads:		
chicken	27.0	3.0
chicken fiesta	35.0	4.0
taco, regular	30.0	7.0
tostada	48.0	13.0
nachos, etc.:		
cheddar melt	17.0	1.0
Mexi-rice	30.0	1.0
nachos	61.0	11.0
nachos deluxe	91.0	17.0
Refritos	44.0	13.0
taco cheeseburger	48.0	7.0
fries:		
cheddar, large	54.0	0
cheddar, medium	40.0	0
cheddar, small	27.0	0

Food and Measure	carb. (gms)	fiber (gms)
Mexi-Fries, large	54.0	0
Mexi-Fries, medium	40.0	0
Mexi-Fries, small	27.0	0
stuffed, large	88.0	6.0
stuffed, medium	50.0	5.0
stuffed, small	34.0	3.0
sauces and dressings:		
green sauce	2.0	<1.0
hot sauce	2.0	0
salsa Fresca	16.0	0
Thousand Island	3.0	0
dessert, *Crustos,* cinnamon	47.0	0
dessert, fruit empanada	37.0	0
Tahini, sesame:		
(*Alma*), ¼ cup	12.0	1.0
(*Arrowhead Mills*), 2 tbsp.	3.0	<1.0
(*Joyva*), 2 tbsp.	3.0	1.0
(*Peloponnese*), 1 tbsp.	2.0	1.0
(*Sesame King*), 2 tbsp.	5.0	3.0
(*Tree of Life*), 2 tbsp.	8.0	5.0
Tamale, canned, 2 pieces, except as noted:		
beef:		
(*Hormel*), 7.5-oz. can	22.0	3.0
(*Hormel* Jumbo)	21.0	3.0
regular or hot-spicy (*Hormel*)	15.0	2.0
chicken (*Hormel*)	15.0	1.0
Tamale, frozen, 1 piece:		
beef (*El Monterey Quick Classics*), 4.5 oz.	26.0	3.0
beef, shredded (*El Monterey Quick Classics*), 4 oz.	24.0	2.0
chicken (*El Monterey Quick Classics*), 4.5 oz.	28.0	2.0
pork (*Goya*)	31.0	2.0
Tamale pie, frozen, meatless (*Amy's* Mexican), 8 oz.	27.0	4.0
Tamari, see "Soy sauce"		
Tamarillo, red or gold (*Frieda's*), 2 pieces, 4.2 oz.	9.0	4.0
Tamarind:		
1 fruit, 3'' × 1''	1.3	.1
pulp, ½ cup	37.5	3.1

Food and Measure	carb. (gms)	fiber (gms)
Tamarind drink:		
(*Foco*), 11.8 fl. oz.	55.0	0
nectar (*Goya*), 12 fl. oz.	59.0	1.0
Tamarind sauce:		
(*Neera's* Asian), 2 tsp.	16.0	0
dipping (*Neera's*), 1 tsp.	3.0	0
Tamarindo (*Frieda's*), 1.1-oz. pod	19.0	2.0
Tandoori paste, see "Curry paste"		
Tangerine, fresh:		
(*Del Monte* Satsuma), 3.8-oz. fruit	15.0	3.0
(*Dole* Tangerine/Mandarin/Tangelo), 1 medium	15.0	3.0
(*Frieda's* Delite/Pixie or Satsuma Mandarin), 1 cup, 5 oz.	16.0	3.0
(*Frieda's* Page Mandarin), 1 cup, 5 oz.	12.0	3.0
(*Sunkist*), 3.8-oz. fruit	15.0	3.0
1 large 2½'' diam., 3.5 oz.	11.0	2.3
sections, 1 cup	21.8	4.5
Tangerine, can or jar (mandarin orange):		
in juice, with liquid, ½ cup	11.9	.9
in juice, lightly sweetened (*S&W* Natural Style), ½ cup	14.0	1.0
in light syrup:		
(*Del Monte*), ½ cup	19.0	<1.0
(*Del Monte*), 4-oz. can	17.0	<1.0
(*Del Monte Fruit Cup*), 4.5 oz.	17.0	<1.0
(*Del Monte Sunfresh*), ½ cup	19.0	<1.0
(*Dole*), ½ cup	19.0	1.0
(*Fanci Food*), ⅓ cup	19.0	1.0
(*S&W*), ½ cup	19.0	<1.0
with liquid, ½ cup	20.4	.9
in orange gelatin (*Del Monte* Lite), 4.5-oz. cup	14.0	0
Tangerine drink (*Ocean Spray* Mandarin Magic), 8 fl. oz.	31.0	0
Tangerine juice, 8 fl. oz.:		
(*Noble* Express)	30.0	0
fresh	25.0	.5
canned, sweetened	29.9	.5
frozen*	26.7	.5
Tannier, see "Malanga"		
Tapenade, see "Olive spread"		

Food and Measure	carb. (gms)	fiber (gms)
Tapioca:		
(*Minute*), 1½ tsp.	5.0	0
(*Reese* Pearls), 1 tbsp.	9.0	0
Tapioca pudding, see "Pudding" and "Pudding and pie filling mix"		
Tapioca flour (*Shiloh Farms*), 1½ tbsp.	11.0	tr.
Taquito, frozen, 3 pieces, 4.5 oz., except as noted:		
corn:		
beef (*El Monterey Quick Classics*), 5 pieces, 5 oz.	31.0	2.0
chicken (*El Monterey*)	31.0	2.0
chicken (*El Monterey Quick Classics*), 5 pieces, 5 oz. ..	37.0	1.0
steak, shredded (*El Monterey*)	31.0	2.0
flour:		
beef and cheese, shredded (*El Monterey*)	37.0	1.0
beef and cheese, shredded (*El Monterey* Fiesta Pack) ..	36.0	1.0
chicken breast, charbroiled (*El Monterey* Mexican Grill), 3 pieces, 5 oz.	36.0	1.0
chicken and cheese (*El Monterey*)	38.0	2.0
chicken and cheese (*El Monterey* Fiesta Pack)	36.0	1.0
chicken, cheese, zesty (*El Monterey* Fiesta Minis), 3 pieces, 4 oz.	41.0	1.0
flour, batter-dipped, 4 pieces, 5.6 oz.:		
beef and cheese, taco (*El Monterey Cruncheros*)	40.0	2.0
chicken, Southwest (*El Monterey Cruncheros*)	52.0	2.0
chicken and cheese (*El Monterey Cruncheros*)	41.0	2.0
Taquito, breakfast, egg, cheese, and bacon (*El Monterey*), 3 pieces, 4.5 oz.	38.0	1.0
Taramosalata (*Krinos*), 1 tbsp.	0	0
Taro, fresh:		
raw (*Frieda's* Taro Root), ⅔ cup, 3 oz.	22.0	3.0
raw, sliced, ½ cup	13.8	2.1
cooked, sliced, ½ cup	22.8	3.4
Tahitian, raw, sliced, ½ cup	4.3	n.a.
Tahitian, cooked, sliced, ½ cup	4.7	n.a.
Taro chips/crisps (see also "Vegetable chips/crisps"):		
(*Terra* Chips), 1 oz.	19.0	4.0
1 oz.	19.3	n.a.

Food and Measure	carb. (gms)	fiber (gms)
½ cup	8.1	n.a.
spiced (*Terra* Chips), 1 oz.	20.0	2.0
Taro leaf:		
raw, ½ cup	.9	.5
steamed, ½ cup	2.9	1.5
Taro shoots:		
raw, sliced, ½ cup	1.0	n.a.
cooked, sliced, ½ cup	2.2	n.a.
Tarragon, ground, 1 tsp.	.8	.1
Tart shell, see "Pastry shell"		
Tartar sauce, 2 tbsp.:		
(*Cains*)	2.0	0
(*Kraft*)	4.0	0
(*Kraft* Fat Free)	5.0	0
(*Litehouse*)	2.0	0
(*Old Bay*)	3.0	0
hot and spicy (*Kraft*)	4.0	0
lemon herb (*Kraft*)	1.0	0
TCBY, ½ cup, except as noted:		
ice cream, hand dip:		
butter pecan	17.0	<1.0
chocolate chocolate	21.0	0
chocolate chunk cookie dough	18.0	0
chocolate fudge	27.0	<1.0
lemon meringue pie	29.0	0
mint chocolate	23.0	<1.0
oatmeal raisin	25.0	0
pralines and cream	22.0	0
strawberry, very berry	19.0	0
vanilla bean	17.0	0
white chunk macadamia	23.0	0
Fruithead Smoothie, with yogurt, 20 oz.:		
Berry Slim or Healthy Balance	95.0	2.0
Holy-Cal	114.0	3.0
A Lotta-Colada	99.0	3.0
Peachy Lean	116.0	<1.0
Raspberry DeLite	85.0	4.0
Raspberry Revitalizer	84.0	3.0

Food and Measure	carb. (gms)	fiber (gms)
Tropical Replenisher	87.0	1.0
Workout Whey	112.0	1.0
Fruithead Smoothie, without yogurt, 20 oz.:		
Berry Slim or Healthy Balance	75.0	2.0
Holy-Cal	94.0	3.0
A Lotta-Colada	69.0	3.0
Peachy Lean	96.0	<1.0
Raspberry DeLite	59.0	3.0
Raspberry Revitalizer	79.0	6.0
Tropical Replenisher	61.0	2.0
Workout Whey	92.0	1.0
sorbet, all flavors	24.0	0
yogurt, soft serve, all flavors, nonfat/96% fat free	23.0	0
yogurt, soft serve, all flavors, nonfat/no sugar	20.0	0
Tea (see also "Tea, iced"), plain, regular or instant, all varieties, 1 bag or 1 tsp.	0	0
Tea, iced, 8 fl. oz., except as noted:		
(*Hood*)	25.0	0
(*SoBe Dragon*)	30.0	0
(*SoBe Zen Tea 3G*)	26.0	0
(*Turkey Hill*)	22.0	0
(*Turkey Hill* Decaf)	20.0	0
all fruit varieties (*Ocean Spray*)	24.0	0
black tea:		
(*AriZona* Botanical)	18.0	0
(*AriZona* Sweet)	23.0	0
with ginseng and herbs (*SoBe*)	27.0	0
with milk (*Thai Kitchen*), 11.5-oz. can	24.0	0
cherry (*Snapple* Very Cherry)	25.0	0
ginseng (*AriZona*)	18.0	0
green tea:		
(*AriZona* Botanical)	16.0	0
(*AriZona* Sweet)	18.0	0
(*Turkey Hill*)	17.0	0
with echinacea and herbs (*SoBe*)	24.0	0
lime (*Snapple*)	25.0	0
herbal:		
(*AriZona* Rx Energy)	31.0	0

Food and Measure	carb. (gms)	fiber (gms)
(*AriZona* Rx Health)	19.0	0
(*AriZona* Rx Memory)	20.0	0
(*AriZona* Rx Stress)	16.0	0
kiwi (*Snapple* Teawi)	26.0	0
lemon:		
(*AriZona*)	25.0	0
(*Nantucket Nectars* Squeezed)	23.0	0
(*Nestea*)	22.0	0
(*Newman's Own* Lemon-Aided)	27.0	0
(*Snapple*)	25.0	0
(*Turkey Hill*)	24.0	0
lemonade:		
(*Minute Maid*)	29.0	0
(*Nantucket Nectars* Squeezed Half and Half)	26.0	0
(*Snapple*)	28.0	0
frozen* (*Minute Maid*)	28.0	0
lime (*Turkey Hill*)	25.0	0
mint (*Snapple*)	27.0	0
mint (*Turkey Hill*)	21.0	0
oolong:		
(*Turkey Hill*)	25.0	0
blueberry (*Turkey Hill*)	24.0	0
with ginseng and herbs (*SoBe*)	25.0	0
orange (*Turkey Hill*)	25.0	0
orange, mandarin (*AriZona*)	19.0	0
peach:		
(*AriZona*)	18.0	0
(*Snapple*)	26.0	0
(*Turkey Hill*)	28.0	0
plum, Asian (*AriZona*)	18.0	0
raspberry:		
(*AriZona*)	25.0	0
(*Snapple*)	26.0	0
(*Turkey Hill*)	28.0	0
red tea (*AriZona* Botanical)	16.0	0
Tea, iced, mix, chai latte (*General Foods International Coffee*), 2 tbsp.	20.0	0
Teff, grain (*Shiloh Farms*), ¼ cup	32.0	6.0

Food and Measure	carb. (gms)	fiber (gms)
Teff flour:		
(*Arrowhead Mills*), 2 oz.	41.0	7.7
(*Shiloh Farms*), ¼ cup	32.0	6.0
Teff seeds (*Arrowhead Mills*), 2 oz.	41.0	7.7
Tekka (*Eden*), 1 tsp.	.5	0
Tempeh:		
(*White Wave* Original), ⅓ block	12.0	8.0
five grain (*White Wave*), ⅓ block	17.0	8.0
sea veggie (*White Wave*), ⅓ block	14.0	12.0
soy rice (*White Wave*), ⅓ block	17.0	5.0
1 oz.	2.7	n.a.
½ cup	7.8	n.a.
Temptation melon (*Frieda's*), ⅒ melon, 4.7 oz.	14.0	1.0
Tempura batter mix, see "Batter and breading mix"		
Tenderizer, see "Meat tenderizer"		
Teriyaki sauce (see also "Marinade"):		
(*Annie Chun's*), 1 tbsp.	5.0	0
(*Sagawa's*), 1 tbsp.	6.0	0
(*San-J*), 1 tbsp.	3.0	0
baste/glaze (*Kikkoman*), 2 tbsp.	11.0	0
baste/glaze, with honey, pineapple (*Kikkoman*), 2 tbsp.	18.0	0
Texas toast, see "Bread, frozen"		
Tex-Mex seasoning (*McCormick 1 Step*), 2 tsp.	3.0	0
Thai entree, pkg., see "Noodle entree, pkg."		
Thai sauce (see also "Peanut sauce" and specific listings):		
(*Neera's*), 1 tsp.	8.0	0
(*World Harbors*), 2 tbsp.	8.0	0
barbecue, spicy (*Thai Kitchen*), 1 tbsp.	<1.0	0
chili:		
(*Kikkoman*), 2 tbsp.	15.0	1.0
sweet red or garlic pepper (*A Taste of Thai*), 1 tsp.	2.0	0
spicy (*Thai Kitchen*), 1 tbsp.	4.0	0
sweet red (*Thai Kitchen*), 1 tbsp.	8.0	0
chili paste, roasted red (*Thai Kitchen*), 1 tbsp.	2.0	0
fish (*A Taste of Thai* Seasoning), 1 tbsp.	1.0	0
fish (*Thai Kitchen*), 1 tbsp.	<1.0	0
pad Thai (*A Taste of Thai*), 2 tbsp.	20.0	1.0
pad Thai (*Thai Kitchen*), 2 tbsp.	22.0	0

Food and Measure	carb. (gms)	fiber (gms)
Thai snack nuggets, frozen (*Health is Wealth Munchees*), 3 oz.	27.0	3.0
Thyme, ground, 1 tsp.	.9	3
Thymus, beef or veal, without added ingredients	0	0
Tilapia, without added ingredients	0	0
Tilapia entree, frozen, stuffed with sun-dried, tomato, shrimp, and lobster (*Oven Poppers*), ½ of 10-oz. pkg.	8.0	0
Tilefish, without added ingredients	0	0
T.J. Cinnamons, 1 serving:		
Cinnachips, 10-oz. bag	157.0	3.0
cinnamon twist	33.0	10.0
The Original Gourmet Cinnamon Roll, without icing	81.0	0
The Original Gourmet Cinnamon Roll, with cream cheese icing	103.0	0
pecan sticky roll	97.0	0
mocha chill, without whipped cream, 12 oz.	48.0	10.0
mocha chill, with whipped cream, 12 oz.	49.0	10.0
mocha chill, with whipped cream, 18 oz.	73.0	15.0
mocha chill, without whipped cream, 18 oz.	72.0	15.0
Tiramisu, see "Cake, frozen"		
Toaster pastry and muffin (see also "Breakfast pocket/sandwich"), 1 piece:		
apple:		
(*Amy's* Toaster Pops)	26.0	<1.0
(*Toaster Strudel*)	26.0	0
iced (*Hot Pockets*)	39.0	2.0
apple cinnamon (*Pop•Tarts*)	37.0	<1.0
berry, mixed (*Pop•Tarts* Wild!Berry)	39.0	<1.0
blueberry:		
(*Pop•Tarts/Pop•Tarts* Frosted)	37.0	1.0
(*Toaster Strudel*)	26.0	0
muffin (*Organic Toaster Classics*)	27.0	<1.0
yogurt (*Pop•Tarts Yogurt Blasts*)	37.0	<1.0
brown sugar cinnamon:		
(*Pop•Tarts*)	35.0	1.0
(*Toaster Strudel*)	28.0	<1.0
frosted (*Pop•Tarts*)	34.0	1.0
frosted (*Pop•Tarts* Low Fat)	39.0	1.0

Food and Measure	carb. (gms)	fiber (gms)
carrot spice muffin (*Organic Toaster Classics*)	29.0	<1.0
cherry (*Toaster Strudel*)	26.0	<1.0
cherry, frosted (*Pop•Tarts*)	38.0	1.0
chocolate chip (*Pop•Tarts*)	35.0	<1.0
chocolate chip, cookie dough (*Pop•Tarts*)	35.0	<1.0
chocolate fudge:		
(*Toaster Strudel*)	25.0	0
frosted (*Pop•Tarts* Low Fat)	39.0	2.0
or vanilla crème, frosted (*Pop•Tarts*)	37.0	1.0
corn (*Awrey's* Toastums)	22.0	0
cranberry corn muffin (*Organic Toaster Classics*)	26.0	1.0
cream cheese:		
(*Toaster Strudel* Danish Style)	23.0	0
raspberry or strawberry (*Toaster Strudel*)	24.0	0
strawberry (*Amy's* Toaster Pops)	24.0	<1.0
strawberry, iced (*Hot Pockets*)	34.0	2.0
grape, frosted, or hot fudge sundae (*Pop•Tarts*)	37.0	<1.0
maple oat muffin (*Organic Toaster Classics*)	29.0	2.0
raspberry (*Toaster Strudel*)	26.0	0
raspberry, frosted (*Pop•Tarts*)	37.0	<1.0
s'mores (*Pop•Tarts*)	36.0	1.0
s'mores (*Toaster Strudel*)	27.0	<1.0
strawberry:		
(*Pop•Tarts*)	37.0	1.0
(*Toaster Strudel*)	25.0	<1.0
iced (*Hot Pockets*)	39.0	2.0
frosted (*Pop•Tarts*)	38.0	1.0
frosted (*Pop•Tarts* Low Fat)	39.0	1.0
yogurt (*Pop•Tarts Yogurt Blasts*)	37.0	<1.0
wild berry (*Toaster Strudel*)	26.0	<1.0
Toffee, see "Candy"		
Toffee baking chips (*Hershey's Bake Shoppe Heath*),		
1 tbsp., .5 oz.	9.0	0
Toffee syrup (*Heath* Sundae), 2 tbsp.	24.0	0
Toffee topping (*Heath* Shell), 2 tbsp.	17.0	<1.0
Tofu (see also "Seitan" and "Tempeh"):		
(*White Wave* Reduced Fat), ⅕ of 1-lb. pkg.	1.0	2.0
fresh, ½ cup	2.3	1.5

Food and Measure	carb. (gms)	fiber (gms)
fresh, extra firm:		
(*Azumaya*), 2.8 oz.	2.0	1.0
(*Azumaya* Lite), 2.8 oz.	3.0	1.0
(*Frieda's*), 3 oz.	1.0	0
(*Frieda's* Organic), 3 oz.	2.0	0
(*White Wave*), 3 oz.	4.0	2.0
fresh, firm:		
(*Azumaya*), 2.8 oz.	2.0	<1.0
(*Frieda's*), 3 oz.	2.0	0
(*Frieda's* Organic), 3 oz.	1.0	0
(*Tree of Life*/Reduced Fat), 3.2 oz.	4.0	2.0
(*Tree of Life* Water Pack), 3.2 oz.	2.0	0
(*White Wave* Box), ⅕ of 1-lb. box	1.0	1.0
(*White Wave* Water Pack), ⅕ of 1-lb. pkg.	4.0	2.0
1 oz.	1.2	.7
½ cup	5.4	2.9
fresh, silken (*Azumaya*), 3.2 oz.	1.0	<1.0
fresh, silken (*Azumaya* Lite), 3.2 oz.	3.0	0
fresh, soft:		
(*Frieda's*), 3 oz.	1.0	0
(*Frieda's* Organic), 3 oz.	2.0	0
(*White Wave* Water Pack), ⅕ of 1-lb. pkg.	4.0	2.0
baked:		
(*Tree of Life*), 2.7 oz.	3.0	0
barbecue, hickory (*White Wave*), 2 oz., ¼ pkg.	2.0	2.0
garlic herb (*Frieda's*), 3 oz.	8.0	1.0
garlic herb Italian (*White Wave*), 2 oz., ¼ pkg.	2.0	2.0
ginger teriyaki (*Frieda's*), 3 oz.	13.0	1.0
lemon pepper (*White Wave* Zesty), 2 oz., ¼ pkg.	2.0	2.0
savory (*Tree of Life*), 2.7 oz.	3.0	0
sesame garlic (*Frieda's*), 3 oz.	10.0	1.0
teriyaki (*White Wave* Oriental), 2 oz., ¼ pkg.	2.0	2.0
Thai style (*White Wave*), 2 oz., ¼ pkg.	2.0	2.0
tomato basil (*White Wave* Roma), 2 oz., ¼ pkg.	2.0	2.0
dried (*Eden*), .4 oz.	0	2.0
salted and fermented (*fuyu*), 1 oz.	1.5	<1.0
seasoned, garlic onion (*Azumaya* Zesty), 3 oz.	3.0	1.0
seasoned, Oriental spice (*Azumaya*), 3 oz.	3.0	1.0

Food and Measure	carb. (gms)	fiber (gms)
smoked, all varieties (*Tree of Life*), 3 oz.	3.0	0
tenders, 4.5 oz.:		
black bean (*TofuTown Tofu Tenders* Havana)	15.0	2.0
sesame ginger teriyaki (*TofuTown Tofu Tenders*)	18.0	3.0
tahini (*Tofu Town Tofu Tenders* Mediterranean)	11.0	2.0
tamari (*Tofu Town Tofu Tenders*)	5.0	2.0
Tofu, ground, frozen, plain or savory garlic (*Tree of Life* Ready Ground), ⅓ of 10-oz. pkg.	2.0	0
Tofu breakfast, frozen, 9-oz. pkg.:		
Rancheros (*Amy's* Meal)	37.0	7.0
scramble (*Amy's* Meal)	19.0	4.0
Tofu dessert, almond or peach mango (*Frieda's*), 3 oz.	9.0	0
Tofu pudding, see "Pudding, nondairy"		
Tofu salad, plain or sun-dried tomato (*Tree of Life* Egg Less Salad), 3 oz.	2.0	<1.0
Tofu scrambler mix (*Fantastic*), 1 tbsp.	7.0	1.0
Tofu seasoning mix (*TofuMate*), ¼ pkg.:		
breakfast scramble	3.0	0
eggless salad	4.0	0
mandarin stir-fry	6.0	0
Mediterranean herb or Texas taco	3.0	0
Szechuan stir-fry	4.0	0
Tom Collins drink mixer (*Holland House*), 4 fl. oz.	49.0	0
Tom and Jerry drink batter (*Trader Vic's*), 1 tbsp.	23.0	0
Tomatillo, fresh:		
(*Frieda's*), ⅔ cup, 3 oz.	5.0	2.0
1 medium, 1⅝'' diam.	2.0	.6
chopped, ½ cup	3.8	1.3
Tomatillo, can or jar:		
whole:		
(*Embasa*), 3 pieces, 2.1 oz.	3.0	2.0
(*La Costeña*), 4 pieces, 4.3 oz.	4.0	4.0
(*La Victoria* Entero), 5 pieces, 4.5 oz.	7.0	5.0
crushed:		
(*Embasa*), ¼ cup	2.0	2.0
(*La Victoria*), 4.5 oz.	8.0	7.0
(*Las Palmas*), ½ cup	7.0	2.0

Food and Measure	carb. (gms)	fiber (gms)
Tomato, fresh, ripe:		
raw:		
(*Del Monte*), 1 medium, 5.2 oz.	7.0	1.0
(*Frieda's* Baby Roma/Teardrop), ⅔ cup, 3 oz.	4.0	1.0
2 ⅜'' tomato	5.7	1.4
chopped, 1 cup	8.4	2.0
boiled, 2 medium, 8.8 oz.	14.3	2.5
boiled, 1 cup	14.0	2.4
orange, 3.9-oz. tomato	3.5	1.0
orange, chopped, 1 cup	5.0	1.4
yellow, 7.8-oz. tomato	6.3	1.5
yellow, chopped, 1 cup	4.1	1.0
Tomato, canned (see also "Tomato paste," "Tomato puree" and "Tomato sauce"), ½ cup, except as noted:		
whole, peeled:		
(*Del Monte*)	6.0	2.0
(*Eden* Organic)	4.0	1.0
(*Hunt's/Hunt's* No Salt)	4.0	1.0
(*Muir Glen* 14.5 oz.)	5.0	1.0
(*Muir Glen* 28 oz.)	9.0	1.0
(*Progresso* Italian Style)	5.0	1.0
(*Red Gold/Red Pack*)	5.0	1.0
(*Red Pack* Plum)	5.0	2.0
(*S&W*)	7.0	2.0
(*Tuttorosso* Pear)	5.0	2.0
with basil (*Eden* Organic)	4.0	1.0
with basil (*Muir Glen*)	9.0	1.0
with basil (*Tuttorosso*)	5.0	1.0
with basil (*Tuttorosso* Pear)	5.0	2.0
fire-roasted (*Muir Glen*)	6.0	1.0
wedges (*Del Monte*)	9.0	2.0
chunky, in puree (*Red Pack*)	6.0	1.0
diced:		
(*Contadina* Recipe Ready)	6.0	1.0
(*Del Monte/Del Monte* Petite/No Salt)	6.0	2.0
(*Eden* Organic)	6.0	2.0
(*Hunt's* Original)	5.0	<1.0
(*Hunt's* Petite)	5.0	1.0

Food and Measure	carb. (gms)	fiber (gms)
(*Muir Glen* 14.5 oz.)	5.0	1.0
(*Muir Glen* 28 oz.)	4.0	1.0
(*Muir Glen* No Salt)	6.0	1.0
(*Red Gold* Chili Ready)	8.0	1.0
(*Red Gold/Red Pack*)	5.0	1.0
(*S&W Petite-Cut* Rich Juice/No Salt)	6.0	2.0
with balsamic vinegar or basil and oil (*Hunt's*)	8.0	1.0
with basil and garlic, garlic and onion, or Italian herbs (*Muir Glen*)	5.0	1.0
with basil, garlic, and oregano (*Del Monte*)	11.0	<1.0
with basil, garlic, and oregano (*Hunt's*)	6.0	1.0
with basil, garlic, and oregano (*Red Pack*)	7.0	1.0
chili style, chunky (*Del Monte*)	8.0	2.0
with chipotle, smoked (*Red Gold* Petite)	8.0	1.0
fire-roasted, regular or green chili (*Muir Glen*)	6.0	1.0
with garlic, roasted (*Contadina* Recipe Ready)	10.0	<1.0
with garlic, roasted (*Hunt's*)	6.0	1.0
with garlic, roasted (*S&W Ready-Cut*)	5.0	<1.0
with garlic, roasted, and onion (*Red Gold/Red Pack*)	5.0	1.0
with garlic and olive oil (*Del Monte* Petite)	10.0	1.0
with garlic and olive oil (*Red Gold/Red Pack* Petite)	9.0	1.0
with garlic and onion (*Del Monte*)	8.0	<1.0
with green chili (*Eden* Organic)	5.0	2.0
with green chili (*Red Gold* Petite)	4.0	1.0
with green chili (*Red Pack* Petite)	5.0	1.0
with green chili (*S&W Ready-Cut*)	6.0	1.0
with green chili, mild (*Del Monte*)	6.0	1.0
with green chili, mild (*Hunt's* Petite)	6.0	2.0
with green pepper, celery, and onions (*Hunt's*)	10.0	1.0
with green pepper and onion (*Del Monte*)	9.0	2.0
Italian (*Red Gold*)	7.0	1.0
Italian (*S&W Ready-Cut*)	4.0	1.0
Italian herbs (*Contadina* Recipe Ready)	10.0	<1.0
with jalapeño (*Del Monte* Petite Cut)	6.0	1.0
with jalapeño (*S&W Petite-Cut*)	7.0	2.0
marinara (*Contadina* Recipe Ready)	13.0	2.0
Mexican (*Red Gold* Fiesta Petite)	5.0	1.0
with mushrooms (*Hunt's* Petite)	6.0	<1.0

Food and Measure	carb. (gms)	fiber (gms)
with mushrooms and garlic (*Del Monte*)	10.0	1.0
with onion (*Red Gold* Chili Ready)	8.0	1.0
with onion, sweet (*Hunt's*)	10.0	<1.0
with onion, sweet (*Red Gold/Red Pack*)	10.0	1.0
with onion and green pepper (*S&W Ready-Cut*)	9.0	2.0
with onion and roasted garlic (*S&W Petite-Cut*)	10.0	1.0
pasta style, chunky (*Del Monte*)	11.0	2.0
primavera (*Contadina* Recipe Ready)	13.0	2.0
with red pepper, roasted (*Contadina* Recipe Ready)	13.0	2.0
in sauce (*Hunt's*)	7.0	1.0
crushed, ¼ cup:		
(*Contadina* Recipe Ready)	4.0	1.0
(*Hunt's*)	7.0	2.0
(*Progresso* Recipe Ready)	3.0	0
(*Eden* Organic)	3.0	1.0
(*Red Gold*)	5.0	1.0
(*Red Pack* All Purpose)	6.0	1.0
(*Red Pack* Puree)	4.0	1.0
with basil (*Muir Glen*)	5.0	1.0
with basil, garlic, oregano (*Red Pack*)	4.0	1.0
with basil, regular or in heavy puree (*Tuttorosso*)	4.0	1.0
fire-roasted (*Muir Glen*)	5.0	1.0
with garlic, roasted (*Contadina* Recipe Ready)	3.0	1.0
with green pepper and mushroom (*Red Gold*)	5.0	0
Italian (*S&W*)	4.0	1.0
Italian herbs (*Contadina* Recipe Ready)	3.0	<1.0
in puree (*S&W*)	4.0	1.0
ground, peeled (*Muir Glen*), ¼ cup	3.0	1.0
ground, peeled (*Red Pack*), ¼ cup	6.0	1.0
stewed:		
(*Contadina*)	9.0	1.0
(*Del Monte/Del Monte* No Salt)	9.0	2.0
(*Hunt's*)	8.0	1.0
(*Hunt's* No Salt)	9.0	1.0
(*Muir Glen*)	7.0	<1.0
(*Red Gold/Red Pack*)	8.0	1.0
(*S&W*)	7.0	2.0
(*S&W* No Salt)	9.0	2.0

Food and Measure	carb. (gms)	fiber (gms)
with basil and oregano (*Red Pack*)	8.0	1.0
Cajun (*Del Monte*)	9.0	2.0
Cajun, Italian, or Mexican (*S&W*)	7.0	2.0
Italian (*Contadina*)	8.0	1.0
Italian (*Del Monte*)	8.0	2.0
Italian (*Red Gold*)	8.0	1.0
Mexican (*Del Monte*)	9.0	2.0
Tomato, dried:		
1 oz.	15.8	3.5
1 piece, 32 pieces per cup	1.1	.3
½ cup	15.3	3.3
chopped or halves (*Frieda's*), ⅓ cup, 1.1 oz.	19.0	2.0
yellow, chopped or halves (*Frieda's*), ½ cup, 3 oz.	47.0	10.0
marinated, in oil:		
julienne or halves (*Frieda's*), 1 tbsp., .4 oz.	4.0	1.0
drained, ½ cup	12.8	3.2
Tomato, dried, blend, seasoned (*Frieda's* Tomato Toss),		
½ cup, 1.1 oz.	19.0	4.0
Tomato, freeze-dried:		
flakes (*AlpineAire*), ½ oz.	10.0	1.0
powder (*AlpineAire*), ⅔ oz.	13.0	0
Tomato, green, raw, 1 large, 6.4 oz.	9.3	2.0
Tomato, pickled:		
(*Ba-Tampte*), ½ piece, 1.5 oz.	1.0	0
halves (*Claussen*), 1 oz.	1.0	0
Tomato, sun-dried, see "Tomato, dried"		
Tomato juice, 8 fl. oz., except as noted:		
(*Campbell's*)	10.0	2.0
(*Campbell's*), 5.5-fl.-oz. can	6.0	1.0
(*Campbell's* Low Sodium)	10.0	1.0
(*Campbell's Healthy Request*)	12.0	1.0
(*Del Monte*)	10.0	1.0
(*Red Gold/Red Gold* No Salt)	10.0	2.0
(*R.W. Knudsen* Organic)	14.0	0
(*Sacramento*)	10.0	2.0
(*S&W*)	10.0	1.0
(*S&W*), 6 fl. oz.	7.0	<1.0
(*Tree of Life Pure Fruit*)	10.0	0

Food and Measure	carb. (gms)	fiber (gms)
Tomato paste, 2 tbsp.:		
(*Contadina*)	6.0	1.0
(*Del Monte*)	7.0	2.0
(*Hunt's/Hunt's* No Salt)	6.0	2.0
(*Muir Glen*)	6.0	1.0
(*Red Gold/Red Pack*)	6.0	1.0
(*S&W*)	6.0	1.0
with basil, garlic, and oregano (*Hunt's*)	6.0	2.0
with Italian seasoning (*Contadina*)	7.0	1.0
with pesto (*Contadina*)	5.0	<1.0
with roasted garlic (*Contadina*)	6.0	1.0
Tomato puree, ¼ cup:		
(*Contadina*)	4.0	<1.0
(*Hunt's*)	7.0	2.0
(*Muir Glen*)	5.0	1.0
(*Progresso*)	5.0	1.0
(*Red Gold/Red Pack*)	5.0	1.0
(*S&W*)	6.0	2.0
plain or with basil (*Tuttorosso*)	5.0	1.0
Tomato relish, 1 tbsp., except as noted:		
(*Heinz* Piccalilli)	4.0	0
hot or mild (*Mrs. Renfro's*)	3.0	0
medium, Indian (*Patak's*)	2.0	0
salsa (*Vlasic* Relish Mixers)	2.0	0
Tomato sauce, can or jar (see also "Pasta sauce," "Pizza sauce," and "Tomato, canned"), ¼ cup:		
(*Contadina*)	3.0	<1.0
(*Contadina* Extra Thick & Zesty)	3.0	1.0
(*Del Monte/Del Monte* No Salt)	4.0	<1.0
(*Goya*)	4.0	1.0
(*Hunt's*)	3.0	<1.0
(*Hunt's* No Salt)	6.0	2.0
(*Muir Glen* Chunky)	4.0	1.0
(*Muir Glen/Muir Glen* No Salt)	5.0	1.0
(*Red Gold/Red Pack/Red Pack* No Salt)	5.0	1.0
(*S&W* Homestyle)	4.0	1.0
(*Tuttorosso*)	5.0	1.0
with basil, garlic, and oregano (*Hunt's*)	3.0	<1.0

Food and Measure	carb. (gms)	fiber (gms)
for chili (*Hunt's* Family Favorites)	5.0	1.0
with garlic, roasted (*Hunt's*)	3.0	<1.0
with garlic and onion (*Contadina*)	4.0	<1.0
with herbs and cheese	6.2	1.3
Italian style (*Contadina*)	4.0	1.0
for lasagna (*Hunt's* Family Favorites)	6.0	1.0
for meat loaf (*Hunt's* Family Favorites)	7.0	2.0
with onion	6.1	1.1
with onion, green pepper, and celery	5.5	.9
with tomato tidbits, no salt added	4.3	.9
Tomato-beef drink (*Beefamato*), 8 fl. oz.	11.0	0
Tomato-chile cocktail:		
(*Snap-E-Tom*), 6 fl. oz.	8.0	1.0
(*Snap-E-Tom*), 8 fl. oz.	13.0	2.0
Tomato-clam drink:		
(*Clamato*), 8 fl. oz.	11.0	0
cocktail (*Chincoteague*), 5 fl. oz.	10.0	0
Tongue, braised:		
beef, 4 oz.	.4	0
lamb, pork, or veal (calves'), 4 oz.	0	0
Tongue lunch meat, beef, corned (*Hebrew National*), 2 oz.	0	0
Topping, dessert (see also specific listings), 2 tbsp.:		
(*Smucker's Magic Shell* Turtle Delight)	17.0	1.0
(*Smucker's Magic Shell Twix*)	18.0	1.0
(*Smucker's Milky Way*)	23.0	1.0
(*Smucker's Sundae Syrup 3 Musketeers*)	23.0	0
Tortellini (see also "Tortelloni"), frozen or refrigerated, 1 cup, except as noted:		
cheese:		
mixed or three (*Buitoni*)	50.0	3.0
three (*DiGiorno*), ⅓ of 9-oz. pkg.	41.0	2.0
whole wheat pasta (*Moneterey*)	48.0	5.0
herb chicken (*Buitoni*)	52.0	2.0
olive, Sicilian, lemon (*Cafferata* Olota)	43.0	1.0
spinach and cheese (*Buitoni*)	49.0	3.0
Tortellini, pkg. (see also "Tortelloni, pkg."), ⅔ cup:		
cheese, three (*Barilla*)	33.0	3.0
cheese and spinach (*Barilla*)	32.0	3.0

Food and Measure	carb. (gms)	fiber (gms)
Tortellini entree, frozen, pesto (*Amy's* Bowls), 9.5-oz. pkg.	58.0	3.0
Tortellini entree, pkg., cheese (*Hormel* Pasta Cup), 1 cont.	23.0	2.0
Tortelloni, frozen or refrigerated (see also "Tortellini"), 1 cup, except as noted:		
cheese and roasted garlic (*Buitoni*)	37.0	2.0
chicken and proscuitto (*Buitoni*)	47.0	2.0
mozzarella and herb (*Buitoni*)	46.0	2.0
mozzarella and pepperoni (*Buitoni*)	45.0	2.0
portobello and cheese (*Buitoni*)	46.0	3.0
sausage, sweet Italian (*Buitoni*)	48.0	3.0
spinach and cheese (*Monterey Carb Smart*), 3.5 oz.	21.0	6.0
tomato, sun-dried (*Buitoni*)	46.0	3.0
Tortelloni, pkg. (see also "Tortellini, pkg."), ¾ cup:		
cheese and garlic (*Barilla*)	31.0	4.0
porcini mushroom (*Barilla*)	32.0	5.0
ricotta and asparagus (*Barilla*)	32.0	4.0
ricotta and spinach (*Barilla*)	32.0	4.0
Tortilla (see also "Wraps"):		
corn (*Garden of Eatin'* Corntillas), 2 pieces, 1.7 oz.	29.0	5.0
corn, blue (*Garden of Eatin'*), 2 pieces, 1.7 oz.	22.0	2.0
flour:		
for burritos (*Old El Paso*), 1.4-oz. piece	21.0	0
for soft tacos (*Old El Paso*), 1.8-oz. piece	26.0	0
for soft tacos (*Taco Bell*), 2 pieces, 2.1 oz.	32.0	1.0
whole wheat (*Garden of Eatin'*), 1.7 oz.	22.0	2.0
Tortilla chips, see "Corn chips/crisps"		
Tostada shell (see also "Taco shell"):		
(*Old El Paso*), 3 pieces	20.0	1.0
(*Zapata*), 2 pieces	14.0	1.0
Triple sec (*Angostura*), 1 tsp.	0	0
Trail mix:		
(*California Trail Mix*), ¼ cup, 1 oz.	18.0	2.0
(*Cape Cod Cranberry Trail Mix*), ¼ cup, 1.1 oz.	17.0	2.0
(*Eden* All Mixed Up), 3 tbsp.	7.0	4.0
(*Eden* All Mixed Up Too), 3 tbsp.	10.0	4.0
(*GeniSoy* Happy Trails), 1 oz.	17.0	2.0

Food and Measure	carb. (gms)	fiber (gms)
(*GeniSoy* Mountain Medley), 1 oz.	16.0	2.0
(*GeniSoy* Tropical Paradise), 1 oz.	18.0	2.0
(*Happy Trails Mix*), ¼ cup, 1.2 oz.	16.0	3.0
(*Kettle* Camping Mix), 1 oz.	11.0	2.0
(*Kettle* Chocolate Lovers Mix), 1 oz.	16.0	2.0
(*Kettle* Deluxe Mix), 1 oz.	6.0	2.0
(*Kettle* Honey Cranberry Mix), 1 oz.	16.0	2.0
(*Kettle* Honey Roast Harvest Mix), 1 oz.	15.0	2.0
(*Kettle* Honey Roast Nuts & Fruit), 1 oz.	16.0	2.0
(*Kettle* Natural Chocolate Lovers Mix), 1 oz.	15.0	2.0
(*Kettle* Raw Hikers Mix), 1 oz.	15.0	2.0
(*Kettle* Southwest BBQ'Mix), 1 oz.	11.0	2.0
(*Kettle* Sporting Mix), 1 oz.	10.0	2.0
(*Kettle* Truffle Trail Mix), 1 oz.	17.0	2.0
(*Kettle* X-Treme Trail Mix), 1 oz.	9.0	2.0
(*New England Naturals* Freedom Trail Mix), 3 tbsp., .9 oz.	10.0	1.0
(*Organic Chocolate Trail Mix*), 3 tbsp., 1 oz.	14.0	2.0
(*Organic Harvest Trail Mix*), ¼ cup, 1.1 oz.	16.0	2.0
(*Planters* Fruit & Nut), 1 oz.	14.0	1.0
(*Planters* Cheese Nips/Mini Ritz*), 1 oz.	9.0	2.0
(*Save the Forest* Fruit & Nut), ¼ cup, 1.1 oz.	19.0	2.0
(*Shiloh Farms* Path Finders), ¼ cup	16.0	2.0
(*Tree of Life* Everyday), 1.1 oz.	14.0	2.0
(*Tree of Life* Organic), ¼ cup	14.0	2.0
(*Vanilla Passion Mix*), ¼ cup, 1.1 oz.	19.0	1.0
chocolate mix (*Save the Forest*), ¼ cup, 1.2 oz.	18.0	2.0
honey nut and caramel (*Planters*), 1.1 oz.	17.0	1.0
macadamia/fruit (*Mauna Loa* Tropical), 1 oz., ¼ cup	23.0	2.0
nut and chocolate (*Planters*), 1.2 oz.	16.0	2.0
nuts, seeds, and raisins (*Planters*), 1 oz.	11.0	3.0
nuts, spicy, and Cajun sticks (*Planters*), 1 oz.	13.0	2.0
soy and mango (*Kettle* Organic Sunrise), 1 oz.	13.0	3.0
tropical (*New England Naturals* Delight), 3 tbsp., 1 oz.	16.0	2.0
Tree fern, cooked, chopped, ½ cup	7.8	2.6
Triticale, whole grain, 1 cup	138.5	34.8
Triticale flour, whole grain, 1 cup	95.1	19.0
Tropical punch, see "Fruit punch"		

Food and Measure	carb. (gms)	fiber (gms)
Trout, fresh or smoked, without added ingredients	0	0
Trout pâté (*Ducktrap River/Ducktrap River* Lowfat), ¼ cup	1.0	0
Trout beans, canned (*Westbrae Natural* Organic Heirloom Beans), ½ cup	18.0	6.0
Tuna, fresh or canned, without added ingredients	0	0
Tuna, freeze-dried, albacore (*AlpineAire*), 1 oz.	0	0
Tuna, smoked (*Acme*), 2 oz.	2.0	0
"Tuna," vegetarian, frozen (*Worthington Tuno*), ½ cup ..	3.0	2.0
Tuna entree, freeze-dried, with noodles and cheese (*AlpineAire*), 1½ cups	41.0	3.0
Tuna entree, frozen, 1 pkg.:		
casserole (*Healthy Choice*), 9 oz.	30.0	5.0
noodle, casserole (*Stouffer's*), 10 oz.	35.0	2.0
noodle, gratin (*Smart Ones*), 9.5 oz.	38.0	3.0
Tuna entree, pkg., albacore steak, 4 oz.:		
ginger and soy (*Bumble Bee*)	3.0	0
lemon cracked pepper or mesquite grilled (*Bumble Bee*) ..	0	0
Tuna entree, mix, 1 cup*		
au gratin or broccoli, cheesy (*Tuna Helper*)	38.0	1.0
broccoli, creamy (*Tuna Helper*)	33.0	1.0
casserole (*Tuna Helper Oven Favorites* Classic)	37.0	1.0
cheddar, garden (*Tuna Helper*)	36.0	1.0
fettuccine Alfredo (*Tuna Helper*)	32.0	1.0
melt (*Tuna Helper*)	34.0	0
Parmesan, creamy (*Tuna Helper*)	32.0	0
pasta, cheesy (*Tuna Helper*)	31.0	1.0
pasta, creamy (*Tuna Helper*)	32.0	2.0
spirals, creamy (*Annie's* Organic Skillet Meal)	30.0	1.0
tetrazzini (*Tuna Helper*)	31.0	1.0
Tuna salad, refrigerated, ⅓ cup:		
(*Wampler*)	9.0	1.0
chunky, with pickle relish (*Wampler*)	8.0	1.0
Tuna salad kit, without crackers, 5 oz.:		
with mayo and onion (*Chicken of the Sea* Single!)	18.0	1.0
with salad dressing and sweet relish (*Chicken of the Sea* Single!)	19.0	1.0

Food and Measure	carb. (gms)	fiber (gms)
Tuna salad lunch kit, with crackers, 1 pkg.:		
(*Bumble Bee*):		
2.9-oz. can salad	6.0	1.0
6 crackers, .6 oz.	12.0	0
(*Bumble Bee* Fat Free):		
2.9-oz. can salad	10.0	0
6 crackers, .6 oz.	14.0	1.0
(*Bumble Bee*), with mayo:		
2.9-oz. can tuna	0	0
6 crackers, .6 oz.	12.0	0
mayo, 3.7-oz. pkt.	12.0	0
(*StarKist Lunch To-Go*), 4.5 oz.	27.0	1.5
Turban squash (*Frieda's*), ¾ cup, 3 oz.	7.0	1.0
Turbot, without added ingredients	0	0
Turkey, fresh or canned, without added ingredients	0	0
Turkey, freeze-dried, cooked, diced (*AlpineAire*), ½ oz.	0	0
Turkey, frozen or refrigerated, raw, 4 oz.:		
all cuts, without added ingredients	0	0
breast, marinated, rotisserie (*Perdue*)	2.0	0
ground, patties, barbecue flavor (*Wampler*)	3.0	0
ground, patties, seasoned (*Wampler*)	1.0	0
tenderloin, marinated:		
(*Shady Brook Farms* Homestyle/Rotisserie)	0	0
honey mustard (*Always Tender*)	4.0	0
teriyaki (*Always Tender*)	6.0	0
Turkey, frozen or refrigerated, cooked, 3 oz., except as noted:		
all cuts, without added ingredients	0	0
whole, Cajun style fried or smoked (*Shady Brook Farms*)	2.0	0
whole, oven roasted (*Shady Brook Farms*)	1.0	0
breast:		
in gravy (*Tyson*), 5 oz.	5.0	0
marinated, rotisserie (*Perdue*)	1.0	0
oven-roasted, bone-in (*Shady Brook Farms*)	1.0	0
roasted, carved (*Perdue Short Cuts*), ½ cup, 2.5 oz.	4.0	0
smoked, bone-in (*Shady Brook Farms*)	2.0	0
and gravy (*Hormel*), 5.7 oz.	4.0	4.0

Food and Measure	carb. (gms)	fiber (gms)
"Turkey," vegetarian:		
canned (*Worthington* Turkee Slices), 3 slices, 3.3 oz.	5.0	0
frozen:		
roast (*Quorn*), ⅕ piece	8.0	6.0
slices (*Yves*), 2.2 oz.	4.0	2.0
smoked (*Worthington*), 3 slices, 2 oz.	4.0	0
Turkey bacon (*Louis Rich*), .5 oz.	0	0
Turkey bologna (*Louis Rich/Oscar Mayer* 50% Less Fat),		
1 oz.	1.0	0
Turkey dinner, frozen, breast, 1 pkg.:		
grilled (*Healthy Choice* Dinners), 10 oz.	31.0	5.0
roasted:		
(*Healthy Choice* Dinners Traditional), 10.5 oz.	50.0	4.0
(*Lean Cuisine Dinnertime Selections*), 14 oz.	50.0	6.0
(*Stouffer's* Homestyle Dinners), 16 oz.	60.0	6.0
Turkey entree, can or pkg.:		
and dressing (*Hormel* Bowl), 10 oz.	33.0	3.0
stew (*Dinty Moore* Can), 1 cup	19.0	2.0
Turkey entree, freeze-dried, 1 serving:		
(*AlpineAire* Wild Tyme)	47.0	7.0
mashed potato and gravy (*AlpineAire*)	56.0	4.0
Romanoff (*AlpineAire*)	35.0	2.0
teriyaki (*AlpineAire*)	50.0	2.0
tetrazzini:		
(*Mountain House* Can), 1 cup	24.0	2.0
(*Mountain House* Double), ½ pouch	30.0	1.0
(*Mountain House* Single)	37.0	2.0
Turkey entree, frozen, 1 pkg., except as noted:		
glazed tenderloins (*Lean Cuisine* Cafe Classics), 9 oz. ...	40.0	4.0
medallions, with mushroom gravy		
(*Smart Ones* Higher Protein), 9 oz.	10.0	3.0
pie/pot pie:		
(*Boston Market*), 1 cup	34.0	2.0
(*Stouffer's*), 10 oz.	52.0	4.0
(*Stouffer's*), ½ of 16-oz. pkg.	42.0	3.0
(*Swanson*), 7 oz.	31.0	5.0
roasted (*Pepperidge Farm*), 1 cup	38.0	2.0

Food and Measure	carb. (gms)	fiber (gms)
roast/roasted:		
(*Lean Cuisine Skillet Sensations* 24 oz.), 6.9 oz.	23.0	3.0
breast (*Healthy Choice*), 8.5 oz.	25.0	4.0
breast (*Lean Cuisine* Cafe Classics), 9.75 oz.	51.0	3.0
breast (*Stouffer's* Homestyle), 9 5/8 oz.	30.0	2.0
with gravy and potato (*Michelina's* Authentico), 8 oz. . .	32.0	2.0
medallions (*Smart Ones*), 9 oz.	33.0	2.0
slow (*Smart Ones Bistro Selections*), 10 oz.	18.0	2.0
slow, breast, and mashed potato (*Healthy Choice*),		
8.5 oz.	19.0	4.0
and vegetables (*Lean Cuisine* Cafe Classics), 8 oz.	12.0	3.0
stuffed (*Smart Ones Bistro Selections*), 10 oz.	37.0	5.0
with stuffing and gravy:		
(*Glory* Savory Singles), 11 oz.	49.0	2.0
potato (*Stouffer's* Family Style Recipes Thanksgiving		
Tonight), 1/4 of 37-oz. pkg.	34.0	2.0
stuffing, baked (*Swanson*), 13.5 oz.	43.0	3.0
tetrazzini (*Stouffer's*), 10 oz.	33.0	2.0
Turkey fat, 2 tbsp.	0	0
Turkey frankfurter, see "Frankfurter"		
Turkey giblets:		
simmered, 4 oz.	2.4	0
simmered, diced, 1 cup	3.0	0
Turkey gravy, can or jar, 1/4 cup:		
(*Campbell's*)	3.0	0
(*Campbell's* Fat Free)	4.0	0
(*Pacific Foods*)	4.0	0
roast, slow (*Franco-American/Franco-American* Fat Free) .	4.0	0
roasted (*Boston Market*)	2.0	0
roasted (*Heinz* Home Style)	3.0	0
Turkey gravy mix, 1/4 cup*:		
(*Lawry's*)	4.0	0
(*McCormick*)	3.0	0
Turkey ham, 2 oz., except as noted:		
(*Healthy Deli*)	2.0	0
(*Louis Rich/Oscar Mayer* 50% Less Fat), 1 oz.	1.0	0
(*Shady Brook Farms*)	0	0

Food and Measure	carb. (gms)	fiber (gms)
Black Forest (*Shady Brook Farms*)	3.0	0
honey-roasted (*Sara Lee*)	2.0	0
smoked (*Louis Rich/Oscar Mayer* 50% Less Fat), 1 oz.	1.0	0
Turkey ham salad (*Wampler*), ⅓ cup	9.0	1.0
Turkey kielbasa, see "Kielbasa"		
Turkey lunch meat (see also "Turkey ham," etc.), breast, 2 oz., except as noted:		
(*Alpine Lace* Fat Free)	1.0	0
(*Boar's Head* Premium 47% Lower Sodium)	0	0
(*Dietz & Watson* Banquet Cater Style/Cater Ready/Gourmet/ Gourmet Lite/Golden Brown/Homestyle Santa Fe)	1.0	0
(*Dietz & Watson* Lite/No Salt)	0	0
(*Hansel 'n' Gretel*)	3.0	0
(*Hatfield Deli Choice* Premium)	1.0	0
(*Louis Rich* 98% Fat Free), 1 oz.	1.0	0
(*Wampler 5 Diamond/4 Diamond*)	0	0
(*Wampler 3 Diamond* Fat Free)	1.0	0
braised (*Dietz & Watson* Cater Ready/Homestyle)	1.0	0
bacon flavor (*Dietz & Watson* Bacon Lovers)	1.0	0
Black Forest:		
(*Boar's Head*)	0	0
(*Dietz & Watson*)	1.0	0
(*Wampler Deli Roast Collection*)	2.0	0
browned, with broth (*Healthy Choice*)	1.0	0
Buffalo style (*Dietz & Watson*)	1.0	0
Buffalo style (*Williams*)	<1.0	0
Cajun style (*Perdue Carving*)	1.0	0
Cajun style, oven-roasted, smoked (*Boar's Head*)	1.0	0
garlic herb (*Williams*)	2.0	0
honey:		
(*Healthy Deli*)	3.0	0
(*Perdue Carving*)	1.0	0
barbecue (*Dietz & Watson*)	1.0	0
or honey maple (*Dietz & Watson*)	3.0	0
maple (*Williams*)	1.0	0
honey-roasted:		
(*Hatfield Deli Choice*)	3.0	0
(*Louis Rich* Fat Free)	3.0	0

Food and Measure	carb. (gms)	fiber (gms)
(*Sara Lee*)	1.0	0
(*Sara Lee* Sliced), 2 slices, 1.6 oz.	1.0	0
(*Tyson* Box), 5 slices, 1.8 oz.	4.0	0
with cracked pepper (*Shady Brook Farms*)	4.0	0
Italian style (*Dietz & Watson*)	1.0	0
London broil (*Dietz & Watson*)	0	0
maple glazed (*Boar's Head Honey Coat*)	2.0	0
oil browned:		
(*Wampler 4 Diamond/3 Diamond*)	1.0	0
skin on (*Wampler 5 Diamond*)	3.0	0
skinless (*Wampler 5 Diamond/3 Diamond*)	1.0	0
oven-browned (*Wampler 4 Diamond*)	1.0	0
oven-roasted:		
(*Boar's Head Ovengold* Skin-on)	1.0	0
(*Boar's Head Ovengold* Skinless/Golden Catering)	0	0
(*Dietz & Watson* Oven Classic)	1.0	0
(*Healthy Choice* Hearty Slices), 1 oz.	1.0	0
(*Healthy Choice* Tub), 5 slices, 1.9 oz.	2.0	0
(*Healthy Choice Deli Thin*), 4 slices, 1.8 oz.	2.0	0
(*Hebrew National* Fat Free)	1.0	0
(*Louis Rich* Fat Free)	1.0	0
(*Louis Rich Carving Board* 98% Fat Free), 2.3 oz.	3.0	0
(*Louis Rich/Oscar Mayer* Fat Free/98% Fat Free), 1 oz.	1.0	0
(*Oscar Mayer* Deli Style Shaved), 1.8 oz.	2.0	0
(*Oscar Mayer* Deli Style Thin Sliced)	2.0	0
(*Perdue/Perdue Carving*)	1.0	0
(*Perdue HealthSense*)	3.0	0
(*Sara Lee*)	0	0
(*Sara Lee* Sliced), 2 slices, 1.6 oz.	2.0	0
(*Shady Brook Farms* Homestyle)	1.0	0
(*Tyson* Bag), 2 slices, 1.6 oz.	1.0	0
(*Tyson* Box), 5 slices, 1.8 oz.	1.0	0
(*Wampler 3 Diamond/2 Diamond/1 Diamond*)	1.0	0
oil braised (*Williams*)	0	0
rotisserie (*Sara Lee*)	1.0	0
skinless (*Healthy Choice* Golden)	1.0	0
white (*Oscar Mayer* 95% Fat Free), 1 oz.	1.0	0

Food and Measure	carb. (gms)	fiber (gms)
pan-roasted:		
(*Perdue Carving Classic*)	0	0
(*Wampler Deli Roast Collection*)	0	0
braised homestyle (*Perdue Carving Classics*)	1.0	0
with broth (*Wampler Deli Roast Collection*)	1.0	0
cracked pepper (*Perdue Carving Classics*)	2.0	0
pepper and garlic (*Dietz & Watson*)	1.0	0
pepper/peppered:		
(*Sara Lee*)	2.0	0
(*Wampler Del Roast Collection*)	1.0	0
cracked (*Sara Lee*)	2.0	0
cracked (*Sara Lee* Sliced), 2 slices, 1.6 oz.	2.0	0
cracked black (*Dietz & Watson*)	1.0	0
cracked pepper (*Williams*)	1.0	0
roasted:		
(*Boar's Head Salsalito*)	1.0	0
(*Hormel*)	0	0
(*Sara Lee* Golden)	0	0
golden (*Tyson* Bag), 2 slices, 2.25 oz.	2.0	0
rotisserie style or spiced (*Wampler Deli Roast Collection*)	1.0	0
smoked:		
(*Boar's Head Cracked Pepper Mill*)	0	0
(*Dietz & Watson* Chef Carved)	1.0	0
(*Healthy Choice Deli Thin*), 4 slices, 1.8 oz.	2.0	0
(*Healthy Deli* Zero Carb Brick Oven)	0	0
(*Hormel*)	1.0	0
(*Louis Rich Carving Board* 98% Fat Free), 2.3 oz.	3.0	0
(*Wampler 4 Diamond/2 Diamond*)	2.0	0
(*Wampler 3 Diamond/1 Diamond*)	1.0	0
hardwood (*Sara Lee*)	1.0	0
hardwood (*Sara Lee* Sliced), 2 slices, 1.6 oz.	1.0	0
hickory (*Louis Rich* Fat Free)	1.0	0
hickory (*Louis Rich/Oscar Mayer* Fat Free), 1 oz.	1.0	0
hickory (*Perdue/Perdue Carving Classics*)	1.0	0
hickory (*Shady Brook Farms*)	1.0	0
hickory (*Tyson*), 2 slices, 2.25 oz.	1.0	0
honey (*Healthy Choice* Heart Slices), 1 oz.	1.0	0
honey (*Healthy Choice Deli Thin*), 4 slices, 1.8 oz.	4.0	0

Food and Measure	carb. (gms)	fiber (gms)
honey (*Hormel*)	3.0	0
honey (*Oscar Mayer* Deli Style Thin Sliced)	2.0	0
honey (*Perdue Carving*)	2.0	0
honey (*Tyson*), 2 slices, 2.25 oz.	5.0	0
honey (*Wampler 4 Diamond/4 Diamond* Petite)	4.0	0
honey, white lean (*Oscar Mayer*), 1 oz.	2.0	0
mesquite (*Boar's Head Mesquite Wood Smoked*)	1.0	0
mesquite (*Healthy Choice*)	2.0	0
mesquite (*Healthy Choice Deli Thin*), 4 slices, 1.8 oz.	2.0	0
mesquite (*Oscar Mayer* Deli Style Thin Sliced)	2.0	0
mesquite (*Perdue Carving*)	0	0
mesquite (*Sara Lee*)	1.0	0
mesquite, honey (*Wampler 4 Diamond*)	4.0	0
mesquite or peppercorn (*Dietz & Watson*)	0	0
skin on (*Wampler 5 Diamond*)	0	0
skinless (*Healthy Choice*)	1.0	0
white (*Louis Rich* 95% Fat Free), 1 oz.	1.0	0
white (*Oscar Mayer* 95% Fat Free), 1 oz.	1.0	0
Southwest grilled (*Healthy Choice*)	2.0	0
Turkey pastrami, 2 oz.:		
(*Boar's Head*)	1.0	0
(*Dietz & Watson*)	1.0	0
(*Healthy Deli*)	2.0	0
dark (*Perdue*)	2.0	0
Turkey pepperoni (*Hormel Pillow Pack*), 17 slices, 1.1 oz.	0	0
Turkey pie, see "Turkey entree, frozen"		
Turkey pocket, frozen, 4.5-oz. piece:		
(*Pot Pie Express*)	45.0	3.0
bacon club (*Croissant Pockets*)	30.0	3.0
broccoli and cheese (*Lean Pockets*)	39.0	3.0
and ham with cheddar (*Lean Pockets*)	43.0	3.0
Turkey salami, 1 oz.:		
cooked	2	0
cotto (*Louis Rich* 50% Less Fat)	0	0
Turkey sausage, see "Sausage"		
Turkey strips, smoked, 1 oz.:		
peppered (*Pemmican* Premium Cut)	5.0	1.0
sweet (*Pemmican* Premium Cut)	5.0	0

Food and Measure	carb. (gms)	fiber (gms)
Turmeric, 1 tsp.	1.4	.5
Turnip:		
raw, 1 large, 6.5 oz.	11.8	3.3
raw, cubed, ½ cup	4.1	1.2
boiled, drained, cubed, ½ cup	3.8	1.6
boiled, drained, mashed, ½ cup	5.6	2.3
Turnip, frozen, boiled, drained, ½ cup	3.4	1.6
Turnip greens, fresh:		
raw, untrimmed, 1 lb.	18.2	7.6
raw, chopped:		
(*Del Monte*), 2 cups	5.0	1.0
(*Glory*), 2 cups	5.0	3.0
chopped, ½ cup	1.6	.7
boiled, chopped, ½ cup	3.1	2.2
Turnip greens, canned, ½ cup:		
(*Allens* No Salt)	3.0	2.0
(*Bush's*)	3.0	2.0
with diced turnip:		
(*Allens* No Salt)	5.0	3.0
(*Bush's*)	5.0	2.0
seasoned (*Allens/Sunshine*)	5.0	2.0
seasoned (*Glory*)	6.0	2.0
seasoned:		
(*Allens/Sunshine*)	5.0	2.0
(*Glory*)	6.0	2.0
(*Sylvia's*)	8.0	3.0
turkey flavor (*Glory*)	5.0	2.0
Turnip greens, frozen:		
boiled, drained, 1 cup	4.7	2.9
seasoned (*Glory* Savory Accents), ½ cup	8.0	2.0
Turnover, frozen, 1 piece:		
apple (*Pepperidge Farm*)	36.0	2.0
apple or cherry (*Pillsbury*)	24.0	0
blueberry (*Pepperidge Farm*)	33.0	1.0
cherry (*Pepperidge Farm*)	34.0	1.0
peach (*Pepperidge Farm*)	35.0	1.0
raspberry (*Pepperidge Farm*)	35.0	2.0
Turtle, green, raw, without added ingredients	0	0

U–V

Food and Measure	carb. (gms)	fiber (gms)
Umeboshi plum (*Eden*), .3-oz. piece	1.0	0
Umeboshi plum paste (*Eden*), 1 tsp.	0	0
Uzbek melon (*Frieda's*), 1 cup, 1.4 oz.	9.0	1.0
Vanilla chai tea, see "Soy beverage"		
Vanilla drink mix (*Nesquik*), 2 tbsp.	21.0	0
Vanilla extract, imitation:		
with alcohol, 1 tbsp.	.3	0
without alcohol, 1 tbsp.	1.8	0
Vanilla syrup (*Ferrara*), 2 oz.	32.0	0
Vanilla topping (*Smucker's PlateScapers*), 2 tbsp.	24.0	0
Veal, meat only, without added ingredients	0	0
Veal dinner, frozen, parmigiana (*Stouffer's* Homestyle Dinners), 17.5-oz. pkg.	62.0	7.0
Veal entree, frozen, parmigiana (*Stouffer's* Homestyle), 11⅝-oz. pkg.	46.0	5.0
Vegetable burger, see "Burger, vegetarian"		
Vegetable chips/crisps (see also specific listings), 1 oz., except as noted:		
(*Eden/Eden* Wasabi Chips), 1.1 oz.	24.0	0
(*Terra* Chips Original)	18.0	3.0
(*Terra Stix*)	16.0	3.0
(*Terra* Chips Mediterranean)	18.0	4.0
all varieties (*Snyder's* Crisps)	18.0	n.a.
mushroom, wild (*Terra Stix* Medley)	16.0	3.0
tomato, zesty (*Terra* Chips)	18.0	4.0
twirls (*Hain PureSnax* Crudités)	22.0	1.0
twirls, sour cream and onion (*Hain PureSnax* Crudités)	21.0	1.0
Vegetable dip (*Cabot Veggie*), 2 tbsp.	2.0	0

Food and Measure	carb. (gms)	fiber (gms)
Vegetable dip mix:		
(*Fantastic* Soup/Dip), 1½ tsp.	5.0	<1.0
(*McCormick*), ½ tsp.	0	0
Vegetable dish, frozen (see also "Vegetable entree, frozen," "Vegetables, mixed, frozen," and specific listings):		
crepes (*Kineret*), 2.2-oz. piece	13.0	1.0
Southern casserole (*Glory* Savory Accents), ½ cup	20.0	2.0
tomato, okra, corn casserole (*Glory* Savory Accents), ½ cup	14.0	2.0
Vegetable entree, frozen (see also "Vegetable entree mix, frozen," "Vegetarian entree, frozen," "Wraps, filled," and specific listings), 1 pkg., except as noted:		
korma (*Ethnic Gourmet*), 12 oz.	52.0	7.0
pie/pot pie:		
(*Amy's*), 7.5 oz.	54.0	4.0
(*Amy's* Country), 7.5 oz.	47.0	4.0
nondairy (*Amy's*), 7.5 oz.	50.0	4.0
stir-fry:		
(*Shanghai* Gourmet), 1 cup	12.0	4.0
with rice (*Michelina's* Zap'ems), 8 oz.	43.0	3.0
teriyaki, with rice (*Uncle Ben's* Rice Bowl), 12 oz.	74.0	4.0
Vegetable entree mix, frozen:		
beefy noodle (*Green Giant Create A Meal!*), 1¼ cups* with ground beef	31.0	3.0
cheesy pasta vegetable (*Green Giant Create A Meal!*), 1¼ cups* with ground beef and milk	29.0	2.0
chicken Alfredo (*Green Giant Create A Meal!*), 1¼ cups* with chicken and milk	36.0	3.0
garlic ginger stir-fry (*Green Giant Create A Meal!*), 1½ cups* with chicken, oil, and water	25.0	4.0
garlic herb chicken (*Green Giant Create A Meal!*), 1¼ cups* with chicken, oil, and water	30.0	3.0
lasagna, skillet (*Green Giant Create A Meal!*), 1¼ cups* with ground beef and water	31.0	3.0
lemon pepper chicken (*Green Giant Create A Meal!*), 1⅔ cups* with chicken and oil	30.0	5.0
lo mein stir-fry (*Green Giant Create A Meal!*), 1¾ cups* with chicken and oil	33.0	3.0

Food and Measure	carb. (gms)	fiber (gms)
Parmesan herb chicken (*Green Giant Create A Meal!*),		
1¾ cups* with chicken and oil	29.0	5.0
stew, homestyle (*Green Giant Create A Meal!*),		
1 cup* with ground beef and water	24.0	3.0
sweet and sour (*Green Giant Create A Meal!*),		
1¼ cups* with chicken and oil	43.0	3.0
Szechuan stir-fry (*Green Giant Create A Meal!*),		
1¼ cups* with chicken and oil	20.0	4.0
teriyaki stir-fry (*Green Giant Create A Meal!*),		
1¼ cups* with chicken and oil	18.0	4.0
Vegetable juice, 8 fl. oz., except as noted:		
(*Bolthouse Farms* Vedge)	11.0	2.0
(*Hain* Veggie)	11.0	0
(*Herdez* Original/Picante Limon), 12 fl. oz.	17.0	2.0
(*Red Gold*)	11.0	2.0
(*R.W. Knudsen Very Veggie* Low Sodium)	11.0	0
(*R.W. Knudsen Very Veggie* Original/Organic/Spicy)	11.0	2.0
(*Sacramento*)	11.0	2.0
(*V8/V8* Essential Antioxidants/Low Sodium)	10.0	2.0
(*V8* Calcium Enriched)	11.0	2.0
(*Walnut Acres*)	12.0	1.0
cocktail	11.0	1.9
lemon twist, picante, or spicy hot (*V8*)	10.0	2.0
Vegetable oyster, see "Salsify"		
Vegetable pie, see "Vegetable entree, frozen"		
Vegetable pocket/sandwich (see also "Wraps, filled"		
and specific listings), frozen, 4.5-oz. piece:		
(*Amy's* Pie)	45.0	3.0
and mozzarella (*Smart Ones Smartwich*)	38.0	3.0
roasted (*Amy's*)	35.0	4.0
Vegetable protein:		
(*AlpineAire*), 2 oz.	17.0	10.0
texturized (*Tree of Life*), 2.8 oz.	24.0	14.0
Vegetable snack rolls (see also specific listings), frozen		
(*Health is Wealth Munchees*), 2 pieces, 1 oz.	9.0	1.0
Vegetables, see specific listings		
Vegetables, mixed, can or jar, ½ cup, except as noted:		
(*Del Monte/Del Monte* No Salt)	8.0	2.0

Food and Measure	carb. (gms)	fiber (gms)
(*Del Monte Savory Sides* Homestyle Medley)	11.0	2.0
(*Freshlike*)	8.0	2.0
(*Green Giant* Garden Medley)	9.0	1.0
(*S&W*)	10.0	2.0
(*Veg-All* Homestyle Large Cut/Hot 'n Spicy/ Original/ No Salt)	8.0	2.0
Cajun (*Veg-All*)	10.0	3.0
with potato (*Del Monte*)	10.0	2.0
stir-fry (*Port Arthur*), ⅓ cup	3.0	0
Vegetables, mixed, freeze-dried, 1 serving:		
(*AlpineAire*)	6.0	1.0
garden (*AlpineAire*)	15.0	3.0
Vegetables, mixed, frozen (see also "Vegetable dishes, frozen" and specific vegetable listings):		
(*Birds Eye* Classic), ⅔ cup	12.0	2.0
(*Cascadian Farm*), ⅔ cup	12.0	2.0
(*Cascadian Farm* Gardener's Blend), ¾ cup	11.0	3.0
(*C&W* Fancy Organic/*Farmer's Harvest* Fancy), ¾ cup	11.0	2.0
(*C&W* Farmer's Harvest Healthy Garden), ¾ cup	4.0	2.0
(*C&W* Ultimate Petite Mixed Vegetables), ¾ cup	11.0	2.0
(*C&W The Ultimate Southwest Blend*), ⅔ cup	15.0	6.0
(*C&W The Ultimate Stir Fry*), ¾ cup	6.0	1.0
(*Dr. Praeger's*), ⅔ cup	12.0	3.0
(*Green Giant*), ¾ cup	10.0	2.0
(*McKenzie's* Garden Fresh), ⅔ cup	4.0	2.0
(*Tree of Life*), ½ cup	13.0	3.0
Alfredo, in sauce (*Green Giant*), 1 cup	8.0	2.0
Alfredo, in sauce (*Green Giant* Boil-in-Bag), ¾ cup	9.0	3.0
Asian, in sesame ginger sauce (*Birds Eye*), 1 cup	12.0	2.0
California blend (*Cascadian Farm*), ⅔ cup	5.0	2.0
in cheese sauce, cheddar, California blend (*Birds Eye*), ½ cup	8.0	1.0
in cheese sauce, winter blend (*Birds Eye*), 1⅓ cups	6.0	3.0
Chinese stir-fry (*Cascadian Farm*), 1 cup	6.0	2.0
gumbo mix (*McKenzie's*), ⅔ cup	8.0	2.0
Italian style, in oil, garlic (*Green Giant*), 1 cup	6.0	2.0
soup mix (*Birds Eye*), ⅔ cup	9.0	2.0

Food and Measure	carb. (gms)	fiber (gms)
soup mix (*McKenzie's*), ⅔ cup	9.0	2.0
stir-fry, 7 vegetable (*Birds Eye*), 1 cup	5.0	2.0
Szechuan, in sauce (*Green Giant*), ⅔ cup	9.0	2.0
Szechuan, in sesame sauce (*Birds Eye*), 1 cup	9.0	2.0
teriyaki (*Green Giant*), 1¼ cups	6.0	2.0
Thai stir-fry (*Cascadian Farm*), ¾ cup	7.0	3.0
Tuscan, in herb tomato sauce (*Birds Eye*), 1 cup	7.0	2.0
Vegetables, mixed, pickled:		
(*Fanci Food* Giardiniera), ⅓ cup	1.0	0
(*Krinos*), 3 oz.	0	2.0
(*Zorba*), ½ cup	2.0	0
hot (*Fanci Food* Medley), ⅓ cup	1.0	0
Vegetarian dish (see also "Vegetarian entree" and specific listings):		
canned:		
(*Loma Linda* Dinner Cuts), 2 slices, 3.3 oz.	4.0	2.0
(*Loma Linda* Tender Bits), 6 pieces, 3 oz.	7.0	3.0
(*Loma Linda* Tender Rounds), 6 pieces, 2.8 oz.	6.0	1.0
(*Worthington* Choplets), 2 slices, 3.3 oz.	4.0	2.0
(*Worthington* Savory Slices), 3 slices, 3 oz.	7.0	0
cutlets, multigrain (*Worthington*), 2 slices, 3.2 oz.	5.0	3.0
frozen:		
(*Worthington* Dinner Roast), ¾" slice, 3 oz.	6.0	3.0
(*Worthington* Fillets), 2 pieces, 3 oz.	8.0	4.0
croquettes (*Worthington* Golden), 4 pieces, 3 oz.	14.0	2.0
patties (*Worthington FriPats*), 2.3-oz. piece	5.0	3.0
Vegetarian entree, frozen (see also "Vegetable entree, frozen," and specific listings), 1 pkg.:		
nuggets, Hawaiian (*Hain Vegetarian Classics*), 10 oz.	55.0	6.0
portobello mushroom barley pilau (*Linda McCartney*), 10 oz.	33.0	8.0
teriyaki (*Ethnic Gourmet*), 12 oz.	71.0	4.0
Vegetarian entree, pkg. (see also specific listings), 1 pkg., except as noted:		
cacciatore (*Linsey Just Add Veggies!*), ¼ pkg.	40.0	5.0
curried garbanzos, potatoes, with rice (*Tamarind Tree* Alu Chole), 9.25 oz.	63.0	9.0
peas and cheese, with rice (*Tasty Bite*), 12 oz.	54.0	11.0

Food and Measure	carb. (gms)	fiber (gms)
peas and greens (*Tasty Bite*), ½ of 10-oz pkg.	9.0	4.0
peas, mushrooms, with rice (*Tamarind Tree*		
Dhingri Mutter), 9.25 oz.	53.0	7.0
pepper steak style (*Linsey Just Add Veggies!*), ¼ pkg. . . .	24.0	4.0
sprouts curry, with rice (*Tasty Bite*), 12 oz.	63.0	12.0
stir-fry, Oriental (*Linsey Just Add Veggies!*), ¼ pkg.	60.0	3.0
stir-fry, teriyaki (*Linsey Just Add Veggies!*), ¼ pkg.	66.0	3.0
vegetables (*Tasty Bite* Jaipur), ½ of 10-oz. pkg.	10.0	4.0
vegetables, with noodles:		
curry, green (*Tasty Bite*), ⅓ pkg.	30.0	0
curry, red (*Tasty Bite*), ⅓ pkg.	31.0	<1.0
curry, yellow (*Tasty Bite*), ⅓ pkg.	33.0	<1.0
vegetables, with rice:		
(*Tasty Bite* Supreme), 12 oz.	55.0	11.0
creamy (*Tamarind Tree* Navratan Korma), 9.25 oz.	60.0	7.0
spicy (*Tamarind Tree* Vegetable Jalfrazi), 9.25 oz.	57.0	7.0
Venison, meat only, without added ingredients	0	0
Vermicelli entree mix, garlic and olive oil (*Near East*),		
2 oz. or 1 cup*	48.0	3.0
Vienna sausage, see "Sausage, canned"		
Vine spinach, raw, untrimmed, 1 lb.	15.4	4.0
Vinegar, 1 tbsp., except as noted:		
all varieties (*S&W*)	0	0
all varieties, except balsamic (*Progresso*)	0	0
apple cider (*Tree of Life*)	1.0	0
apple cider or red wine (*Eden*)	0	0
balsamic:		
(*Hain*)	2.0	0
(*Pompeian*)	2.0	0
(*Progresso*)	2.0	0
(*Regina*)	2.0	0
(*Zabar's*)	1.0	0
malt, tarragon, or red/white wine (*Fanci Food*)	0	0
red wine (*Pompeian*)	0	0
red wine (*Regina*)	<1.0	0
red or white wine (*Hain*)	0	0
rice, brown (*Eden*)	0	0

Food and Measure	carb. (gms)	fiber (gms)
rice, seasoned (*Marukan*)	6.0	0
sushi (*Sushi Chef*)	6.0	0
ume plum (*Eden*), 1 tsp.	0	0
white wine (*Regina*)	<1.0	0
white wine, raspberry (*Fanci Food*)	2.0	0

W

Food and Measure	carb. (gms)	fiber (gms)
Waffle, frozen, 2 pieces, except as noted:		
(*Aunt Jemima* Homestyle)	32.0	1.0
(*Aunt Jemima* Low Fat)	30.0	1.0
(*Eggo* Homestyle)	29.0	1.0
(*Eggo* Homestyle Minis), 3 sets of 4 pieces	38.0	1.0
(*Eggo* Froot Loops)	30.0	1.0
(*Eggo Special K* 99% Fat Free)	37.0	1.0
(*Eggo Special K* Low Carb)	15.0	7.0
(*GoLean* Original)	33.0	6.0
(*Pillsbury* Homestyle)	29.0	<1.0
(*Belgian Chef*)	34.0	2.0
apple cinnamon (*Eggo*)	30.0	1.0
banana bread (*Eggo*)	30.0	2.0
blueberry:		
(*Aunt Jemima*)	32.0	<1.0
(*Eggo*)	30.0	1.0
(*GoLean*)	33.0	6.0
(*Hungry Jack*)	33.0	<1.0
buttermilk:		
(*Aunt Jemima*)	33.0	1.0
(*Eggo*)	26.0	1.0
(*Pillsbury*)	28.0	<1.0
chocolate chip (*Eggo*)	32.0	1.0
cinnamon toast (*Eggo*), 3 sets of 4 pieces	46.0	1.0
honey oat (*Heart to Heart*)	31.0	3.0
strawberry (*Eggo*)	32.0	1.0
whole wheat (*Eggo Nutri-Grain*/Low Fat)	28.0	3.0
Waffle, filled, apple cinnamon, blueberry, or		
strawberry (*Eggo Waf-fulls*), 1 piece	25.0	<1.0

Food and Measure	carb. (gms)	fiber (gms)
Waffle mix, see "Pancake mix"		
Waffle sticks, 6 pieces with syrup:		
(*Pillsbury* Homestyle)	60.0	1.0
blueberry (*Pillsbury*)	64.0	<1.0
chocolate chip (*Pillsbury*)	68.0	1.0
cinnamon (*Pillsbury*)	62.0	1.0
Walnut, dried:		
(*Fisher*), 1 oz.	3.0	3.0
(*Planters*), 1.2 oz.	6.0	2.0
black:		
(*Planters*), 2-oz. pkg.	8.0	3.0
shelled, 1 oz.	3.4	1.4
chopped, 1 cup	15.1	6.3
English or Persian:		
shelled, 1 oz.	5.2	1.4
pieces, 1 cup	22.0	5.8
halves, 1 cup	18.3	4.8
glazed, see "Candy"		
pieces (*Planters*), 1 oz.	5.0	1.0
Walnut topping, in syrup (*Smucker's*), 2 tbsp.	20.0	1.0
Wasabi, root, fresh, sliced, ½ cup	15.3	5.0
Wasabi chips, see "Vegetable chips/crisps"		
Wasabi powder (*Eden*), 1 tsp.	1.0	.5
Wasabi sauce, 1 tsp.:		
(*S&B* Tube)	3.0	0
with ginger (*Gold's*)	1.0	0
Water chestnut, fresh:		
(*Frieda's*), 1 tbsp., 1.1 oz.	7.0	1.0
4 medium, 1.3 oz.	8.6	1.1
sliced, ½ cup	14.8	1.9
Water chestnut, can or jar:		
whole (*Port Arthur*), ½ cup	9.0	1.0
whole, 4 pieces, 1 oz.	3.5	.7
sliced, with liquid, ½ cup	8.7	1.8
Watercress:		
(*Frieda's*), 1 cup, 3 oz.	1.0	2.0
10 sprigs, 11¼''	.3	.6
chopped, ½ cup	.2	.4

Food and Measure	carb. (gms)	fiber (gms)
Watermelon, fresh:		
1'' slice, 10'' diam.	34.6	2.4
diced, (*Del Monte*), 2 cups, 9.9 oz.	27.0	2.0
diced, ½ cup	5.7	.4
yellow seedless (*Frieda's*), ½ cup, 3 oz.	6.0	0
Watermelon drink blend, 8 fl. oz.:		
(*AriZona*)	27.0	0
(*Snapple* What-a-Melon)	25.0	0
strawberry (*Nantucket Nectars*)	30.0	0
Watermelon juice blend (*Juicy Juice*), 8 fl. oz.	31.0	0
Watermelon rind, pickled, sweet:		
(*Old South*), 2 cubes, 1 oz.	17.0	0
(*Reese*), 2 cubes	17.0	0
Watermelon seeds, dried, 1 oz.	4.4	n.a.
Wax beans, fresh, see "Green beans"		
Wax beans, canned, golden (*Del Monte*), ½ cup	4.0	2.0
Wax gourd:		
raw, cubed, 1 cup	4.0	3.8
boiled, drained, cubed, 1 cup	5.3	1.8
Welsh rarebit, frozen (*Stouffer's*), ¼ cup	6.0	1.0
Wendy's, 1 serving:		
chicken nuggets:		
4 pieces	10.0	0
5 pieces	13.0	0
barbecue sauce	11.0	0
honey mustard	6.0	0
sweet and sour	12.0	0
chicken strips:		
3 pieces	33.0	0
chipotle sauce	4.0	0
honey mustard	6.0	0
ranch sauce	1.0	0
sandwiches:		
Big Bacon Classic	46.0	3.0
cheeseburger, kids' meal	34.0	1.0
cheeseburger, Monterey ranch	42.0	2.0
cheeseburger Jr.	34.0	1.0
cheeseburger Jr., with bacon	34.0	2.0

Food and Measure	carb. (gms)	fiber (gms)
cheeseburger Jr. deluxe	37.0	2.0
chicken fillet, home style or spicy	57.0	2.0
chicken fillet, ultimate grill	44.0	2.0
hamburger, kids' meal	33.0	1.0
hamburger Jr.	34.0	1.0
Classic Single, with everything	37.0	2.0
Classic Triple/Double, with everything	38.0	2.0
salad, *Garden Sensations:*		
chicken BLT	10.0	4.0
add garlic croutons	9.0	2.0
add honey mustard dressing	11.0	1.0
chicken strips	33.0	5.0
add ranch dressing	5.0	0
fresh fruit bowl	33.0	3.0
add strawberry yogurt	16.0	0
Mandarin Chicken	17.0	4.0
add almonds	4.0	2.0
add noodles	10.0	0
add sesame dressing	19.0	0
spring mix	11.0	5.0
add honey pecans	5.0	2.0
add vinaigrette	8.0	0
taco supreme	31.0	9.0
add salsa	6.0	0
add sour cream	2.0	0
add taco chips	29.0	2.0
salad dressing, light:		
French, fat free	19.0	0
honey mustard, low fat	21.0	0
ranch, reduced fat	6.0	1.0
sides:		
chili, large	35.0	8.0
chili, small	23.0	5.0
add cheddar	1.0	0
add hot seasoning	2.0	0
add saltines, 2 pieces	5.0	0
fries:		
Biggie	65.0	6.0

Food and Measure	carb. (gms)	fiber (gms)
Great Biggie	77.0	7.0
kids' meal	37.0	3.0
medium	58.0	5.0
fruit cup	20.0	2.0
mandarin orange cup	20.0	1.0
potato, baked, plain or with *Country Crock* spread	61.0	7.0
potato, baked, with:		
bacon and cheese	69.0	8.0
broccoli and cheese	69.0	9.0
sour cream and chive	62.0	7.0
side salad	7.0	3.0
side salad, Caesar	3.0	2.0
add garlic croutons	9.0	0
add Caesar dressing	1.0	0
Frosty cup:		
junior, 6 oz.	28.0	0
medium, 16 oz.	74.0	0
small. 12 oz.	56.0	0
Wheat, whole grain:		
(*Arrowhead Mills*), ¼ cup	31.0	5.0
durum, 1 cup	136.6	n.a.
hard red:		
(*Shiloh Farms*), ¼ cup	34.0	7.0
spring, 1 cup	130.6	24.2
winter, 1 cup	136.7	24.2
hard white, 1 cup	145.7	n.a.
hard white, spring (*Shiloh Farms*), ¼ cup	33.0	11.0
soft red winter, 1 cup	124.7	21.0
soft white, 1 cup	126.6	21.3
Wheat, parboiled, see "Bulgur"		
Wheat, sprouted, 1 cup	45.9	1.2
Wheat berries, see "Wheat kernels"		
Wheat bran (see also "Cereal"):		
coarse (*Shiloh Farms*), ¼ cup	10.0	6.0
crude (*Hodgson Mill* Unprocessed), ¼ cup	10.0	7.0
crude, 2 tbsp.	4.5	3.0
fine (*Shiloh Farms*), ¼ cup	7.0	6.0

Food and Measure	carb. (gms)	fiber (gms)
toasted (*Kretschmer*), ¼ cup	10.0	7.0
untoasted (*Hodgson Mill*), 2 tbsp.	7.0	4.0
Wheat flakes, ⅓ cup:		
(*Shiloh Farms*)	24.0	5.0
rolled (*Arrowhead Mills*)	24.0	5.0
Wheat flour, ¼ cup, except as noted:		
(*Hodgson Mill* 50/50), <¼ cup	21.0	2.0
biscuit (*Gold Medal Baker's Blend*)	23.0	1.0
bread:		
(*Gold Medal Baker's Blend*)	25.0	1.0
(*Gold Medal Better for Bread*)	22.0	<1.0
(*Hodgson Mill* Best for Bread)	22.0	1.0
wheat (*Gold Medal Better for Bread*)	21.0	1.0
cake (*Swans Down*)	22.0	0
cake, self-rising (*Presto*)	20.0	1.0
cookie (*Gold Medal Baker's Blend*)	25.0	1.0
gluten, see "Wheat gluten"		
graham, whole wheat (*Hodgson Mill*), <¼ cup	22.0	3.0
pasta, see "Semolina flour"		
pastry (*Arrowhead Mills*), ⅓ cup	23.0	3.0
pastry, whole wheat (*Hodgson Mill*), <¼ cup	22.0	3.0
seasoned (*Kentucky Kernel*), 4 tsp.	8.0	0
self-rising (*Gold Medal*)	22.0	<1.0
self-rising, 1 cup	92.8	4.0
tortilla mix, 1 cup	74.5	n.a.
white, all-purpose (*Gold Medal/Gold Medal* Organic)	22.0	<1.0
white, all purpose, presifted (*Wondra*)	23.0	<1.0
white, unbleached:		
(*Arrowhead Mills*)	26.0	<1.0
(*Hodgson Mill*), <¼ cup	23.0	1.0
(*Hodgson Mill* Organic)	23.0	1.0
(*Shiloh Farms*), ⅓ cup	33.0	0
white, whole wheat (*Hodgson Mill*)	21.0	3.0
whole grain, 1 cup	87.1	15.1
whole wheat:		
(*Arrowhead Mills*)	26.0	4.0
(*Gold Medal*)	21.0	3.0
(*Shiloh Farms*)	25.0	4.0

Food and Measure	carb. (gms)	fiber (gms)
Wheat germ:		
(*Hodgson Mill* Untoasted), 2 tbsp.	7.0	4.0
(*Kretschmer*), 2 tbsp.	6.0	2.0
crude, 1 oz.	14.7	3.7
raw or flake (*Shiloh Farms*), 3 tbsp.	10.0	2.0
honey crunch (*Kretschmer*), 1⅔ tbsp.	8.0	1.0
toasted:		
(*Shiloh Farms* Glass), 3 tbsp.	12.0	3.0
(*Tree of Life*), 3 tbsp.	12.0	3.0
1 oz.	14.1	3.7
Wheat gluten, vital:		
(*Hodgson Mill*), 4 tsp.	3.0	1.0
(*Shiloh Farms*), 3 tsp.	1.0	0
Wheat kernels, ¼ cup:		
(*Purity Foods* Berries)	34.0	7.0
(*Shiloh Farms* Soft)	35.0	7.0
Wheat malt syrup, see "Malt syrup"		
Wheat pilaf mix (*Near East*), 2 oz. or 1 cup*	40.0	9.0
Wheat salad, cracked (*Cedar's*), 3.5 oz.	26.0	2.0
Whelk, meat only:		
raw, 4 oz.	8.8	0
boiled, steamed, or poached, 4 oz.	17.6	0
Whey, fluid, acid or sweet, 1 cup	12.6	0
Whipped topping, see "Cream topping"		
Whiskey, see "Liquor"		
White beans, mature:		
boiled, ½ cup	22.6	5.7
small, dry (*Jack Rabbit*), ¼ cup	22.0	14.0
small, boiled, ½ cup	22.5	5.6
White beans, canned:		
(*S&W*), ½ cup	19.0	6.0
with liquid, ½ cup	28.7	6.3
Spanish style (*Goya*), 7.5 oz.	29.0	12.0
White Castle, 1 serving:		
breakfast sandwich	17.0	0
burgers:		
cheeseburger, regular or bacon	13.0	<1.0
cheeseburger, double	19.0	1.0

Food and Measure	carb. (gms)	fiber (gms)
hamburger	13.0	<1.0
hamburger, double	19.0	1.0
chicken ring sandwich, with cheese	17.0	<1.0
fish sandwich, with cheese	18.0	<1.0
sides:		
cheese sticks, 5 pieces	37.0	2.0
fries, small	37.0	4.0
onion rings, 8 pieces	28.0	1.0
White sauce mix:		
(*Knorr*), 2 tsp.	4.0	0
(*McCormick*), 2 tsp.	3.0	0
Whitefish, fresh or smoked, without added		
ingredients	0	0
Whitefish salad, smoked (*Acme*), 4 tbsp.	3.0	1.0
Whiting, without added ingredients	0	0
Wiener, see "Frankfurter"		
Wild rice:		
raw, ¼ cup:		
(*Fanci Food*)	35.0	2.0
(*Lundberg* Organic)	34.0	3.0
(*Shiloh Farms*)	34.0	3.0
cracked (*Gourmet House*)	35.0	2.0
raw, quick (*Fanci Food*), ½ cup	25.0	2.0
raw, quick (*Gourmet House*), ½ cup	25.0	2.0
cooked, 1 cup	35.0	1.5
Wild rice blends, see "Rice"		
Wild rice dishes, see "Rice dishes"		
Wine, 3.5 fl. oz., except as noted:		
dessert or apertif[1]	12.2	0
dry or table[2]:		
red	1.8	0
rose	1.4	0
white	.8	0
sake, 1 fl. oz.	.1	0

[1] Includes fortified wines containing more than 15% alcohol, such as port, sherry, vermouth, etc.
[2] Includes wines containing less than 15% alcohol, such as Burgundy, Chablis, champagne, etc.

Food and Measure	carb. (gms)	fiber (gms)
Wine, cooking, 2 tbsp., except as noted:		
Burgundy or Chablis (*Fanci Food*)	0	0
Burgundy or Sauterne (*Regina*)	3.0	0
Marsala (*Holland House*)	4.0	0
red (*Holland House*)	1.0	0
rice (*Eden* Marin), 1 tbsp.	7.0	0
rice (*Sun Luck* Mirin), 1 tbsp.	5.0	0
sherry:		
(*Fanci Food*)	2.0	0
(*Holland House*)	5.0	0
(*Regina*)	5.0	0
white, plain or with lemon (*Holland House*)	0	0
Wine cooler (*Bartles & Jaymes*), 12 fl. oz.:		
berry, exotic	34.0	0
blackberry, luscious	40.0	0
blue Hawaiian	31.0	0
classic original	29.0	0
fuzzy navel	43.0	0
kiwi strawberry or hard raspberry lemonade	37.0	0
lemonade, hard, or strawberry daiquiri	38.0	0
tropical burst	39.0	0
Wing sauce (*Ott's*), 2 tbsp.	0	0
Winged beans, fresh, raw or boiled, drained, ½ cup	1.0	n.a.
Winged beans, mature:		
dry, ½ cup	38.0	14.1
boiled, ½ cup	12.8	n.a.
Winged bean leaves, trimmed, 1 oz.	4.0	n.a.
Winged bean tuber, trimmed, 1 oz.	8.0	n.a.
Winter squash (see also specific listings), all varieties:		
raw, cubed, 1 cup	10.2	1.7
boiled, drained, cubed, 1 cup	17.9	5.7
Winter squash, frozen, ½ cup:		
(*Cascadian Farm*), ½ cup	19.0	2.0
cooked (*Birds Eye*), ½ cup	11.0	2.0
Witloof, see "Chicory, witloof"		
Wolf fish, without added ingredients	0	0
Wonton wrapper (see also "Wrappers") (*Frieda's* Fiesta), 4 pieces, 1 oz.	17.0	1.0

Food and Measure	carb. (gms)	fiber (gms)
Worcestershire sauce:		
(*Annie's Naturals* Organic), 2 tbsp.	5.0	0
(*Lea & Perrins*), 1 tsp.	1.0	0
(*World Harbors Angostura*), 1 tbsp.	1.0	0
white wine (*Lea & Perrins*), 1 tsp.	.7	0
Wrappers (see also "Egg roll wrapper" and "Wonton wrapper"):		
round (*Azumaya*), 10 pieces	31.0	1.0
square (*Azumaya*), 8 pieces	31.0	1.0
square, large (*Azumaya*), 3 pieces	31.0	1.0
Wraps (see also "Tortilla"), unfilled, 1 piece:		
(*Cedar's* Low Carb), 1.5 oz.	14.0	9.0
garlic pesto (*Aladdin* Gourmet), 3.5 oz.	53.0	5.0
roasted red pepper (*Aladdin* Gourmet), 3.5 oz.	52.0	5.0
spinach (*Cedar's*), 2.5 oz.	34.0	3.0
wheat (*Cedar's*), 2.5 oz.	38.0	3.0
wheat (*Sahara*), 2.1 oz.	27.0	4.0
white (*Cedar's*), 2.5 oz.	27.0	1.0
white (*Sahara*), 2.1 oz.	29.0	<1.0
Wraps, filled (see also "Breakfast pocket/sandwich"), frozen, 1 piece:		
chicken tikka (*Ethnic Gourmet*), 8 oz.	45.0	3.0
couscous vegetable (*Cedarlane* Veggie Wraps), 6 oz.	36.0	3.0
Indian samosa vegetable (*Amy's*), 5 oz.	38.0	4.0
kung pao tofu (*Ethnic Gourmet*), 8 oz.	48.0	4.0
peanut satay, vegetarian (*Ethnic Gourmet*), 8 oz.	49.0	6.0
pizza veggie (*Cedarlane* Veggie Wraps), 6 oz.	32.0	2.0
vegetable paneer (*Ethnic Gourmet*), 8 oz.	42.0	4.0
vegetable and rice teriyaki (*Cedarlane*), 6 oz.	56.0	2.0
veggie "ham" and cheese (*Cedarlane* Veggie Wraps), 6 oz.	36.0	1.0
Wraps, filled kit, refrigerated (*South Beach Diet*), 1 pkg.:		
chicken, Southwestern style	26.0	15.0
chicken Caesar, grilled or ham and turkey, deli	24.0	15.0
turkey and bacon club	25.0	15.0

Y

Food and Measure	carb. (gms)	fiber (gms)
Yachtwurst, with pistachios, cooked, 2 oz.	.8	0
Yam (see also "Name yam"), cubed:		
raw, ½ cup	20.9	3.1
baked or boiled, ½ cup	18.8	2.7
Yam, canned or frozen, see "Sweet potato"		
Yam, mountain, Hawaiian, ½ cup:		
raw, cubed	11.1	n.a.
steamed, cubed	14.4	n.a.
Yam beans, tuber:		
raw (*Frieda's* Jicama), ¾ cup, 3 oz.	7.0	1.0
raw, sliced, ½ cup	5.3	2.9
boiled, drained, 4 oz.	10.0	n.a.
Yard-long beans, fresh:		
raw (*Frieda's* Dow Gok), ¾ cup, 3 oz.	7.0	0
boiled, drained, sliced, ½ cup	4.8	n.a.
Yard-long beans, mature:		
dry, ½ cup	52.0	4.0
boiled, ½ cup	18.1	1.4
Yautia root, see "Malanga"		
Yeast, baker's:		
active, dry (*Hodgson Mill*), 5/16 oz.	3.0	1.0
active, dry, 1 tbsp.	4.6	.3
compressed, .6-oz.	1.1	<.1
fast rise (*Hodgson Mill*), 5/16 oz.	4.0	1.0
Yellow beans, dried, boiled, ½ cup	22.2	9.2
Yellow squash, fresh, see "Crookneck squash"		
Yellow squash, canned, sliced (*Sunshine*), ½ cup	5.0	2.0
Yellowtail, without added ingredients	0	0

Food and Measure	carb. (gms)	fiber (gms)
Yogurt, 8 oz., except as noted:		
plain:		
(*Cabot* Nonfat)	19.0	0
(*Dannon* Lowfat)	14.0	0
(*Dannon* Lowfat/Nonfat), 6 oz.	14.0	0
(*Darigold* Lowfat)	21.0	0
(*Stonyfield* Lowfat)	17.0	3.0
(*Stonyfield* Lowfat), 6 oz.	13.0	2.0
(*Stonyfield* Nonfat)	18.0	3.0
(*Stonyfield* Nonfat), 6 oz.	14.0	2.0
(*Yoplait* Grande! Nonfat)	19.0	0
all flavors:		
(*Breyers* Light Nonfat)	22.0	0
(*Breyers* Creme Savers)	45.0	0
(*Cabot* Nonfat)	24.0	0
(*Danimals XL*), 5.75 oz.	29.0	0
(*Dannon* Natural Flavors), 6 oz.	26.0	0
(*Dannon Light 'n Fit* with Fiber), 4 oz.	13.0	3.0
(*Dannon Light 'n Fit Carb Control*), 4 oz.	3.0	0
(*Dannon Sprinkl'ins*), 4.1 oz.	22.0	0
(*Go-Gurt*), 2.25 oz.	13.0	0
(*Trix*), 4 oz.	23.0	0
(*Yoplait* Light 6-Pack), 4 oz.	13.0	0
(*Yoplait* 99% Fat Free 6-Pack), 4 oz.	22.0	0
(*Yoplait* Thick & Creamy), 6 oz.	32.0	0
(*Yoplait Ultra*), 6 oz.	8.0	0
(*Yoplait Whips*), 4 oz.	25.0	0
(*Yumsters*), 4 oz.	21.0	0
except banana crème pie, Boston crème pie, lemon crème pie, and vanilla (*Yoplait* Light), 6 oz.	19.0	0
except cherry, raspberry, and strawberry-banana (*Darigold* Lowfat)	45.0	0
except coconut crème pie and lemon (*Yoplait*), 6 oz.	33.0	0
except raspberry (*Dannon Light 'n Fit* Creamy), 6 oz.	16.0	0
except vanilla, French (*Hood Carb Countdown*), 6 oz.	4.0	0
apple cinnamon (*Dannon* Fruit on the Bottom), 6 oz.	31.0	<1.0
apple cobbler (*Breyers* Smooth & Creamy)	46.0	0

Food and Measure	carb. (gms)	fiber (gms)
apricot mango (*Stonyfield* Nonfat), 6 oz.	26.0	2.0
banana cream (*la Crème*), 4 oz.	21.0	0
banana cream pie (*Yoplait* Light), 6 oz.	20.0	0
banana vanilla (*Stonyfield* Lowfat Banilla)	38.0	4.0
berry:		
(*Stonyfield* Nonfat Bash), 6 oz.	25.0	2.0
mixed (*Breyers* Fruit on the Bottom)	46.0	0
mixed (*Dannon* Fruit on the Bottom), 6 oz.	28.0	0
berry-banana (*Cabot* Nonfat)	24.0	0
blackberry (*Stonyfield* Nonfat), 6 oz.	29.0	2.0
blackberry pie (*Dannon Light 'n Fit*), 6 oz.	16.0	0
blueberry:		
(*Breyers* Fruit on the Bottom)	44.0	0
(*Dannon* Fruit on the Bottom), 6 oz.	29.0	0
(*Dannon Creamy Fruit Blends*), 6 oz.	33.0	0
(*Dannon Light 'n Fit*), 6 oz.	17.0	0
(*Stonyfield* Lowfat), 6 oz.	25.0	2.0
(*Stonyfield* Nonfat), 6 oz.	26.0	2.0
Boston crème pie (*Yoplait* Light), 6 oz.	20.0	0
boysenberry (*Dannon* Fruit on the Bottom), 6 oz.	28.0	0
caramel (*Stonyfield* Lowfat), 6 oz.	38.0	2.0
cherry:		
(*Dannon* Fruit on the Bottom), 6 oz.	29.0	<1.0
(*Dannon Creamy Fruit Blends*), 6 oz.	31.0	0
(*Darigold* Lowfat)	44.0	0
black (*Breyers* Fruit on the Bottom)	46.0	0
black (*Stonyfield* Nonfat), 6 oz.	26.0	2.0
cherry parfait, black (*Breyers* Smooth & Creamy)	46.0	0
cherry parfait, black (*Breyers* Smooth & Creamy), 4 oz. ..	23.0	0
cherry vanilla (*Dannon Light 'n Fit*), 6 oz.	17.0	0
chocolate (*Stonyfield* Nonfat Underground), 6 oz.	29.0	2.0
chocolate, white, raspberry (*Dannon Light 'n Fit*), 6 oz. ..	16.0	0
coconut crème pie (*Yoplait*), 6 oz.	34.0	0
coffee (*Dannon* Natural), 6 oz.	26.0	0
lemon:		
(*Stonyfield* Lowfat Luscious), 6 oz.	25.0	3.0
(*Stonyfield* Nonfat Lotsa), 6 oz.	28.0	2.0
(*Yoplait* Burst), 6 oz.	36.0	0

Food and Measure	carb. (gms)	fiber (gms)
chiffon (*Dannon Light 'n Fit*), 6 oz.	16.0	0
créme pie (*Yoplait* Light), 6 oz.	20.0	0
lime, key (*Stonyfield* Nonfat), 6 oz.	29.0	2.0
maple vanilla (*Stonyfield* Lowfat), 6 oz.	23.0	2.0
mocha latte (*Stonyfield* Lowfat), 6 oz.	25.0	2.0
orange (*la Crème* Mousse), 2.6 oz.	15.0	0
orange mango (*Dannon Light 'n Fit*), 6 oz.	16.0	0
peach:		
(*Breyers* Fruit on the Bottom)	45.0	0
(*la Crème*), 4 oz.	21.0	0
(*Dannon* Fruit on the Bottom), 6 oz.	29.0	0
(*Dannon Creamy Fruit Blends*), 6 oz.	33.0	0
(*Dannon Light 'n Fit*), 6 oz.	16.0	0
(*Stonyfield* Lowfat/Nonfat), 6 oz.	25.0	2.0
peaches and cream (*Breyers* Smooth & Creamy)	48.0	0
peaches and cream (*Breyers* Smooth & Creamy), 4 oz. ..	24.0	0
pineapple (*Breyers* Fruit on the Bottom)	46.0	0
raspberries and cream (*Breyers* Smooth & Creamy)	48.0	0
raspberries and cream (*Breyers* Smooth & Creamy), 4 oz.	24.0	0
raspberry:		
(*Breyers* Fruit on the Bottom)	46.0	0
(*la Crème*), 4 oz.	20.0	0
(*Dannon* Fruit on the Bottom), 6 oz.	29.0	0
(*Dannon Creamy Fruit Blends*), 6 oz.	32.0	<1.0
(*Dannon Light 'n Fit* Creamy), 6 oz.	17.0	0
(*Darigold* Lowfat)	44.0	0
(*Stonyfield* Lowfat), 6 oz.	25.0	3.0
(*Stonyfield* Nonfat), 6 oz.	25.0	2.0
strawberries and cream (*Breyers* Smooth & Creamy), 4 oz.	24.0	0
strawberry:		
(*Breyers* Fruit on the Bottom)	46.0	0
(*Breyers* Smooth & Creamy)	46.0	0
(*Breyers* Smooth & Creamy), 4 oz.	23.0	0
(*la Crème*), 4 oz.	20.0	0
(*la Crème* Mousse), 2.6 oz.	15.0	0
(*Dannon* Fruit on the Bottom), 6 oz.	30.0	0
(*Dannon Creamy Fruit Blends*), 6 oz.	31.0	0

Food and Measure	carb. (gms)	fiber (gms)
(*Dannon Light 'n Fit*), 6 oz.	17.0	0
(*Stonyfield* Lowfat)	17.0	3.0
(*Stonyfield* Lowfat), 6 oz.	25.0	2.0
(*Stonyfield* Nonfat)	36.0	3.0
(*Stonyfield* Nonfat), 6 oz.	26.0	2.0
(*Yoplait* Grande! 99% Fat Free)	48.0	0
strawberry-banana:		
(*Breyers* Fruit on the Bottom)	46.0	0
(*Breyers* Smooth & Creamy)	49.0	0
(*Breyers* Smooth & Creamy), 4 oz.	24.0	0
(*Dannon* Fruit on the Bottom), 6 oz.	30.0	0
(*Dannon Creamy Fruit Blends*), 6 oz.	32.0	0
(*Dannon Light 'n Fit*), 6 oz.	17.0	0
(*Darigold* Lowfat)	46.0	0
strawberry cheesecake (*Breyers* Smooth & Creamy)	47.0	0
strawberry cheesecake (*Stonyfield* Nonfat), 6 oz.	29.0	2.0
strawberry-kiwi (*Dannon Light 'n Fit*), 6 oz.	17.0	0
vanilla:		
(*Breyers* Smooth & Creamy)	47.0	0
(*Cabot* Nonfat)	24.0	0
(*la Crème*), 4 oz.	20.0	0
(*Dannon Light 'n Fit*), 6 oz.	16.0	0
(*Stonyfield* Lowfat)	34.0	3.0
(*Stonyfield* Lowfat), 6 oz.	25.0	2.0
(*Yoplait* Grande! 99% Fat Free)	48.0	0
(*Yoplait* Light Very), 6 oz.	20.0	0
vanilla, French:		
(*la Crème* Mousse), 2.6 oz.	15.0	0
(*Hood Carb Countdown*), 6 oz.	3.0	0
(*Stonyfield* Nonfat)	36.0	3.0
(*Stonyfield* Nonfat), 6 oz.	28.0	2.0
Yogurt, frozen, ½ cup:		
(*Ben & Jerry's half baked*)	35.0	<1.0
black cherry vanilla swirl (*Dreyer's/Edy's* Nonfat)	20.0	0
blueberry (*Turkey Hill* Muffin)	23.0	2.0
caramel brownie sundae (*Hood* Nonfat)	28.0	0
caramel praline swirl (*Dreyer's/Edy's* Nonfat)	23.0	0
cherry chocolate chip (*Ben & Jerry's Cherry Garcia*)	32.0	<1.0

Food and Measure	carb. (gms)	fiber (gms)
chocolate (*Stonyfield* Nonfat)	19.0	<1.0
chocolate almond praline (*Hood*)	24.0	0
chocolate cherry cordial (*Turkey Hill* Nonfat)	23.0	1.0
chocolate chip cookie dough (*Turkey Hill*)	22.0	3.0
chocolate fudge brownie (*Ben & Jerry's*)	35.0	1.0
chocolate fudge brownie (*Häagen-Dazs*)	35.0	2.0
chocolate marshmallow (*Turkey Hill* Nonfat)	25.0	1.0
chocolate marshmallow caramel (*Ben & Jerry's* Phish Food*)	41.0	1.0
chocolate mint chip (*Stonyfield* Lowfat)	22.0	<1.0
coffee (*Häagen-Dazs*)	31.0	0
coffee (*Stonyfield* Nonfat Decaf)	19.0	0
cookies and cream (*Dreyer's/Edy's*)	19.0	0
cookies and cream (*Hood*)	25.0	0
crème caramel (*Stonyfield* Lowfat)	23.0	0
dulce de leche (*Häagen-Dazs*)	35.0	0
graham, with peanut butter (*Turkey Hill* Graham Canyon)	23.0	3.0
lemon (*Turkey Hill* Nonfat Southern Pie)	25.0	0
mint cookies and cream (*Turkey Hill*)	22.0	1.0
mocha fudge (*Hood* Nonfat)	27.0	0
mocha fudge, almond (*Stonyfield* Lowfat)	23.0	1.0
Neapolitan (*Turkey Hill* Nonfat)	19.0	1.0
peach (*Green's* Lowfat)	22.0	0
peach (*Green's* Nonfat)	23.0	0
peanut butter marshmallow (*Turkey Hill*)	25.0	2.0
raspberry (*Stonyfield* Nonfat)	21.0	0
raspberry, double (*Hood* Nonfat)	26.0	0
raspberry vanilla (*Dreyer's/Edy's*)	16.0	0
strawberry (*Häagen-Dazs*)	31.0	0
strawberry (*Hood* Nonfat)	23.0	0
coffee crunch (*Dreyer's/Edy's Heath*)	18.0	0
vanilla:		
(*Dreyer's/Edy's*)	17.0	0
(*Dreyer's/Edy's* Nonfat)	19.0	0
(*Green's* Lowfat)	20.0	0
(*Green's* Nonfat)	22.0	0
(*Hood* Nonfat)	24.0	0
(*Stonyfield* Nonfat)	19.0	0

Food and Measure	carb. (gms)	fiber (gms)
vanilla bean (*Turkey Hill*)	19.0	3.0
vanilla chocolate swirl (*Dreyer's/Edy's* Nonfat)	19.0	0
vanilla, chocolate, strawberry (*Hood Classic Trio*)	22.0	0
vanilla fudge swirl:		
(*Green's* Nonfat)	25.0	0
(*Stonyfield* Nonfat)	23.0	0
(*Turkey Hill* Nonfat Fudge Ripple)	22.0	0
vanilla Swiss almond (*Hood*)	25.0	0
"Yogurt," soy, 6 oz., except as noted:		
plain (*Silk*), 8 oz.	22.0	1.0
apricot mango, key lime, or raspberry (*Silk*)	30.0	1.0
banana-strawberry, blueberry, or black cherry (*Silk*)	29.0	1.0
lemon or strawberry (*Silk*)	31.0	1.0
peach (*Silk*)	32.0	1.0
vanilla (*Silk*)	25.0	1.0
Yogurt bar, frozen, 1 piece:		
all flavors, chocolate coated (*Yoplait* Triple Dipped)	11.0	0
all flavors, with fruit pieces (*Yoplait* Double Smoothies) ..	11.0	0
sorbet and, see "Sorbet bar"		
strawberry, with cereal (*Yoplait* Breakfast)	23.0	<1.0
vanilla, with cereal (*Yoplait* Breakfast)	24.0	<1.0
Yogurt drink (see also "Kefir"):		
(*DanActive* Original), 3.3 fl. oz.	16.0	0
all flavors:		
(*Breyers Creme Savers* Smoothie), 10 fl. oz.	32.0	0
(*DanActive*), 3.3 fl. oz.	18.0	5
(*Danimals*), 3.1 fl. oz.	16.0	0
(*Dannon Light 'n Fit Carb Control* Smoothie); 7 fl. oz. .	4.0	0
(*Hood Carb Countdown* Smoothie), 10 fl. oz.	4.0	0
(*Yoplait Nouriche* Breakfast Smoothie), 11 fl. oz.	60.0	6.0
(*Yoplait Nouriche* Breakfast Smoothie Light), 11 fl. oz. .	33.0	5.0
banana-berry (*Dannon Fusion*), 10 fl. oz.	52.0	0
berry, mixed (*Dannon Light 'n Fit* Smoothie), 7 fl. oz. ...	15.0	0
berry, wild (*Dannon Fusion*), 10 fl. oz.	53.0	0
cherry berry (*Dannon Fusion*), 10 fl. oz.	53.0	<1.0
peach passion fruit (*Dannon Fusion*), 10 fl. oz.	51.0	0
peach passion fruit (*Dannon Light 'n Fit* Smoothie),		
7 fl. oz.	15.0	0

Food and Measure	carb. (gms)	fiber (gms)
raspberry (*Dannon Light 'n Fit* Smoothie), 7 fl. oz.	15.0	<1.0
strawberry (*DanActive*), 3.3 fl. oz.	18.0	0
strawberry (*Dannon Light 'n Fit* Smoothie), 7 fl. oz.	14.0	0
strawberry-banana or tropical fruit (*Dannon Light 'n Fit* Smoothie), 7 fl. oz.	15.0	0
strawberry-kiwi or tropical fruit (*Dannon Fusion*), 10 fl. oz.	52.0	0
vanilla (*DanActive*), 3.3 fl. oz.	18.0	0
Yogurt sandwich, frozen, 1 piece:		
orange vanilla, with cereal waffles (*Yoplait* Breakfast)	33.0	0
vanilla (*Turkey Hill*)	30.0	3.0
Yogurt seasoning (*Neera's*), 1 tsp.	2.0	0
Yogurt smoothie, see "Yogurt drink"		
Youngberry juice, (*Ceres*), 8 fl. oz.	30.0	0
Yu choy sum (*Frieda's*), 1 cup, 3 oz.	3.0	0
Yuca root (*Frieda's*), ⅔ cup, 3 oz.	23.0	1.0

Z

Food and Measure	carb. (gms)	fiber (gms)
Ziti pasta entree, frozen, three cheese (*Smart Ones*), 10-oz. pkg.	47.0	5.0
Zucchini, fresh, with skin:		
raw:		
chopped, ½ cup	1.8	.7
sliced, ½ cup	1.6	.7
baby (*Frieda's*), ⅔ cup, 3 oz.	3.0	0
baby, 1 large, 3⅛"	.5	<.1
boiled, drained, sliced, ½ cup	3.5	1.3
boiled, drained, mashed, ½ cup	4.7	1.7
Zucchini, canned, Italian style:		
(*Del Monte*), ½ cup	7.0	1.0
with tomato juice, ½ cup	7.8	1.0
Zucchini, frozen:		
with skin, boiled, drained, 1 cup	7.9	2.9
yellow and green (*C&W*), ⅔ cup	2.0	1.0
Zucchini, breaded, frozen (*Empire Kosher*), 7 pieces, 3 oz.	18.0	1.0
Zucchini, marinated, sun-dried, in jars (*Antica Italia*), 1 oz.	2.0	1.0